D1373956

ANNALS OF THE NEW YORK ACADEMY OF SCIENCES

Volume 527

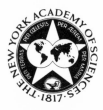

EDITORIAL STAFF

Executive Editor
BILL BOLAND

Managing Editor
JUSTINE CULLINAN

Associate Editor
LINDA H. MEHTA

The New York Academy of Sciences
2 East 63rd Street
New York, New York 10021

VASOACTIVE INTESTINAL
PEPTIDE AND RELATED PEPTIDES

ANNALS OF THE NEW YORK ACADEMY OF SCIENCES
Volume 527

VASOACTIVE INTESTINAL PEPTIDE AND RELATED PEPTIDES

Edited by Sami I. Said and Viktor Mutt

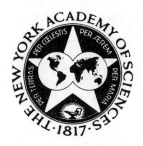

The New York Academy of Sciences
New York, New York
1988

Library of Congress Cataloging-in-Publication Data

Vasoactive intestinal peptide and related peptides.

(Annals of the New York Academy of Sciences, ISSN 0077-8923 ; v. 527)
Result of a conference held by the New York Academy of Sciences on Mar. 2-4, 1987, in New York City.
Includes bibliographies and index.
1. Vasoactive intestinal peptides—Congresses. 2. Peptide hormones—Congresses. 3. Neuropeptides—Congresses.
I. Saʻīd, Sāmi. II. Mutt, Viktor. III. New York Academy of Sciences. IV. Series. [DNLM: 1. Vasoactive Intestinal Peptide—congresses. W1 AN626YL v.527 / WK 170 V3343 1987]
Q11.N5 vol. 527   500 s   88-15199
[QP572.V28]   [612′.33]
ISBN 0-89766-449-3
ISBN 0-89766-450-7 (pbk.)

PCP
Printed in the United States of America
ISBN 0-89766-449-3 (cloth)
ISBN 0-89766-450-7 (paper)
ISSN 0077-8923

ANNALS OF THE NEW YORK ACADEMY OF SCIENCES

Volume 527
June 17, 1988

VASOACTIVE INTESTINAL PEPTIDE AND RELATED PEPTIDES[a]

Editors
SAMI I. SAID AND VIKTOR MUTT

CONTENTS

[a]This volume is the result of a conference entitled Vasoactive Intestinal Peptide and Related Peptides, which was held by the New York Academy of Sciences on March 2-4, 1987, in New York City.

Financial assistance was received from:

- MEIJI SEIKA KAISHA, LTD. (JAPAN)
- MERCK SHARP AND DOHME RESEARCH LABORATORIES
- MERRELL DOW RESEARCH INSTITUTE
- MILES LABORATORIES
- SANDOZ PHARMACEUTICALS
- UNIVERSITY OF OKLAHOMA, COLLEGE OF MEDICINE
- NATIONAL INSTITUTE OF NEUROLOGICAL AND COMMUNI-
  CATIVE DISORDERS AND STROKE (NEUROSCIENCES PRO-
  GRAM)
- NATIONAL INSTITUTE OF ALLERGY AND INFECTIOUS DIS-
  EASES (ASTHMA & ALLERGY BRANCH)

- NATIONAL INSTITUTE OF CHILD HEALTH & HUMAN DEVELOPMENT
- NATIONAL INSTITUTE OF ARTHRITIS, DIABETES, DIGESTIVE AND KIDNEY DISEASES (UROLOGY PROGRAM)
- NATIONAL INSTITUTE OF DIABETES, DIGESTIVE, AND KIDNEY DISEASES (DIGESTIVE DISEASES BRANCH)
- BACHEM INC.
- KABIGEN AB (SWEDEN)

Preface

SAMI I. SAID

Department of Medicine
University of Illinois College of Medicine
and West Side VA Medical Center
Chicago, Illinois 60612

The discovery and isolation of the vasoactive intestinal peptide (VIP) in 1970 culminated the search for a vasodilator peptide, first in lung extracts, then in intestinal extracts. For the following few years, VIP was considered a candidate gastrointestinal hormone, but its physiological release into the general circulation—a prime requisite for hormonal status—could not be documented. The rediscovery of VIP in the brain and in peripheral nerves established its true identity as a neuropeptide with neurotransmitter and neuromodulator properties.

VIP has been shown to be widely present in animal species, with considerable conservation of its amino-acid composition. The "family" of VIP-related peptides, originally thought to be limited to secretin and glucagon, is now known to include at least eleven other peptides: PHI (peptide with NH_2-terminal histidine and COOH-terminal isoleucine amide), PHM (the counterpart of PHI in human tissues, peptide with NH_2-terminal histidine and COOH-terminal methionine amide), secretin, glucagon, corticotropin-releasing factor (CRF), growth hormone-releasing factor (GRF), sauvagine, urotensin I, helodermin, helospectin, and gastric inhibitory peptide.

Much has been learned about the biology of VIP in health and disease. In addition to its vasodilator activity, which guided its isolation and gave it its name, VIP has important activities on a variety of cells and tissues throughout the body, including epithelial cells, secretory acini and ducts, vascular and nonvascular smooth muscle, T-lymphocytes, myocardium, osteoclasts, and certain neurons, endocrine cells and other specialized cells. As a result of these activities, and the presence of VIP-containing nerves in close proximity to these structures as well as the presence of specific binding sites, VIP probably helps regulate a number of major physiological functions, including regional blood flow, cardiovascular dynamics, smooth muscle tone, secretion of water, anions and macromolecules, immune and neuroendocrine function, brain metabolism, and bone resorption.

The biosynthesis of VIP (together with PHI or, in humans, PHM) has been clarified and the VIP gene has been sequenced and its chromosomal localization determined.

Specific membrane receptors for VIP, coupled to adenylate cyclase, have been demonstrated in almost all target cells and tissues. Recent evidence suggests that VIP also binds to nuclear receptors, and that some of its actions may be mediated by the Ca^{2+} messenger—the inositol phospholipid system.

Hypersecretion of VIP by certain tumors results in a distinct clinical entity, which now can be moderated by appropriate inhibitors, such as somatostatin analogues. And VIP has been linked to several other diseases, including several intestinal disorders, hepatic cirrhosis, bronchial asthma, cystic fibrosis, and the acquired immunodeficiency syndrome (AIDS).

Despite these advances, many gaps in our knowledge of VIP physiology and pathophysiology remain to be filled. Among these are: the nature and significance of its interactions with other neurotransmitters and peptides; the control of its local release in different tissues and organs; the properties and regulation of its receptors; the full intracellular mechanisms mediating its actions; and its precise role in human disease. The answers will no doubt be forthcoming in the next few years, provided the research on VIP maintains its lively pace of the recent past.

This volume, the proceedings of the first international conference on VIP and related peptides held in the United States, is organized in five parts dealing with: chemistry, synthesis, biosynthesis, and structure–activity relationships; VIP as a neuropeptide in the central and peripheral nervous systems; mechanisms of action and receptors; physiological role; and relationship to human disease. Speakers and discussants, numbering 72, came from the United States and 14 other countries (Australia, Belgium, Canada, Denmark, Federal Republic of Germany, France, Israel, Italy, Japan, Mexico, Norway, Sweden, Switzerland, and the United Kingdom). One sad note was the sudden death, shortly before the conference, of the young French investigator Jacqueline Besson, a pioneer in VIP research. The news shocked her many friends and colleagues, who miss her deeply.

Finally, it is a pleasure to acknowledge the help of those individuals and organizations who made the conference possible: the contributing scientists; the advisory committee and the staff of the conference and editorial departments of the Academy, especially Ms. Ellen A. Marks, Ms. Cindy Wishengrad, Ms. Sheila Kane, and Ms. Linda H. Mehta; my assistant Ms. Brenda Hansel; the National Institutes of Health and other institutions and corporations who gave their financial support; and my associate and mentor, Viktor Mutt, cochairman of the conference.

Vasoactive Intestinal Polypeptide and Related Peptides

Isolation and Chemistry[a]

VIKTOR MUTT

Department of Biochemistry II
Karolinska Institute
S-104 01 Stockholm, Sweden

In his treatise "Mémoire sur Le Pancréas" of 1856, an English translation of which, by Dr. John Henderson, appeared in 1985,[1] Claude Bernard published a colored drawing of the pancreas of a dog that had not received food for 36 hours and of one that had just been fed. In the first case the pancreas is seen to be pale, almost bloodless, while in the second it is reddish, with vessels engorged with blood. Today we know that this difference is, at least in part, due to the action of the vasoactive intestinal polypeptide (VIP).[2]

VIP, porcine VIP, to be specific, was isolated 17 years ago,[3] and its complete amino acid sequence was disclosed four years later.[4] Some work has also been carried out on its higher order structures,[5,6] but here much more remains to be done.

Isolation of a peptide is here taken to mean that the peptide has been brought to an "essentially pure" state, in practice meaning pure enough for unambiguous determination of amino acid sequence to be possible. This might seem obvious but is not, since as discussed elsewhere[7] the term "isolation" may be used with a different meaning by different authors. For instance, it is claimed in an important recent publication[8] that "Substance P was first isolated from brain and intestine more than 50 years ago." The work referred to in this case is the article by v. Euler and Gaddum[9] entitled "An Unidentified Depressor Substance in Certain Tissue Extracts." Many such examples may be found.

In the 1960s we had, from pig intestine, isolated the hormones secretin,[10,11] discovered by Bayliss and Starling,[12] cholecystokinin, discovered by Ivy and Oldberg,[13] and pancreozymin, discovered by Harper and Raper.[14] The cholecystokinetic and pancreozyminic activities were unexpectedly[15] found to be exerted by one and the same substance. Nowadays, the articles by Ivy and Oldberg[13] and by Harper and Raper[14] are sometimes referred to as supposedly showing that cholecystokinin has both cholecystokinetic and pancreozyminic activity (e.g., Hays *et al.*[16] and Cantor[17]). There is, however, no mention of pancreatic enzyme secretion in the article by Ivy and Oldberg, and none of gallbladder contraction in that by Harper and Raper.

[a]This study was supported by grants from the Medical Research Council of Sweden (No. 13X-01010), KabiGen AB, Skandigen AB, and the Karolinska Institute.

Through our work with gastrointestinal hormones, we came in contact with others interested in these and other hormonal peptides. In particular Sami I. Said from Richmond, and John C. Brown from Vancouver came in the late 1960s to work in our laboratory, each on his own problem. This resulted in the isolation of VIP on the one hand, and of motilin and GIP (the gastric inhibitory [or glucose-dependent insulinotropic] polypeptide) on the other.

Sami Said and coworkers had earlier made observations suggesting that the vasoactivity exhibited by lung extracts might to a substantial degree be due to substances of peptide nature.[18] That this was indeed so could be confirmed.[19] However, it was also found that certain peptide side-fractions from the isolation of secretin from pig upper small intestine were strongly vasoactive, and from one of them, eluting after secretin on cation-exchange chromatography on carboxymethyl cellulose, VIP was isolated.[3]

John Brown and his coworkers had found that partially purified preparations of CCK contained, in addition to CCK, a nonCCK inhibitor of gastric acid secretion.[20] From a side fraction from the isolation of CCK, GIP was then isolated[21] in our laboratory. Brown further found that a commercially available pancreozymin (CCK) preparation contained a nonCCK stimulant of gastric motor activity.[22] Such a stimulant was isolated, from a side fraction from the isolation in our laboratory of secretin, that eluted before secretin during chromatography on carboxymethyl cellulose, and was subsequently named motilin.[23] The term motilin had indeed already been used earlier, in another connection,[24] but we were unaware of this at the time.

ISOLATION OF VIP FROM DIFFERENT SPECIES: ISOLATION METHODOLOGY

VIP from pig small intestine was isolated starting with large amounts—hundreds of kilograms—of tissue.[3] The same is true for the isolation of VIP from pig brain,[25] ox small intestine,[26] and chicken intestine.[27] More recently VIP has been isolated also from human colonic[28] and ganglioneuroblastoma[29] tissues, rat intestine,[30] goat colonic tissue,[31] dog intestine,[32] guinea pig intestine,[33] and dogfish intestine.[34] In these latter cases very much smaller amounts of tissues have been used than in the former. Partly this reflects advances in separatory methodology, as when dog VIP was isolated from the intestine of a single dog,[32] partly advances in analytical methodology, particularly in the determination of the amino acid compositions of peptides and of their sequences, and also in part advances in methodology of peptide synthesis. The amino acid composition of dog VIP was determined by Wang et al.[32] using 100 picomoles of VIP, and its sequence using 800 picomoles, that is, all in all about 3 micrograms. Even if it had been possible for us 17 years ago to isolate VIP from an equally small quantity of pig intestine, this would have been a rather meaningless undertaking since it had hardly been possible, with the methodology then known, to elucidate its sequence using the minute amount of VIP obtained. It is obvious that today it is possible to isolate a hormonal peptide from only a small amount of tissue, determine its amino acid sequence, and then synthesize its replicate for pharmacological experimentation. Does this then mean that the need to extract peptides from large amounts of tissue is a thing of the past? An affirmative answer appears reasonable; however, extraction on a large scale may yield the purified peptide in such quantity that its sequence can also be determined in a laboratory not equipped with vastly expensive semiautomatic microsequencing equipment. Also, the amount produced may be sufficient for pharmacological experimentation before synthetic material becomes available. When it is available, the high yield of large-scale extractions can be used, to carry out comparisons, chemical and pharmacological, between the natural and synthetic preparations. This is of course especially important when a previously unknown peptide has been isolated, and such peptides may be found in side-fractions obtained on the isolation of already known peptides, as was the case with VIP. Also with known peptides there may exist variant forms of considerable interest, which occur in much smaller amounts in the tissue extract than the peptide originally described. In such cases work with small amounts of tissue may be fraught with difficulties even when using the most sophisticated separatory and analytical methodology available. In practice, work on a large scale means that tissue material must be freely available as a side fraction from some industrial process. There are cases when work with large amounts of tissue is precluded, for instance when working on the identification of human forms of hormonal peptides or tracing peptide evolution in endangered wildlife species. Several years ago Dimaline and Dockray found that extracts of human colonic tissue as well as of dog, rat, and pig gut and brain contained different forms of VIP-immunoreactive material. In addition to what appeared to be the known octacosapeptide, forms existed that appeared to be of the same size but less basic, as evidenced by their elution patterns on cation-exchange chromatography.[35] Together with Dimaline and coworkers, we have found VIP-immunoreactive material present also in types of fractions other than those from which the octacosapeptide has been isolated. We (G. Gafvelin, M. Andersson, and H. Jörnvall) are currently working on the isolation of the peptide(s) responsible for this immunoreactivity.

These VIP-immunoreactive fractions are obtained from the same type of crude peptide concentrate, concentrate of thermostable intestinal peptides (CTIP) described by us long ago.[36] CTIP has been prepared by extracting heat-denatured small intestinal tissue with 0.5 M acetic acid at about 4–10°C, filtering, adsorbing the peptides from the filtrate to alginic acid, eluting with cold 0.2 M HCl and salting out of the peptides with NaCl. Recently we have added the additional step of raising the pH of the filtrate to about 3 with sodium acetate before salting out with NaCl. To prepare CTIP is of course not a perfect way to obtain a peptide concentrate from which to isolate different peptides. It has, for instance, been pointed out[37] that reactivation of proteolytic enzymes may take place during the extraction step. It has, nevertheless, the important advantage that CTIP can easily be prepared from large quantities of tissue, which is not the case, in laboratory surroundings, if toxic and/or inflammable water-miscible organic solvents are to be used for the extraction step. Besides for secretin, CCK, VIP, motilin, and GIP, as mentioned above, CTIP has also been used for the isolation of the hormonal peptides somatostatin-28,[38] PHI (peptide with NH_2-terminal histidine and COOH-terminal isoleucine amide),[39] PYY (peptide with NH_2-terminal tyrosine and COOH-terminal tyrosine amide),[40,41] NPY (neuropeptide Y),[42] GRP (gastrin releasing peptide),[43] galanin,[44] as well as two peptides of less clear function, valosin[45] and prosomatostatin$_{1-32}$.[46]

Peptides may, of course, be isolated from CTIP in different ways. Since each peptide in it is diluted with a multitude of other, different, peptides, a subfractionation of CTIP is advisable before the application of various chromatographic procedures for the isolation of any individual peptide in it. We have long used fractionation of aqueous solutions of CTIP with ethanol.[47] Recently we have found that preliminary fractionation using isopropanol might give a more efficient preliminary concentration of at least VIP and secretin. It may be remembered that extraction of gastrin from solution in strong aqueous dipotassium hydrogen phosphate into isopropanol was an important step in the isolation of gastrin by Gregory and Tracy.[48] Our fractionation scheme is briefly outlined in TABLE 1. The fraction F3 usually weighs about 1.5 g (wet weight, as also for CTIP) and is a convenient peptide concentrate for the isolation of, particularly, VIP and secretin.

The amino acid sequence of the common mammalian form of VIP is

His-Ser-Asp-Ala-Val-Phe-Thr-Asp-Asn-Tyr-Thr-Arg-Leu-Arg-Lys-Gln-Met-Ala-Val-Lys-Lys-Tyr-Leu-Asn-Ser-Ile-Leu-Asn-NH$_2$.[4,33]

Guinea pig VIP differs from it by having Leu-5, Thr-9, Met-19, and Val-26 (instead of Val-5, Asn-9, Val-19, and Ile-26),[33] and chicken VIP by having Ser-11, Phe-13, Val-26, and COOH-terminal threonine amide (instead of Thr-11, Leu-13, Ile-26, and COOH-terminal asparagine amide).[27,85] The substitution in position 26 is consequently the same for guinea pig and chicken whereas the remaining three substitutions, in each of these two species, are different.

The correctness of the amino acid sequence established at the protein level for

TABLE 1. CTIP Fractionation

	Protocol	Precipitate
1.	500 g CTIP in 4 1 water, 18 1 isopropanol added (room temp.)	F0
2.	Filtrate: 18 1 isopropanol added (−20°C)	F1
3.	Filtrate: pH to 6 ± 0.1^a	F2
	Filtrate: Peptides transferred into water. Precipitated with NaCl$_{sat.}$	F3

^{a} Adjusted with potassium acetate, (acetic acid). Measured on aliquots of solution diluted 1 : 5 with water.

human VIP has been confirmed by deduction from the nucleotide sequences established for the corresponding cDNA[49,50] and also from the gene nucleotide sequence.[51-53]

VIP is structurally related to five other types of mammalian peptides, and, in addition, to two as yet isolated only from a nonmammalian species. The mammalian ones are PHI, secretin, GIP, the growth hormone releasing factor GRP or somatocrinin, and glucagon. The nonmammalian ones are helodermin and helospectin.

PHI

This heptacosapeptide was first isolated from a side-fraction from the purification of secretin from pig intestine, which on chromatography on carboxymethyl cellulose eluted before secretin. It was discovered by way of its COOH-terminal isoleucine amide structure and its isolation was monitored using this structural detail as an analytical marker.[39,54] Subsequently it has been isolated from pig brain,[55] ox intestine,[56] and human colonic tissue.[57] PHI from pig brain and intestine was found to be identical but, in contrast to VIP, the human, pig, and ox PHIs were all found to differ in amino acid sequences, albeit only slightly. Already, before the sequence of human PHI had been determined on the isolated peptide, it had been deduced from the corresponding cDNA sequence.[49,50] It was found that the PHI was in the same preprohormone as was VIP. The VIP sequence was COOH-terminal to the PHI sequence and separated from it by a heptadecapeptide sequence with Gly-Lys-Arg NH$_2$-terminally and Lys-Arg COOH-terminally.

The amino acid sequence of human PHI is

His-Ala-Asp-Gly-Val-Phe-Thr-Ser-Asp-Phe-Ser-Lys-Leu-Leu-Gly-Gln-Leu-Ser-Ala-Lys-Lys-Tyr-Leu-Glu-Ser-Leu-Met-NH$_2$

Consequently human PHI may also, correctly, be named PHM, unless, of course, PHI is taken to be a generic name, once given no longer dependent on the reason for constructing it.

Pig PHI differs from the human by having Arg-12 and COOH-terminal isoleucine amide (instead of Lys-12 and COOH-terminal methionine amide).

Ox PHI differs from pig PHI only by having Tyr-10 (instead of Phe-10).

Lundberg and Tatemoto[58] found that although pig PHI and pig VIP both caused vasodilation in the submandibular gland of the anesthetized cat, the VIP was about a thousand times more potent in this action than was the PHI. However, in their relaxing effects on human submandibulary salivary gland arteries, *in vitro* human VIP and human PHI (PHM) were found to have the same potency.[59] Larsson *et al.*[59] point to the possibility that cat PHI may, perhaps, differ from porcine PHI in some detail essential for stimulating cat vasodilation.

Yiangou *et al.*[60] obtained immunochemical evidence for the presence in extracts of pig stomach of a larger form of PHI than the heptacosapeptide originally isolated. More recently these workers, now working with extracts of human tissues, have provided evidence that this form is PHI, or PHM, extended COOH-terminally by the heptadecapeptide, which in the preprohormone connects the PHI sequence to the VIP sequence.[61] If the COOH-terminal Lys-Arg sequence of the connecting peptide were removed the "big PHM" would, like GIP, have a chain length of 42 amino acid residues.

THE GROWTH HORMONE RELEASING FACTOR OR SOMATOCRININ

When PHI had been isolated and sequenced, the similarity of its sequence to the sequences of VIP, secretin, GIP, and glucagon was obvious.

Wholly unexpectedly came the revelation that it was also strikingly similar to the sequence of the growth hormone releasing factor (GRF), alternatively named somatocrinin.[62] (The rational term somatoliberin has also been used, but possibly for another, not yet isolated, peptide.[63])

GRF, the human form of it, was first isolated from pancreatic, acromegaly-causing, tumor tissue by Guillemin *et al.*[64] and Rivier *et al.*[65]

Guillemin[64] found the amino acid sequence

Tyr-Ala-Asp-Ala-Ile-Phe-Thr-Asn-Ser-Tyr-Arg-Lys-Val-Leu-Gly-Gln-Leu-Ser-Ala-
Arg-Lys-Leu-Leu-Gln-Asp-Ile-Met-Ser-Arg-Gln-Gln-Gly-Glu-Ser-Asn-Gln-Glu-
Arg-Gly-Ala-Arg-Ala-Arg-Leu-NH$_2$

for the GRF that they had isolated, while Rivier et al.[65] found the same sequence, except for the lack of the COOH-terminal tetrapeptide for the GRF that they had isolated.

A comparison of this sequence with the sequence of PHM, the human form of PHI, on alignment of the peptides from their NH$_2$-termini, shows that there are identical amino acid residues in no fewer than 14 of the 27 possible positions. GRF has subsequently been isolated from pig, ox, sheep, goat (references in Brazeau et al.[66]) and rat[67] hypothalamic tissue. The goat and ox CRFs are mutually identical, but none of these five CRFs is identical to human CRF. Except for rat CRF, the differences are, however, modest and with one exception (a substitution of Val-13 for Ile-13 in sheep CRF) located COOH-terminally to the NH$_2$-terminal hexacosapeptide sequences of the CRFs, that is, to a region that seems to be of less importance for hormonal activity[62] than the NH$_2$-terminal.

Rat GRF, with its 43 amino acid residues, differs from the human in no fewer than 14 positions, spread across the length of the peptide chain. Of functional importance is the substitution of the Tyr-1 of the human CRF for His-1 in the rat. Laburthe et al.[68] have found that rat GRF has a much higher affinity than human GRF for VIP receptors in human and rat intestinal epithelial cell membranes, and that for stimulation of adenylate cyclase in these membranes rat GRF acted as a full agonist, but human GRF acted only as a partial agonist.

The amino acid sequence for human preproGRF has been deduced from the cDNA[69–71] and gene nucleotide sequences.

GIP

Although originally named "gastric inhibitory polypeptide" because of its ability to inhibit gastric acid secretion, at least under certain experimental conditions, interest for GIP has mainly focused on its ability to release insulin. Because of this it is also known as glucose-dependent insulinotropic polypeptide.[72]

Like PHI, GIP has been, to date, isolated from three mammalian species and the three GIPs have been found to be nonidentical, although highly similar.

The amino acid sequence of human GIP is[73]

Tyr-Ala-Glu-Gly-Thr-Phe-Ile-Ser-Asp-Tyr-Ser-Ile-Ala-Met-Asp-Lys-Ile-His-Gln-
Gln-Asp-Phe-Val-Asn-Trp-Leu-Leu-Ala-Gln-Lys-Gly-Lys-Lys-Asn-Asp-Trp-Lys-
His-Asn-Ile-Thr-Gln.

The pig dotetracontapeptide differs from it by having Arg-18 and Ser-34 (instead of His-18 and Asn-34).[74,75]

The ox dotetracontapeptide is identical to the porcine except for having Ile-37 (instead of Lys-37).[76]

It has been pointed out[77] that of the four types of structurally related intestinal polypeptides, secretin, VIP, PHI, and GIP, the three former each consists of about 30 amino acid residues, while GIP consists of 42 residues, and that the Gly_{31}-Lys-Lys sequence of GIP is a sequence that, if it occurred in a prohormone, would be cleaved enzymatically so that the amino group of the glycine residue in the mature hormone would be retained in the COOH-terminal carboxamido group of its COOH-terminal amino acid residue.[78,79] In all mammalian peptide hormones with COOH-terminal α-amide structures hitherto isolated, the COOH-terminal amino acid has, however, been found to have an uncharged sidechain, reflecting the substrate requirements of the "amidating enzyme."[80,81] Consequently the occurrence of the basic lysine residue in position 30 of all the known forms of GIP_{1-42} may explain why cleavage of the Lys_{30}-Gly_{31} bond in GIP either does not occur or occurs in such low yield that GIP-30 has not been detected in extracts of intestinal tissue. Recently M. Carlquist in our laboratory has synthesized the replicate of GIP_{1-31}[82] and in collaboration with others found that it has substantial insulin-releasing activity.[83]

The amino acid sequence of preproGIP seems not to have been elucidated yet.

SECRETIN

When chicken secretin was being isolated, the sequences of the related chicken glucagon[84] and chicken VIP[85] were already known. Chicken glucagon differs in one position from pig glucagon and differs from chicken VIP in four positions. By analogy it was expected that chicken secretin too would differ in only a few positions from pig secretin. Unexpectedly, however, chicken secretin proved to differ from pig secretin in no fewer than 13 positions of the 27 possible.[86] Chicken secretin was the second secretin to be isolated after pig secretin and the minimal statistical sample suggested that secretin might prove to show greater species variability than either glucagon or VIP. This was not brought out by the third secretin to be isolated, ox secretin, which was found to be identical to pig secretin.[87] The fourth secretin, the human, did indeed differ from ox-pig secretin in two positions,[88] while with the exception of guinea pig glucagon and VIP, all previously isolated mammalian glucagons have been found to be identical, as have all the VIPs.

The amino acid sequence of human secretin is

His-Ser-Asp-Gly-Thr-Phe-Thr-Ser-Glu-Leu-Ser-Arg-Leu-Arg-Glu-Gly-Ala-Arg-
Leu-Gln-Arg-Leu-Leu-Gln-Gly-Leu-Val-NH$_2$

and ox-pig secretin differs from the human by having Asp-15 and Ser-16 (instead of Glu-15 and Gly-16).

A comparison of the sequences of ox-pig secretin and chicken secretin shows, in one-letter code for amino acid residues:

ox–pig secretin: H S D G T F T S E L S R L R D S A R L Q R L L Q G L V ■
chicken secretin: H S D G L F T S E Y S K M R G N A Q V Q K F I Q N L M■

The symbol ■ indicates that the COOH-terminal amino acid is amidated. Because of its COOH-terminal α-amide structure, porcine secretin could have been expected to be cleaved out from a precursor protein in which its sequence is followed by a glycine residue, in turn, presumably followed either by a pair of basic amino acid residues as are the sequences of VIP and PHI in their precursor[49,50] or by a single basic residue, as is the sequence of GRF in its precursor.[69,70] It has indeed been possible to isolate, from extracts of porcine small intestinal tissue, an octacosapeptide that has the sequence of secretin except that it does not terminate COOH-terminally by valine amide but by valyl-glycine. This peptide was found to exhibit secretin-like bioactivity on the pancreatic secretin of the anesthetized cat,[89] but its potency was not determined. Later work has led to the isolation of a triacontapeptide in which the secretin sequence is extended by a glycyl-lysyl-arginine sequence.[90] This triacontapeptide was found to be appreciably more potent than secretin in the above-mentioned bioassay system. It could be of interest to compare the bioactivities of other COOH-terminally amidated gastrointestinal hormones with those forms that are extended COOH-terminally by short peptide sequences. The presence of such extended forms has been demonstrated in tissue extracts by immunochemical methods, for example, both gastrin and CCK,[91-93] but except for secretin no such form seems to have actually been isolated and bioassayed.

GLUCAGON SUBGROUP

Pig pancreatic glucagon was the first member of the group of peptides to which VIP also belongs to be isolated and sequenced.[94]

However, for years there was no evidence, or even suggestion, that glucagon might belong to any kind of group. That it could be so classified became evident only when secretin was isolated.[11] Because of this the term "secretin-glucagon" (or "glucagon-secretin") group appears to be the appropriate designation for the group of peptides discussed here.

It was soon recognized that compared to many other peptide hormones, glucagon has been strongly conserved during evolution. The human, pig, and ox insulins, for instance, are all different[95] while the corresponding glucagons are identical.[96] Indeed with the exception of guinea pig glucagon, all mammalian glucagons that have hitherto been isolated (human, pig, ox, camel, rabbit, rat)[97] or had their amino acid sequences deduced from the corresponding cDNA or gene nucleotide sequences (human,[98] ox,[99] hamster,[100] rat[101] glucagon) are, or appear to be, identical (the isolated rabbit, rat, and camel glucagons were not actually sequenced, but their composition was found to be identical to that of pig glucagon).

The amino acid sequence of the common mammalian glucagon is:

His-Ser-Gln-Gly-Thr-Phe-Thr-Ser-Asp-Tyr-Ser-Lys-Tyr-Leu-Asp-Ser-Arg-Arg-Ala
Gln-Asp-Phe-Val-Gln-Trp-Leu-Met-Asn-Thr.

Guinea pig glucagon has, in exactly the same sequence, 20 amino acid residues counting from the NH_2-terminus, but then has five substitutions in the COOH-terminal nonapeptide (Gln-21, Leu-23, Lys-24, Leu-27, and Val-29 instead of Asp-21, Val-23, Gln-24, Met-27, and Thr-29).[102,103]

No nonmammalian glucagon seems yet to have been found that is identical to the common mammalian glucagon, but in several species the differences to it are small, often smaller than for guinea pig glucagon.

The mutually identical chicken and turkey glucagons differ from the mammalian only by having Ser-28 (instead of Asn-28),[96] while the mutually identical duck[96] and alligator[104] glucagons are identical to chicken/turkey glucagon (except for having Thr-16 instead of Ser-16).

Recently, glucagon has been isolated from the pancreas of an elasmobranchian fish, the *Torpedo marmorata*,[105] and was found to differ from mammalian glucagon in three positions only (Glu-3, Asn-16, and Lys-20, instead of Gln-3, Ser-16, and Gln-20). Teleostean fish glucagon seems to have diverged further: Coho salmon glucagon differs from the mammalian in eight positions,[106] catfish glucagon in six (possibly seven) positions,[107] and the two anglerfish glucagons in seven resp. nine positions.[108] The finding that the anglerfish had two different glucagons instead of one[109,110] led to a dramatic increase in interest in the biosynthesis of glucagon. Unexpectedly the anglerfish preproglucagon was found to contain the sequence of an additional glucagon-like peptide GLP, highly similar to each other in the two preproglucagons but not identical and separated from the respective glucagon sequences by intervening peptide sequences with pairs of basic amino acid residues at their NH_2- and COOH-termini.[108] Later it was found that mammalian preproglucagons too contain GLPs, and not only one but two that are different, but similar, designated GLP-1 and GLP-2 in each preproglucagon.[98–101] On the other hand mammals apparently have only one preproglucagon each. The possible evolutionary developments underlying this difference between fish and mammals has been discussed by Lopez *et al.*[111] The two anglerfish glucagon amino acid sequences, as deduced from the corresponding cDNA sequences,[108] are identical over their NH_2-terminal 15 residues but exhibit six differences over the COOH-terminal residues:

AFG I   H S E G T F S N D Y S K Y L E D R K A Q E F V R W L M N N
AFG II   H S E G T F S N D Y S K Y L E T R R A Q D F V Q W L K N S

This resembles the sequence conservation between the guinea pig and the common mammalian glucagons. However, on comparing the two anglerfish glucagon sequences with the sequence of the common mammalian glucagon, no exceptional conservations of their NH_2-terminal parts is evident

AFG I   H S E G T F S N D Y S K Y L E D R K A Q E F V R W L M N N
Mammalian glucagon   H S Q G T F T S D Y S K Y L D S R R A Q D F V Q W L M N T

AFG II   H S E G T F S N D Y S K Y L E T R R A Q D F V Q W L K N S
Mammalian glucagon   H S Q G T F T S D Y S K Y L D S R R A Q D F V Q W L M N T

The conservation of the position 17-26 sequence of anglerfish glucagon II and mammalian glucagon appears, if anything, more impressive than any conserved sequence in the NH_2-terminal halves of the peptide. It may also be noticed that in the COOH-terminal tetradecapeptides the variations between mammalian glucagon and the two anglerfish glucagons occur exclusively in those positions where the two latter also show variations between each other.

The presence of presumptive hormonal sequences in proteins, however interesting, does not by itself show that such sequences actually represent hormones released under physiological conditions. The probability that GLPs do play some hormonal role(s) has been greatly increased by the isolation from catfish pancreatic tissue of one such GLP, with the sequence

H A D G T Y T S D V S S Y L Q D Q A A K D F I T W L K S G Q P K P E

This sequence shows homology in varying degrees to the various GLP sequences known to occur in preproglucagons. The degree of homology is, for instance, higher to the GLP sequence in anglerfish preproglucagon II than to that in anglerfish preproglucagon I and higher to hamster GLP-1 than to hamster GLP-2. A peculiar feature (*vide infra*) of the catfish GLP, and of the GLP sequence in anglerfish pre-proglucagon II is the occurrence of a residue of tyrosine instead of one of phenylalanine in position 6.[107] More recently another GLP has been isolated from Coho salmon[106] and found to be an untriacontapeptide showing differences in six positions to catfish GLP (an alignment of the peptides from their NH_2-termini). Also this GLP was found to have tyrosine in position six.

Recently Andrews *et al.*[112] carried out a careful study of the products formed on *in vivo* processing of anglerfish preproglucagon II. Among other interesting findings was that the GLP was obtained in three different forms, one a tetratriacontapeptide with the COOH-terminal sequence -Gly-Arg-Gly-Arg-Arg-Glu, the other an untria-contapeptide that lacks the COOH-terminal-Arg-Arg-Glu sequence of the former, and finally a triacontapeptide with COOH-terminal arginine amide, obviously formed from the untriacontapeptide by the action of the amidating enzyme. As these authors point out, peptides with COOH-terminal basic amino acid amides have very seldom been found in nature. Investigation of how glucagon is biosynthesized in mammals did not start with recombinant DNA methodology but with the isolation by Tager and Steiner[113] from a commercially available preparation of bovine-porcine glucagon of a polypeptide consisting of glucagon extended by an octapeptide from its COOH-ter-minus. When Thim and Moody[114] determined the amino acid sequence of glicentin, a glucagon-immunoreactive peptide from pig intestinal tissue,[115] it was evident that in glicentin the glucagon sequence was extended COOH-terminally by the octapeptide described by Tager and Steiner,[113] although a minor revision of the sequence found by them was necessary. The correct sequence was Lys-Arg-Asn-Lys-Asn-Asn-Ile-Ala. NH_2-terminally in glicentin, glucagon is extended over a lysyl-arginine sequence by the triacontapeptide GRPP (glicentin-related pancreatic peptide). The sequence of GRPP is

R S L Q N T E E K S R S F P A P Q T D P L D D P D Q M T E D K R.

The position 33-69 sequence of glicentin, that is, the proglucagon fragment of Tager and Steiner, has been isolated from porcine lower small intestine and named oxyn-tomodulin because of the stimulatory activity it was found to be able to exert on adenylate cyclase, especially in the oxyntic gland area of the rat stomach.[116] As to the release or nonrelease of the GLPs in mammals: Patzelt and Schiltz[117] found that in rat pancreatic islets *in vitro* a "major proglucagon fragment" (MPGF), which no longer contained glucagon but still contained GLP-1 and GLP-2 united by their intervening peptide, was formed from preproglucagon and evidently was not processed further in the islets. In accordance with these findings, Ørskov *et al.*[118] found that GLP-1 and GLP-2 are secreted separately from pig small intestine but not from pig pancreas.

Recently Mojsov *et al.*[119] found that rat preproglucagon is the same in rat intestine and pancreas, but that it was processed somewhat differently, at least quantitatively, into its component peptides in the two tissues. An interesting finding (*vide infra*) was that in intestine and pancreas alike part of the GLP_{1-37} released was converted into GLP_{7-37}. Also, the peptide intervening between the GLP-1 -Lys-Arg and the Gly-Arg-Arg- GLP-2 sequences was released in COOH-terminally α-amidated forms. All hitherto isolated mammalian peptides with COOH-terminal α-amide structures have been found to exhibit some hormonal activity or other. They further drew attention to some other potential processing sites in the preproglucagon sequence, among them the -Lys-Gly-Arg-Gly at the COOH-terminus of the GLP-1 sequence; this being particularly interesting in view of the finding by Andrews *et al.*[112] of the anglerfish GLP with COOH-terminal arginine amide.

It should be remembered that glucagon is the only one of the secretin-glucagon group of peptides to have been crystallized and to have its three-dimensional structure determined by X-ray crystallography. Blundell *et al.*[120] have discussed possible three-dimensional structures of other members of the group against the background of the glucagon structure.

HELOSPECTIN AND HELODERMIN

Raufman *et al.*[121] found that peptide(s) in Gila monster (*Heloderma horridum* or *Heloderma suspectum*) venom reacted with VIP receptors on dispersed acini from guinea pig pancreas to activate adenylate cyclase and stimulate enzyme secretion.

These observations have been followed by the isolation of three peptides from the venom:

1. helospectin I with the sequence

His-Ser-Asp-Ala-Thr-Phe-Thr-Ala-Glu-Tyr-Ser-Lys-Leu-Leu-Ala-Lys-Leu-Ala-Leu-Gln-Lys-Tyr-Leu-Glu-Ser-Ile-Leu-Gly-Ser-Ser-Thr-Ser-Pro-Arg-Pro-Pro-Ser-Ser;

2. helospectin II, identical to helospectin I except for the lack of Ser-38;[122]
3. helodermin with the sequence

His-Ser-Asp-Ala-Ile-Phe-Thr-Gln-Gln-Tyr-Ser-Lys-Leu-Leu-Ala-Lys-Leu-Ala-Leu-Gln-Lys-Tyr-Leu-Ala-Ser-Ile-Leu-Gly-Ser-Arg-Thr-Ser-Pro-Pro-Pro-NH$_2$.[123]

Robberecht *et al.*[124] have provided immunochemical evidence for the presence of helodermin-like immunoreactivity in certain mammalian tissue extracts. In collaboration with the Belgian workers, we have also obtained evidence for helodermin-like immunoreactivity in certain of our pig intestinal peptide fractions.

DISCUSSION

No peptide of the secretin-glucagon group, to which VIP belongs, contains any residue of cysteine, and these peptides are consequently without disulfide bridges. Cysteine is indeed absent from the whole of human preproVIP/PHI (PHM) and from human preproglucagon. Proline is absent from glucagon, GIP, GRF, secretin, and from the amidated forms of PHI and VIP, although, as is evident from preproVIP/PHI (PHM), it could occur in long, COOH-terminally extended forms of these peptides. Proline does occur in the helospectins and in helodermin, although so far only COOH-terminally. It also is present in glicentin NH$_2$-terminally to the glucagon sequence. VIP is conspicuous by the absence of glycine, which commonly occurs in peptides.

Several years ago it was pointed out[125] that although VIP contains a residue of methionine, which is easily oxidized to the sulfoxide, such oxidation does not inactivate VIP, at least not in its stimulatory effect on cat pancreatic bicarbonate secretion. This is in contrast to the reversible inactivation that many other hormones (for instance, CCK[126] or corticotropin[127]) undergo upon oxidation of their methionine residues.

In view of the finding[33] that there are two residues of methionine in guinea pig VIP, instead of one as in the common mammalian VIP, it could be of interest to find out whether or not the activity of guinea pig VIP is influenced by oxidation.

Since oxidation does not affect the activity of the common mammalian VIP, it might be that this residue does not interact with the VIP receptor surface. If so, it might be a useful point for attaching VIP to an insoluble matrix so as to obtain an affinity column for receptor purification. (M. Andersson in our laboratory is currently carrying out work in this direction.)

When we had determined the amino acid sequence of pig VIP,[4] we pointed out that since VIP and secretin stimulated pancreatic bicarbonate secretion whereas glucagon did not, an investigation of the possible importance of such amino acid residues that have identical positions in secretin and VIP but different positions in glucagon might help to clarify which amino acid residues in secretin and VIP are of particular importance for the stimulation of pancreatic secretion. One such residue is obviously the Asp-3 of VIP and secretin, which contrasts to the Gln-3 of glucagon. Indeed, synthetic work by M. Bodanszky (referred to in Mutt and Jorpes[128] and by Wünsch et al.[129]) has shown that this aspartic acid residue is indeed important for this activity of secretin and of VIP.

On comparing the amino acid sequences of the pig forms of PHI (which has negligible pancreatic stimulatory activity), secretin, and VIP (both of which are strongly stimulatory), it is evident that there are only two positions in which the amino acid residues are identical in secretin and VIP but different in PHI:

```
PHI        H A D G V F T S D F S R L L G Q L S A K K Y L E S L I
VIP        H S D A V F T D N Y T R L R K Q M A V K K Y L N S I L N
Secretin   H S D G T F T S E L S R L R D S A R L Q R L L Q G L V
```

Consequently it might be of interest to investigate what effect substitution of the Ala-2 and Leu-14 of PHI by serine and arginine, respectively, may have on the ability of the peptide to stimulate pancreatic secretion.

A conspicuous feature of the peptides of the secretin-glucagon group is the occurrence of a phenylalanine residue in position six from the NH_2-terminus.

This is found in glucagon, secretin, VIP, PHI, GIP, and GRF and, as may be seen from the amino acid sequences of the preprohormones, should be so also in the GLP from anglerfish preproglucagon I and in all known mammalian GLP-2s. (In the GLP from anglerfish preproglucagon-II and in some other fish GLPs, a residue of tyrosine is in this position.) As was pointed out previously,[130] there is, however, no phenylalanine residue in mammalian GLP-1, in the form GLP-1$_{1-37}$ this peptide is commonly assumed to have. However on removal of the NH_2-terminal hexapeptide from the heptatriacontapeptide, the resulting GLP-1$_{7-37}$ would have such a structure. Consequently GLP-1$_{1-37}$ is perhaps actually an inactive prohormone to GLP-1$_{7-37}$.

It is difficult to believe that the constancy with which phenylalanine occurs in position six in the secretin-glucagon group of peptides does not have any functional importance. However, at the present stage of our knowledge it cannot be stated that it has.

[**Note added in proof:** In the recently discovered magainins, or PGSs, antimicrobial peptides from the skin of *Zenopus laevis* (M. Zasloff, Proc. Natl. Acad. Sci. **84:** 5449-5453, 1987; M. G. Giovannini, L. Poulter, B. W. Gibson & D. H. Williams, Biochem. J. **243:** 113-120, 1987) residues of histidine and of phenylalanine are spaced relative to each other as they are in the secretin-glucagon group of peptides, although the histine residues are here not NH$_2$-terminally situated.]

REFERENCES

1. BERNARD, C. 1985. Memoir on The Pancreas. Translated by John Henderson. Monographs of the Physiological Society No. 42. Academic Press. London, England.
2. FINKE, U. & J. SEIFERT. 1986. Differential effects of gastrointestinal hormones on the blood flow of the alimentary tract of the dog. Res. Exp. Med. **186:** 151-165.
3. SAID, S. I. & V. MUTT. 1970. Polypeptide with broad biological activity: Isolation from small intestine. Science **169:** 1217-1218.
4. MUTT, V. & S. I. SAID. 1974. Structure of the porcine vasoactive intestinal octacosapeptide. Eur. J. Biochem. **42:** 581-589.
5. BODANSZKY, M., A. BODANSZKY, Y. S. KLAUSNER & S. I. SAID. 1974. A preferred conformation in the vasoactive intestinal peptide (VIP). Molecular architecture of gastrointestinal hormones. Bioorg. Chem. **3:** 133-140.
6. FOURNIER, A., J. K. SAUNDERS & S. ST-PIERRE. 1982. 400 MHz NMR study on the C-terminal fragment 21-28 of vasoactive intestinal peptide. Peptides **3:** 345-352.
7. MUTT, V. 1986. Isolation and chemical characterization of hormonal (poly) peptides. *In* Biological Regulation of Cell Proliferation. R. Baserga, P. Goa, D. Metcalf & E. E. Polli, Eds. **34:** 327-342. Raven Press. New York.
8. NAWA, H., T. HIROSE, H. TAKASHIMA, S. INAYAMA & S. NAKANISHI. 1983. Nucleotide sequences of cloned cDNAs for two types of bovine brain substance P precursor. Nature **306:** 32-36.
9. V. EULER, U. S. & J. H. GADDUM. 1931. An unidentified depressor substance in certain tissue extracts. J. Physiol. **72:** 74-87.
10. JORPES, J. E. & V. MUTT. 1961. On the biological activity and amino acid composition of secretin. Acta Chem. Scand. **15:** 1790-1791.
11. JORPES, J. E., V. MUTT, S. MAGNUSSON & B. B. STEELE. 1962. Amino acid composition and N-terminal amino acid sequence of porcine secretin. Biochem. Biophys. Res. Commun. **9:** 275-279.
12. BAYLISS, W. M. & E. H. STARLING. 1902. On the causation of the so-called "peripheral reflex secretion" of the pancreas. Proc. R. Soc. London **69:** 352-353.
13. IVY, A. C. & E. OLDBERG. A hormone mechanism for gall-bladder contraction and evacuation. Am. J. Physiol. **86:** 599-613.
14. HARPER, A. A. & H. S. RAPER. 1943. Pancreozymin, a stimulant of the secretion of pancreatic enzymes in extracts of the small intestine. J. Physiol. **102:** 115-125.
15. JORPES, J. E. & V. MUTT. 1966. Cholecystokinin and pancreozymin, one single hormone? Acta Physiol. Scand. **66:** 196-202.
16. HAYS, S. E., M. C. BEINFELD, R. T. JENSEN, F. K. GOODWIN & S. M. PAUL. 1980. Demonstration of a putative receptor site for cholecystokinin in rat brain. Neuropeptides **1:** 53-62.
17. CANTOR, P. 1986. Evaluation of a radioimmunoassay for cholecystokinin in human plasma. Scand. J. Clin. Lab. Invest. **46:** 213-221.
18. SAID, S. I., H. L. ESTEP, M. E. WEBSTER & H. A. KONTOS. 1968. Potent vasodepressor substance in normal lung. J. Clin. Invest. **47:** 85a-86a.
19. SAID, S. I. & V. MUTT. 1969. Long acting vasodilator peptide from lung tissue. Nature **224:** 699-700.
20. BROWN, J. C. & R. A. PEDERSON. 1970. A multiparameter study on the action of

preparations containing cholecystokinin-pancreozymin. Scand. J. Gastroenterol. **5:** 537-541.

21. BROWN, J. C., V. MUTT & R. A. PEDERSON. 1970. Further purification of a polypeptide demonstrating enterogastrone activity. J. Physiol. **209:** 57-64.

22. BROWN, J. C. 1967. Presence of a gastric motor-stimulating property in duodenal extracts. Gastroenterology **52:** 225-229.

23. BROWN, J. C., V. MUTT & J. R. DRYBURGH. 1971. The further purification of motilin, a gastric motor activity stimulating polypeptide from the mucosa of the small intestine of hogs. Can. J. Physiol. Pharmacol. **49:** 399-405.

24. HALLION, M. 1904. Discussion. *In* La Sécrétion physiologique du su intestinal. Action de l'acide chlorohydrique sur la sécrétion duodénale, by C. Delezenne and A. Frouin. Compt. Rend. Soc. Biol. **56:** 322.

25. CARLQUIST, M., H. JÖRNVALL, K. TATEMOTO & V. MUTT. 1982. A porcine brain polypeptide is identical to the vasoactive intestinal polypeptide. Gastroenterology **83:** 245-249.

26. CARLQUIST, M., V. MUTT & H. JÖRNVALL. 1979. Isolation and characterization of bovine vasoactive intestinal peptide (VIP). FEBS Lett. **108:** 457-460.

27. NILSSON, A. 1974. Isolation, amino acid composition and terminal amino acid residues of the vasoactive octacosapeptide from chicken intestine. Partial purification of chicken secretin. FEBS Lett. **47:** 284-289.

28. CARLQUIST, M., T. J. MCDONALD, V. L. W. GO, D. BATAILLE, C. JOHANSSON & V. MUTT. 1982. Isolation and amino acid composition of human vasoactive intestinal polypeptide (VIP). Horm. Metab. Res. **14:** 28-29.

29. BUNNETT, N. W., J. R. REEVE, JR., R. DIMALINE, J. E. SHIVELY, D. HAWKE & J. H. WALSH. 1984. The isolation and sequence analysis of vasoactive intestinal peptide from a ganglioneuroblastoma. J. Clin. Endocrinol. Metab. **59:** 1133-1137.

30. DIMALINE, R., J. R. REEVE, JR., J. E. SHIVELY & D. HAWKE. 1984. Isolation and characterization of rat vasoactive intestinal peptide. Peptides **5:** 183-187.

31. ENG, J., B. H. DU, J. P. RAUFMAN & R. S. YALOW. 1986. Purification and amino acid sequences of dog, goat and guinea pig VIPs. Peptides 7(Suppl. 1): 17-20.

32. WANG, S. C., B. H. DU., J. ENG, M. CHANG, J. D. HULMES, Y.-C. E. PAN & R. S. YALOW. 1985. Purification of dog VIP from a single animal. Life Sci. **37:** 979-983.

33. DU, B.-H., J. ENG, J. D. HULMES, M. CHANG, Y.-C. E. PAN & R. S. YALOW. 1985. Guinea pig has a unique mammalian VIP. Biochem. Biophys. Res. Commun. **128:** 1093-1098.

34. DIMALINE, R., M. C. THORNDYKE & J. YOUNG. 1986. Isolation and partial sequence of elasmobranch VIP. Regul. Pept. **14:** 1-10.

35. DIMALINE, R. & G. J. DOCKRAY. 1979. Molecular variants of vasoactive intestinal polypeptide in dog, rat and hog. Life Sci. **25:** 1893-1899.

36. JORPES, J. E. & V. MUTT. 1961. Process for the production of gastrointestinal hormones and hormone concentrate. U. S. Patent 3,013,944. December 1961.

37. NEWGARD, C. B. & J. J. HOLST. 1981. Heterogeneity of somatostatin like immunoreactivity (SLI) in extracts of porcine, canine and human pancreas. Acta Endocrinol. **98:** 564-572.

38. PRADAYROL, L., H. JÖRNVALL, V. MUTT & A. RIBET. 1980. N-terminally extended somatostatin: The primary structure of somatostatin-28. FEBS Lett. **109:** 55-58.

39. TATEMOTO, K. & V. MUTT. 1981. Isolation and characterization of the intestinal peptide porcine PHI (PHI-27), a new member of the glucagon-secretin family. Proc. Natl. Acad. Sci. USA **78:** 6603-6607.

40. TATEMOTO, K. & V. MUTT. 1980. Isolation of two novel candidate hormones using a chemical method for finding naturally occurring polypeptides. Nature **285:** 417-418.

41. TATEMOTO, K. 1982. Isolation and characterization of peptide YY (PYY), a candidate gut hormone that inhibits pancreatic exocrine secretion. Proc. Natl. Acad. Sci. USA **79:** 2514-2518.

42. TATEMOTO, K., S. SIIMESMAA, H. JÖRNVALL, J. M. ALLEN, J. M. POLAK, S. R. BLOOM & V. MUTT. 1985. Isolation and characterization of neuropeptide Y from porcine intestine. FEBS Lett. **179:** 181-184.

43. McDONALD, T. J., H. JÖRNVALL, G. NILSSON, M. VAGNE, M. GHATEI, S. R. BLOOM & V. MUTT. 1979. Characterization of a gastrin releasing peptide from porcine non-antral gastric tissue. Biochem. Biophys. Res. Commun. **90:** 227-233.
44. TATEMOTO, K., Å. RÖKAEUS, H. JÖRNVALL, T. J. McDONALD & V. MUTT. 1983. Galanin—a novel biologically active peptide from porcine intestine. FEBS Lett. **164:** 124-128.
45. SCHMIDT, W. E., V. MUTT, M. CARLQUIST, H. KRATZIN, J. M. CONLON & W. CREUTZFELDT. 1985. Valosin: Isolation and characterization of a novel peptide from porcine intestine. FEBS Lett. **191:** 264-268.
46. SCHMIDT, W. E., V. MUTT, H. KRATZIN, M. CARLQUIST, J. M. CONLON & W. CREUTZFELDT. 1985. Isolation and characterization of proSS$_{1-32}$, a peptide derived from the N-terminal region of porcine preprosomatostatin. FEBS Lett. **192:** 141-146.
47. MUTT, V. 1959. Preparation of highly purified secretin. Arkiv Kemi **15:** 69-74.
48. GREGORY, R. A. & H. J. TRACY. 1964. The constitution and properties of two gastrins extracted from hog antral mucosa. Gut **5:** 103-117.
49. ITOH, N., K.-I. OBATA, N. YANAIHARA & H. OKAMOTO. 1983. Human preprovasoactive intestinal polypeptide contains a novel PHI-27-like peptide, PHM-27. Nature **304:** 547-549.
50. BLOOM, S. R., J. DELAMARTER, E. KAWASHIMA, N. D. CHRISTOFIDES, G. BUELL & J. M. POLAK. 1983. Diarrhoea in vipoma patients associated with cosecretion of a second active peptide (peptide histidine isoleucine) explained by single coding gene. Lancet **II:** 1163-1165.
51. TSUKADA, T., S. J. HOROVITCH, M. R. MONTMINY, G. MANDEL & R. H. GOODMAN. 1985. Structure of the human vasoactive intestinal polypeptide gene. DNA **4:** 293-300.
52. BODNER, M., M. FRIDKIN & I. GOZES. 1985. Coding sequences for vasoactive intestinal peptide and PHM-27 peptide are located on two adjacent exons in the human genome. Proc. Natl. Acad. Sci. USA **82:** 3548-3551.
53. LINDER, S., T. BARKHEM, A. NORBERG, H. PERSSON, M. SCHALLING, T. HÖKFELT & G. MAGNUSSON. 1987. Structure and expression of the gene encoding the vasoactive intestinal peptide precursor. Proc. Natl. Acad. Sci. USA **84:** 605-609.
54. TATEMOTO, K. & V. MUTT. 1978. Chemical determination of polypeptide hormones. Proc. Natl. Acad. Sci. USA **75:** 4115-4119.
55. TATEMOTO, K., M. CARLQUIST, T. J. McDONALD & V. MUTT. 1983. Isolation of a brain peptide identical to the intestinal PHI (peptide HI). FEBS Lett. **153:** 248-252.
56. CARLQUIST, M., R. KAISER, K. TATEMOTO, H. JÖRNVALL & V. MUTT. 1984. A novel form of the polypeptide PHI isolated in high yield from bovine upper intestine. Eur. J. Biochem. **144:** 243-247.
57. TATEMOTO, K., H. JÖRNVALL, T. J. McDONALD, M. CARLQUIST, V. L. W. GO, C. JOHANSSON & V. MUTT. 1984. Isolation and primary structure of human PHI (peptide HI). FEBS Lett. **174:** 258-261.
58. LUNDBERG, J. M. & K. TATEMOTO. 1982. Vascular effects of the peptides PYY and PHI: Comparison with APP and VIP. Eur. J. Pharmacol. **83:** 143-146.
59. LARSSON, O., M. DUNÉR-ENGSTRÖM, J. M. LUNDBERG, B. B. FREDHOLM & A. ÅNGGÅRD. 1986. Effects of VIP, PHM and substance P on blood vessels and secretory elements of the human submandibular gland. Regul. Pept. **13:** 319-326.
60. YIANGOU, Y., N. D. CHRISTOFIDES, M. A. BLANK, N. YANAIHARA, K. TATEMOTO, A. E. BISHOP, J. M. POLAK & S. R. BLOOM. 1985. Molecular forms of peptide histidine isoleucine-like immunoreactivity in the gastrointestinal tract. Gastroenterology **89:** 516-524.
61. YIANGOU, Y., F. REQUEJO, J. M. POLAK & S. R. BLOOM. 1986. Characterization of a novel prepro VIP derived peptide. Biochem. Biophys. Res. Commun. **139:** 1142-1149.
62. LING, N., F. ESCH, P. BÖHLEN, P. BRAZEAU, W. B. WEHRENBERG & R. GUILLEMIN. 1984. Isolation, primary structure, and synthesis of human hypothalamic somatocrinin: Growth hormone-releasing factor. Proc. Natl. Acad. Sci. USA **81:** 4302-4306.
63. SYKES, J. E. C. & P. J. LOWRY. 1983. Purification of a high-molecular-weight somatoliberin (growth-hormone-releasing factor) from pig hypothalami. Biochem. J. **209:** 643-651.
64. GUILLEMIN, R., P. BRAZEAU, P. BÖHLEN, F. ESCH, N. LING & W. B. WEHRENBERG.

1982. Growth hormone-releasing factor from a human pancreatic tumor that caused acromegaly. Science **218**: 585-587.

65. RIVIER, J., J. SPIESS, M. THORNER & W. VALE. 1982. Characterization of a growth hormone-releasing factor from a human pancreatic islet tumour. Nature **300**: 276-278.

66. BRAZEAU, P., P. BÖHLEN, F. ESCH, N. LING, W. B. WEHRENBERG & R. GUILLEMIN. 1984. Growth hormone-releasing factor from ovine and caprine hypothalamus: Isolation, sequence analysis and total synthesis. Biochem. Biophys. Res. Commun. **125**: 606-614.

67. SPIESS, J., J. RIVIER & W. VALE. 1983. Characterization of rat hypothalamic growth hormone-releasing factor. Nature **303**: 532-535.

68. LABURTHE, M., A. COUVINEAU & C. ROUYER-FESSARD. 1986. Study of species specificity in growth hormone-releasing factor (GRF) interaction with vasoactive intestinal peptide (VIP) receptors using GRF and intestinal VIP receptors from rat and human: Evidence that Ac-Tyr¹hGRF is a competitive VIP antagonist in the rat. Mol. Pharmacol. **29**: 23-27.

69. GUBLER, U., J. J. MONAHAN, P. T. LOMEDICO, R. S. BHATT, K. J. COLLIER, B. J. HOFFMAN, P. BÖHLEN, F. ESCH, N. LING, F. ZEYTIN, P. BRAZEAU, M. S. POONIAN & L. P. GAGE. 1983. Cloning and sequence analysis of cDNA for the precursor of human growth hormone-releasing factor, somatocrinin. Proc. Natl. Acad. Sci. USA **80**: 4311-4314.

70. MAYO, K. E., G. M. CERELLI, R. V. LEBO, B. D. BRUCE, M. G. ROSENFELD & R. M. EVANS. 1985. Gene encoding human growth hormone-releasing factor precursor: Structure, sequence, and chromosomal assignment. Proc. Natl. Acad. Sci. USA **82**: 63-67.

71. MAYO, K. E., W. VALE, J. RIVIER, M. G. ROSENFELD & R. M. EVANS. 1983. Expression-cloning and sequence of a cDNA encoding human growth hormone-releasing factor. Nature **306**: 86-88.

72. BROWN, J. C. & R. A. PEDERSON. 1976. GI hormones and insulin secretion. In Endocrinology. V. H. T. James, Ed. Vol. **2**: 568-570. Excerpta Medica. Amsterdam, the Netherlands.

73. MOODY, A. J., L. THIM & I. VALVERDE. 1984. The isolation and sequencing of human gastric inhibitory peptide (GIP). FEBS Lett. **172**: 142-148.

74. JÖRNVALL, H., M. CARLQUIST, S. KWAUK, S. C. OTTE, C. H. S. McINTOSH, J. C. BROWN & V. MUTT. 1981. Amino acid sequence and heterogeneity of gastric inhibitory polypeptide (GIP). FEBS Lett. **123**: 205-210.

75. BROWN, J. C. & J. R. DRYBURGH. 1971. A gastric inhibitory polypeptide II: The complete amino acid sequence. Can. J. Biochem. **49**: 867-872.

76. CARLQUIST, M., M. MALETTI, H. JÖRNVALL & V. MUTT. 1984. A novel form of gastric inhibitory polypeptide (GIP) isolated from bovine intestine using a radioreceptor assay. Eur. J. Biochem. **145**: 573-577.

77. CARLQUIST, M. 1984. Isolation and chemical characterization of gastrointestinal hormones. Thesis. Sundt Offset Stockholm. Sweden.

78. ZIMMERMAN, M., R. A. MUMFORD & D. F. STEINER, Eds. 1980. Precursor Processing in the Biosynthesis of Proteins. Vol. 343. Ann. N.Y. Acad. Sci. New York.

79. KREIL, G. 1984. Occurrence, detection, and biosynthesis of carboxy-terminal amides. Methods Enzymol. **106**(Part A): 218-223.

80. BRADBURY, A. F. & D. G. SMYTH. 1983. Substrate specificity of an amidating enzyme in porcine pituitary. Biochem. Biophys. Res. Commun. **112**: 372-377.

81. EIPPER, B. A., R. E. MAINS & C. C. GLEMBOTSKI. 1983. Identification in pituitary tissue of a peptide α-amidation activity that acts on glycine-extended peptides and requires molecular oxygen, copper, and ascorbic acid. Proc. Natl. Acad. Sci. USA **80**: 5144-5148.

82. CARLQUIST, M. 1987. Solid phase synthesis of a 31-residue fragment of human glucose-dependent insulinotropic polypeptide (GIP) by the continuous flow polyamide method. Acta Chem. Scand. **B41**: 494-498.

83. MALETTI, M., J. J. ALTMAN, D. HUI BON HOA, M. CARLQUIST & G. ROSSELIN. 1986. Evidence of functional gastric inhibitory polypeptide receptors in human insulinoma. Adenylyl cyclasic activity of the synthetic human 1-31 gastric inhibitory polypeptide. Diabetologia **29**: A568/319.

84. POLLOCK, H. G. & J. R. KIMMEL. 1975. Chicken glucagon. J. Biol. Chem. **250**: 9377-9380.

85. NILSSON, A. 1975. Structure of the vasoactive intestinal octacosapeptide from chicken intestine. The amino acid sequence. FEBS Lett. **60:** 322-325.
86. NILSSON, A., M. CARLQUIST, H. JÖRNVALL & V. MUTT. 1980. Isolation and characterization of chicken secretin. Eur. J. Biochem. **112:** 383-388.
87. CARLQUIST, M., H. JÖRNVALL & V. MUTT. 1981. Isolation and amino acid sequence of bovine secretin. FEBS Lett. **127:** 71-74.
88. CARLQUIST, M., H. JÖRNVALL, W.-G. FORSSMANN, L. THULIN, C. JOHANSSON & V. MUTT. 1985. Human secretin is not identical to the porcine/bovine hormone. IRCS Med. Sci. Biochem. **13:** 217-218.
89. CARLQUIST, M. & Å. RÖKAEUS. 1984. Isolation of a proform of porcine secretin by ion-exchange and reversed-phase high-performance liquid chromatography. J. Chromatogr. **296:** 143-151.
90. GAFVELIN, G., M. CARLQUIST & V. MUTT. 1985. A proform of secretin with high secretin-like bioactivity. FEBS Lett. **184:** 347-352.
91. DELVALLE, J., K. SUGANO & T. YAMADA. 1985. Release of glycine-extended processing intermediates of cholecystokinin into human plasma by intraduodenal fat infusion. Gastroenterology **88:** 1362.
92. ALLARD, L. R. & M. C. BEINFELD. 1985. The subcellular distribution of peptides immunoreactive for the carboxyl-terminal extension of cholecystokinin in rat brain. Neuropeptides **6:** 239-245.
93. REHFELD, J. F. 1986. Accumulation of nonamidated preprogastrin and preprocholecystokinin products in porcine pituitary corticotrophs. J. Biol. Chem. **261:** 5841-5847.
94. BROMER, W. W., L. G. SINN, A. STAUB & O. K. BEHRENS. 1956. The amino acid sequence of glucagon. J. Am. Chem. Soc. **78:** 3858-3860.
95. SMITH, L. F. 1966. Species variations in the amino acid sequence of insulin. Am. J. Med. **40:** 662-666.
96. SUNDBY, F. 1976. Species variations in the primary structure of glucagon. Metabolism **25**(Suppl. 1): 1319-1321.
97. CONLON, J. M., H. F. HANSEN & T. W. SCHWARTZ. 1985. Primary structure of glucagon and a partial sequence of oxyntomodulin (glucagon-37) from the guinea pig. Regul. Pept. **11:** 309-320.
98. BELL, G. I., R. SANCHEZ-PESCADOR, P. J. LAYBOURN & R. C. NAJARIAN. 1983. Exon duplication and divergence in the human preproglucagon gene. Nature **304:** 368-371.
99. LOPEZ, L. C., M. L. FRAZIER, C.-J. SU, A. KUMAR & G. F. SAUNDERS. 1983. Mammalian pancreatic preproglucagon contains three glucagon-related peptides. Proc. Natl. Acad. Sci. USA **80:** 5485-5489.
100. BELL, G. I., R. F. SANTERRE & G. T. MULLENBACH. 1983. Hamster preproglucagon contains the sequence of glucagon and two related peptides. Nature **302:** 716-718.
101. HEINRICH, G., P. GROS & J. F. HABENER. 1984. Glucagon gene sequence. J. Biol. Chem. **259:** 14082-14087.
102. CONLON, J. M., H. F. HANSEN & T. W. SCHWARTZ. 1985. Primary structure of glucagon and a partial sequence of oxyntomodulin (glucagon-37) from the guinea pig. Regul. Pept. **11:** 309-320.
103. HUANG, C. G., J. ENG, Y.-C. E. PAN, J. D. HULMES & R. S. YALOW. 1986. Guinea pig glucagon differs from other mammalian glucagons. Diabetes **35:** 508-512.
104. LANCE, V., J. W. HAMILTON, J. B. ROUSE, J. R. KIMMEL & H. G. POLLOCK. 1984. Isolation and characterization of reptilian insulin, glucagon, and pancreatic polypeptide: Complete amino acid sequence of alligator (*Alligator mississippiensis*) insulin and pancreatic polypeptide. Gen. Comp. Endocrinol. **55:** 112-124.
105. CONLON, J. M. & L. THIM. 1985. Primary structure of glucagon from an elasmobranchian fish *Torpedo marmorata.* Gen. Comp. Endocrinol. **60:** 398-405.
106. PLISETSKAYA, E., H. G. POLLOCK, J. B. ROUSE, J. W. HAMILTON, J. R. KIMMEL & A. GORBMAN. 1986. Isolation and structures of coho salmon (*Oncorhynchus kisutch*) glucagon and glucagon-like peptide. Regul. Pept. **14:** 57-67.
107. ANDREWS, P. C. & P. RONNER. 1985. Isolation and structures of glucagon and glucagon-like peptide from catfish pancreas. J. Biol. Chem. **260:** 3910-3914.
108. LUND, P. K., R. H. GOODMAN, M. R. MONTMINY, P. C. DEE & J. F. HABENER. 1983.

Anglerfish islet pre-proglucagon II. J. Biol. Chem. **258:** 3280-3284.

109. SHIELDS, D., T. G. WARREN, S. E. ROTH & M. J. BRENNER. 1981. Cell-free synthesis and processing of multiple precursors to glucagon. Nature **289:** 511-514.

110. LUND, P. K., R. H. GOODMAN & J. F. HABENER. 1981. Pancreatic pre-proglucagons are encoded by two separate mRNAs. J. Biol. Chem. **256:** 6515-6518.

111. LOPEZ, L. C., W.-H. LI, M. L. FRAZIER, C.-C. LUO & G. F. SAUNDERS. 1984. Evolution of glucagon genes. Mol. Biol. Evol. **1:** 335-344.

112. ANDREWS, P. C., D. H. HAWKE, T. D. LEE, K. LEGESSE, B. D. NOE & J. E. SHIVELY. 1986. Isolation and structure of the principal products of preproglucagon processing, including an amidated glucagon-like peptide. J. Biol. Chem. **261:** 8128-8133.

113. TAGER, H. S. & D. F. STEINER. 1973. Isolation of a glucagon-containing peptide: Primary structure of a possible fragment of proglucagon. Proc. Natl. Acad. Sci. USA **70:** 2321-2325.

114. THIM, L. & A. J. MOODY. 1981. The primary structure of porcine glicentin (proglucagon). Regul. Pept. **2:** 139-150.

115. SUNDBY, F., H. JACOBSEN & A. J. MOODY. 1976. Purification and characterization of protein from porcine gut with glucagon-like immunoreactivity. Horm. Metab. Res. **8:** 366-371.

116. BATAILLE, D., K. TATEMOTO, C. GESPACH, H. JÖRNVALL, G. ROSSELIN & V. MUTT. 1982. Isolation of glucagon-37 (bioactive enteroglucagon/oxyntomodulin) from porcine jejuno-ileum. FEBS Lett. **146:** 79-86.

117. PATZELT, C. & E. SCHILTZ. 1984. Conversion of proglucagon in pancreatic alpha cells: The major endproducts are glucagon and a single peptide, the major proglucagon fragment, that contains two glucagon-like sequences. Proc. Natl. Acad. Sci. USA **81:** 5007-5011.

118. ØRSKOV, C., J. J. HOLST, S. KNUHTSEN, F. G. A. BALDISSERA, S. S. POULSEN & O. V. NIELSEN. 1986. Glucagon-like peptides GLP-1 and GLP-2, predicted products of the glucagon gene, are secreted separately from pig small intestine but not pancreas. Endocrinology **119:** 1467-1475.

119. MOJSOV, S., G. HEINRICH, I. B. WILSON, M. RAVAZZOLA, L. ORCI & J. F. HABENER. 1986. Preproglucagon gene expression in pancreas and intestine diversifies at the level of post-translational processing. J. Biol. Chem. **261:** 11880-11889.

120. BLUNDELL, T. L., S. DOCKERILL, K. SASAKI, I. J. TICKLE & S. P. WOOD. 1976. The relation of structure to storage and receptor binding of glucagon. Metabolism **25**(Suppl. 1): 1331-1339.

121. RAUFMAN, J.-P., R. T. JENSEN, V. E. SUTLIFF, J. J. PISANO & J. D. GARDNER. 1982. Actions of Gila monster venom on dispersed acini from guinea pig pancreas. Am. J. Physiol. **242:** G470-G474.

122. PARKER, D. S., J.-P. RAUFMAN, T. L. O'DONOHUE, M. BLEDSOE, H. YOSHIDA & J. J. PISANO. 1984. Amino acid sequences of helospectins, new members of the glucagon superfamily, found in Gila monster venom. J. Biol. Chem. **259:** 11751-11755.

123. HOSHINO, M., C. YANAIHARA, Y.-M. HONG, S. KISHIDA, Y. KATSUMARU, A. VANDERMEERS, M.-C. VANDERMEERS-PIRET, P. ROBBERECHT, J. CHRISTOPHE & N. YANAIHARA. 1984. Primary structure of helodermin, a VIP-secretin-like peptide isolated from Gila monster venom. FEBS Lett. **178:** 233-239.

124. ROBBERECHT, P., J. DE GRAEF, M.-C. WOUSSEN, M.-C. VANDERMEERS-PIRET, A. VANDERMEERS, P. DE NEEF, A. CAUVIN, C. YANAIHARA, N. YANAIHARA & J. CHRISTOPHE. 1985. Immunoreactive helodermin-like peptides in rat: A new class of mammalian neuropeptides related to secretin and VIP. Biochem. Biophys. Res. Commun. **130:** 333-342.

125. MUTT, V. 1981. Additional observations on cholecystokinin and the vasoactive intestinal polypeptide. Peptides **2**(Suppl. 2): 209-214.

126. MUTT, V. 1964. Behaviour of secretin, cholecystokinin and pancreozymin to oxidation with hydrogen peroxide. Acta Chem. Scand. **18:** 2185-2186.

127. DEDMAN, M. L., T. H. FARMER & C. J. O. R. MORRIS. 1961. Studies on pituitary adenocorticotrophin. 3. Identification of the oxidation-reduction centre. Biochem. J. **78:** 348-352.

128. MUTT, V. & J. E. JORPES. 1967. Contemporary developments in the biochemistry of the gastrointestinal hormones. Rec. Progr. Horm. Res. **23:** 483-503.
129. WÜNSCH, E., E. JAEGER & L. MORODER. 1977. Progress in the problem of structure-activity relations of gastrointestinal hormones. *In* Hormonal Receptors in Digestive Tract Physiology. S. Bonfils, P. Fromageot, G. Rosselin, Eds.: 19-27. North-Holland Publ. Co. Amsterdam, New York, Oxford.
130. MUTT, V. 1986. Questions answered and raised by work on the chemistry of gastrointestinal and cerebrogastrointestinal hormonal polypeptides. Chemica Scripta **26B:** 191-207.

Synthesis of Vasoactive Intestinal Peptide and Related Peptides

MIKLOS BODANSZKY

Department of Chemistry
Case Western Reserve University
Cleveland, Ohio 44106

Twenty years have elapsed since the publication of the first synthesis[1,2] of a gastrointestinal hormone, porcine secretin. Therefore, it might be timely to assess the work accomplished in this area during the last two decades. Yet, the exponential growth of research and the rapid emergence of new, biologically active peptides render it nearly impossible to write a concise and still comprehensive review on the entire secretin-VIP-glucagon family of peptides. Instead of an exhaustive treatment, we will discuss here only a few aspects of peptide synthesis with emphasis mainly on studies concerning secretin and VIP.

The principal objectives of peptide synthesis are (a) proof of structure derived from degradation, (b) preparation of biologically active peptides in amounts sufficient for diagnosis and therapy, and (c) elucidation, with the help of synthetic analogues, of the relationships between structure (including architecture) and activity. These aims were vigorously pursued when the sequences of secretin,[3] glucagon,[4] VIP,[5] the gastric inhibitory polypeptide, or glucose-dependent insulinotropic polypeptide (GIP)[6] and of the peptide known by the acronym PHI[7] (peptide with histidine at the NH_2-terminus and isoleucine amide at the COOH-terminus) became known. The results of the synthetic studies will be discussed separately for each individual peptide. The less closely related somatocrinins[8,9] lie outside the limited scope of this review.

SECRETIN

A preliminary report by Professor Mutt on the amino acid sequence of porcine secretin allowed us to begin work on the synthesis of the hormone in 1964, even before the final structure was published.[3] The chain of 27 amino acids was built according to the stepwise strategy,[10] through incorporation of single amino acid residues, starting with the COOH-terminal valine amide. Comparison of the synthetic COOH-terminal hexapeptide and 13-peptide amides with the corresponding tryptic fragments by paper chromatography, electrophoresis, and side by side enzymatic degradation followed by a similar examination of the final product provided rigorous evidence for the correctness of the sequence of porcine secretin:

His- Ser- Asp- Gly- Thr- Phe- Thr- Ser- Glu- Leu- Ser- Arg- Leu- Arg-
1   2   3   4   5   6   7   8   9   10   11   12   13   14

Asp-Ser- Ala- Arg-Leu-Gln-Arg-Leu-Leu-Gln-Gly-Leu- Val- NH$_2$
15   16   17   18   19   20   21   22   23   24   25   26   27

The synthetic 27-peptide amide[2] was indistinguishable from the natural hormone in a series of tests including its effectiveness in the release of bicarbonate from the pancreas. Soon a second synthesis of secretin was carried out[11] via condensation of partially blocked segments of the chain and the pure peptide could be secured in fairly large amounts (several grams).

In subsequent years several laboratories embarked on the synthesis of secretin, obviously to develop approaches for industrial production. The chain of the porcine hormone was assembled from segments by Wünsch and his associates[12] and also by the Höchst group led by Geiger.[13] The latter effort was continued and afforded a process by which secretin is produced on a commercial scale. A return to stepwise chain building is the synthesis reported by Van Zon and Beyerman.[14,15] They proceeded through the same intermediates that were described in the first synthesis[1,2] of the hormone except that mixed anhydrides rather than active esters were applied in the coupling steps. The stepwise strategy[10] was followed in the syntheses of secretin by the solid-phase technique of Merrifield.[16] The difficulties encountered in the separation of the peptide chain from the insoluble polymeric support in the form of the amide[17] could be overcome by improvements in the execution of ammonolysis.[18] In the meantime the problem was circumvented by application of benzhydrylamine-type resins[19] that permit the separation of peptide amides via acidolysis. Thus Hemmassi and Bayer[20] reported the first synthesis of secretin by the solid-phase method. The same approach was applied by Coy and his associates.[21]

In recent years an increase in the interest in practical methods for the production of secretin could be noted. Publications concerning syntheses through the condensation of segments[22–24] and numerous patent applications[25] covering similar avenues are complemented by reports concerning production in bacterial cells with the help of synthetic DNA molecules coding for the secretin sequence. Some attempts of biogenetic engineering[26,27] are obviously inconclusive, because the peptide produced by them is not secretin itself but its inactive 27-desamido derivative, that is, a 27-peptide ending with valine rather than valine amide. A more sophisticated approach by König et al.[28] yields secretylglycine, which is then converted to secretin by a specific enzyme. The primary product of fermentation is β-galactosidasyl-methionyl-secretyl-glycine, which is first cleaved with cyanogen bromide at the methionine residue to afford secretyl-glycine. The reported yields are fairly modest: From 10 g of the protein, 50 mg of the secretin derivative could be obtained and conversion of the latter to the desired amide produced only 1.2 mg of the hormone. While it seems to be quite possible to improve the process, it might be even more practical to synthesize the gene corresponding to the proform of secretin,[29] which, instead of valine amide, has the sequence valyl-glycyl-lysyl-arginine at the COOH-terminus. This 32-peptide is at least as potent as the 27-peptide amide. It should be noted however, that since the 28-peptide secretyl-glycine is also active,[30] its conversion to the 27-peptide amide could turn out to be unnecessary.

The sequence of bovine secretin[31] is identical to that of the porcine hormone, but human secretin[32] is different from it at two points: It has an aspartyl residue at position 15 and serine at position 16. At the time of writing this article, only one year after publication of its sequence, synthetic human secretin is already commercially available. Improvements in the methods of peptide synthesis and peptide purification led to this interesting situation. Chicken secretin[33] in which positions 15 and 18 are occupied by neutral residues has also been synthesized and is marketed for research purposes.

Analogues of secretin were prepared in order to study the side reactions that often accompany the process of synthesis. Thus, the 3-β-aspartyl and 3-aminosuccinyl analogues were synthesized[34] because the aspartyl-glycine partial sequence in positions three and four is prone to rearrangement, which yields these undesired analogues. For similar reasons analogues containing D-residues instead of the natural L-residue in selected positions were prepared[35] to assist the scrutiny of synthetic preparations in which such diastereoisomers can be present, albeit in minor amounts, as a consequence of racemization during the condensation of peptide segments.

In a study[36] of the structure-biological activity relationship, a secretin analogue with pyrazolylalanine replacing histidine in position one and others with D-tryptophan and D-alanine in position four and with D-phenylalanine in position six were prepared,[36] the last one being somewhat more potent than the parent hormone. Hybrid molecules in which the COOH-terminal hexapeptide sequence of secretin was replaced by the corresponding sequences of VIP, GIP, or glucagon were synthesized[37] as were secretin-glucagon hybrids in which positions 3, 9, 10, 13, 22, and 25 were studied.[38] Secretin-VIP hybrids remain to be objectives of synthesis.[39,40]

Exploration of the three-dimensional structure of secretin with the help of synthetic analogues provided some information. Thus, a folded and partially helical character of the chain could be established by examination of the entire molecule of the hormone and of the deblocked intermediates of its first syntheses.[1,2,11] Analogues in which the side-chain carboxyl groups are replaced by carboxamides were designed and secured to establish the role of ion pairs in the final determination of the architecture.[41] Also, in order to obtain experimental evidence for the position of the helical stretch, an analogue with aspartic acid replacing glutamic acid in position nine was prepared and studied.[42] These and related investigations were recently reviewed.[43] Interesting supporting evidence for a compact architecture comes from the examination of secretin by dark-field electron microscopy.[44]

VASOACTIVE INTESTINAL PEPTIDE

The first synthesis[45,46] of vasoactive intestinal peptide (VIP) closely followed the determination of the sequence[5] of its amino acid constituents. The synthetic material was compared with natural porcine VIP through side by side degradation with proteolytic enzymes and similar comparisons were carried out between tryptic and chymotryptic fragments of VIP and the corresponding synthetic peptides. The sequence proposed by Mutt and Said[5] for porcine VIP,

His- Ser- Asp-Ala-Val-Phe-Thr-Asp-Asn- Tyr- Thr-Arg-Phe-Arg-
 1   2   3   4   5   6   7   8   9   10 11 12 13 14

Lys-Gln-Met-Ala-Val-Lys- Lys- Tyr- Leu- Asn-Ser-Ile-Leu-Asn-NH$_2$
15 16 17 18 19 20 21 22 23 24 25 26 27 28

was fully confirmed in these investigations. The synthetic 28-peptide amide had all the characteristic biological activities of porcine VIP and was equipotent with it. Chiroptical properties of the complete chain and of shorter segments revealed a folded, partially helical molecule similar to the one found in studies of secretin[48] except that the conformational freedom in VIP seems to be less restricted than in secretin. In fact, the ord-cd spectra of VIP were closest to those of a secretin analogue without structure-stabilizing ion pairs.[49] Studies by Fournier et al.[50] gave results that were in harmony with this general description of the geometry of the VIP molecule. A more detailed account of their work is included in this volume.

The first synthesis of VIP[46] was complicated by the poor solubility of the blocked intermediates in organic solvents including dimethylformamide. Therefore the initially attempted stepwise strategy[10] was abandoned and the segment condensation approach followed. It might be possible to overcome the solubility problem by reducing the tendency of the intermediates for aggregation (self association).[51] This could be achieved[52] by the replacement of the COOH-terminal asparagine amide with an ester of asparagine and conversion to the amide at a later stage. The synthesis of chicken VIP[53] in which the COOH-terminal residue is threoninamide appeared less problematic and its chain could indeed be assembled through stepwise incorporation of amino acids in the form of their active esters by the *in situ* technique.[54] The synthetic material was fully active.[55] Synthesis of chicken VIP by segment condensation was achieved by Yajima and his associates,[56] who prepared the porcine peptide as well.[57]

In solid-phase peptide synthesis, the solubility of the intermediates has no immediate effect on the course of the process; it is enough if the peptidyl resin swells in dichloromethane or dimethylformamide. Synthesis of porcine VIP could indeed be accomplished[58] by this technique. Subsequently an advanced version of solid-phase synthesis was applied for the preparation of the same 28-peptide amide by Colombo[59] who used the base-sensitive 9-fluorenylmethyloxycarbonyl (Fmoc) blocking group[60] for the protection of the α-amino function of the individual amino acids that were activated in the form of their symmetrical anhydrides. Deblocking after each chain-lengthening step with piperidine in dimethylformamide and removal of the tertiary butyl-based semipermanent blocking groups by acidolysis could be carried out under mild conditions and the results are encouraging in regard to the synthesis of peptides of similar size. The analogous application of Fmoc amino acids in an attempt[61] to prepare chicken VIP in solution proceeded well until the poor solubility of the blocked intermediates in dimethylformamide interfered with the removal of the Fmoc group.

The biosynthetic pathway leading to VIP seems to be more complex than that of secretin. The generally used method of separating the target peptide from an adjacent protein by incorporating a residue between them and cleaving with cyanogen bromide cannot be applied because VIP contains methioinine in position 17 and its chain would be split into two fragments in the process. Of course, this obstacle can be overcome by targeting, instead of VIP, rather its analogue in which the methionine residue is replaced, for example by leucine. The 17-norleucine analogue of the COOH-terminal 15-peptide sequence was found[62] to have the activities of the unaltered peptide. Thus the methionine residue is not essential for the biological effects of VIP. This finding was corroborated[63] by the synthesis and examination of the complete 28-peptide amide molecule. It seems to be likely that leucine will provide an equally effective replacement for methionine. A gene coding for the unaltered sequence has been synthesized.[64]

Structure-activity relationships were explored with the help of synthetic analogues of VIP. A 28-peptide amide in which aspartic acid in position eight was replaced by a glutamic acid residue was prepared[65] by segment condensation in solution while a series of biologically active analogues with multiple substitutions were obtained[66] by solid-phase peptide synthesis. The intriguing questions about the activity of smaller peptides with partial sequences of VIP were the subject of several investigations. Synthesis of VIP_{16-28} with pyroglutamic acid instead of glutamine was carried out[67] in the assumption that this 13-peptide amide might be the product of a process in which the VIP molecule plays the role of a prohormone and is cleaved at Arg-Lys in position 14-15. Quite interestingly, peptide amides encompassing residues 11-23, secured[68] both by solid-phase synthesis and by synthesis in solution, were found to promote colonic motility and to have antiulcer activity. The less than rigid structural requirement for biological activity in the VIP molecule was already indicated in the weak but measurable potency of the NH_2-terminal decapeptide[69] and even more in the VIP-like activity of the secretin analogue in which a single residue, aspartic acid in position 15, was exchanged for lysine, the characteristic VIP residue in this position.[70]

A more comprehensive treatment of structure-activity relationships and the synthesis of VIP antagonists is the subject of Dr. Rivier's contribution to this volume.

GLUCAGON

The amino acid sequence of glucagon, isolated from porcine pancreas, was published[4] in 1957:

His- Ser-Gln-Gly- Thr- Phe-Thr-Ser-Asp-Tyr-Ser-Lys-Tyr-Leu-
 1   2   3   4   5   6   7   8   9   10   11   12   13   14

Asp-Ser-Arg-Arg- Ala- Gln- Asp-Phe-Val-Gln-Trp-Leu-Met-Asn-Thr-
15   16   17   18   19   20   21   22   23   24   25   26   27   28   29

While several laboratories reported syntheses of peptides corresponding to partial sequences of the 29-peptide chain, its first total synthesis was announced by Wünsch[71] ten years later and was rightly regarded as a major accomplishment. Several syntheses, also from segments condensed in solution, followed yielding the porcine[72] and the avian[73] glucagon. The hormone was obtained by segment condensation on an insoluble polymeric support as well.[74] The ready availability of glucagon from the pancreas of the pork renders its synthesis less imperative than that of other gastrointestinal peptides, and major efforts aimed mainly at the elucidation of the relationship between structure and hormonal activity. This topic is discussed in more detail by Dr. Bataille elsewhere in this volume. We merely mention the concentrated efforts of the group led by Hruby[75-78] toward the conformational aspects of biological activity with the help of numerous analogues of glucagon, all prepared by solid-phase peptide synthesis.

As noted at the last VIP symposium,[43] the biologically relevant conformation of glucagon remains elusive. The expectation voiced there that studies on rigid cyclic analogues might solve the difficulties caused by the considerable conformational freedom of the chain and the tendency of the glucagon molecule for self-association in various forms must be tempered in view of the results from X-ray crystallography[79,80] of desamino-oxytocin and pressinoic acid. These relatively small and simple molecules have, in spite of their cyclic structure and solid state, more than one conformation. Desamino-oxytocin is present in two conformers in the same crystal.

GASTRIC INHIBITORY POLYPEPTIDE OR GLUCOSE-DEPENDENT INSULINOTROPIC POLYPEPTIDE

Elucidation of the amino acid sequence of porcine gastric inhibitory polypeptide (GIP) revealed[81] a 43-residue peptide that was soon synthesized.[82] A subsequent reexamination[6] showed that the chain of GIP consists of 42 rather than 43 residues:

Tyr-Ala-Glu-Gly-Thr-Phe-Ile-Ser-Asp-Tyr-Ser-Ile-Ala-Met-
 1   2   3   4   5   6   7   8   9   10 11 12 13 14

Asp-Lys-Ile-Arg-Gln-Gln-Asp-Phe-Val-Asn-Trp-Leu-Leu-Ala-
15 16 17 18 19 20 21 22 23 24 25 26 27 28

Gln-Lys-Gly-Lys-Lys-Ser-Asp-Trp-Lys-His-Asn-Ile-Thr-Gln-
29 30 31 32 33 34 35 36 37 38 39 40 41 42

A glutamine residue following position 29 in the originally published sequence had to be deleted. Synthesis[83] of the revised structure by segment condensation in solution and the similar synthesis of the human hormone[84] demonstrated the usefulness of several improvements in protection and deprotection.

PEPTIDE HAVING NH$_2$-TERMINAL HISTIDINE AND COOH-TERMINAL ISOLEUCINE AMIDE (PHI-27 or PHI)

The sequence of this recently discovered[7] member of the secretin family

His-Ser-Asp-Gly-Val-Phe-Thr-Ser-Asp-Phe-Ser-Arg-Leu-Leu-
 1   2   3   4   5   6   7   8   9   10 11 12 13 14

Gly-Gln-Leu-Ser-Ala-Lys-Lys-Tyr-Leu-Glu-Ser-Leu-Ile-NH$_2$
15 16 17 18 19 20 21 22 23 24 25 26 27

has already been confirmed by syntheses[85,86] through segment condensation carried out in solution. An analogue in which glutamic acid in position 24 was replaced by glutamine was also prepared[87] because this position is occupied by glutamine or by asparagine in the other members of the secretin family and in the related growth hormone releasing factor[8,9] as well. The question of whether a glutamine to glutamic acid conversion took place during isolation of PHI could not be answered by this experiment because the two peptides were equipotent.

PERSPECTIVES

The methods of peptide synthesis have advanced considerably in recent years and this progress in conjunction with improvements in purification processes (high-pressure liquid chromatography, affinity chromatography) has made it possible to prepare medium-sized peptides such as the members of the secretin-VIP-glucagon family almost routinely by solid-phase peptide synthesis or by synthesis in solution. The ensuing availability of small samples from commercial sources facilitated research on structure-activity relationships. Exploration of conformations remains an arduous task. A word of caution must be added here. The methods applied in the preparation of peptides in research quantities are not necessarily satisfactory when larger amounts are needed, as for therapy. Therefore, further development of the method of peptide synthesis remains a valid challenge.

REFERENCES

1. BODANSZKY, M. & N. J. WILLIAMS. 1967. J. Am. Chem. Soc. **89:** 685-689.
2. BODANSZKY, M., M. A. ONDETTI, S. D. LEVINE & N. J. WILLIAMS. 1967. J. Am. Chem. Soc. **89:** 6753-6757.
3. MUTT, V., J. E. JORPES & S. MAGNUSSON. 1970. Eur. J. Biochem. **15:** 513-519.
4. BROMER, W. W., L. G. SINN & O. K. BEHRENS. 1957. J. Am. Chem. Soc. **79:** 2807-2810.
5. MUTT, V. & S. I. SAID. 1974. Eur. J. Biochem. **42:** 581-589.
6. JOERNVALL, H., M. CARLQUIST, S. KWAUK, S. C. OTTE, C. H. S. MCINTOSH, J. C. BROWN & V. MUTT. 1981. FEBS Lett. **123:** 205-210.
7. TATEMOTO, K. & V. MUTT. 1981. Proc. Natl. Acad. Sci. USA **78:** 6603-6607.
8. GUILLEMIN, R., P. BRAZEAU, P. BÖHLEN, F. ESCH, N. LING & W. B. WEHRENBERG. 1982. Science **218:** 585-587.
9. RIVIER, J., J. SPIESS, M. THORNER & W. VALE. 1982. Nature **300:** 276-278.
10. BODANSZKY, M. 1960. Ann. N.Y. Acad. Sci. **88:** 655-664.
11. ONDETTI, M. A., V. L. NARAYANAN, M. VON SALZA, J. T. SHEEHAN, E. F. SABO & M. BODANSZKY. 1968. J. Am. Chem. Soc. **90:** 4711-4716.
12. WÜNSCH, E. 1971. Naturwissenschaften **59:** 239-246.
13. JÄGER, G., W. KÖNIG, H. WISSMANN & R. GEIGER. 1974. Chem. Ber. **107:** 215-231.
14. VAN ZON, A. & H. C. BEYERMAN. 1973. Helv. Chim. Acta **56:** 1729-1740.
15. VAN ZON, A. & H. C. BEYERMAN. 1976. Helv. Chim. Acta. **59:** 1112-1126.
16. MERRIFIELD, R. B. 1963. J. Am. Chem. Soc. **85:** 2149-2154.
17. BODANSZKY, M. & J. T. SHEEHAN. 1966. Chem. Ind. 1597-1598.
18. WRIGHT, D. E., D. S. AGARWAL & V. J. HRUBY. 1980. Int. J. Peptide Protein Res. **15:** 271-278.
19. PIETTA, P. G. & G. R. MARSHALL. 1970. J. Chem. Soc. D: 650-651.
20. HEMASSI, B. & E. BAYER. 1977. Int. J. Pept. Protein Res. **9:** 63-70.
21. COY, D. H., K. Y. LEE & W. Y. CHEY. 1982. Peptides **3:** 137-141.
22. UCHIYAMA, M., T. SATO, H. YOSHINO, Y. TSUCHIYA, T. TSUDA, M. KONISHI, Y. HISATAKE & A. KOIWA. 1985. Chem. Pharm. Bull. **33:** 1990-1999; C.A. **103:** 142360.
23. UCHIYAMA, M., T. SATO, H. YOSHINO, Y. TSUCHIYA, T. TSUDA, M. KONISHI, M. TSUJII, Y. HISATAKE & A. KOIWA. 1985. Chem. Pharm. Bull. **33:** 2000-2005; C.A. **103:** 142361.
24. KIYAMA, S., K. KITTAGAWA, T. AKITA, W. Y. CHEY, A. AYALP, A. OTSUKI, S. FUNAKOSHI, N. FUJII & H. YAJIMA. 1985. Chem. Pharm.. Bull. **33:** 3205-3217.
25. Chem. Abstr. **96:** 200177, 200178; **97:** 145285; **100:** 139625, 139626, 139627, 139628, 192279; **101:** 91431.
26. MIYOSHI, K., A. HASEGAWA, M. TOMIYAMA & T. MIYAKE. 1981. Nucleic Acid Symp. Ser. **10:** 197-200; Chem. Abstr. **96:** 63642. (*cf.* also Chem. Abstr. **98:** 138434 and Chem. Abstr. **99:** 51847.)
27. SUMI, S., F. NAGAWA, T. HAYASHI & H. AMAGASE. 1984. Gene **29:** 125-134.
28. KÖNIG, W., J. ENGELS, E. UHLMANN & W. WETEKAM. 1985. Chem. Abstr. **103:** 82727.
29. GAFVELIN, G., M. CARLQUIST & V. MUTT. 1985. FEBS Lett. **184:** 347-352.
30. MUTT, V. 1986. Chem. Scr. **26B:** 191-207.
31. CARLQUIST, M., H. JÖRNVALL & V. MUTT. 1981. FEBS Lett. **127:** 71-74.
32. CARLQUIST, M., H. JÖRNVALL, W. G. FORSSMANN, L. THULIN, C. JOHANSSON & V. MUTT. 1985. IRCS Med. Sci. Biochem. **13:** 217-218.
33. NILSSON, A., M. CARLQUIST, H. JÖRNVALL & V. MUTT. 1981. Eur. J. Biochem. **112:** 383-388.
34. VOSKAMP, D. & H. C. BEYERMAN. 1981. Int. J. Pept. Protein Res. **18:** 284-288.
35. KÖNIG, W., M. BICKEL, K. KARCH, V. TEETZ & R. UHLMANN. 1984. Peptides **5:** 189-193.
36. YANAIHARA, N., C. YANAIHARA, M. KUBOTA, M. SAKAGAMI, Z. ITOH, M. OTSUKI, S. BABA & M. SHIGA. 1979. Proc. 6th Am. Pept. Symp. E. Gross & J. Meienhofer, Eds.: 539-542. Pierce Chemical Co. Rockford, IL.
37. MORODER, L., E. JAEGER, F. DREES, M. GEMEINER, S. KNOF, H. P. STENZEL, P. THAMM, D. BATAILLE, S. DOMSCHKE, W. SCHLEGEL, I. SCHULZ & E. WÜNSCH. Bioorg. Chem. **9:** 27-54.

38. ANDREAU, D. & R. B. MERRIFIELD. 1985. Proc. 9th Am. Pept. Symp. C. M. Deber, V. Hruby, K. D. Kopple, Eds.: 595-598. Pierce Chemical Co. Rockford, IL.
39. BEYERMAN, H. C., A. W. VAN WEELDEREN, T. M. BUIJEN, W. Y. CHEY, M. I. GROSSMAN, P. KRANENBURG, T. SCRATCHERD, T. E. SOLOMON & D. VOSKAMP. 1981. Life Sci. 29: 895-902.
40. KÖNIG, W., M. BICKEL, H. WISSMANN & J. SANDOW. 1986. Peptides 7: 61-65.
41. FINK, M. L. & M. BODANSZKY. 1975. J. Am. Chem. Soc. 98: 974-977.
42. BODANSZKY, M. & M. L. FINK. 1976. Bioorg. Chem. 5: 275-282.
43. BODANSZKY, M. & A. BODANSZKY. 1986. Peptides 7(Suppl.1): 43-48.
44. KORN, A. P. & F. P. OTTENSMEYER. 1982. J. Ultrastruct. Res. 79: 142-157.
45. BODANSZKY, M., Y. S. KLAUSNER & S. I. SAID. 1973. Proc. Natl. Acad. Sci. USA 70: 382-384.
46. BODANSZKY, M., Y. S. KLAUSNER, C. Y. LIN, V. MUTT & S. I. SAID. 1974. J. Am. Chem. Soc. 96: 4973-4978.
47. BODANSZKY, M., A. BODANSZKY, Y. S. KLAUSNER & S. I. SAID. 1974. Bioorg. Chem. 3: 133-140.
48. BODANSZKY, A., M. A. ONDETTI, V. MUTT & M. BODANSZKY. 1969. J. Am. Chem. Soc. 91: 944-949.
49. BODANSZKY, M., M. L. FINK, K. W. FUNK & S. I. SAID. 1976. Clin. Endocrinol. 5(Suppl): 195_s-200_s.
50. FOURNIER, A., J. K. SAUNDERS & S. ST.-PIERRE. 1984. Peptides 5: 169-177.
51. TONIOLO, C., G. M. BONORA & W. M. M. SCHAAPER. 1984. Int. J. Pept. Protein Res. 23: 389-393.
52. SCHAAPER, W. M. M. & D. VOSKAMP. 1983. Proc. 17th Eur. Pept. Symp. K. Blaha & P. Malon, Eds.: 141-144. De Gruyter. Berlin, Germany.
53. NILSSON, A. 1975. FEBS Lett. 60: 322-325.
54. BODANSZKY, M., K. W. FUNK & M. L. FINK. 1973. J. Org. Chem. 38: 3565-3570.
55. BODANSZKY, M., A. BODANSZKY & S. I. SAID. 1978. Unpublished observations. cf. Fed. Proc. 37: 1829.
56. YAJIMA, H., M. TAKEYAMA, K. KOYAMA, T. TOBE, K. INOUE, T. KAWANO & H. ADACHI. 1980. J. Pept. Protein Res. 16: 33-34.
57. TAKEYAMA, M., K. KOYAMA, K. INOUE, T. KAWANO, H. ADACHI, T. TOBE & H. YAJIMA. 1980. Cham. Pharm. Bull. 28: 1873-1883.
58. COY, D. & J. GARDNER. 1980. Int. J. Pept. Protein Res. 15: 73-78.
59. COLOMBO, R. 1982. Int. J. Pept. Protein Res. 19: 71-78.
60. CARPINO, L. A. & G. Y. HAN. 1972. J. Org. Chem. 37: 3404-3409.
61. BODANSZKY, A., M. BODANSZKY, N. CHANDRAMOULI, J. Z. KWEI, J. MARTINEZ & J. C. TOLLE. 1980. J. Org. Chem. 45: 72-76.
62. BODANSZKY, M.,C. YANG LIN & S. I. SAID. 1974. Bioorg. Chem. 3: 320-323.
63. WÜNSCH, E. & G. WENDELBERGER. 1986. Wien. Tierärztl. Wochenschr. 73: 164-168.
64. THERIAULT, N. Y., C. S. C. TOMICH & W. WIERENGA. 1986. Nucleosides Nucleotides 5: 15-32.
65. TAKEYAMA, M., K. KOYAMA, H. YAJIMA, M. MORIGA, M. MITSURU & M. MURAKAMI. 1980. Chem. Pharm. Bull. 28: 2265-2269.
66. U.S. PATENT 4605-641-A.
67. BODANSZKY, M., A. BODANSZKY, S. S. DESHMANE, J. MARTINEZ & S. I. SAID. 1979. Bioorg. Chem. 8: 399-407.
68. SUMMERS, C., G. WOOTTON & E. A. WATTS. 1986. Eur. Pat. Appl. EP 184302-A2; Chem. Abstr. 105: 97961.
69. BODANSZKY, M., J. B. HENES, A. E. YIOTAKIS & S. I. SAID. 1977. J. Med. Chem. 20: 1461-1464.
70. BODANSZKY, M., S. NATARAJAN, J. D. GARDNER, G. MAKHLOUF & S. I. SAID. 1978. J. Med. Chem. 21: 1171-1173.
71. WÜNSCH, E. 1967. Naturwissenschaften 22b: 1270-1276.
72. FUJINO, M., M. WAKIMASU, S. SHINAGAWA, C. KITADA & H. YAJIMA. 1978. Chem. Pharm. Bull. 26: 539-548.
73. OGAWA, H., M. SUGIURA, H. YAJIMA, H. SAKURAI & K. TSUDA. 1978. Chem. Pharm. Bull. 26: 1549-1557.

74. SYNTHETIC RESEARCH GROUP, CHINA BIOCHEM. INST. 1975. Acta Biochim. Biophys. Sinica 7: 119. (cf. Ogawa et al.[73])
75. HRUBY, V. J., J. KRSTENANSKY, B. GYSIN, J. T. PELTON, D. TRIVEDI & R. L. MCKEE. 1986. Biopolymers 25: s135-s155.
76. MCKEE, R. L., J. T. PELTON, D. TRIVEDI, D. G. JOHNSON, D. C. COY, J. SUEIRAZ-DIAZ & V. J. HRUBY. 1986. Biochemistry 25: 1650-1656.
77. KRSTENANSKY, J. L., D. TRIVEDI & V. J. HRUBY. 1986. Biochemistry 25: 3833-3839.
78. KRSTENANSKY, J. L., D. TRIVEDI, D. JOHNSON & V. J. HRUBY. 1986. J. Am. Chem. Soc. 108: 1696-1698.
79. WOOD, S. P., I. J. TICKLE, A. M. TREHARNE, J. E. PITTS, Y. MASCARENHAS, J. Y. LI, J. HUSAIN, S. COOPER, T. L. BLUNDELL, V. J. HRUBY, A. BUKU, A. J. FISCHMAN & H. R. WYSSBROD. 1986. Science 232: 633-636.
80. LANGS, D. A., G. D. SMITH, J. J. STEZOWSKI & R. E. HUGHES. 1986. Science 232: 1140-1142.
81. BROWN, J. C. & J. R. DRYBURGH. 1971. Can J. Biochem. 49: 867-872.
82. OGAWA, H., M. KUBOTA, H. YAJIMA, T. TOBO, M. FUJIMURA, K. HENMI, K. TORIZUKA, H. ADACHI, H. IMURA & T. TAMINATO. 1976. Chem. Pharm. Bull. 24: 2447-2456.
83. SAKURAI, M., K. AKAJI, N. FUJII, M. MORIGA, M. AONO, K. MIZUTA, M. NOGUCHI, K. INOUE, R. HOSOTANI, T. TOBE & H. YAJIMA. 1986. Chem. Pharm. Bull. 34: 3447-3453.
84. FUJII, N., M. SAKURAI, K. AKAJI, M. NOMIZU, H. YAJIMA, K. MIZUTA, M. AONO, M. MORIGA, K. INOUE, R. HOSOTANI & T. TOBE. 1986. Chem. Pharm. Bull. 34: 2397-2410.
85. MORODER, L., P. GÖHRING, P. THAMM & E. WÜNSCH. 1982. Z. Naturforsch. 37b: 772-780.
86. FUJII, N., W. LEE, H. YAJIMA, M. MORIGA & K. MIZUTA. 1983. Chem. Pharm. Bull. 31: 3503-3514.
87. MORODER, L., W. GÖHRING, P. LUCIETTO, J. MUSIOL, R. SCHARF, P. THAMM, G. BOVERMANN & E. WÜNSCH. 1983. Z. Physiol. Chem. 364: 1563-1584.

Immunochemical and Biochemical Properties of Purposely Designed Synthetic Peptides

NOBORU YANAIHARA,[a,b] CHIZUKO YANAIHARA,[a]
MINORU HOSHINO,[b] TOHRU MOCHIZUKI,[a] AND
KAZUAKI IGUCHI[a]

[a]Laboratory of Bioorganic Chemistry
Shizuoka College of Pharmacy
Shizuoka, Japan
[b]Laboratory of Cellular Metabolism
National Institute for Physiological Sciences
Okazaki, Aichi, Japan

Recent rapid advances in methods for cloning and sequencing mRNAs and genes have provided a flood of information about biologically important peptides and their precursor proteins. However, this information can be fully appreciated and applied to biological problems only by synthesis of these new structures, as well as fragments and analogues. Fortunately, progress in methods of peptide synthesis has made it possible to prepare the needed materials in quantities sufficient for a wide variety of studies.

Synthetic peptides related to a regulatory peptide or its precursor provide us with important substrates not only for the investigation on the molecular basis of the physiological roles of the regulatory peptide, but also for the production of region-specific antisera against the peptide.

This report provides information from some of our immunochemical and functional studies with use of synthetic peptides in special reference to PHI (peptide histidine isoleucine) and galanin.

IMMUNOCHEMICAL APPLICATIONS OF SYNTHETIC PEPTIDES

The discovery of the common precursor for vasoactive intestinal polypeptide (VIP) and PHM (human PHI)[1] followed by immunocytochemical demonstration of the coexistence of PHI with VIP in mammalian intestinal nerves[2] spawned a great interest in the relationship between the two peptides in terms of physiological significance.

Region-specific antisera, directed against PHI and related peptides, have been used in our previous study to characterize the molecular forms of the peptide present in mammalian tissues[3,4] and in the human neuroblastoma NB-OK-1 cell line[5,6] as compared with those of VIP. Defining the immunologic determinants of an antiserum against a peptide to be used is an essential step in interpreting properly the information obtained with the antiserum. On the other hand, antisera against one specific peptide may have different immunologic determinants. These different antisera are useful for analysis of multiple chemical and biological aspects of the peptide. In this context, we have used peptides purposely synthesized as haptenic immunogens to obtain a variety of region-specific PHI antisera. As shown in FIGURE 1, eight different PHI-related peptides have been used as immunogens for this purpose. It has been our principle in the production of antisera against a peptide, especially regulatory peptide, to use the peptide itself as an immunogen without conjugating it to any macromolecular carrier, as long as the peptide is large enough to be an effective immunogen.[3,7,8] Since the purity of the synthetic peptide used as an immunogen is always carefully assessed before use, there would be little possibility of antibody production against modified forms of the peptide molecule. Along this line, synthetic human and porcine PHIs were used for immunization without conjugation. On the other hand, in order to produce region-specific antisera, we have used as haptenic immunogens fragments of PHI such as porcine PHI (20-27), (14-27), and (1-15); human PHI (13-27) and

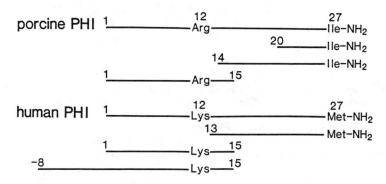

FIGURE 1. Synthetic PHI-related peptides used as immunogens to produce PHI antisera.

(1-15); and a tricosapeptide, human PHI (1-15) with an octapeptide extension at the amino-terminus of the next eight residues in the pro-PHI sequence. Immunization with such peptides allowed us to produce antisera specific for the amino-terminal or carboxyl-terminal region of PHI. Among more than ten antisera raised, we used three in this study: one specific for the amino-terminal region of PHI and two specific for the carboxy-terminal region.

Immunochemical Characterization of PHI-Related Peptides Released by Vagal Stimulation in Dogs

Coexistence of the structures of VIP and PHI in one common precursor implies production and release of the two biologically active peptides in equimolar amounts. Our previous study on the synthesis and release of PHI in the human neuroblastoma cultured cells, however, provided data inconsistent with the stoichiometric formation of PHI and VIP in the cells.[5] We have examined[9,10] PHI release on electrical vagal stimulation in anesthetized dogs as well as VIP release under the condition described by Fahrenkrug *et al.*[11,12]

Portal plasma levels of immunoreactive (IR) PHI as well as IR-VIP increased upon electrical stimulation (2.5, 5, and 10 Hz) of both vagi. Atropine failed to suppress the vagal release of IR-PHI and IR-VIP, whereas hexamethonium abolished the increase of both peptide immunoreactivities, suggesting that PHI and VIP are coreleased by vagal stimulation via a nicotinic ganglionic mechanism. Plasma levels of IR-PHI measured by the carboxyl-terminal specific antiserum were similar to those of IR-VIP. On the other hand, IR-PHI measured by the amino-terminal specific antiserum was 2.5 times higher. The amount of IR-PHI released depended upon the frequency of stimulation applied. The difference in PHI concentration as determined by the different antisera was most remarkable at 10 Hz. The discrepancy in the apparent concentrations of IR-PHI was explained by the existence of an extra component of a larger molecular form of IR-PHI in the portal plasma that was detected at a K_{av} of 0.30 in gel filtration of the plasma on a Sephadex G50 column. This large form was recognized only by the amino-terminal specific antiserum. With the currently used amino-terminal-specific antiserum, the large form of IR-PHI, as found in the portal plasma, was detected in dog stomach tissue extracts. The presence of this large molecular weight form together with a PHI-27-like component was also demonstrated with the amino-terminal specific antiserum in tissue extracts of the entire length of the intestine.

On the basis of the cross-reactivities, the large form of IR-PHI is most likely a molecule containing the amino-terminal portion of PHI-27 but lacking part of its carboxyl region or having its carboxyl region modified so as to lose cross-reactivity to the carboxyl-terminal-specific antiserum. The predominant presence of this large form of PHI in gastrointestinal tissues and its release into the circulation by vagal stimulation suggest the physiological significance of this PHI-related component, although there is no direct evidence for its identity.

Immunochemical Characterization of PHI-Related Peptides in Human Neuroblastoma Cells

The amino- and carboxyl-terminal specific PHI antisera were also useful for characterization of PHI-related peptides in human neuroblastoma cells.

We have reported[5,6] that human neuroblastoma NB-OK-1 cells are stimulated by dibutyryl cAMP to produce and release IR-PHI as well as IR-VIP. The rates of production and release of the immunoreactivities were significantly different from each other. Especially interesting is the difference between production and release of amino- and carboxy-terminal immunoreactivities of PHI (FIG. 2). TPA (12-*O*-tetradecanoylphorbol-13-acetate; 0.16 nM-1.6 µM), itself had no effect on the NB-OK-1 cells, not only morphologically but also biochemically. However, in combination with dibutyryl cAMP (1 mM), the phorbol ester (16 nM) synergistically enhanced differentiation of the cells and, at the same time, increased the production of IR-VIP and IR-PHI, which was measured with the amino-terminal-specific PHI antiserum (FIG. 3).[13] IR-PHI concentration in extract of the cells as measured with the carboxyl-specific antiserum was not elevated by the combined addition of TPA with the cAMP derivative. Gel filtration profiles of IR-VIP and IR-PHI in extract of the cells that

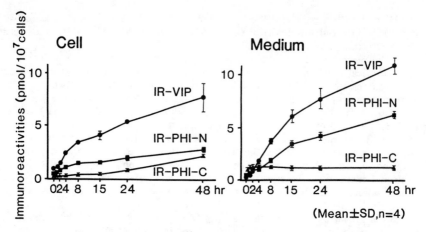

FIGURE 2. Immunoreactive (IR) VIP and PHI in human neuroblastoma NB-OK-1 cells and the culture medium. IR-PHI-N and IR-PHI-C represent PHI measured with amino- and carboxyl-terminal-specific PHI radioimmunoassays, respectively.

had been cultured in the presence of dibutyryl cAMP with or without TPA revealed that the combined addition of TPA with the cAMP derivative stimulated more markedly the production of larger forms of IR-VIP (10K and 18K daltons) and IR-PHI (10K and 18K daltons), which cross-reacted only with the amino-terminal specific PHI antiserum (FIG. 4). The increased larger forms of IR-PHI components are likely to correspond to those of IR-VIP. The enhanced formation of PHI-27 by dibutyryl cAMP was little affected by the addition of TPA. TPA with dibutyryl cAMP as well

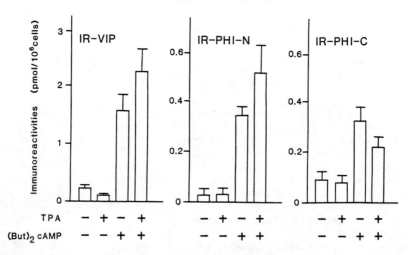

FIGURE 3. Effect of TPA and dibutyryl cAMP on the production of immunoreactive (IR) VIP and PHI in human neuroblastoma NB-OK-1 cells. IR-PHI-N and IR-PHI-C represent PHI measured with amino- and carboxyl-terminal-specific PHI radioimmunoassays, respectively. Dibutyryl cAMP was used in 1 mM concentration and TPA 16 nM.

as the cAMP derivative alone[14] seem to stimulate the production of a VIP/PHI precursor protein that cannot be converted to matured VIP-28 and PHI-27 because of its modified structure or a possible defect in the enzyme systems for its posttranslational processing.

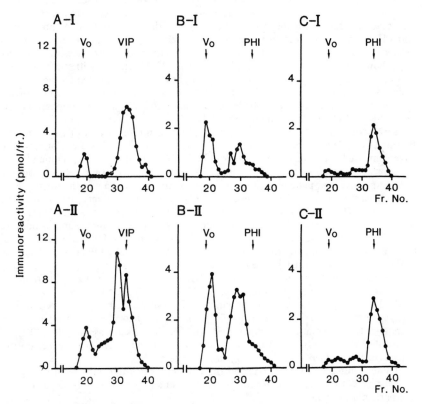

FIGURE 4. Gel filtration profiles of immunoreactive (IR) VIP (A) and PHI (B and C) produced in human neuroblastoma NB-OK-1 cells in the presence of 1 mM dibutyryl cAMP (I) or in the presence of 1 mM dibutyryl cAMP and 16 nM TPA (II). Crude extract of the cells (4 × 10^7) was chromatographed on a Sephadex G50 superfine column (1 × 100 cm) with 3 M acetic acid as eluent. Each fraction (2 ml) was divided into three portions and measured by (A) VIP specific, (B) PHI amino-terminal, and (C) carboxyl-terminal specific PHI radioimmunoassays, respectively.

These results support the necessity of the use of antisera recognizing different portions of a peptide of interest and strongly suggest that not only quantitation of nucleotides and protein products but also characterization of their structures are necessary to elucidate the mechanism of protein synthesis stimulated by exogenous reagents such as cyclic nucleotides and phorbol esters.

FUNCTIONAL STUDIES WITH SYNTHETIC PEPTIDES

Peptide Histidine Isoleucine

The amino-terminal portion of PHI displays the highest sequence homology with VIP, secretin, glucagon, GRF, and helodermin, and the amino-terminal portion is known to be essential for the biological activities of these peptides.[15–18] Although PHI and VIP are biosynthesized in a common precursor, the amino acid sequences of PHI in mammals, in contrast to VIP, show species variation; the differences are not very large, however (FIG. 5). Using a Beckman Model 990B peptide synthesizer, we have carried out the synthesis of rat PHI by a solid-phase technique, based on the deduced amino acid sequence of rat VIP precursor.[19] The synthetic peptide was extensively purified by gel filtration on a Sephadex G25 column followed by reverse-phase HPLC on a TSK Gel ODS-125T column in 0.01 N HCl/CH$_3$CN.

Szecowka *et al.* have proposed a role for PHI in the regulation of pancreatic A, B, and D cell function on the basis of *in vitro*[20] and *in vivo*[21,22] studies in rats. We have compared the potencies of three synthetic PHIs having porcine,[4] human,[23] and rat sequences for stimulation of glucose (250 mg%) induced insulin release from the isolated perfused rat pancreas. In this system, synthetic PHI having the rat sequence at a concentration of 10^{-9} M showed a potency, significantly higher than that of the other two PHIs (FIG. 6), indicating that rat PHI receptors may have a very high selectivity for hormone sequence recognition. The amino acid residues in positions 10 and 17 are substituted with Tyr and Ile, respectively, in rat PHI. Either or both of the two residues are apparently involved significantly in attaining full biological activity in the rat pancreas perfusion assay system.

We have previously shown[24] that the PHI carboxyl-terminal (14-27) fragment (10^{-8} M) opposes the potentiating effect of PHI-27 (10^{-9} M) on glucose (250 mg%) induced insulin release in isolated rat pancreas. In contrast with this observation, VIP carboxyl-terminal (16-28) fragment (10^{-8} M), which by itself is inactive was found to enhance the potentiating activity of PHI (10^{-9} M) in the same assay system (TABLE 1). Neither PHI$_{14-27}$ (10^{-8} M) nor VIP$_{16-28}$ (10^{-8} M) had a significant effect on the potentiating activity of VIP (10^{-9} M) in the system.

These results, with three PHIs and the PHI and VIP fragments, seem to suggest the existence of receptor binding sites for PHI distinct from those for VIP at least in this particular system.

Galanin

Galanin is a 29-residue peptide isolated from porcine upper small intestine.[25] The carboxyl-terminal portion of galanin is structurally more or less similar to those of substance P, substance K (neurokinin A), gastrin-releasing peptide (GRP), and other tachykinins (FIG. 7). Immunohistochemical and radioimmunological studies showed that IR-galanin is widely distributed in the mammalian peripheral and central nervous systems, indicating that galanin is a novel brain-gut peptide.

We have synthesized porcine galanin[26,27] and several related peptides using solid-phase technology with the Beckman peptide synthesizer, Model 990B. The peptides

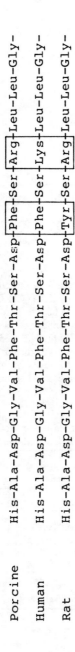
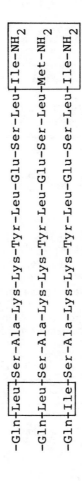

Porcine	His-Ala-Asp-Gly-Val-Phe-Thr-Ser-Asp-Phe-Ser-Arg-Leu-Leu-Gly-
Human	His-Ala-Asp-Gly-Val-Phe-Thr-Ser-Asp-Phe-Ser-Lys-Leu-Leu-Gly-
Rat	His-Ala-Asp-Gly-Val-Phe-Thr-Ser-Asp-Tyr-Ser-Arg-Leu-Leu-Gly-

-Gln-Leu-Ser-Ala-Lys-Lys-Tyr-Leu-Glu-Ser-Leu-Ile-NH$_2$

-Gln-Leu-Ser-Ala-Lys-Lys-Tyr-Leu-Glu-Ser-Leu-Met-NH$_2$

-Gln-Ile-Ser-Ala-Lys-Lys-Tyr-Leu-Glu-Ser-Leu-Ile-NH$_2$

FIGURE 5. Amino acid sequences of porcine, human, and rat PHIs.

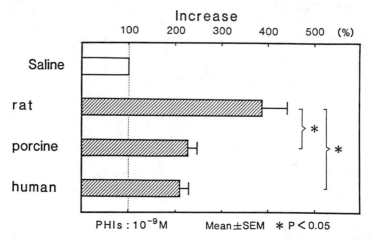

FIGURE 6. Potentiating effects of rat, porcine, and human PHIs on glucose (250 mg%) induced insulin release in isolated rat pancreas.

were purified by gel filtration on a BioGel P-6 column followed by reverse-phase HPLC on a TSK Gel ODS-125T column in 0.01 N HCl/CH$_3$CN. Purity of the products was assessed by routine analytical criteria. The effects of galanin on spinal reflexes were then studied with use of the synthetic replica.[26,28] In the isolated hemisected spinal cord of the newborn rat, galanin (0.1-5 μM) depressed the monosynaptic reflex induced by dorsal root stimulation and recorded from the corresponding ventral root. In the isolated spinal cord tail preparation of the newborn rat, galanin (0.3-0.6 μM) depressed the nociceptive reflex evoked by application of capsaicin to the tail

TABLE 1. Effects of PHI and VIP Fragments on Potentiating Activities of PHI and VIP on Glucose (250 mg%) Induced Insulin Release in Isolated, Perfused Rat Pancreas

PHI	VIP	Fragment	Fragment Conc.	Released IR-Insulin[a] (ng equivalent)
—	—	—	—	127.9 ± 52.3
10^{-9} M	—	—	—	293.3 ± 22.6[b]
10^{-9} M	—	PHI$_{14-27}$	10^{-9} M	287.2 ± 139.4
10^{-9} M	—	—	10^{-8} M	180.8 ± 24.7[c]
10^{-9} M	—	VIP$_{16-28}$	10^{-8} M	503.7 ± 61.5[c]
10^{-9} M	—	PHI$_{1-15}$	10^{-8} M	248.8 ± 47.1
—	10^{-9} M	—	—	560.6 ± 68.1
—	10^{-9} M	PHI$_{14-27}$	10^{-8} M	635.7 ± 179.2
—	10^{-9} M	VIP$_{16-28}$	10^{-8} M	454.1 ± 61.5

[a] Mean ± SEM (n = 5-9).
[b] p < 0.01.
[c] Significantly different from b (p < 0.01).

```
                        1                                    10
Galanin          H-Gly-Trp-Thr-Leu-Asn-Ser-Ala-Gly-Tyr-Leu-Leu-Gly-Pro-His-Ala-
                                         20                                  29
                 -Ile-Asp-Asn-His-Arg-Ser-Phe-His-Asp-Lys-Tyr-Gly-Leu-Ala-OH


Substance P      H-Arg-Pro-Lys-Pro-Gln-Gln-Phe-Phe-Gly-Leu-Met-NH₂

Substance K      H-His-Lys-Thr-Asp-Ser-Phe-Val-Gly-Leu-Met-NH₂

Neurokinin B     H-Asp-Met-His-Asp-Phe-Phe-Val-Gly-Leu-Met-NH₂

pGRP             -----Gly-Asn-His-Trp-Ala-Val-Gly-His-Leu-Met-NH₂

Neuromedin B     H-Gly-Asn-Leu-Trp-Ala-Thr-Gly-His-Phe-Met-NH₂
```

FIGURE 7. Amino acid sequence of porcine galanin and structure comparison of its carboxyl-portion with some tacykinins.

and recorded from a lumbar ventral root. The depressant effect of galanin on the monosynaptic reflex was much stronger than that of [Met⁵]enkephalin or somatostatin.

Synthetic galanin (10^{-9}-10^{-7} M) also caused significant suppression of glucose (300 mg%) induced insulin release in the isolated rat pancreas.[27] We have done structure-function studies of galanin with use of synthetic galanin-related peptides in the same pancreas preparation. As can be seen in FIGURE 8, removal of the first amino acid, Gly, caused complete loss of the suppressing effect. Further shortening the peptide chain gave peptides that conversely showed potentiating effects, with maximum potency at the (15-29) length. This is, as far as we are aware, the first demonstration that a peptide and its fragments possess opposite effects in action on a single biological system. The results suggest that the second amino acid, Trp, is vitally involved in this reversal of the galanin effect.

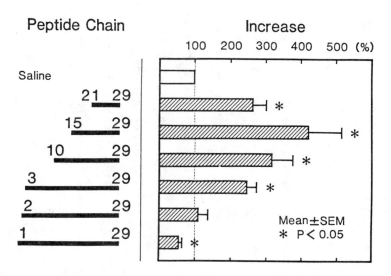

FIGURE 8. Effects of galanin$_{1-29}$ and its fragments on glucose (300 mg%) induced insulin release in isolated, perfused rat pancreas.

Substitution of the Trp residue with D-Trp or Phe did not cause a substantial change in the galanin effect on glucose-induced insulin release (FIGS. 9 and 11). On the contrary, the Ala-substituted galanin was found to possess a potentiating effect on insulin release similar to that of the shorter fragments. These results demonstrated the crucial role of the aromatic ring of the amino acid residue in position two for the galanin effect. From the secondary structures predicted by the Chou-Fasman method[29,30] (FIG. 10), high incidence of β-sheet structure in the amino-terminal region of galanin seems to be essential for the suppressing effect on glucose-induced insulin release in isolated rat pancreas. [Ala²]galanin and galanin-related peptides lacking the amino-terminal amino acid sequence were predicted to have little β-sheet structure in the amino-terminal portion by the Chou-Fasman method.

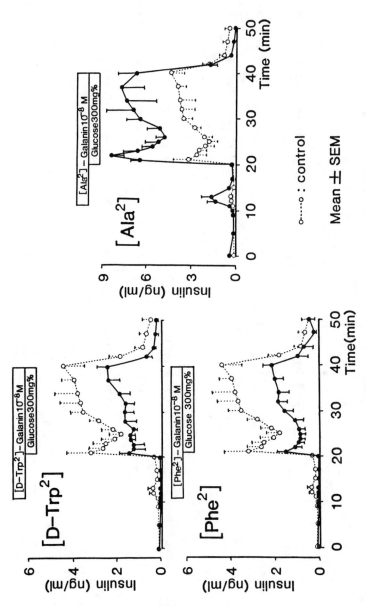

FIGURE 9. Effects of galanin analogues substituted in position two with [D-Trp], [Phe], or [Ala] on glucose-induced insulin release in isolated, perfused rat pancreas.

```
                   1                 10                  20              29
                   G-W-T-L-N-S-A-G-L-L-G-P-H-A-I-D-N-H-R-S-F-H-D-K-Y-G-L-A

Galanin            e e e e e c e e e e e c c c c c c c c c c c c c c c c c c
Galanin(2-29)        e e e e e e e e e e c c c c c c c c c c c c c c c c c c
Galanin(3-29)          c c c c e e e e e c c c c c c c c c c c c c c c c c c

(Phe2)-Galanin     c e e e e e e e e e e c c c c c c c c c c c c c c c c c c
(Ala2)-Galanin     c c c c c c e e e e e c c c c c c c c c c c c c c c c c c
```

FIGURE 10. Secondary structures of galanin$_{1-29}$ and its fragments and analogues predicted by the Chou-Fasman method. e: β-sheet structure c: random coil structure.

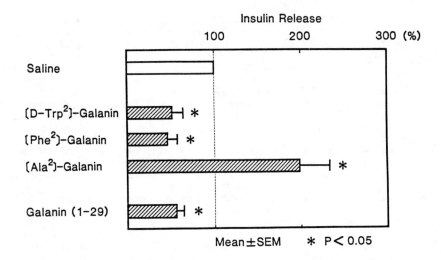

FIGURE 11. Relative potencies of galanin analogues in effect on glucose (300 mg%) induced insulin release in isolated, perfused rat pancreas.

CONCLUSION

With these results we have demonstrated the usefulness of purposely synthesized peptides for exploration of complex biological systems.

REFERENCES

1. ITOH, N., K. OBATA, N. YANAIHARA & H. OKAMOTO. 1983. Human preprovasoactive intestinal polypeptide contains a novel PHI-27-like peptide, PHM-27. Nature **304**: 547-549.
2. YANAIHARA, N., K. NOKIHARA, C. YANAIHARA, T. IWANAGA & T. FUJITA. 1983. Immunocytochemical demonstration of PHI and its coexistence with VIP in intestinal nerves of the rat and pig. Arch. Histol. Jpn. **46**: 575-581.
3. YANAIHARA, N., C. YANAIHARA, K. NOKIHARA, K. IGUCHI, S. FUKATA, M. TANAKA, Y. YAMAMOTO & T. MOCHIZUKI. 1984. Immunochemical study on PHI/PHM with use of synthetic peptides. Peptides **5**: 247-254.
4. NOKIHARA, K., C. YANAIHARA, K. IGUCHI, S. FUKATA, M. TANAKA, T. MOCHIZUKI, K. TATEMOTO, J. M. LUNDBERG, V. MUTT & N. YANAIHARA. 1984. Synthesis of PHI (peptide histidine isoleucine) and related peptides on immunochemical confirmation of amino acid residue in position 24 of PHI with use of the synthetic peptides. J. Am. Chem. Soc. **106**: 7909-7916.
5. HOSHINO, M., C. YANAIHARA, K. OGINO, K. IGUCHI, H. SATO, T. SUZUKI & N. YANAIHARA. 1984. Production of VIP- and PHM (human PHI)-related peptides in human neuroblastoma cells. Peptides **5**: 155-160.

6. OGINO, K., M. HOSHINO, K. NOKIHARA, K. IGUCHI, C. YANAIHARA & N. YANAIHARA. 1986. Processing products of VIP/PHM precursor in human neuroblastoma cultured cells. *In* Peptide Chemistry. 1985. Y. Kiso, Ed.: 385-390. Protein Research Foundation. Osaka, Japan.

7. YANAIHARA, N., M. SAKAGAMI, H. SATO, K. YAMAMOTO, T. HASHIMOTO, C. YANAIHARA, Z. ITO, K. YAMAGUCHI & K. ABE. 1977. Immunological aspects of secretin, substance P, and VIP. Gastroenterology **72:** 803-810.

8. YANAIHARA, C., T. MOCHIZUKI, T. INOUE, K. IGUCHI, M. TOYOSHIGE, M. HOSHINO, T. IWANAGA, T. FUJITA, S. IZUMI, K. NAKANE & N. YANAIHARA. Immunochemical approach to insulin receptor with use of synthetic peptides. Acta Histochem. Cytochem. **20:** 245-250.

9. YASUI, A., S. NARUSE, C. YANAIHARA, S. SHIONOYA & N. YANAIHARA. 1986. The larger form of immunoreactive peptide histidine isoleucine is released on electrical vagal stimulation in the dog. Can. J. Physiol. Pharmacol.: 38. Proceedings of the 6th Symposium on Gastrointestinal Hormones. Vancouver, Canada.

10. YASUI, A., S. NARUSE, C. YANAIHARA, T. OZAKI, M. HOSHINO, T. MOCHIZUKI, E. E. DANIEL & N. YANAIHARA. Co-release of PHI and VIP by vagal stimulation in the dog. Am. J. Physiol. **253:** G13-G19.

11. FARENKRUG, J., H. GALBO, J. J. HOLST & O. B. SCHAFFALITZKY DE MUKADELL. 1978. Influence of the autonomic nervous system on the release of vasoactive intestinal polypeptide from the porcine gastrointestinal tract. J. Physiol. **280:** 405-422.

12. FARENKRUG, J., U. HAGLUND, M. JODAL, O. LUNDGREN, L. OLBE & O. B. SCHAFFALITZKY DE MUKADELL. 1978. Nervous release of vasoactive intestinal polypeptide in the gastrointestinal tract of cats: Possible physiological implications. J. Physiol. **284:** 291-305.

13. HOSHINO, M., C. YANAIHARA, K. OGINO, K. IGUCHI, T. SUZUKI & N. YANAIHARA. 1986. Phorbol ester stimulation of biosynthesis of VIP- and PHM-related peptides in a human neuroblastoma. Biomed. Res. 7(Suppl. 2): 137-140.

14. YANAIHARA, N., T. SUZUKI, H. SATO, M. HOSHINO, Y. OKARU & C. YANAIHARA. 1981. Dibutyryl cAMP stimulation of production and release of VIP-like immunoreactivity in a human neuroblastoma cell line. Biomed. Res. **2:** 728-734.

15. BREGMAN, M. D., D. TRIVEDI & V. J. HRUBY. 1980. Glucagon amino groups. Evaluation of modifications leading to antagonism and agonism. J. Biol. Chem. **255:** 11725-11731.

16. ROBBERECHT, P., T. P. CONLON & J. D. GARDNER. 1976. Interaction of porcine vasoactive intestinal peptide with dispersed pancreatic acinar cells from the guinea pig. Structural requirements for effects of vasoactive intestinal peptide and secretin on cellular adenosine 3':5'-monophosphate. J. Biol. Chem. **251:** 4635-4639.

17. CHRISTOPHE, J. P., T. P. CONLON & J. D. GARDNER. 1976. Interaction of porcine vasoactive intestinal peptide with dispersed pancreatic acinar cells from the guinea pig. Binding of radioiodinated peptide. J. Biol. Chem. **251:** 4629-4634.

18. COUVINEAU, A., C. ROUYER-FESSARD, A. FOURNIER, S. ST-PIERRE, R. PIPKORN & M. LABURTHE. 1984. Structural requirements for VIP interaction with specific receptors in human and rat intestinal membranes: Effect of nine partial sequences. Biochem. Biophys. Res. Commun. **121:** 493-498.

19. NISHIZAWA, M., Y. HAYAKAWA, N. YANAIHARA & H. OKAMOTO. 1985. Nucleotide sequence divergence and functional constraint in VIP precursor mRNA evolution between human and rat. FEBS Lett. **183:** 55-59.

20. SZECOWKA, J., E. SANDBERG & S. EFENDIC. 1980. The interaction of vasoactive intestinal polypeptide (VIP), glucagon and arginine on the secretion of insulin, glucagon and somatostatin in the perfused rat pancreas. Diabetologia **19:** 137-142.

21. SZECÓWKA, J., P. E. LINS, K. TATEMOTO & S. EFENDIC. 1983. Effects of porcine intestinal heptacosapeptide (PHI) and vasoactive intestinal polypeptide (VIP) on insulin and glucagon secretion in rat. Endocrinology **112:** 1469-1473.

22. SZECÓWKA, J, K. TATEMOTO, V. MUTT & S. EFENDIC. 1980. Interaction of a newly isolated intestinal polypeptide (PHI) with glucose and arginine to affect the secretion of insulin and glucagon. Life Sci. **26:** 435-438.

23. NOKIHARA, K., Y. YAMAMOTO, M. TANAKA, T. MOCHIZUKI, C. YANAIHARA & N. YANAIHARA. 1984. Syntheses of PHM (human PHI) and its related peptides. *In* Peptide Chemistry 1983. E. Munekata, Ed.: 303-308. Protein Research Foundation, Osaka, Japan.

24. YANAIHARA, C., Y. HASHIMOTO, Y. TAKEDA, I. KATO, N. S. TRACK, K. NOKIHARA, H. MANAKA, T. IWANAGA, T. FUJITA, H. OKAMOTO & N. YANAIHARA. 1986. PHI structural requirements for potentiation of glucose-induced insulin release. Peptide 7(Suppl. 1): 83-88.
25. TATEMOTO, K., A. RÖKAEUS, H. JORNVALL, T. J. MCDONALD & V. MUTT. 1983. Galanin—a novel biologically active peptide from porcine intestine. FEBS Lett. 164: 124-128.
26. YANAIHARA, C., H. YAGI, H. OKAMURA, Y. IBATA, M. YANAGISAWA, M. OTSUKA & N. YANAIHARA. 1986. Galanin in spinal cord. Can. J. Physiol. Pharmacol.: 161. Proceedings of the 6th Symposium on Gastrointestinal Hormones. Vancouver, Canada.
27. TAKEDA, Y., C. YANAIHARA, Y. HASHIMOTO, Y. YAMAMOTO, R. TAKEDA, K. TATEMOTO, V. MUTT & N. YANAIHARA. 1986. Galanin effect on insulin and C-peptide release. Can. J. Physiol. Pharmacol.: 95. Proceedings of the 6th Symposium on Gastrointestinal Hormones. Vancouver, Canada.
28. YANAGISAWA, M., N. YAGI, M. OTSUKA, C. YANAIHARA & N. YANAIHARA. 1986. Inhibitory effects of galanin on the isolated spinal cord of the newborn rat. Neurosci. Lett. 70: 278-282.
29. CHOU, P. Y. & G. D. FASMAN. 1974. Conformational parameters for amino acids in helical, β-sheet, and random coil regions calculated from proteins. Biochemistry 13: 211-221.
30. CHOU, P. Y. & G. D. FASMAN. 1974. Prediction of protein conformation. Biochemistry 13: 222-245.

Potent Long-Acting Growth Hormone Releasing Factor Analogues[a]

J. RIVIER, C. RIVIER, R. GALYEAN, G. YAMAMOTO,
AND W. VALE

Clayton Foundation Laboratories for Peptide Biology
The Salk Institute
San Diego, California

INTRODUCTION

It is now well established that the neuroregulation of growth hormone (GH) secretion is mediated by somatostatin, an inhibitory 14-peptide, and a stimulatory growth hormone releasing factor (GRF), which was isolated as a 37-,[1] 40-,[1,2] or 44-NH$_2$[1] peptide. Both biological activities and potency of GRF were found to reside in the first 29 amino acids of the sequence.[2] This original observation was later confirmed by several investigators.[3,4] Interestingly, all GRFs characterized to date from different species are structurally homologous to vasoactive intestinal 28-peptide amide (VIP), a 27-peptide with NH$_2$-terminus histidine and COOH-terminus isoleucine amide (PHI), glucagon, secretin, helodermin, helospectin, and a gastrointestinal 43-peptide (GIP). Several investigations have addressed the problem of specificity of these different structures for their respective receptors; a study by Pandol *et al.*,[5] for example, has shown rat GRF (rGRF) to have a VIP-like bioactivity on guinea pig pancreatic islets to secrete amylase, while human GRF (hGRF) was at least 100 times less potent than rGRF in that assay. While efforts are directed toward the understanding of the mechanism of action,[6] clinical significance,[7] and specificity[5] of GRF, other efforts are directed toward the understanding of structure–activity relationships (SAR).[1,3,4] Structurally, an amphiphilic π-helical stretch encompassing residues 1-22, for example, has been proposed by Kezdy and Kaiser[8] on the basis of the strong binding of GRF to liposomes. Others[3,9,10] have suggested an α-helix stretch between residues 10-30 on the basis of statistical analysis using Chou and Fasman's[11] parameters. Additional SAR studies evaluated the role of single amino acids by introducing specific substitutions in a systematic[4] or less systematic fashion.[3,4,9,11,12] Increased potency is generally obtained by introducing amino acid substitutions that bear on the receptors' ability to recognize better and/or bind more tightly the designed analogue. This is generally achieved by altering the conformation of the peptide in such a way as to stabilize the

[a]This research was supported in part by National Institutes of Health Grant AM26741 and The Clayton Foundation of Research, California Division. Drs. W. Vale and C. Rivier are Clayton Foundation investigators.

active conformation or by introducing residues (naturally occurring or unnatural) that allow tighter binding to the receptor and/or confer resistance to enzymatic attack.

We report here on the synthesis of eight GRF_{1-29} analogues with modifications in positions 1, 27, 28, and 29. Four of the analogues substituted at the three or four positions, such as ([NMeTyr^1,Nle^{27},Asn^{28}]hGRF$_{1-29}$NHEt) (4SG-29), were found to be approximately ten times as potent as $GRF_{1-40}OH$ *in vitro* and to be long acting in urethane-anesthetized rats. This latter analogue was synthesized in gram quantities, tested for short-term toxicity in the rat and is currently being investigated for its clinical potential.

RESULTS AND DISCUSSION

Solid-phase peptide synthesis[13] in tandem with reversed-phase HPLC for purification of unprotected peptides[14,15] has allowed the synthesis of a large number of peptides used to generate antibodies, to study SAR of biologically active peptides, to build models of all types for testing biochemical or biophysical hypotheses, or to generate large quantities of peptides for clinical investigation. It is now accepted that highly purified peptides up to 50 residues long can be obtained using these conventional techniques. Hence, when the structure of GRF became available, a synthetic replica could be tested and compared with the native substance. At the same time, a strong program for the study of SAR was initiated. Indeed, GRF and its analogues have been shown to be potent promoters of GH release in animals and humans resulting in noticeable increased structural growth as compared to controls.[7] Short duration of action and poor oral or nasal adsorption however, have triggered our interest in developing analogues with greater resistance to endo- and exopeptidases. This report is limited to our study of the role of exopeptidases in the degradation of GRF. Conferring exopeptidase resistance to GRF should be possible by introducing modifications at the NH$_2$- and COOH-terminus that would render these native residues unrecognizable by enzymes. We concentrated our efforts on blocking the NH$_2$-terminus by introduction of the unnatural amino acid NCH$_3$Tyr in position one or NMeDAla in position two. Both modifications could theoretically protect the Tyr^1-Ala^2 bond. Introduction of the COOH-terminal ethylamide could similarly protect the COOH-terminus against degradation by carboxy peptidases.[16] TABLE 1 describes the structures that were synthesized, a physical constant ($[\alpha]D$), the retention times of these analogues under standard HPLC conditions, and their relative potency *in vitro*. Peptides, after purification,[17] were isolated as the trifluoroacetate salts and were shown to be greater than 95% pure using two different HPLC systems. Their amino acid composition after acid hydrolysis gave the expected ratios. Mass spectrometric analysis of one of the analogues (4SG-29) confirmed the expected molecular weight. *In vitro,* the peptides were tested for their ability to stimulate the release of GH from cultured pituitary cells.[18] Potencies of GRF analogues were expressed relative to a standard, [hGRF(1-40)OH]. *In vivo,* peptides were tested as described in the FIGURE 1 legend.

Substitution by Nle in position 27 resulted in a peptide that was significantly more stable chemically because of the substitution of the oxygen-susceptible methionine residue by the aliphatic isosteric amino acid norleucine and increased the potency of hGRF$_{1-29}$NH$_2$ by a factor of three (see TABLE 1). It is apparent that substitution of Tyr by NMeTyr in position one or of Ala by NMeDAla in position two further

TABLE 1. Characterization of GRF Analogues

Compound	$[\alpha]D^a$	HPLC[b] RT	Relative Potency in Vitro[c]
hGRF$_{1-40}$ OH	−64.3°	14.2	1.00
hGRF$_{1-29}$ NH$_2$	−46.3°	17.9	1.34 (1.1-1.7)
[Nle^{27}] hGRF$_{1-29}$ NH$_2$	−60.9°	19.2	3.02 (2.0-4.5)
[NMeTyr^1, Nle^{27}] hGRF$_{1-29}$ NH$_2$	−58.2°	19.3	3.30 (1.7-6.4)
[NMeTyr^1, Nle^{27}, Asn^{28}] hGRF$_{1-29}$ NH$_2$	−60.4°	18.4	10.39 (7.4-14.5)
[NMeTyr^1, Nle^{27}, Asn^{28}] hGRF$_{1-29}$ NHEt	−60.5°	21.1	9.27 (7.0-12.4)
[NMeDAla^2 Nle^{27}] hGRF$_{1-29}$ NHEt	−51.5°	23.2	9.03 (5.3-14.9)
[NMeDAla^2, Nle^{27}, Asn^{28}] hGRF$_{1-29}$ NH$_2$	−51.9°	18.7	9.34 (6.6-13.2)
[NMeDAla^2, Nle^{27}, Asn^{28}] hGRF$_{1-29}$ NHEt	−50.6°	21.4	10.27 (6.2-16.5)

[a] c = 1 in 1% AcOH.

[b] RT = retention time expressed in minutes on Vydac analytical C$_{18}$ column (0.46 × 25 cm) 5 μm particle size, detection at 210 nm, [A] = 1% TFA, gradient was 28.8 to 40.8% CH$_3$CN in 20 minutes, 2.0 ml/min flow rate.

[c] Potency expressed relative to hGRF$_{1-40}$ OH = 1. Compounds at several doses were incubated for three hours on dispersed rat pituitary cells after three days in culture. Medium was tested for GH by RIA. Dose-response curves were plotted and a relative potency is derived: 95% confidence limits are given in parentheses.

improved potency. Introduction of Asn in position 28 resulted in analogues 10-fold more potent than the standard. However, it should be noted that Asn^{28} is the original residue in the rat structure.[19] As a result, the observed high biopotency may be species specific as both assays used either rats or rat tissues. Addition of the NHEt substitution at the COOH-terminus did not result in increased potency *in vitro*. FIGURE 1 shows the time course of action of [NMeTyr^1,-Nle^{27},Asn^{28}]hGRF$_{1-29}$NHEt as compared to that of hGRF$_{1-40}$OH. The highest dose of GRF$_{1-40}$OH (10 μg) gave only minimal growth hormone release at 30 minutes, while both the 2.0 and 10.0 μg doses of the analogue still released GH significantly. Similarly, [NMeDAla^2,Nle^{27},Asn^{28}]-hGRF$_{1-29}$NHEt showed extended duration of action (data not shown). However, [NMeTyr^1,Nle^{27},-Asn^{28}]-hGRF$_{1-29}$NH$_2$ and [NMeDAla^2,Nle^{27},Asn^{28}]-hGRF$_{1-29}$NH$_2$, which do not contain the COOH-terminus ethylamide block, were also longer acting than hGRF$_{1-40}$OH, thus suggesting that amino peptidase may play a much more significant role than carboxy peptidases in the processing of GRF. An argument that may color this statement stems from the observation[2,4] that GRF$_{1-29}$OH is less potent *in vitro* than the corresponding peptide amide. Whether this decrease in potency is due to enzymatic instability (resulting from removal of the amide block) or lowered affinity for the GRF receptor has not been fully addressed for lack of the appropriate assay systems. We are presently investigating the effect of endopeptidases in the degradation process of GRF in an effort to generate analogues with significantly greater duration of action. The preliminary results presented here strongly support the validity of such an approach.

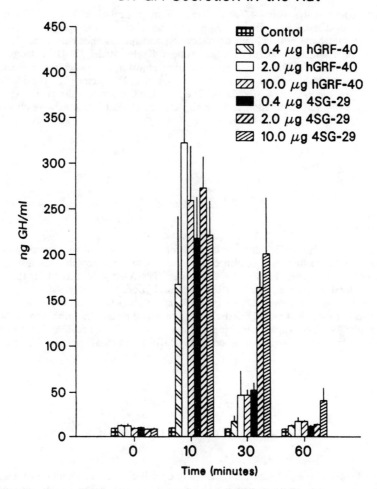

FIGURE 1. Adult male Sprague-Dawley rats (230-250 g) were anesthetized with urethane (1.5 g/kg body weight, i.p. at −2 h). Blood samples were obtained at t = 0, 10, 30, and 60 minutes. The treatments were injected into the jugular vein in a volume of 1 ml. Plasma were separated and kept frozen. GH levels were measured by RIA, using materials provided by the NIADDK distribution program. Each bar represents the mean ± SEM of five rats.

EXPERIMENTAL

Instruments

Amino acid analyses after 4.0 N methane sulfonic hydrolysis at 110°C for 24 hours were performed on a Perkin-Elmer high-pressure liquid chromatograph (HPLC) using orthophthalaldehyde post column derivatization and fluorescence detection. HPLCs were run on a Waters Associates gradient system, Kratos model 757 UV detector, an Omniscribe Series D500 dual pen recorder from Houston Instruments, a Shimadzu Chromatopac EIA integrator and a rheodyne model 7125 injector. The peptide synthesizer used was Beckman Model 990. The HF cleavage line was designed in-house and allowed for HF elimination under high vacuum. Optical rotations were obtained on a Perkin-Elmer model 141 polarimeter.

Starting Materials

The methyl benzhydrylamine resin used for the synthesis of the peptide amides was obtained according to a published procedure[20] using p-toluoylchloride instead of benzoyl chloride during the Friedel-Crafts step. The N-ethyl resin used for the synthesis of the peptide N-ethylamide was synthesized in our laboratory according to the procedure of Kornreich et al.[21] Resins with substitution 0.3 meq/g to 0.6 meq/g were used. Boc-NCH$_3$Tyr(0-2,6Cl$_2$Bzl) was synthesized using the procedure of Shuman et al.[22] Boc amino acids were brought from Bachem (Torrance, CA). All solvents were reagent grade; diisopropylcarbodiimide (DIIC) was obtained from Aldrich.

Synthesis, Purification, and Characterization

Analogues were synthesized automatically on a Beckman 990 Peptide Synthesizer using a previously described protocol.[23] Briefly, t-butyloxycarbonyl (Boc) was used for NH$_2$-terminal protection with NH$_2$-terminal deblocking achieved with 60% TFA in CH$_2$Cl$_2$ and 1-2% ethanedithiol. Washes included isopropanol, CH$_2$Cl$_2$, and MeOH. Triethylamine (10% in CH$_2$Cl$_2$) was used for neutralization. Couplings were mediated by DIIC in CH$_2$Cl$_2$ or 50% DMF/CH$_2$Cl$_2$ depending on the solubility of the Boc-amino acids. HF cleavages were carried out under different conditions depending on the desired products. Peptide amides were cleaved for one hour at 0°C while peptide ethylamides required an extended period (2-3 h) at room temperature.

SUMMARY

Amidated fragments 1 to 29 of human growth hormone releasing factor, $(GRF_{1-29}NH_2)$, were designed to encompass modifications that could prevent degradation by exopeptidases. The NH_2-terminus was blocked by either N-methylation of Tyr^1 or by introduction of $NMeDAla^2$ while the COOH-terminus was blocked by an N-ethylamide. Other substitutions such as Nle in position 27 for methionine conferred stability toward air oxidation while Asn^{28}, an amino acid substitution found in rat GRF, seemed to confer stronger binding affinity to the GRF receptor. Potency *in vitro* and duration of action *in vivo* of $[NMeTyr^1,Nle^{27},Asn^{28}]hGRF_{1-29}NHEt$ (4SG-29) were compared to those of $hGRF_{1-40}OH$. 4SG-29 was found to be both ten times more potent than $hGRF_{1-40}OH$ and exhibit significantly extended duration of action.

ACKNOWLEDGMENTS

We thank Dr. J. Varga for the synthesis of Boc-NCH$_3$Tyr(0-2,6Cl$_2$Bzl), R. Kaiser and J. Dykert for technical assistance in the synthesis and characterization of the peptides, S. Cappel and D. Jolley for GH RIA, G. Morgan and G. Berg for help with the bioassays, and R. Hensley for manuscript preparation.

REFERENCES

1. GUILLEMIN, R., P. BRAZEAU, P. BOHLEN, F. ESCH, N. LING & W. B. WEHRENBERG. 1982. Science **218:** 585.
2. RIVIER, J., J. SPIESS, M. THORNER & W. VALE. 1982. Nature **300:** 276.
3. COY, D. H., W. A. MURPHY, J. SUEIRAS-DIAZ, E. J. COY & V. A. LANCE. 1985. J. Med. Chem. **28:** 181.
4. LING, N., A. BAIRD, W. A. WEHRENBERG, N. UENO, T. MUNEGUMI & P. BRAZEAU. 1984. Biochem. Biophys. Res. Commun. **123:** 854.
5. PANDOL, S. J., H. SEIFERT, M. W. THOMAS, J. RIVIER & W. VALE. 1984. Science **225:** 326-328.
6. VALE, W., L. BILEZIKJIAN, N. BILLESTRUP, P. PLOTSKY, H. SEIFERT, M. PERRIN, J. VAUGHAN, J. SPIESS & J. RIVIER. 1985. *In* Neuroendocrine Perspectives. E. E. Muller & R. M. MacLeod, Eds. Vol. **5:** 13-22. Elsevier. Amsterdam, the Netherlands.
7. THORNER, M. O., M. L. VANCE, K. Y. HO, W. S. EVANS, R. M. BLIZZARD, A. D. ROGOL, C. BROOK, P. SMITH, G. J. KLINGENSMITH, I. BURR, J. NAJJAR, R. FURLANETTO, J. RIVIER & W. VALE. 1987. *In* Proceedings of the Meeting of the International Society of Neuroendocrinology in San Francisco. R. I. Weiner & S. M. McCann, Eds.: 212-219. Karger Publishing Company. Basel, Switzerland.
8. KAISER, E. T. & F. J. KEZDY. 1984. Science **23:** 249.
9. COY, D. H., W. A. MURPHY, V. A. LANCE & M. L. HEIMAN. 1987. J. Med. Chem. **30:** 219-222.
10. VELICELEBI, G., S. PATTHI & E. T. KAISER. 1986. Proc. Natl. Acad. Sci. USA **83:** 5397-5399.
11. CHOU, P. Y. & G. D. FASMAN. 1974. Biochemistry **13:** 222.

12. LING, N., A. BAIRD, W. B. WEHRENBERG, N. UENO, T. MUNEGUMI, T-C. CHIANG, M. REGNO & P. BRAZEAU. 1984. Biochem. Biophys. Res. Commun. **122:** 304-310.
13. MERRIFIELD, R. B. 1963. J. Am. Chem. Soc. **85:** 2149.
14. BURGUS, R. & J. RIVIER. 1976. *In* Peptides 1976. A. Loffet, Ed.: 85-94. Editions de l'Universite de Bruxelles. Brussels, Belgium.
15. RIVIER, J. 1978. J. Liquid Chromatogr. **1:** 343-367.
16. FUJINO, M., S. KOBAYASHI, M. OBAYASHI, *et al.* 1972. Biochem. Biophys. Res. Commun. **49:** 863-869.
17. RIVIER, J., R. MCCLINTOCK, R. GALYEAN & H. ANDERSON. 1984. J. Chromatogr. **288:** 303-328.
18. VALE, W. & G. GRANT. 1984. *In* Methods in Enzymology, Hormones and Cyclic Nucleotides. B. W. O'Malley & J. G. Hardman, Eds.: 213-19. Academic Press. New York.
19. SPIESS, J., J. RIVIER & W. VALE. 1983. Nature **303:** 532-535.
20. RIVIER, J., W. VALE, R. BURGUS, N. LING, M. AMOSS, R. BLACKWELL & R. GUILLEMIN. 1973. J. Med. Chem. **16:** 545-549.
21. KORNREICH, W., H. ANDERSON, J. PORTER, W. VALE & J. RIVIER. 1984. Int. J. Pept. Protein Res. **25:** 414-420.
22. SHUMAN, R. T., E. L. SMITHWICK, D. L. SMILEY, G. S. BROOKS & P. D. GESELICHEN. 1983. *In* Peptides Structure and Function. Proceedings of the 8th American Peptide Symposium. V. J. Hruby and D. H. Rich, Eds.: 143-146. Pierce Chemical Co. Rockford, IL.
23. MARKI, W., J. SPIESS, Y. TACHE, M. BROWN & J. E. RIVIER. 1981. J. Am. Chem. Soc. **103:** 3178-3185.

Conformational Analysis of Vasoactive Intestinal Peptide and Related Fragments[a]

ALAIN FOURNIER,[b,c] JOHN K. SAUNDERS,[d] YVAN
BOULANGER,[e] AND SERGE A. St-PIERRE[b]

[b]Institut National de la Recherche Scientifique-Santé,
Université du Québec
Pointe-Claire, Québec, Canada

[d]National Research Council of Canada
Ottawa, Ontario, Canada

[e]Institut de Génie Biomédical
Faculté de Médecine
Université de Montréal
Montréal, Québec, Canada

INTRODUCTION

The conformation adopted by polypeptides is responsible of their high specificity for receptors and is the main determinant governing the expression of the biological activity. Therefore, conformational analysis together with structure-activity studies are most valuable to correlate the biological activity and the three-dimensional structure of peptides. As shown by the classical denaturation-restructuration experiments,[1,2] all of the information required to produce the final structure of most polypeptides is contained in the amino acid sequence. Thus, it is possible using theoretical analysis of the primary structure[3–6] to evaluate the structural potential of each segment of a peptide chain and to predict its prevailing spatial arrangement. Among those empirical conformational calculations, the Chou and Fasman procedure[3,5] has been the most used because of its simple rules and quite acceptable level of accuracy. On the other hand, spectroscopic studies using circular dichroism (CD) and high-resolution NMR can provide invaluable information about the secondary and tertiary structures of polypeptides. CD is particularly useful in estimating the helical content of the peptide structure. That latter value becomes extremely important with the development of the amphiphilic concept.[7,8] High-resolution NMR spectroscopy has become the most powerful technique for peptide conformational studies in solution, as it can provide direct information about the interactions between various chemical functions of the peptide and the folding pattern of the chain.

[a]This work was supported by the Medical Research Council of Canada and the Fonds de la Recherche en Santé du Québec.
[c]Recipient of a Medical Research Council of Canada Fellowship.

Several structure-activity studies were carried out with vasoactive intestinal peptide (VIP),[9-11] allowing the identification of important chemical groups in the molecule. However, the conformational requirements remain unclear because the number of structural analyses of VIP is actually very small.[12-16] In this paper, we report conformational characteristics of VIP and some related fragments evaluated by means of CD and 400-MHz NMR spectroscopies.

METHODS

The circular dichroism spectra were recorded with a Cary 60 instrument equipped with a Model 6001 attachment. A 0.01-cm cell and concentrations of 0.05 mg/ml were used for the measurements. Peptides were studied in 1,1,1,3,3,3-hexafluoro-2-propanol (HFIP) and water mixture and the molar ellipticities $[\theta]_\lambda$ ($[\theta]_\lambda = \theta \times$ MRW/10 $\times$ c $\times$ d) are reported in degree-cm^2-dmole^{-1} using the mean residue weight (MRW) of each peptide.

The [^{1}H]NMR spectra were recorded at 400 MHz with a Bruker spectrometer operating in the FT mode. The peptide was dissolved in water and mixed with anion exchange resin (AG2-X8, chloride form, Bio-Rad Laboratories). The filtrate was lyophilized and the compound was dried *in vacuo* over P_2O_5. NMR studies were performed in D_2O (99.996%) or d_6-DMSO (99.5%) at 20°C.

RESULTS AND DISCUSSION

Spectroscopic Study by CD

Circular dichroism spectra of VIP and various NH$_2$- and COOH-terminal fragments show that these molecules do not adopt, as seen with most linear peptides,[17] a well-defined secondary structure when dissolved in water. With the addition of increasing concentrations of HFIP, an excellent structure-promoting cosolvent,[18] the far-UV spectra (250-190 nm) indicate an important helical content in the secondary structure of VIP and its COOH-terminal fragments 2-28 and 14-28 (FIG. 1). Similar observations were made by Bodanszky *et al.*[12] by means of optical rotatory dispersion and by Robinson *et al.*,[13] using CD spectroscopy with lipidic solutions of VIP. The helical content increases proportionally with the concentration of HFIP in the solution, up to a limit between 60% and 80%. As shown in FIGURE 1, peptides are less helical in the mixture containing 80% of cosolvent. A decreased solubility of the peptides at that concentration is probably responsible for that observation. FIGURE 1D shows the curves measured at 40% HFIP/H$_2$O. This allows the visualization of the differences between the helical content of the various peptides. First, it appears that the overall content in the 14-28 fragment is approximately the same as the one observed in the octacosapeptide. A different result has been presented by Bodanszky *et al.*[12] who estimated a larger helical content in VIP than in the 14-28 fragment. Since the fragment contains the helical nucleus, as calculated from the Chou and Fasman[3,5] predictive method, it has been concluded that the NH$_2$-terminal segment of the molecule protects the helical portion of the peptide chain from hydration.[19] Our results at 40% are not in agreement with that conclusion. However, comparison of the ellipticity curves of VIP and VIP$_{14-28}$ measured at 20% HFIP (FIGS. 1A and 1C), which is closer to the concentration of cosolvent used by Bodanszky *et al.*[12] (25% TFE/H$_2$O), shows this time a larger helical content in the octacosapeptide ($[\theta]_{222}$ of VIP: $-26,200$ degree-cm^2-dmole^{-1}; $[\theta]_{222}$ of VIP$_{14-28}$: $-19,200$ degree-cm^2-dmole^{-1}), which suggests that the secondary structure of this fragment is effectively more vulnerable to the hydration than the entire molecule. Therefore, a decrease in the water content in the mixture, as seen at 40% HFIP, favors the adoption of the α-helix.

The spectral characteristics of VIP$_{2-28}$ indicate a larger helical content in this fragment than in the entire sequence. The absence of the histidine residue is mainly responsible since that aromatic chromophore gives a positive signal at 215 nm.[20] This hides the real helix content in the molecule and largely contributes to the difference observed between the two curves. However, another factor might be involved in this result. Predictive Chou and Fasman calculations strongly suggest the presence of a β-turn in position 1-4. In absence of His^1, the β-turn structure cannot exist. In such a case, this would delete the positive absorbance coming from that secondary structure and would give rise to an increase of the global helical content.

Experiments were performed in nonbuffered solutions resulting in the pH of the HFIP/H$_2$O mixture as slightly acidic (VIP, 0.05 mg/ml in 40% HFIP/H$_2$O, pH $= 4.2$). Therefore, the curve of ellipticity was measured in water at pH 4.2 in order to verify whether or not the pH had any effect on the induction of the secondary structure of VIP. It has been demonstrated that the slightly acidic pH of the solution does not contribute to the adoption of the helical structure of VIP. This conclusion can also be applied to the full scale of pH, since no major modifications were observed in the ellipticity curves measured at pH ranging from 2.8 to 11.7.

Among the other fragments investigated, none showed any characteristic spectra reflecting a particular secondary structure at the HFIP concentrations used. Even the 1-14 fragment exhibits a spectral pattern in the far-UV suggesting the absence in this peptide of the two β-turns (1-4 and 7-10)[15] theoretically estimated by the Chou and Fasman calculations. However, as seen in FIGURE 1D, a bathochromic shift is observed for VIP$_{1-14}$ and not for VIP$_{2-14}$, which indicates that the presence of the histidine residue in the NH$_2$-terminal fragment favors the adoption of a folded structure giving rise to that shift. For the reasons discussed previously, the intensity of that absorbance observed at 208 nm is probably more accentuated than the one measured, because of the presence of the chromophore histidine.

Spectroscopic Study by NMR

Spectrum of VIP in D$_2$O

The NMR spectrum of VIP was recorded in deuterated water at its pH of dissolution. Its analysis has been carried out by comparing the resonances to the ones identified by means of the NH$_2$- and COOH-terminal fragments, using two-dimensional correlation NMR spectroscopy (FIG. 2), selective homonuclear irradiation (FIG. 3), chemical shifts versus pH or temperature experiments,[14] and so forth. As illustrated in FIGURE 4, the methyl groups belonging to the threonine residues 7 and 11 are practically chemically equivalent in fragments 1-14 and 6-14 while a difference of

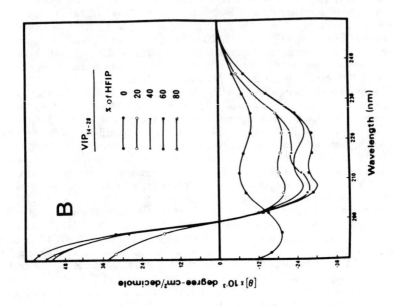

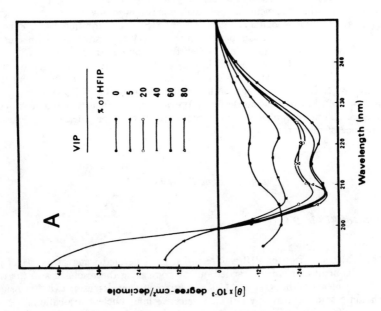

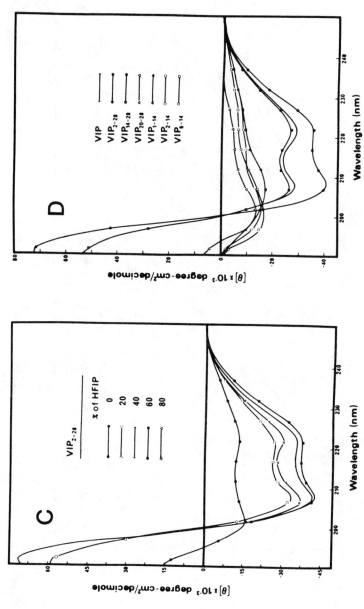

FIGURE 1. Circular dichroism spectra of VIP and related fragments in HFIP (c = 0.05 mg/ml, d = 0.1 cm). (A) VIP, (B) VIP$_{14-28}$, (C) VIP$_{2-28}$, (D) related fragments at 40% HFIP/H$_2$O.

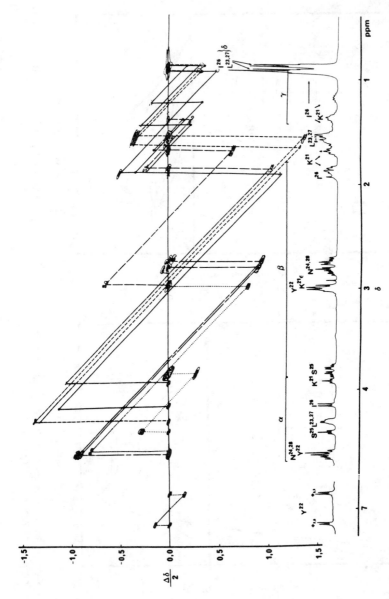

FIGURE 2. 400 MHz [¹H]NMR two-dimensional spin-echo correlation spectroscopy (SECSY) spectrum of VIP$_{21-28}$ dissolved in water.

0.04 ppm separates these signals for the octacosapeptide and its 2–28 fragment, showing that the COOH-terminal portion of the molecule exerts some effects on the structure adopted by the other segment of the peptide chain. The multiplet found at 0.9 ppm corresponds to the absorbances of the aliphatic protons of leucine, valine, and isoleucine residues. The similarity of the pattern observed for VIP and VIP$_{2-28}$ suggests the absence of any interaction between the imidazole group of His[1] and the side chains of the aliphatic residues of the sequence.

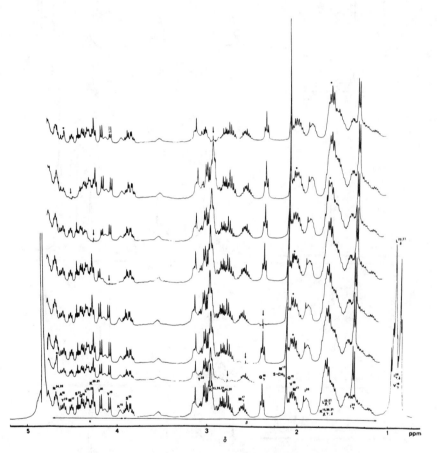

FIGURE 3. Selective homonuclear decoupling experiments of VIP$_{15-28}$ in water. Irradiation sites are identified by arrows and the modified resonances by (●).

The region between 6.8 and 8.0 ppm shows the nonequivalence of the aromatic protons of tyrosine 10 and 22. The first AA′BB′ spin system is observed at $\simeq$7.0 ppm (6.8 and 7.1 ppm) while the second one is at $\simeq$7.8 ppm (7.6 and 7.9 ppm). This situation is not found in the fragment 2–28, which clearly demonstrates the important role played by the histidine-1 residue on the conformation. Although the identity of

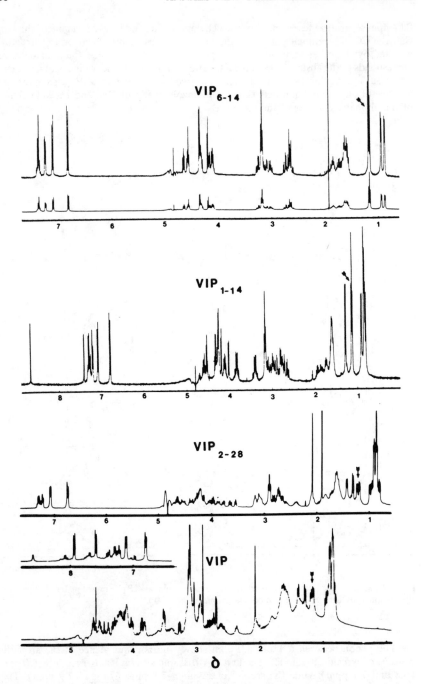

FIGURE 4. 400 MHz [^{1}H]NMR spectrum of VIP and fragments 6-14, 1-14, and 2-28 in water. The arrows indicate the $C^\gamma H_3$ resonances of threonine residues 7 and 11.

this tyrosine has not been demonstrated, it is likely, considering the structural potential of VIP as estimated with the predictive method, that the side chain of Tyr[10] comes under the influence of the imidazole group. The multiplet at $\simeq$7.3 ppm results from the aromatic protons of phenylalanine-6. The pattern indicates a complex spin system in which the *ortho* protons are more shielded. The chemical shift values, consistent with the ones found in the literature, and the chemical equivalence of the *ortho* protons as well as of the *meta* protons, show the absence of any major interaction susceptible to slow down the rotation of the aromatic ring along the C^β-C^1 bond. Resonances from the nonlabile protons of the imidazole nucleus are observed at 8.67 ppm (C^2H) and 7.39 ppm (C^4H). NMR studies by Tanokura *et al.,*[21] who evaluated various dipeptides containing histidine, interpreted these chemical shifts for a histidine residue followed by serine (e.g. octacosapeptide VIP) to mean that the His[1] side chain is in the imidazolium form.

Spectrum of VIP in d_6-DMSO

FIGURE 5 shows the 400 MHz [^{1}H]NMR spectrum of VIP in d_6-DMSO. In spite of its complexity, some resonances can be immediately identified. For instance, the two phenolic rings of tyrosines 10 and 22 (values in ppm, H2,H6: 8.17, H3,H5: 7.82; H2,H6: 7.13, H3,H5: 6.74) which are, as in water, magnetically nonequivalent. The multiplet at 7.31 ppm results from the aromatic protons of Phe,[6] and the singlet at 2.10 ppm corresponds to the S-CH$_3$ group of methionine. As shown in FIGURE 6, the region of the aromatic protons shows interesting modifications in function of the length of the peptide chain. As a matter of fact, the phenolic protons of tyrosine generally appear at approximately 7.0 ppm, as seen in fragments 21-28 and 1-14. Nevertheless, an important nonequivalence is observed for the tyrosine residues of VIP. This is explained by the presence of histidine-1 in the sequence, as demonstrated by the comparison of the VIP and VIP$_{2-28}$ spectra. When the peptide is dissolved in dimethylsulfoxide, the deshielding effect on the phenolic protons located at approximately 7.8 ppm (7.6 and 7.9 ppm) in water is increased by 0.25 ppm. This increase is also observed in the 2-28 fragment, which shows that the imidazole group is not involved in this additional interaction. This suggests that DMSO induces a more structured conformation of the peptides that could be related to the three-dimensional arrangement of VIP in contact with its receptor.

The spin-spin coupling patterns of phenylalanine-6 are also influenced by the size of the peptide and the choice of the solvent. For instance, the aromatic protons of Phe[6] in the 6-14 fragment shows a A_2B_2X spin system when the peptide is dissolved in water and a more complex system when the peptide is in DMSO. According to London *et al.,*[22] who observed a similar pattern during the NMR study of bradykinin, a Phe residue showing that spin system has its side chain well exposed to the solvent. By increasing the length of the NH$_2$-terminal fragment, the coupling pattern, as seen in VIP$_{1-14}$, reassembles to a A_2M_2X system. This particular spin-spin coupling pattern is found in the octacosapeptide, which indicates that the aromatic nucleus is relatively free to rotate along the C^β-C^1 bond[23] but each type of proton comes under the influence of a characteristic microenvironment specific to each one.

Aliphatic protons are also disturbed by the elongation of the peptide chain and the medium in which the spectra are recorded (FIG. 7). Previously, it has been shown for fragments 6-14 and 1-14 that in water the methyl groups of threonine 7 and 11

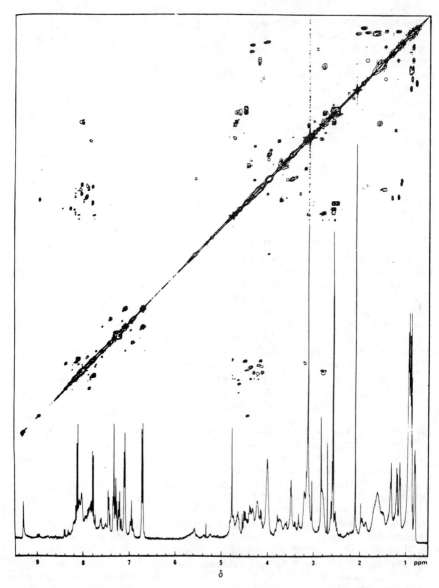

FIGURE 5. 400 MHz [¹H]NMR two-dimensional correlated spectroscopy (COSY) spectrum of VIP dissolved in DMSO.

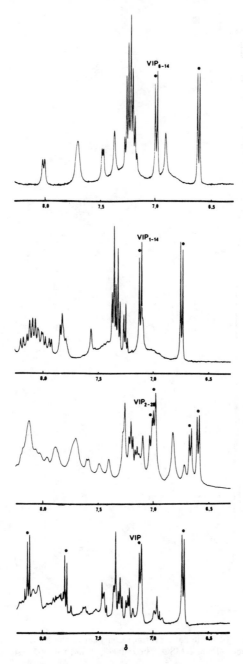

FIGURE 6. Region of the aromatic proton resonances in the NMR spectra of VIP fragments 6-14, 1-14, 2-28, and VIP in DMSO. Tyrosine resonances are identified by (●).

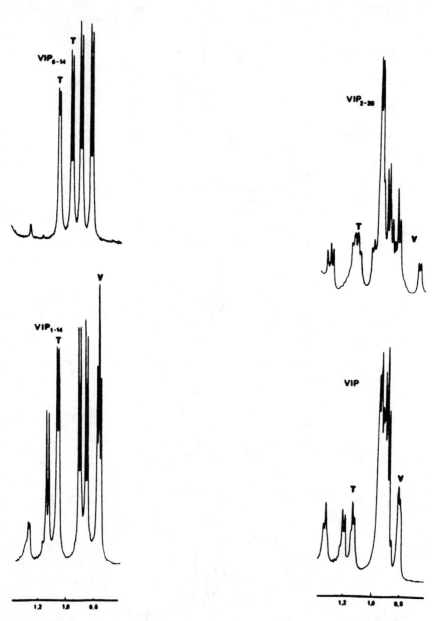

FIGURE 7. Region of the aliphatic proton resonances in the NMR spectra of VIP fragments 6-14, 1-14, 2-28, and VIP in DMSO. Threonine-7,11 and valine-5 residues are identified by T and V.

are almost chemically equivalent. However, this is no longer the case when these peptides are dissolved in DMSO. For instance, the methyl protons of one of the threonine residues of VIP_{6-14} are located at a standard position (1.02 ppm), while those of the second residue are found at a higher field. On the contrary, the chemical equivalence of these two residues is more accentuated in the 1-14 fragment, and this time this is in favor of the standard position. That condition appears to be maintained in VIP, suggesting that the environment of the threonine residues is very similar in these two peptides.

Valine side chain resonances are also modified under the influence of the peptide chain elongation. As seen in FIGURE 7, the chemical shift corresponding to the $C^\gamma H_3$ protons of valine 5 is found at a standard position[23] in the 1-14 fragment. This is also the case for Val^{19} in the 15-28 fragment (FIG. 8). However, in VIP_{2-28} and VIP (FIG. 7), one of the valine residues gives rise to resonances in the high field of the spectrum, which suggests that the three-dimensional structure of one portion of the VIP molecule modulates the conformation adopted by the second segment. A similar conclusion was reached after the study of the aromatic protons of tyrosines 10 and 22. In fact, those protons are observed at approximately 7.0 ppm in NH_2- and COOH-terminal fragments. In VIP_{2-28} and especially VIP, an important chemical shift is measured for one of the residues showing once again the mutual influence exerted by both portions of the octacosapeptide.

Attempts were made to precisely identify the resonances obtained from the tyrosine 10 and 22 by means of two-dimensional nuclear Overhauser enhancement spectroscopy (NOESY). Successive experiments made with different mixing times did not allow the identification of the residues. However, as seen in FIGURE 9, a NOE effect was observed between the *ortho* and *meta* aromatic protons of phenylalanine-6 and the *trans* amide proton of an asparagine side chain. Among the asparagine residues found in VIP (asparagine 9, 24, and 28), Asn^9 is the most probable candidate, since the Chou and Fasman calculations suggest a folding of the NH_2-terminal segment of VIP, which could bring the asparagine-9 side chain to proximity with the aromatic nucleus of Phe.[6]

CONCLUSION

The pattern of the ellipticity curve obtained by circular dichroism of VIP in water suggests that the peptide is predominantly in a random coil structure. However, even under such conditions a spatial arrangement can exist in the molecule and give rise to particular spectral manifestations. For instance, it has been demonstrated by high-resolution NMR that the introduction of histidine-1 creates important shifts toward the low field for the aromatic protons of a tyrosine residue. A folding of the peptide chain is likely in order to bring the tyrosine side chain in close proximity to a site able to induce such effect (most likely a strong positively charged environment). Calculations using the Chou and Fasman parameters strongly suggest a β-turn structure for the segments 1-4 and 7-10 of the molecule, with potentials $<P_t>$ of 1.13 ($<p_t> = 2.02 \times 10^{-4}$) and 1.28 ($<p_t> = 2.26 \times 10^{-4}$), respectively. Assuming the folding of the NH_2-terminal portion of VIP according to the predictive estimations, the aromatic nucleus of Tyr^{10} can come close to the histidine residue and be influenced by the N^α-ammonium group as well as the imidazolium moiety.

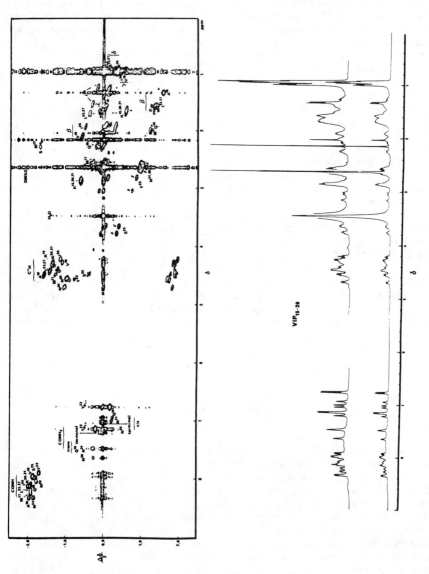

FIGURE 8. 400 MHz [^{1}H]NMR two-dimensional spin-echo correlation spectroscopy (SECSY) spectrum of VIP $_{15-28}$ dissolved in DMSO.

The orientation of the tyrosine-10 side chain and its interaction with histidine would imply for VIP an important biological significance since most members of the VIP/secretin family have this aromatic residue at position 10. As a matter of fact, a secretin analogue in which the leucine-10 is replaced by a tyrosine residue recognizes the high-affinity receptors for VIP,[24,25] showing the participation of Tyr[10] for the affinity of the peptide. NMR experiments demonstrated that the interaction involving the tyrosine residue is more defined in DMSO than in water. This situation would be a consequence of the conformation adopted by the segment 7-10 of VIP when the peptide is in a solvent of lower dielectric constant. This is suggested by the shielding of the $C^{\gamma}H_3$ of valine-5 and the nuclear Overhauser effect between the aromatic protons of Phe[6] and the *trans* amide proton of an asparagine residue assumed to be Asn[9].

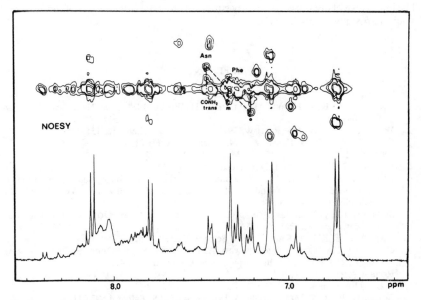

FIGURE 9. Region of amide and aromatic proton resonances in the 400 MHz [¹H]NMR two-dimensional nuclear Overhauser enhancement spectroscopy (NOESY) spectrum of VIP in DMSO.

The β-turn involving the residues 7 to 10 can serve as initiation site for an α-helix.[26,27] As estimated with the theoretical calculations, residues 12 to 23 have a strong propensity to adopt a helical structure ($p = 1.13$). This is confirmed by the circular dichroism data that show that the 14-28 fragment gives the characteristic α-helix spectral pattern with the addition of increasing amounts of fluorinated alcohol to the aqueous solution. This helical nucleus is maintained in the octacosapeptide confirming the previous observations of Bodanszky *et al.*[12] and Robinson *et al.*[13] It is also the case with VIP$_{2-28}$ in which the overall helical content is significantly higher than in VIP itself and supports the existence of a turn in position 1-4. It is worth while to note that this turn would not be absolutely necessary for the expression of the biological activity of VIP since *in vivo* and *in vitro* bioassays showed that the 2-28 fragment still retains some activity.[15,16]

The axial projection of the helical segment clearly shows the amphiphilic character[28] of this secondary structure in VIP. That characteristic would be extremely important for the mechanism of recognition of VIP by its receptors and for the induction of the biological response. However, this structure needs the NH_2-terminal portion of the molecule to be fully expressed since the 14-28 fragment, which is able to form a α-helix, is not recognized by the receptor when used as an agonist or antagonist in pharmacological preparations.[15,16] A similar conclusion is reached with the NH_2-terminal segment of the molecule. As shown by NMR, the 1-14 fragment is unable to adopt the structure giving rise to the particular chemical shifts observed with the octacosapeptide. Therefore, it is tempting to postulate that the α-helical structure adopted by the COOH-terminal portion of VIP might be necessary to stabilize the NH_2-terminal segment of the molecule and favor the formation of the β-turns. The low degree of organized secondary structure observed from the CD of this fragment would also support this hypothesis.

REFERENCES

1. ANFINSEN, C. B., E. HABER, M. SELA & F. H. WHITE. 1961. Proc. Natl. Acad. Sci. USA **47:** 1309-1314.
2. WETLAUFER, D. B. & S. RISTOW. 1973. Ann. Rev. Biochem. **42:** 135-158.
3. CHOU, P. Y. & G. D. FASMAN. 1974. Biochemistry **13:** 211-222.
4. LEVITT, M. & J. GREER. 1977. J. Mol. Biol. **114:** 181-239.
5. FASMAN, G. D. 1980. Ann. N.Y. Acad. Sci. **348:** 147-159.
6. ZIMMERMAN, S. S. 1985. Theoretical methods in the analysis of peptide conformation. *In* The Peptides. S. Udenfriend, J. Meienhofer & V. J. Hruby, Eds. Vol. **7:** 165-212. Academic Press. New York.
7. SEGREST, J. P., R. L. JACKSON, J. D. MORRISETT & A. M. GOTTO. 1974. Fed. Eur. Biochem. Soc. Lett. **38:** 247-253.
8. KAISER, E. T. & F. J. KEZDY. 1984. Science **223:** 249-255.
9. COUVINEAU, A., C. ROUYER-FESSARD, A. FOURNIER, S. ST-PIERRE, R. PIPKORN & M. LABURTHE. 1984. Biochem. Biophys. Res. Commun. **121:** 493-498.
10. ROBBERECHT, P., D. H. COY, P. DE NEEF, J.-C. CAMUS, A. CAUVIN, M. WAELBROECK & J. CHRISTOPHE. 1986. Eur. J. Biochem. **159:** 45-49.
11. BOLIN, D. R., J. A. MEIENHOFER & I.-I. SYTWU. U.S. Patent 4,605,641.
12. BODANSZKY, M., A. BODANSZKY, Y. S. KLAUSNER & S. I. SAID. 1974. Bioorg. Chem. **3:** 133-140.
13. ROBINSON, R. M., E. W. BLAKENEY & W. L. MATTICE. 1982. Biopolymers **21:** 1217-1228.
14. FOURNIER, A., J. K. SAUNDERS & S. ST-PIERRE. 1982. Peptides **3:** 345-352.
15. FOURNIER, A., J. K. SAUNDERS & S. ST-PIERRE. 1984. Peptides **5:** 169-177.
16. FOURNIER, A. 1984. Ph.D. Thesis. University of Sherbrooke. Quebec, Canada.
17. ROQUES, B. P., C. GARBAY-JAUREGUIBERRY, S. BAJUSZ & B. MAIGRET. 1980. Eur. J. Biochem. **113:** 105-119.
18. GRIFF, D., S. FERMANDJIAN, P. FROMAGEOT, M. C. KHOSLA, R. R. SMEBY & F. M. BUMPUS. 1976. Eur. J. Biochem. **61:** 297-305.
19. BODANSZKY, M. & A. BODANSZKY. 1982. Synthesis of VIP and related peptides: Structure-activity relationships. *In* Vasoactive Intestinal Peptide. S. I. Said, Ed.: 11-22. Raven Press. New York.
20. LINTNER, K., S. FERMANDJIAN, P. FROMAGEOT, M. C. KHOSLA, R. R. SMEBY & F. M. BUMPUS. 1977. Biochemistry **16:** 806-812.
21. TANOKURA, M., M. TASUMI & T. MIYAZAWA. 1976. Biopolymers **15:** 393-401.

22. LONDON, R. E., J. M. STEWART, J. R. CANN & N. A. MATWIYOFF. 1978. Biochemistry
    17: 2270-2277.
23. WÜTHRICH, K. 1976. Proton NMR of amino acids—An introduction to high-resolution
    NMR spectroscopy. *In* NMR in Biological Research: Peptides and Protein.: 15-64.
    American Elsevier Publishing Co. New York.
24. GARDNER, J. D., T. P. CONLON, H. C. BEYERMAN & A. VAN ZON. 1977. Gastroenterology
    73: 52-56.
25. MORODER, L., E. JAEGER, F. DREES, M. GEMEINER, S. KNOF, H.-P. STELZEL, P. THAMM,
    D. BATAILLE, S. DOMSCHKE, W. SCHLEGEL, I. SCHULZ & E. WUNSCH. 1980. Bioorg.
    Chem. **9:** 27-54.
26. CHOU, P. Y. & G. D. FASMAN. 1974. Biochemistry **13:** 222-245.
27. SMITH, J. A. & L. G. PEASE. 1980. CRC Crit. Rev. Biochem. **8:** 315-399.
28. KAISER, E. T. & F. J. KEZDY. 1983. Proc. Natl. Acad. Sci. USA **80:** 1137-1143.

The Regulation of Vasoactive Intestinal Peptide Synthesis in Neuroblastoma and Chromaffin Cells[a]

MARGERY C. BEINFELD,[b] PHILLIP L. BRICK,
ALLYN C. HOWLETT, AND I. LEE HOLT

Department of Pharmacology
St. Louis University Medical Center
St. Louis, Missouri 63104

REBECCA M. PRUSS

Merrell Dow Research Institute
Cincinnati, Ohio 45215

JOSEPH R. MOSKAL

Departments of Neurosurgery and Neuroscience
Albert Einstein College of Medicine
Montefiore Hospital
Bronx, New York 10467

LEE E. EIDEN

Laboratory of Cell Biology
National Institute of Mental Health
Bethesda, Maryland 20892

[a] This research was supported in part by National Institutes of Health Grants NS 18667 (to MCB), NS 16513 and NS 00868 (to ACH), and RR 05388 (to St. Louis University).

[b] Address for correspondence: Department of Pharmacology, St. Louis University Medical Center, 1402 South Grand Boulevard, St. Louis, MO 63104.

INTRODUCTION

Vasoactive intestinal polypeptide (VIP) is a basic 28 amino acid peptide isolated originally from porcine intestine[1] now known also to be distributed in the central and peripheral nervous system. A VIP-related peptide called PHI (peptide histidine iso-leucine amide) was subsequently isolated from porcine intestine,[2] and cloning of the cDNA for the mRNA encoding the VIP precursor protein has revealed that both VIP and PHM (the human equivalent of PHI) are contained in the same precursor.[3,4] A PHI-like peptide was also found in the rat VIP precursor.[5] The distribution of VIP and PHI overlap completely, although the ratio of the concentration of PHI to VIP is not always unity in every tissue in which it is measured.[6]

Studies on the regulation of VIP biosynthesis have made use of several cell types that make VIP: murine and human neuroblastoma, neuroblastoma-glioma hybrids, bovine and human adrenal chromaffin cells in short-term culture, and human pheo-chromocytoma in culture.

Regulation of VIP biosynthesis by cyclic nucleotides, phorbol esters, and ascorbate in these biological systems will be compared and discussed.

PHEOCHROMOCYTOMAS

Some, but not all, human pheochromocytomas have been reported to produce or contain VIP.[7-10] In some cases, these tumors may produce sufficient VIP to cause a severe diarrheal syndrome.[7] This VIP production is "ectopic" because VIP is not usually detectable in normal human adrenal gland.[11]

Pheochromocytoma cells dissociated and grown in cultures express VIP and exhibit neurite-like processes. Nerve growth factor (NGF) enhances the outgrowth of these processes and increases VIP production, while dexamethasone inhibits both neurite extension and VIP production.[10]

HUMAN ADRENAL CHROMAFFIN CELLS IN CULTURE

Chromaffin cells dissociated from normal human adrenal glands express VIP after some time in culture. They also make neurite extensions, and, like cultured pheo-chromocytomas, their extension activity and VIP production is increased by NGF and decreased by dexamethasone.[12]

BOVINE CHROMAFFIN CELLS

Bovine adrenal, like human, does not produce detectable VIP *in vivo*.[8,13] However, after 24 hours in culture, bovine chromaffin cells produce immunoreactive VIP that was judged to be identical to porcine VIP_{1-28} based on elution on reversed-phase chromatography.[13] The number of cells expressing VIP immunoreactivity under these conditions is about 1%.[14] This appearance of VIP represents an induction of VIP expression, not a proliferation of a VIP-producing cell since the cultures are grown in the presence of a mitotic inhibitor.[13]

A high percentage of the VIP stored in these cells (up to 65%) can be released by a 15-minute incubation with high potassium, veratridine, or by the cholinergic agonists nicotine and carbachol. The release induced by these agents is Ca^{2+}-dependent.[15]

Exposure of these cells for 17 hours to agents that mimic or raise intracellular levels of cAMP produced a dramatic increase in VIP concentration in the cells and the media. This increase represents *de novo* biosynthesis because it was blocked by addition of cycloheximide.[15]

Culturing the cells under depolarizing conditions or in the presence of nicotine, in addition to increasing VIP release, results in an increase in VIP in the cells.[16] This increase in cellular levels of VIP accompanying evoked release strongly suggests that biosynthesis is tightly coupled to release. The increase in VIP synthesis by agents that stimulate release is similar to that seen following forskolin treatment.

The tumor-producing phorbol esters have been used to investigate how activation of protein kinase C and the subsequent phosphorylation of cellular proteins influences synthesis and release of neuropeptides and hormones.[17,18] The action of phorbol esters has significant physiological relevance because phorbol esters mimic the action of diacylglycerol, a product of inositol phospholipid metabolism. Diacylglycerol, as well as inositol trisphosphate are considered to be important cellular mediators in many hormone and neurotransmitter systems.[19,20] Phorbol esters sometimes have complex actions and can be stimulatory or inhibitory. Because phorbol esters are not as readily metabolized as diacylglycerol, they produced a sustained activation of protein kinase C. In some systems, sustained activation of protein kinase C results in inhibition of agonist activity.

Treatment of chromaffin cells with the active phorbol ester TPA (12-0-tetradecanoyl-phorbol-13-acetate) for one to three days elevated the concentration of VIP and PHI in the cells and the media, while the inactive phorbol had no effect on VIP or PHI.[21] When added together, the effect of forskolin and TPA on VIP levels was roughly additive. The large increase in VIP due to TPA and forskolin treatment was due to the appearance of proportionately more VIP-immunoreactive cells in the cultures. The combined effect of TPA and forskolin on the number of cells staining positive for VIP was also additive.[21]

HUMAN NEUROBLASTOMA CELLS

A human neuroblastoma cell line that produces VIP[22] and a PHM-like peptide[23] has been used as the source of mRNA to determine the sequence of the cDNA coding pro-VIP/PHM[3] and has been used in several studies on the regulation of VIP biosynthesis.

Using a pulse-chase paradigm, the conversion of immunoprecipitable pro-VIP/PHM to VIP was demonstrated when a three-hour pulse was followed by a three-hour chase.[24] Elevation of cAMP in cultures of these cells causes them to differentiate and send out neurites. When cultured for 48 hours in dibutyryl cAMP, the synthesis of pro-VIP/PHM and VIP/PHM mRNA was increased about 11-fold, with only small increases in total RNA and protein synthesis. The VIP gene was not amplified by the cyclic nucleotide treatment. It appears that the action of cyclic nucleotides in this system is at the transcriptional level and is achieved by increasing the rate of transcription of pre-pro-VIP/PHM mRNA.[25]

Five hours after the addition of the active phorbol TPA, the VIP/PHM mRNA levels increased five-fold; a similar treatment with dibutyryl cAMP produced a 10-fold increase. When both agents are added together, a 38-fold increase occurs, indicating a synergistic action of the two agents on VIP/PHM mRNA transcription. These agents either alone or together did not amplify the VIP/PHM gene in these cells.[26]

MURINE NEUROBLASTOMA CELLS

VIP-like immunoreactivity was reported to be present in several neuroblastoma cell lines descended from the C1300 transplantable tumor,[27] in neuroblastoma × glioma hybrids, but not in glioma cells.[28]

Another cell line descended from the C1300 tumor, N18TG2, reported by Glaser et al.[28] to make moderate amounts of VIP-like material, was used to study the regulation of VIP biosynthesis. Based on elution of this immunoreactive VIP-like material in cells and media from high-pressure liquid chromatography, it appears to be identical to porcine VIP.[29]

This cell line, in addition to making VIP, has a high density of secretin receptors[30] and will respond to secretin and VIP by making cAMP. In this cell line, the VIP and secretin appear to act on the same receptor, with secretin being about 10 times more potent than VIP in stimulating adenylate cyclase and about 100 times more potent in inhibiting labeled secretin binding.

As in the human neuroblastoma, agents that elevate intracellular cAMP cause the cells to differentiate and send out neurites. Forskolin treatment (in the presence of a phosphodiesterase inhibitor) causes the VIP content of the cells and media to increase four- to fivefold. Treatment with secretin and dibutyryl cAMP also increases the VIP content of cells and media.

Ascorbate is thought to be a cofactor for the enzyme responsible for amidating many neuropeptides during posttranslational processing.[31,32] Addition of 10 μM ascorbate causes about a twofold increase in VIP in the media. This indicates that ascorbate may be a rate-limiting factor in VIP biosynthesis under these experimental conditions. Addition of both forskolin and ascorbate resulted in about a 10-fold increase in VIP in the media, demonstrating that their actions are synergistic. That the actions of ascorbate and forskolin are synergistic suggests that they are operating by different mechanisms, forskolin by increasing VIP mRNA transcription, while ascorbate may be increasing subsequent posttranslational processing of VIP such that it is reactive in the radioimmunoassay.[29]

At the ultrastructural level, it is possible to observe that some of these cells clearly contain abundant VIP immunostaining, while some adjacent cells are not stained with VIP antisera (FIG. 1). Within the immunostained cells, the reaction product is widely dispersed in the cytoplasm and does not appear to be restricted to any clearly identifiable subcellular organelle. Since authentic VIP$_{1-28}$ is detected in both cell and medium extracts, the cells are clearly capable of correct processing of pro-VIP to

VIP_{1-28} (FIG. 2). It will be of interest to know in what subcellular organelle the processing occurs.

The synthesis of VIP in these cells appears to be a function of their state of differentiation, because drug treatments that increase differentiation (like forskolin) also increase VIP synthesis. Conversely, when these cells were injected into nude mice, they grew at a fast rate into a large solid tumor. When this tumor was removed and assayed for VIP immunoreactivity with the VIP RIA, none was detectable.

It was not possible to elicit release of VIP from these cells under depolarizing conditions, such as treatment with 60 mM K$^+$ or veratridine, even when they had been stimulated by ascorbate or had previously been differentiated with forskolin. The reason for this is not clear and is still under investigation.

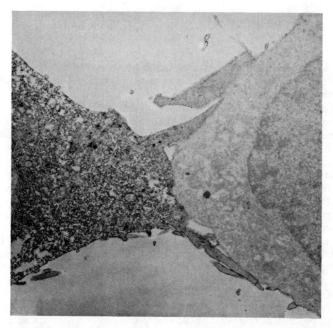

FIGURE 1. A VIP immunopositive murine neuroblastoma cell (left) in contact with a non-immunoreactive cell. EM courtesy of Stuart Hendry, University of California at Irvine.

These cells did not produce detectable PHI immunoreactivity under any of the conditions in which VIP was detectable. To insure that murine PHI was detectable with the PHI RIA that was used,[6] brain regions of the A/J mouse (in which the tumor arose originally) were assayed for PHI immunoreactivity and were found to have levels of PHI similar to rat and pig brain.[6] Whether the failure to detect PHI in these cells is a defect in mRNA splicing or in peptide processing is unclear, but it is most likely that the PHI in these cells is incompletely processed, so the PHI antiserum doesn't detect it. Aberrant forms of PHI have been reported in human neuroblastoma cells[23] and in VIPoma tumors.[33]

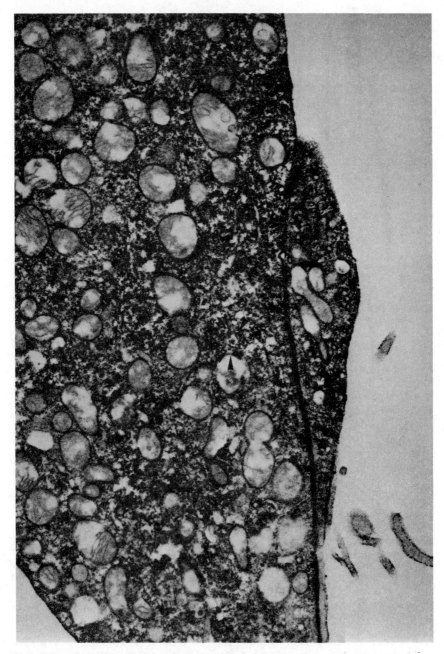

FIGURE 2. A higher magnification of a VIP immunoreactive cell. The arrows surround what appears to be a coated vesicle surrounded by VIP reaction product. EM courtesy of Stuart Hendry, University of California at Irvine.

SUMMARY

What is clear from these studies is that, in general, VIP biosynthesis is easily stimulated in a number of different cell types. The factors that modify VIP biosynthesis (summarized in TABLE 1) act through a variety of second messengers. These factors include agents like cyclic nucleotides, phorbol esters, ascorbate, NGF, dexamethasone, and nicotine.

TABLE 1. Factors that Modulate VIP Biosynthesis

Factor	Human Endocrine Cells	Murine Neuroblastomas	Bovine Chromaffin Cells
Agents that raise intracellular cAMP	↑ pro VIP/PHM[a] ↑ VIP mRNA[b]	↑ VIP in cells + medium[f]	↑ VIP in cells + medium[g]
Phorbol esters	↑ VIP mRNA[c] synergistic with cAMP[c] gene not amplified[c]	?	↑ VIP in cells + medium[h] additive with cAMP
Ascorbic acid	?	↑ VIP in cells + medium Synergistic with cAMP[f]	?
NGF	↑ VIP accompanies neurite extension[d,e]	?	?
Dexamethasone	↓ VIP accompanies decreased neurite extension[d,e]	?	?
High potassium, veratridine, nicotine	?	?	↑ VIP in cells + medium[i]

[a] Human neuroblastoma; Obata et al.[24]
[b] Human neuroblastoma; Hayakawa et al.[25]
[c] Human neuroblastoma; Ohsawa et al.[26]
[d] Human pheochromcytoma; Tischler et al.[10]
[e] Human chromaffin cells; Tischler et al.[12]
[f] Brick et al.[29]
[g] Eiden and Hotchkiss.[15]
[h] Pruss et al.[21]
[i] Waschek et al.[16]

Several cellular mechanisms appear to act to regulate VIP biosynthesis: (1) Cyclic nucleotides, acting by a Ca^{2+}-independent mechanism involving cAMP-dependent protein kinase works at the level of VIP mRNA transcription to increase VIP biosynthesis. (2) Phorbol esters (mimicking the action of diacylglycerol), acting through a Ca^{2+}-independent mechanism involving activation of protein kinase C, increase VIP mRNA transcription to increase VIP biosynthesis. That the effect of cyclic nucleotides and phorbols is additive or synergistic suggests that these agents act independently via their respective kinase to increase VIP mRNA transcription. (3) VIP biosynthesis appears to be tightly coupled to release by a process that does require Ca^{2+}. What mechanism is involved in the coupling of synthesis and secretion is unclear. (4) Ascorbate appears to be required as a cofactor for the processing of VIP and may be rate-limiting in some cell culture media, although the requirement for ascorbate may be difficult to demonstrate *in vivo,* because it is hard to make most animals deficient in ascorbate. In summary, multiple factors appear to be able to modify VIP biosynthesis. The precise mechanism for regulation of VIP biosynthesis in any given type of neural or endocrine cell may involve a combination of these mechanisms.

REFERENCES

1. SAID, S. I. & V. MUTT. 1970. Polypeptide with broad biological activity: Isolation from small intestine. Science **169:** 1217-1218.
2. TATEMOTO, K. & V. MUTT. 1981. Isolation and characterization of the intestinal peptide porcine PHI (PHI-27), a new member of the glucagon-secretin family. Proc. Natl. Acad. Sci. USA **78:** 6603-6607.
3. ITOH, N., K.-I. OBATA, N. YANAIHARA & H. OKAMOTO. 1983. Human pre-provasoactive intestinal peptide contains a novel PHI-27-like peptide, PHM-27. Nature **304:** 547-549.
4. BLOOM, S. R., J. DELAMARTER, E. KAWASHIMA, N. D. CHRISTOFIDES, G. BUELL & J. M. POLAK. 1983. Diarrhea in VIPoma patients associated with co-secretion of a second active peptide (peptide histidine isoleucine) explained by single coding gene. Lancet **1:** 1163-1165.
5. NISHIZAWA, M., Y. HAYAKAWA, N. YANAIHARA & H. OKAMOTO. 1985. Nucleotide sequence divergence and functional constraint in VIP precursor mRNA evolution between human and rat. FEBS Lett. **183:** 55-59.
6. BEINFELD, M. C., D. M. KORCHAK, B. L. ROTH & T. L. O'DONOHUE. 1984. The distribution and chromatographic characterization of PHI (peptide histidine isoleucine amide)-27-like peptides in rat and porcine brain. J. Neurosci. **4:** 2681-2688.
7. SAID, S. I. 1976. Evidence for secretion of vasoactive intestinal peptide by tumors of pancreas, adrenal medulla, thyroid and lung: Support for unifying APUD concept. J. Clin. Endocrinol. **5:** 201S-204S.
8. EIDEN, L. E., P. GIRAUD, A. HOTCHKISS & M. J. BROWNSTEIN. 1982. Enkephalins and VIP in human pheochromocytomas and bovine adrenal chromaffin cells. *In* Regulatory Peptides: From Molecular Biology to Function. E. Costa & M. Trabuchi, Eds.: 387-395. Raven Press. New York.
9. HASSOUN, J., G. MONGES, P. GIRAUD, J. F. HENRY, C. CHARPIN, H. PAYAN & M. TOGA. 1984. Immunohistochemical study of pheochromocytomas, an investigation of methionine-enkephalin, vasoactive intestinal peptide, somatostatin, corticotropin, β-endorphin, and calcitonin in 16 tumors. Am. J. Pathol. **114:** 56-63.
10. TISCHLER, A. S., Y. C. LEE, R. L. PERLMAN, D. COSTOPOULOS, V. W. SLAYTON & S. R. BLOOM. 1984. Production of "ectopic" vasoactive intestinal peptide-like and neurotensin-like immunoreactivity in human pheochromocytoma cell cultures. J. Neurosci. **4:** 1398-1404.
11. LINNOILA, R. I., R. P. DIAGUSTINE, A. HERVONEN & R. J. MILLER. 1980. Distribution of [Met^5]- and [Leu^5]enkephalin, VIP, and substance P-like immunoreactivity in human adrenal glands. Neuroscience **5:** 2247-2259.
12. TISCHLER, A. S., Y. C. LEE, R. L. PERLMAN, D. COSTOPOULOS & S. R. BLOOM. 1985. Production of "ectopic" vasoactive intestinal peptide-like immunoreactivity in normal human chromaffin cell cultures. Life Sci. **37:** 1881-1886.
13. EIDEN, L. E., R. L. ESKAY, J. SCOTT, H. POLLARD & A. J. HOTCHKISS. 1983. Primary cultures of bovine chromaffin cells synthesize and secrete vasoactive intestinal polypeptide (VIP). Life Sci. **33:** 687-693.

14. SIEGEL, R. E., L. E. EIDEN & R. M. PRUSS. 1985. Multiple populations of neuropeptide-containing cells in cultures of the bovine adrenal medulla. Dev. Brain Res. **17:** 267-270.

15. EIDEN, L. E. & A. J. HOTCHKISS. 1983. Cyclic adenosine monophosphate regulates vasoactive intestinal polypeptide and enkephalin biosynthesis in cultured bovine chromaffin cells. Neuropeptides **4:** 1-9.

16. WASCHEK, J. A., R. M. PRUSS, R. E. SIEGEL, L. E. EIDEN, M. F. BADER & D. AUNIS. 1987. Regulation of enkephalin, VIP and chromagranin biosynthesis in actively secreting chromaffin cells: Multiple strategies for multiple peptides. Ann. N. Y. Acad. Sci. **493:** 308-323.

17. HUTTON, J. C., M. PESHAVARIA & K. W. BROCKLEHURST. 1984. Phorbol ester stimulation of insulin release and secretory-granule protein phosphorylation in a transplantable rat insulinoma. Biochem. J. **224:** 483-490.

18. SUGANO, K., J. PARK, A. SOLL & T. YAMADA. 1986. Phorbol esters stimulate somatostatin release from cultured cells. Am. J. Physiol. **250:** G686-G690.

19. NISHIZUKA, Y. 1984. Turnover of inositol phospholipids and signal transduction. Science **225:** 1365-1370.

20. BELL, R. M. 1986. Protein kinase C activation by diacylglycerol second messengers. Cell **45:** 631-632.

21. PRUSS, R. M., J. R. MOSKAL, L. E. EIDEN & M. C. BEINFELD. 1985. Specific regulation of vasoactive intestinal polypeptide biosynthesis by phorbol ester in bovine chromaffin cells. Endocrinology **117:** 1020-1026.

22. YANAIHARA, N., T. SUZUKI, H. SATO, M. HOSHION, Y. OKARU & C. YANAIHARA. 1981. Dibutyryl cAMP stimulation of production and release of VIP-like immunoreactivity in a human neuroblastoma cell line. Biomed. Res. **2:** 728-734.

23. HOSHINO, M., C. YANAIHARA, K. OGINO, K. IGUCHI, H. SATO, T. SUZUKI & N. YANAIHARA. 1984. Production of VIP- and PHM(human PHI)-related peptides in human neuroblastoma cells. Peptides **5:** 155-160.

24. OBATA, K-I., N. ITOH, H. OKAMOTO, C. YANAIHARA, N. YANAIHARA & T. SUZUKI. 1981. Identification and processing of biosynthetic precursors to vasoactive intestinal polypeptide in human neuroblastoma cells. FEBS Lett. **136:** 123-126.

25. HAYAKAWA, Y., K-I. OBATA, N. ITOH, N. YANAIHARA & H. OKAMOTO. 1984. Cyclic AMP regulation of pro-vasoactive intestinal polypeptide/PHM-27 synthesis in human neuroblastoma cells. J. Biol. Chem. **259:** 9207-9211.

26. OHSAWA, K., Y. HAYAKAWA, M. NISHIZAWA, T. YAMAGAMI, H. YAMAMOTO, N. YANAIHARA & H. OKAMOTO. 1985. Synergistic stimulation of VIP/PHM-27 gene expression by cyclic AMP and phorbol esters in human neuroblastoma cells. Biochem. Biophys. Res. Commun. **132:** 885-891.

27. SAID, S. I. & R. N. ROSENBERG. 1976. Vasoactive intestinal polypeptide: Abundant immunoreactivity in neural cell lines and normal nervous tissue. Science **192:** 907-908.

28. GLASER, T., J. BESSON, G. ROSSELIN & B. HAMPRECHT. 1983. Vasoactive intestinal polypeptide: Presence in neuroblastoma × glioma hybrid cells. Eur. J. Pharmacol. **90:** 121-123.

29. BRICK, P. L., A. C. HOWLETT & M. C. BEINFELD. 1985. Synthesis and release of vasoactive intestinal polypeptide (VIP) by mouse neuroblastoma cells: Modulation by cyclic nucleotides and ascorbic acid. Peptides **6:** 1075-1078.

30. ROTH, B. L., M. C. BEINFELD & A. C. HOWLETT. 1984. Secretin receptors on neuroblastoma cell membranes: Characterization with ^{125}I-labeled secretin binding and association with adenylate cyclase. J. Neurochem. **42:** 1145-1152.

31. BRADBURY, A. F., M. D. A. FINNEY & D. G. SMYTHE. 1982. Mechanism of C-terminal amide formation by pituitary enzymes. Nature **298:** 686-690.

32. EIPPER, B. A., C. G. GLEMBOTSKI & R. E. MAINS. 1983. Bovine intermediate pituitary α-amidation enzyme, preliminary characterization. Peptides **4:** 921-928.

33. FAHRENKRUG, J. 1985. Evidence for common precursors but differential processing of VIP and PHM in VIP-producing tumors. Peptides **6:** 357-361.

Biosynthesis and Regulation of Expression

The Vasoactive Intestinal Peptide Gene

ILLANA GOZES

Department of Hormone Research
The Weizmann Institute of Science
Rehovot, 76100, Israel.

INTRODUCTION

In view of the functional importance of VIP, it is of substantial interest to follow the mechanisms regulating its biosynthetic pathways. Our studies toward the understanding of the regulation of VIP gene expression were divided into four stages of research including:

A. Isolation, sequencing, and chromosomal localization of the human VIP gene. This gene was found to contain seven exons, each encoding a distinct functional domain on the VIP precursor or its mRNA. The VIP gene was located on human chromosome 6(6q24).

B. Detection and characterization of multiple RNA forms containing VIP-encoding sequences including a stable mRNA precursor. Our results suggest posttranscriptional regulation of VIP-gene activity.

C. Ontogenic regulation of VIP-gene expression. The developmental patterns of VIP-gene expression imply a differentiation factor role for VIP.

D. Hormonal modulation of VIP-gene transcription. VIP-gene activity was found to be regulated by circulating steroids such as corticosterone.

These studies lay out the foundations for future investigations focused on the elucidation of the molecular mechanisms controlling VIP-gene activation and VIP-gene function. In the future, these experiments can be coupled to investigations of the VIP receptor. As the peptide exerts its function in conjunction with the appropriate receptor, understanding both the peptide and its receptor should complement each other elucidating the physiological roles of VIP in particular and the operation of complicated cellular arrays that are crucial for maintaining physiological homeostasis. Moreover, these studies can serve as a model for a general approach to investigations of neuroendocrine-specific peptides that should lead to a better comprehension of the neuroendocrine network.

77

THE VIP GENE AND ITS EXPRESSION

Cloning, Sequencing, and Chromosomal Localization of the Human VIP Gene

We have isolated the human VIP gene, using synthetic oligodeoxynucleotides. These specific hybridization probes were constructed according to the human VIP-cDNA sequence[1,2] and were synthesized using the deoxynucleotide phosphoramidite approach[3,4] to a length of up to 20 bases. When longer probes were needed, two short probes were ligated.[5] Screening a recombinant phage genomic library, followed by Southern blot analysis, resulted in the successful isolation of a chimeric phage containing the single human VIP gene.[5,6] This gene (~9000 base-pairs long) was found to contain seven exons, each encoding a distinct functional domain of the VIP-precursor or its mRNA: the 5′ untranslated region of the mRNA, putative signal peptide, NH_2-terminal peptide, PHM (peptide histidine-methionine amide), VIP, COOH-terminal peptide and 3′-untranslated region of the mRNA. PHM is a 27 amino acid peptide (with NH_2-terminal histidine and COOH-terminal methionine amide) closely related in sequence and activity to VIP. The VIP and the PHM exons encode both the hormone amino acid residues as well as the posttranslational processing signal sequences. The 3′ splice sites of the two exons contain an identical stretch of nine nucleotides. The occurrence of VIP and PHM coding sequences on two separate exons of the human genome and the identity of their 3′ splice site may allow alternative RNA processing.[5] This possibility is now being studied, utilizing RNA hybridization (see below). Our results on VIP-gene organization were corroborated by Tsukuda *et al.*[7]

In its intron-exon organization the VIP gene is similar to genes coding for VIP-related peptides that include the glucagon gene[8,9] and the growth hormone releasing factor gene.[6,10] In the case of the glucagon gene, the presence of three exons possessing internal homology (i.e., the glucagon and the two glucagon-like peptide-coding exons) may be a consequence of tandem exon duplication.[8] A similar mechanism may account for the evolution of the VIP and PHM coding exons. The high degree of VIP conservation among various species[11,13] underscores its important physiological roles. The segregation of the exons of the VIP-gene family into distinct functional domains and the amino acid similarities of the peptide products[12] suggests evolution from common ancestral genes.[6]

By means of chromosomal mapping using rodent × human somatic cell hybrids,[14] we localized the VIP gene to human chromosome 6 (6p21 to 6qter). Furthermore, by *in situ* hybridization, we have localized the VIP gene more precisely to 6q24.[15] This assignment of the VIP gene to its specific site on the chromosome should contribute to the understanding of its function. A deficient VIP-innervation of sweat glands was recently described as a possible pathogenic factor in sweating abnormalities characteristic for patients suffering from the prevalent hereditary disease, cystic fibrosis.[16] Since a close linkage of the cystic fibrosis trait was found with genes at the human chromosome locus 7cen-7q22,[17–20] our findings exclude the possibility of a defective VIP gene as a primary cause of cystic fibrosis. This does not, of course, exclude other genes that might affect VIP innervation from consideration for a primary role in this disease.

The assignment of the VIP-gene locus to chromosome 6 is interesting from several viewpoints. VIP and VIP-like peptides have been implicated as candidates for the prolactin-releasing factors,[21–26] and the prolactin gene itself has been mapped to the human chromosome region 6p23-6q12.[27]

Genes found in close proximity on the same chromosome are often functionally related. The chromosome region 6q24, which was demonstrated to contain the VIP-gene region[15] has been previously shown to contain the nuclear proto-oncogene c-myb,[28] which is the cellular homologue of the transforming gene v-myb. As VIP is primarily expressed in the nervous system, we investigated whether c-myb can be correlated with VIP in neuronal tissue. A sharp peak of c-myb-mRNA in the hippocampus of three-day-old rats was discovered, preceding the peak of VIP-mRNA that occurs at eight days of age.[15] Thus, the function of the proto-oncogene c-myb may be associated with brain development events expressed before the appearance of accentuated concentrations of VIP.

Detection of VIP-Gene Transcripts Using the Cloned VIP Gene

Our initial model system for VIP-gene expression studies was the human buccal tumor that we found to be a VIP overproducer. This tumor (HEp3) is a human carcinoma, primary in the buccal mucosa, originally obtained from a 62-year-old patient several years before the discovery of VIP.[29] By a combination of chromatographic procedures (molecular sieving, ion-exchange chromatography, and high-pressure liquid chromatography) and radioimmunoassay, we found that this tumor contains 0.67 ± 0.05 ng VIP/μg protein, concentrations that are greater than the richest source in brain.[4]

To characterize VIP-gene transcripts, we used three independent but complementary approaches, namely, RNA blot hybridization, S_1-nuclease analysis, and cDNA cloning. Our hybridization results show that a major transcript of the VIP-gene is an intron containing, $\sim 7,000$-base RNA.[6,30] This RNA is probably a precursor-RNA form, as the VIP-gene is ~ 9000-base-pairs long, containing 90% intron sequences. By means of S_1-nuclease analysis,[6] we determined the relative amounts of intron-hybridizing RNA to mature (exon specific) RNA and obtained a ratio $\geq 3 : 1$, in the tumor cells.

For cDNA preparations, the combined method using oligo-dT primed reverse transcription and RNase H-DNA polymerase I-mediated second-strand synthesis was applied.[30] Double-stranded cDNA was then subjected to EcoRI digestion followed by ligation to similarly restricted λgt10-phage DNA.[31] Recombinant phages were screened using VIP-specific synthetic oligodeoxynucleotides.[30] When the isolated clones were subjected to restriction analysis, complete identity between the EcoRI cDNA insert and the EcoRI gene fragment containing the VIP-encoding exon was observed. Sequence analysis of the established cDNA clones revealed complete identity with the cloned gene.[30]

In conclusion, we suggest that the control of VIP-gene expression resides, in part, in RNA-processing mechanisms. We found elevated amounts of this precursor RNA in the human tumor, indeed, most clones isolated were of the precursor type. Moreover, our results with rat brain RNA suggest a $\sim 7,000$-base VIP precursor RNA, enriched in nuclear preparations.[30] Thus, in contrast to most genes in which the primary RNA transcript is labile and protein-coding sequences are almost exclusively found in the mature mRNA form, an intron-containing transcript of the VIP-gene ($\sim 7,000$-base RNA) can be stable. This regulation may offer a mechanism for cellular storage, or cellular memory. In a broader sense, it is interesting that high molecular weight precursor RNA species were found also for other peptides such as calcitonin,[32] proen-

kephalin,[33] and vasopressin.[34] Our cloning of such a precursor cDNA verifies unequivocally previous hybridization results. Indeed, in the case of peptide hormones,
which play a central role in cellular communication,[35] multiple mechanisms are required to regulate their production. These mechanisms combine to generate the diversity of controls characteristic of the nervous system.

Detection and Partial Purification of a Mature-mRNA Containing VIP Coding Sequence from a Human Buccal Tumor

To characterize the mature VIP-mRNA, we devised three types of exon-specific
probes. Originally, mixtures of synthetic oligodeoxynucleotides with nucleotide sequences complementary to a relatively unambiguous part of the presumptive sequence
of VIP-mRNA[3,4] were synthesized using the deoxynucleoside phosphoramidite approach. As the sequence of the VIP-mRNA and gene was discovered,[5] we designed
probes with unique specific sequences.[30] Lastly, a set of RNA detection probes derived
by insertion of four of the exons of the VIP-gene into transcription plasmid vector
(pGEM™-1, Promega Biotec) were used. This plasmid contains a multiple cloning
site and two RNA polymerase promotors SP6 and T7 that allow transcription of
either of the inserted DNA strands to obtain uniformly labeled RNA hybridization
probes (riboprobes). The availability of exon-specific hybridization probes should
contribute to the precision of the identification of the corresponding mRNA.[15,30,36–40]

When mixtures of synthetic oligodeoxynucleotides were employed, we identified
a $\sim$1,600-base poly(A)-rich mRNA containing VIP-related sequences. This mRNA
was identified in rat brain[3] and in the human buccal tumor.[4]

To increase the sensitivity of detection, we synthesized DNA probes of unique
sequences corresponding to both DNA strands (sense and anti-sense) of the VIP and
PHM-encoding segments. These probes were made with the anti-sense probe extending
over only a part of the sense probe, allowing enzymatic addition of radioactive deoxy-
nucleotides, to yield very high specific activity labeled hybridization probes.[30] For
preferential detection of the mature messenger RNA, a probe was designed to contain
the junction of the VIP exon and its following exon. This probe hybridized to the
mature 1,600-base tumor RNA; however, the $\sim$7,000-base tumor RNA was detected
as well, representing partial hybridization (as the $\sim$7,000-base RNA contains
introns[30]). When a probe corresponding to the PHM exon was used on the same
RNA preparation, it apparently hybridized only to the high molecular weight precursor
RNA. Similar results were obtained with VIP and PHM exon specific riboprobes,
thus, the $\sim$1,600-base RNA hybridized only to the VIP-riboprobe while the $\sim$7,000-
base RNA hybridized to both riboprobes. Thus, it is possible that alternative processing
and exon exclusion occurs in this particular tumor state.

The 1,600-base VIP-related mRNA was further characterized by partial purification on sucrose gradients followed by in vitro translation in a reticulocyte-lysate
cell-free system. Among the newly synthesized proteins, an 11,000-dalton protein
exhibited VIP immunoreactivity, representing a VIP precursor protein.[4] It is interesting
to note that a similar molecular mass protein (11,000 daltons) was proposed as the
VIP precursor by pulse-labeling experiments in human neuroblastoma cells.[41] cDNA
cloning indicates a somewhat higher molecular weight precursor. As suggested above,
the 1,600-base mRNA may not contain all the exons of the gene, due to exon exclusion
during RNA processing, which will result in a lower molecular mass protein product.

At the posttranslational level, the VIP-precursor has a glycosylation site located at amino acid residues 68-70.[1] Glycosylation may alter the apparent molecular weight of the protein. Indeed, high molecular weight proteins containing VIP-like sequences have been identified using immunological probes such as monoclonal and polyclonal antibodies.[42-45]

VIP-mRNA in Rat Brain

As VIP is a major neuropeptide, regulation of its synthesis in the nervous system is of importance. We used rat brain as a model system, which facilitated developmental studies and experimental manipulations. The high degree of homology (80-90%) between rat and human VIP-encoding sequences[11] permitted the use of the human exon-specific riboprobes to detect rat brain mRNA. A major RNA species of ~2,000 bases hybridized with four VIP-specific riboprobes corresponding to the exon sequences for the signal peptide, PHM, VIP and the 3' exon. The identity of this RNA was verified using synthetic oligodeoxynucleotides containing rat-specific VIP-encoding sequences. These probes were also used to characterize the mature ~2,000-base VIP mRNA in polyribosomal RNA preparations.[38] Other minor RNA species were apparent as well, one of ~7,000 bases and a smaller form of ~5,000 bases. These RNA species probably contain intron sequences (see above). The ~1,600-base RNA detected previously[3] represented a minor population of VIP-related RNA molecules in the rat brain.[38]

Developmental Regulation of VIP-Gene Expression

Next we investigated whether the dramatic increase of VIP concentration in the developing rat brain[46-48] is a result of enhanced VIP-mRNA levels. We found that in the developing frontal cortex, the ~2,000-base VIP-mRNA increased at least fivefold from birth to three to four days postnatally, showing a maximal content at 14-16 days (an order of magnitude higher than 3-4 days). VIP-mRNA synthesis therefore apparently precedes by several days peptide synthesis, as VIP in the rat cortex begins to increase only at about seven days of age. Similarly, in the parietal cortex, VIP-mRNA was detected by three days of age. However, the increase in the mRNA content from 3 to 14 days of age was greater than in the frontal cortex (~14-fold) while almost no VIP-mRNA was detected in the newborn rat parietal cortex. In contrast, the hypothalamus contained significant quantities of VIP-mRNA at birth, the levels in the newborn being much higher than anticipated compared to the peptide levels. In the hippocampus, the major peak of VIP-mRNA occurred at eight days of age showing an ~30-fold increase over the levels in the newborn. The high molecular weight VIP-related RNA forms (~7,000 bases and ~5,000 bases) showed developmental regulation as well. For example, in the frontal cortex, at birth, they represented up to 80% of the total VIP RNA species, reducing gradually to about 30% at 14 days and to about 20% at 30 days. To verify the integrity of the mRNA preparations and accuracy of the measurements, the same blots were hybridized with β-actin cDNA.[49] Actin content has been shown to gradually decrease during brain maturation,[50] and the expected reduction was apparent at the mRNA level.[38]

In conclusion, the increase in the ~2,000-base VIP-mRNA with brain maturation implies regulation at the transcriptional level. According to Emson et al.,[46] VIP immunoreactivity is ontogenically increasing within single neurons. Our results indicate that this increase is due to enhancement in the specific gene transcriptions. Moreover, the differential onset of VIP-gene expression in various brain regions implies local environmental controls in different neuronal populations. The ontogenically related change in the ratio of the high molecular weight VIP-RNA to the mature mRNA suggests an additional control operating at the RNA processing level. These different control mechanisms should allow fine-tuning of VIP-gene expression in response to environmental stimuli. The finding of large quantities of a VIP-mRNA preceeding the appearance of the peptide is intriguing; it is of interest to investigate whether other peptide products of the VIP-gene appear at an early age.

In the peripheral nervous system, the intestine is densely innervated by VIP-neurons that may be associated with differential secretory processes and with gastrointestinal peristalsis.[12] In contrast to the brain, VIP is detected in the rat embryonal intestine at 16 days' gestation.[46] Developmental studies revealed substantial amounts of the ~2,000-base VIP-mRNA in 16-day-old rat embryos,[40] coinciding with the establishment of the fetal circulatory system at this age.[51] After birth, high levels of the ~2,000-base VIP-mRNA were found in the intestine of newborn rats, decreasing somewhat during postnatal development and then increasing threefold in the adult. The increase in the adult is correlated with weaning and a change in the diet that may alter the hormonal regulation of VIP-gene transcription.[38] As for hormonal regulation in brain, Nobou et al.[48] suggested that hypercorticism and hypocorticism modify the postnatal levels of immunoreactive VIP, implying a role for corticoids in the developmental patterns of VIP. Our results show changes in VIP-mRNA levels in the developing rat brain, following corticosterone administration. In the developing hypothalamus, the ~2,000-base VIP-mRNA increased following corticosterone treatment[39] in agreement with an increase at the peptide level.[48]

Hormonal Modulation of VIP-Gene Transcripts

VIP was shown to be involved in neuroendocrine regulation and to modify the release of various hormones both in vivo and in vitro.[12] Indeed, VIP affects prolactin release.[21–26,52] Prolactin is a key pituitary hormone associated with milk secretion and fertility control. In lactating animals, many neurons in the hypothalamic paraventricular nucleus that regulates pituitary action[52] become VIP immunopositive. To investigate whether there is indeed an increase of VIP synthesis in the rat hypothalamus during lactation, we have used our exon-specific RNA probes to detect and quantify VIP-mRNA in the hypothalamus. When lactating mothers were compared to "normal" female rats, an approximately twofold increase in VIP-mRNA was detected.[37] Thus, the VIP-gene can be transcriptionally regulated by hormonal events associated with suckling and elevated prolactin secretion. An increase in VIP-gene activity during lactation may be reflected in the finding of elevated secretion of VIP in milk,[53] associated with the peptide's putative function as a differentiation factor.[13]

The regulation of VIP-mRNA during lactation may be modulated by changes in circulating steroids that occur at that period. Our preliminary data show that injection of corticosterone and estrogen into immature rats can induce an increase in the VIP-mRNA in the hypothalamus.[39,54]

Interestingly, VIP enhances progestin and estrogen production by granulosa cells of hypophysectomized estrogen-treated rats implying mutual interactions between VIP and estrogen. We have discovered VIP-mRNA in ovaries, indicating local synthesis in this organ.[36] The concentration of VIP-mRNA did not seem to alter significantly upon induction of ovulation with human chorionic gonadotropin (hCG) although the latter seemed to induce a reduction in the high molecular weight VIP-mRNA, indicating an increased rate of processing toward the mature mRNA.[36] Thus, steroid hormones may affect VIP-gene activity and VIP-mRNA content and other hormones (hCG) may be involved in the regulation of posttranscriptional events such as RNA processing.[36]

IN CONCLUSION

We have isolated the human VIP-gene and determined its structure and chromosomal location. At the RNA level, we found a developmental regulation of VIP-gene expression in the brain. The mechanisms underlying the VIP-gene regulation may reside, in part, on the concentrations of circulating steroid hormones that exert a differential effect on the various neuronal populations. Protein hormones, such as prolactin and human chorionic gonadotropin, may directly or indirectly affect VIP-mRNA levels as well. We have obtained evidence that VIP-gene expression can be controlled also at the level of RNA processing as we discovered elevated levels of high molecular weight RNA in a human tumor, in the developing brain and in ovaries. In the tumor, the mature VIP-mRNA is somewhat smaller than the brain's most abundant mature VIP-mRNA that may indicate additional regulation at the RNA structure level. The developmental patterns of VIP-gene expression suggest a crucial role for the peptide products in the maturation and maintenance of the nervous system.

OVERVIEW: PAST, PRESENT, AND PROJECTED RESEARCH

Our interest is in neuronal specific molecules and neuroendocrine regulations. VIP is expressed in a variety of neuronal cell types, and we now ask what are the mechanisms responsible for *VIP*-gene activation. This question is a central one in molecular neuroendocrinology in relation to any neuroendocrine-specific peptide.

Stages of Future Research

In general, factors that lead to a change in VIP content are now being discovered. Many neuroactive substances may influence VIP-gene activity[13] and studies at the mRNA level may also pave the path for neuronal circuit studies and identification of the specific neurons innervating the VIP-cell. The sensitive techniques for identification of VIP-mRNA will further facilitate the examination of VIP-gene activity *in situ*, in various brain neurons at the single cell level as well as in isolated nuclei. The determination of control sequences on the VIP-gene, which interact with factors that stimulate transcription, should follow. The isolated VIP-gene fragments make such studies feasible, utilizing transfection experiments with various constructs containing defined regions of the VIP-gene.

In order to study the biological role associated with a known peptide transmitter, it is possible to design antibodies against it and inject them into the animal, or to use specific antagonists. Antibodies may not neutralize all the peptide synthesized and antagonists may have side effects. To date, there are not many antagonists that block all the VIP activities described above. One antagonist is an analogue of growth hormone releasing factor,[55] which inhibits VIP-stimulated adenylate cyclase activity in rat pancreatic membranes. Such an antagonist should be tested in different systems where VIP exerts an effect, to discern the physiological significance of the multiple functions attributed to VIP. In addition, a strategy for specific inhibition of the expression *in vivo* of known gene sequences has been developed.[56] An anti-sense transcript (noncoding DNA strand) that has a sequence complementary to the target mRNA can presumably anneal with the mRNA and disrupt the normal processing leading to efficient translation. Such a plasmid specifically inhibited expression of the cognate sense thymidine kinase (TK) plasmid after both plasmids were microinjected into cells.[56] The results with this model system suggest that anti-sense RNA can provide an additional methodology for genetic analysis in eukaryotic systems that are not readily amenable to standard mutational analysis. Inhibition of function by anti-sense RNA is a regulatory strategy in prokaryotes where it has been found to control translation, as well as the activity of RNA primers for initiating episome DNA replication.

With the availability of mechanical and viral methods for introducing anti-sense DNA and RNA into cells, the procedure described above can be used to study VIP function. Developing this technique for VIP can be expanded to other transmitter hormones yielding better understanding of neuronal activity. This approach could be first used at the cellular level and thereafter applied to the whole animal.

Finally, studies of receptor gene expression and mapping functional domains of the receptor molecule are expected to complement investigations of the neuropeptide gene expression eventually leading to the elucidation of neuroendocrine homeostasis.

REFERENCES

1. ITOH, N., K.-I. OBATA, N. YANAIHARA & H. OKAMOTO. 1983. Nature **304:** 547-549.
2. BLOOM, S. R., N. D. CRISTOFIDES, J. DELAMARTER, G. BUELL, E. KAWACHIMA & J. M. POLAK. 1983. Lancet ii: 1163-1165.
3. GOZES, I., M. BODNER, Y. SHANI & M. FRIDKIN. 1984. J. Cell Biochem. **26:** 147-156.
4. GOZES, I., M. BODNER, H. SHWARTZ, Y. SHANI & M. FRIDKIN. 1984. Peptides **5:** 161-166.
5. BODNER, M., M. FRIDKIN & I. GOZES. 1985. Proc. Natl. Acad. Sci. USA **82:** 3548-3551.
6. GOZES, I., M. BODNER, Y. SHANI & M. FRIDKIN. 1986. Peptides **7:** 1-6.
7. TSUKADA, T., S. J. HOROVITCH, M. R. MONTMINY, G. MANDEL & R. H. GOODMAN. 1985. DNA **4:** 293-300.
8. BELL, G. I., R. SANCHEZ-PESCADOR, P. J. LAYBOURN & R. C. NAJARIAN. 1983. Nature **304:** 368-371.
9. HEINRICH, G., P. GROS & J. F. HABENER. 1984. J. Biol. Chem. **259:** 14082-14087.
10. MAYO, K. E., G. M. CERELLI, R. V. LEBO, B. D. BRUCE, M. G. ROSENFELD & R. M. EVANS. 1985. Proc. Natl. Acad. Sci. USA **82:** 63-67.

11. NISHIZAWA, N., Y. HAYAKAWA, N. YANAIHARA & H. OKAMOTO. 1985. FEBS Lett. 183: 55-59.
12. SAID, S. I. 1986. J. Endocr. Invest. 9: 191-200.
13. GOZES, I. 1986. VIP gene expression. Chapter 10. In Brain Peptides, Update. Volume 1. J. B. Martin, M. J. Brownstein & D. T. Krieger, Eds.: 141-162. John Wiley. New York.
14. GOZES, I., R. AVIDOR, D. KATZNELSON, Y. YAHAV, C. CROCE & K. HUEBNER. 1987. Human Genetics. 75: 41-44.
15. GOZES, I., H. NAKAI, M. BYERS, R. AVIDOR, Y. WEINSTEIN, Y. SHANI & T. B. SHOWS. 1987. Somatic Cell Mol. Gen. 13: 305-313.
16. HEINZ-ERIAN, P., R. D. DEY, M. FLUX & S. I. SAID. 1985. Science 229: 1407-1408.
17. KNOWLTON, R. G., O. COHEN-HAGUENAUER, N. BAN CONG, J. FRÉZAL, V. A. BROWN, D. BARKER, J. C. BRAMAN, J. W. SCHUMM, L.-C. TSUI, M. BUCHWALD & H. DONIS-KELLER. 1985. Nature 318: 380-382.
18. TSUI, L. C., M. BUCHWALD, D. BARKER, J. C. BRAMAN, R. KNOWLTON, J. W. SCHUMM, H. EIBERG, J. MOHR, D. KENNEDY, N. PLAVSIC, M. ZSIGA, D. MARKIEWITZ, G. AKOTS, V. BROWN, C. HELMS, T. GRAVIERS, C. PARKER, K. REDIKER & H. DONIS-KELLER. 1985. Science 230: 1054-1057.
19. WAINWRIGHT, B. J., P. J. SCAMBLER, J. SCHMIDTKE, E. A. WATSON, H. Y. LAW, M. FARRALL, H. J. COOKE, H. EIBERG & R. WILLIAMSON. 1985. Nature 318: 384-387.
20. WHITE, R., S. WOODWARD, M. LEPPERT, P. O'CONNELL, M. HOFF, J. HERBST, J. M. LALOUEL, M. DEAN & G. VANDE WOUDE. 1985. Nature 318: 382-385.
21. ABE, H., D. ENGLER, M. E. MOLITCH, J. BOLLINGER-GRUBER & S. REICHLIN. 1985. Endocrinology 116: 1383-1390.
22. FINK, G. 1985. Nature 316: 487-488.
23. HÖKFELT, T., J. FAHRENKRUG, K. TATEMOTO, V. MUTT, N. WERNER, A.-L. HULTING, L. TERENIUS & K. J. CHANG. 1983. Proc. Natl. Acad. Sci. USA 80: 895-898.
24. RUBERG, M., W. ROTSZTEJN, S. ARANCIBIA, J. BESSON & A. ENALBERT. 1978. Eur. J. Pharmacol. 51: 319-320.
25. VIJAYAN, E., W. SAMSON, S. I. SAID & S. M. MCCANN. 1979. Endocrinology 104: 53-57.
26. GOURDJI, D., D. BATAILLE, N. VANCLIN, D. GROUSELLE, G. ROSSELIN & A. TIXIER-VIDAL. 1979. FEBS Lett. 104: 165-168.
27. OWERBACH, D., W. J. RUTTER, N. E. COOKE, J. A. MARTIAL & T. B. SHOWS. 1981. Science 212: 815-816.
28. HARPER, M. E., G. FRANCHINI, J. LOVE, M. I. SIMON, R. C. GALLO & F. WONG-STAAL. 1983. Nature 304: 169-171.
29. TOOLAN, H. W. 1954. Cancer Res. 14: 660-666.
30. GOZES, I., E. GILADI & Y. SHANI. 1987. J. Neurochem. 48: 1136-1141.
31. GLOVER, D., ED. 1985. DNA cloning techniques, a practical approach. IRL Press. London, U.K.
32. AMARA, S. G., B. JONES, M. G. ROSENFELD, E. S. ONG & R. M. EVANS. 1982. Nature 298: 240-244.
33. SCHWARTZ, J. P., I. MOCCHETTI, O. GIORGI & T. T. QUACH. 1984. J. Cell. Biochem. Suppl. 8B: 110.
34. SAUSVILLE, E., D. CARNEY & J. BATTEY. 1985. J. Biol. Chem. 260: 10236-10241.
35. BLOOM, F. E., E. BATTENBERG, A. FERRON, J. MANCILLAS, R. J. MILNER, G. R. SIGGINS & J. G. SUTCLIFFE. 1985. Neuropeptides: Interactions and diversities. In Recent Progress in Hormone Research. R. Greep, Ed. 41: 339-367. Academic Press. New York.
36. GOZES, I. & A. TSAFRIRI. 1986. Endocrinology 119: 2606-2610.
37. GOZES, I. & Y. SHANI. 1986. Endocrinology 119: 2497-2501.
38. GOZES, I., Y. SHANI & W. H. ROSTÉNE. 1987. Mol. Brain Res. 2: 137-148.
39. GILADI, E., Y. SHANI & I. GOZES. 1987. Isr. J. Med. Sci. 23: 924.
40. GOZES, I., P. SCHÄCHTER, Y. SHANI & E. GILADI. 1988. Neuroendocrinology 47: 27-31.
41. HIOKI, Y., M. HOSHINO, C. YANAIHARA, K. OGINO, H. SATO & N. YANAIHARA. 1983. Characterization of VIP-like immunoreactivity in a human neuroblastoma cell line. In Peptide Chemistry. 1982. S. Sakakibara, Ed.: 263-266. Osaka: Protein Research Foundation. Osaka, Japan.
42. GOZES, I., D. T. O'CONNOR & F. E. BLOOM. 1983. Reg. Peptides 6: 111-119.

43. GOZES, I., R. J. MILNER, F.-T. LIU, E. JOHNSON, E. L. F. BATTENBERG, D. KATZ & F.
    E. BLOOM. 1983. J. Neurochem. **41:** 549-556.
44. GOZES, I. 1984. Molecular aspects of vasoactive intestinal polypeptide biosynthesis. *In*
    Molecular Biology Approach to the Neurosciences IBRO Handbook Series. Methods in
    the Neurosciences. H. Soreq, Ed. **7:** 133-140. J. Wiley & Sons. New York.
45. GOZES, I. 1985. Vasoactive intestinal polypeptide—from gene to peptide. *In* Gene Expres-
    sion in Brain C. Zomzely-Neurath & W. A. Walker, Eds.: 275-296. John Wiley & Sons.
    New York.
46. EMSON, P. C., R. F. T. GILBERT, I. LOREN, J. FAHRENKRUG, F. SUNDLER, & O. B.
    SCHAFFALITZKY DE MUCKADELL. 1979. Brain Res. **177:** 437-444.
47. McGREGOR, G. P., P. L. WOODHAMS, D. J. O'SHAUGHNESSY, M. S. GHATEI, J. M.
    POLAK & S. R. BLOOM. 1982. Neurosci. Lett. **28:** 21-28.
48. NOBOU, F., J. BESSON, W. ROSTÉNE & G. ROSSELIN. 1985. Dev. Brain Res. **20:** 296-301.
49. GINZBURG, I. & U. Z. LITTAUER. 1984. The expression and cellular organization of
    microtubule proteins: Brain-specific probes in the study of differential expression during
    development. *In* Molecular Biology of the Cytoskeleton. G. G. Borisy, D. W. Cleveland
    & D. B. Murphy, Eds.: 357-366. Cold Spring Harbor Laboratory. Cold Spring Harbor,
    NY.
50. SCHMITT, H., I. GOZES & U. Z. LITTAUER. 1977. Brain Res. **121:** 327-342.
51. ALTMAN, P. L. & D. S. DITTMER. 1962. Growth, Including Reproduction and Morphol-
    ogical Development. Prepared under the auspices of the committee on Biological Hand-
    books Federation of American Societies for Experimental Biology, Washington, D.C.
52. MEZEY, E. & J. Z. KISS. 1985. Proc. Natl. Acad. Sci. USA **82:** 245-247.
53. WERNER, H., Y. KOCH, M. FRIDKIN, J. FAHRENKRUG & I. GOZES. 1985. Biochem.
    Biophys. Res. Commun. **133:** 228-232.
54. WERNER, H., Y. KOCH, F. BALDINO, JR. & I. GOZES. 1987. Soc. Neurosci. Abstr. **13:**
    1286.
55. WAELBROECK, M., P. ROBBERECHT, D. H. COY, J.-C. CAMUS, P. DE NEEF & J. CHRIS-
    TOPHE. 1985. Endocrinology **116:** 2643-2649.
56. IZANT, J. G. & H. WEINTRAUB. 1985. Science **229:** 345-352.

Complete Nucleotide Sequence of Human Vasoactive Intestinal Peptide/PHM-27 Gene and Its Inducible Promoter[a]

TAKASHI YAMAGAMI,[b] KENZO OHSAWA,[b] MIKIO NISHIZAWA,[b] CHIYOKO INOUE,[b] EISUKE GOTOH,[b] NOBORU YANAIHARA,[c] HIROSHI YAMAMOTO,[b] AND HIROSHI OKAMOTO[b,d]

[b]Department of Biochemistry
Tohoku University School of Medicine
Sendai 980, Miyagi, Japan

[c]Laboratory of Bioorganic Chemistry
Shizuoka College of Pharmacy
Shizuoka 422, Shizuoka, Japan

INTRODUCTION

Vasoactive intestinal peptide (VIP), a 28 amino acid peptide originally isolated from porcine upper intestinal tissues,[1] is present not only in gastrointestinal tissues but also in neural and other tissues and exhibits a variety of physiological functions.[2]

In 1983, we determined the DNA sequence complementary to the mRNA coding for human VIP precursor.[3] The entire amino acid sequence of the precursor, deduced from the nucleotide sequence, indicated that the precursor protein contained not only VIP but also a novel PHI-27-like peptide, PHM-27. We also reported that synthesis of pro-VIP/PHM-27 was induced by dibutyryl cyclic AMP (Bt_2cAMP) in human neuroblastoma cells,[4] and that this was due to an increase in the rate of transcription of the VIP/PHM-27 gene.[5] Recently, we demonstrated that tumor-promoting phorbol esters also increased the synthesis of prepro-VIP/PHM-27 mRNA in the human neuroblastoma cells.[6]

To elucidate the organization of the VIP/PHM-27 gene and the regulatory mechanism of its expression by Bt_2cAMP and phorbol esters, we have determined the complete nucleotide sequence of the human VIP/PHM-27 gene including 1.9 kilobase pairs (kb) of the 5' flanking region. The VIP/PHM-27 gene spanned 8,837 base pairs (bp) containing seven exons and six introns, and the VIP and PHM-27 sequences

[a]This work was supported in part by Grants-in-Aid for Scientific Research and for Cancer Research from the Ministry of Education, Science and Culture, Japan.

[d]Author to whom correspondence should be addressed.

87

were encoded in different exons. In the 5' flanking region, four TATA-box sequences were present, but only the TATA-box sequence 28 bp upstream from the 5' end of the first exon was identified as the promoter inducible by cAMP and phorbol esters.

MATERIALS AND METHODS

Isolation of the Human VIP/PHM-27 Gene

A Charon 4A genomic library containing human fetal liver DNA[7] was screened with ^{32}P-labeled human prepro-VIP/PHM-27 cDNA[3] according to Benton and Davis.[8] Two clones, λHV1 and λHV2 (FIG. 1), were identified from about 5 × 10[6] recombinants. Each clone contained a 12-kb insert. To see whether these clones covered the entire VIP/PHM-27 gene, Southern blot hybridization of EcoRI-digested λHV1 and λHV2 DNA was done[9] using the 110-bp PstI-Sau3AI fragment of the 5' portion, the 410 bp Sau3AI-EcoRI fragment of the middle portion and the 730 bp EcoRI-PstI fragment of the 3' portion of the human prepro-VIP/PHM-27 cDNA[5] as probes. λHV1 contained the 5' portion of the VIP/PHM-27 gene, λHV2 contained the 3' portion, and they overlapped (FIG. 1). The restriction map of EcoRI and XbaI digests of λHV1 and λHV2 DNA is shown in FIGURE 1.

Subcloning and DNA Sequence Analysis

EcoRI fragments measuring 2.3, 1.3, 1.1, 2.2, 3.2, and 5.2 kb and 1.1, 3.2, and 3.5 kb XbaI fragments of λHV1 and λHV2 (FIG. 1) were subcloned into pUC8 and pUC18 (Pharmacia, Sweden). A more detailed restriction map was made and the

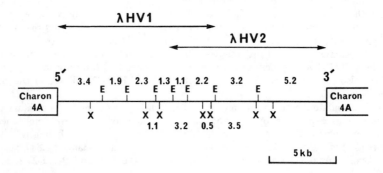

FIGURE 1. Restriction map of λHV1 and λHV2. The middle line indicates human genome and the boxes on both sides indicate the vector DNA. The genomic DNA inserts of λHV1 and λHV2 DNA are shown as arrows. Numbers indicate the size of EcoRI and XbaI fragments in kb. E, EcoRI; X, XbaI.

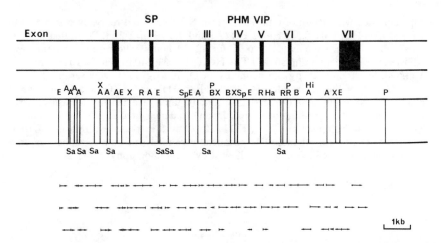

FIGURE 2. Restriction map of the human VIP/PHM-27 gene and sequencing strategy. The top portion indicates the organization of exons and introns of the human VIP/PHM-27 gene. Exons and introns are shown as filled boxes and open boxes, respectively. SP indicates the signal peptide. The middle portion indicates the restriction map. The bottom indicates the strategy for sequencing. Arrows indicate the direction and extent of the nucleotide sequence determined. For arrows starting with a vertical bar, the universal M13 primer (Takara) was used for sequencing. For arrows starting with a closed circle, synthetic oligonucleotides were used as primers. E, *Eco*RI; A, *Alu*I; Sa, *Sac*I; X, *Xba*I; R, *Rsa*I; Sp, *Sph*I; B, *Bam*HI; Ha, *Hae*III; Hi, *Hin*dIII; P, *Pst*I.

DNA sequence was determined by the dideoxynucleotide chain termination method[10] according to the sequencing strategy (FIG. 2).

Cell Culture and RNA Isolation

A human neuroblastoma cell line, NB-1, was originally established by Miyake *et al.*[11] Cells were grown in RPMI 1640 medium supplemented by 10% fetal bovine serum (Gibco) and 0.005% kanamycin (Meiji Seika, Japan).[6] In the logarithmic growth phase, NB-1 cells were incubated with 32 nM 12-*O*-tetra-decanoylphorbol-13-acetate (TPA) and 1 mM Bt$_2$cAMP for nine hours and total RNA was isolated from the cells by the guanidinium thiocyanate–CsCl method.[12]

Primer Extension Analysis

Primer extension analysis was performed as described by Leonald *et al.*[13] with slight modifications. A synthetic oligodeoxyribonucleotide complementary to the first 50 nucleotides of exon II was end-labeled with [γ-^{32}P] ATP (Amersham, UK) and T4 polynucleotide kinase (Takara, Japan). The labeled oligodeoxyribonucleotide was coprecipitated with 40 μg of total RNA from NB-1 cells and redissolved in 5.5 μl of 10 mM Tris-HCl (pH 8.3)/1 mM EDTA, and 4.5 μl of 2 M KCl, heated at 65°C for 5 min, and then incubated at 60°C for 12–13 hours. The reaction mixture was adjusted to 60 μl containing 50 mM Tris-HCl (pH 8.3); 140 mM KCl; 10 mM MgCl$_2$; 5 mM dithiothreitol; 25 μg/ml actinomycin D; 100 μg/ml bovine serum albumin; 0.2 mM each of the nucleotides dATP, dCTP, dGTP, and dTTP; 0.5 U/μl human placental RNase inhibitor (Amersham); and 10 units of avian myeloblastosis virus reverse transcriptase (Seikagaku Kogyo, Japan), and incubated at 42°C for 90 minutes. The reaction was stopped by adding EDTA to 20 mM, extracted with phenol/CHCl$_3$ and precipitated with ethanol. The products were analyzed by electrophoresis on a 5% polyacrylamide/8 M urea gel followed by autoradiography.

Exon Mapping

An *Eco*RI fragment spanning $-1,929$ to 356 was inserted into a plasmid carrying T7 and SP6 promoters, pGEM3 (Promega Biotec), and transcribed in the anti-sense orientation in the presence of [α-^{32}P]CTP (Amersham) and other NTPs using T7 RNA polymerase. The resultant ^{32}P-labeled anti-sense RNA (10^6cpm) was hybridized to 20 μg of total RNA from NB-1 cells in 20 μl of 80% formamide, 40 mM Hepes (pH 6.7), 0.4 M NaCl, and 1 mM EDTA at 45°C for 12–13 hours. Following hybridization, RNase digestion was performed as described by Melton *et al.*[14] The product was analyzed by electrophoresis on a 5% polyacrylamide/8 M urea gel followed by autoradiography.

Mung Bean Nuclease Mapping

Mung bean nuclease mapping was performed mainly as described previously.[15] This nuclease was preferred to S1 nuclease for its lack of accessory reactions. A 2.2-kb *Hpa*II fragment containing $-1,929$ to 143 of the VIP/PHM-27 gene was isolated from a recombinant plasmid, labeled at the 5' end with [γ-^{32}P]ATP and T4 polynucleotide kinase, and digested with *Sau*3AI. The resultant 830-bp *Sau*3AI-*Hpa*II fragment (-689 to 143) was isolated by 5% polyacrylamide gel electrophoresis. One hundred and twenty nanograms of this fragment and 40 μg of RNA from TPA- and Bt$_2$cAMP-treated NB-1 cells were lyophilized and dissolved in 20 μl of 80% formamide, 0.4 M NaCl, 40 mM Pipes (pH 6.4), and 1 mM EDTA. The solution was heated at 70°C for 10 minutes and incubated at 60°C for 12–13 hours in a sealed capillary tube. Hybridization was terminated by rapidly diluting the reaction mixture in 400 μl of ice-cold mung bean nuclease buffer containing 0.24 M NaCl, 30 mM CH$_3$COONa (pH 4.5), and 2 mM ZnSO$_4$. The sample was incubated with 250 units of mung bean nuclease (Takara) at 37°C for two hours and precipitated with ethanol. The product was analyzed by electrophoresis on a 6% polyacrylamide/8.3 M urea gel followed by autoradiography.

RESULTS

Primary Structure of the Human PreproVIP/PHM-27 Gene

FIGURE 3 shows the complete nucleotide sequence of the human VIP/PHM-27 gene and its 5' and 3' flanking regions. The organization of exons and introns was determined by the comparison of the genomic DNA sequence and the human prepro-VIP/PHM-27 cDNA sequence. The length and position of exon I was determined as described later. It was found that the human VIP/PHM-27 gene spans 8,837 bp and consists of seven exons and six introns. Exon I comprises 165 bp and encodes the 5' untranslated region of the gene. Exon II comprises 117 bp and encodes the rest of the 5' untranslated region, the signal peptide of the preproVIP/PHM-27 and a part of the amino-terminal region. Exon III comprises 123 bp and encodes most of the amino-terminal region. Exon IV comprises 105 bp and encodes the PHM-27 sequence and a portion of the region that separates PHM-27 and VIP. Exon V comprises 132 bp and encodes the rest of the intervening region, the sequence of VIP, and a small part of the carboxy-terminal region. Exon VI comprises 89 bp and encodes most of the carboxy-terminal region and a part of the 3' untranslated region of the gene. Exon VII comprises 724 bp and encodes the rest of the 3' untranslated region.

The nucleotide sequence of each exon completely corresponded to that of the human preproVIP/PHM-27 cDNA[3] except for exon VII, which possessed minor changes; four substitutions, two insertions, and one deletion of nucleotides compared with the cDNA sequence (FIG. 3). It was supposed that these changes were due to the difference in the materials from which the cDNA and the gene had been isolated (neuroblastoma cells and fetal liver, respectively).

We next compared sequences around each splice junction. As shown in FIGURE 4, 5' and 3' splice sites of each exon-intron boundary were homologous with the consensus sequence.[16] In particular, the 5' splice sites of introns IV and V downstream of PHM-27-encoding exon IV and VIP-encoding exon V contained an identical stretch of nine nucleotides (AGGTAAAGA). The 3' splice sites of these introns also contained an identical stretch of six nucleotides (AGCAGT). In addition, both introns IV and V fell after the second nucleotide of the serine codon, AGC.

In the 1,929-bp sequence of the 5' flanking region, four TATA-box sequences were found at 28, 145, 772, and 900 bp upstream from the cap site, but there were no CAAT- or GC-box sequences.

Identification of the Inducible Promoter

To see which TATA-box sequence is the promoter inducible by Bt_2cAMP and TPA, primer extension, exon mapping, and mung bean nuclease mapping analyses were performed. FIGURE 5 shows the result of primer extension study. Using a 50-base oligodeoxyribonucleotide complementary to the first 50 nucleotides of exon II as primer and RNA from TPA- or Bt_2cAMP-treated NB-1 cells as template, 220-base and 140-base reverse transcripts were found to be synthesized (lanes 2 and 3). The amounts of these transcripts were significantly increased with RNA from NB-1 cells that had been treated with both Bt_2cAMP and TPA (lane 4). The transcripts

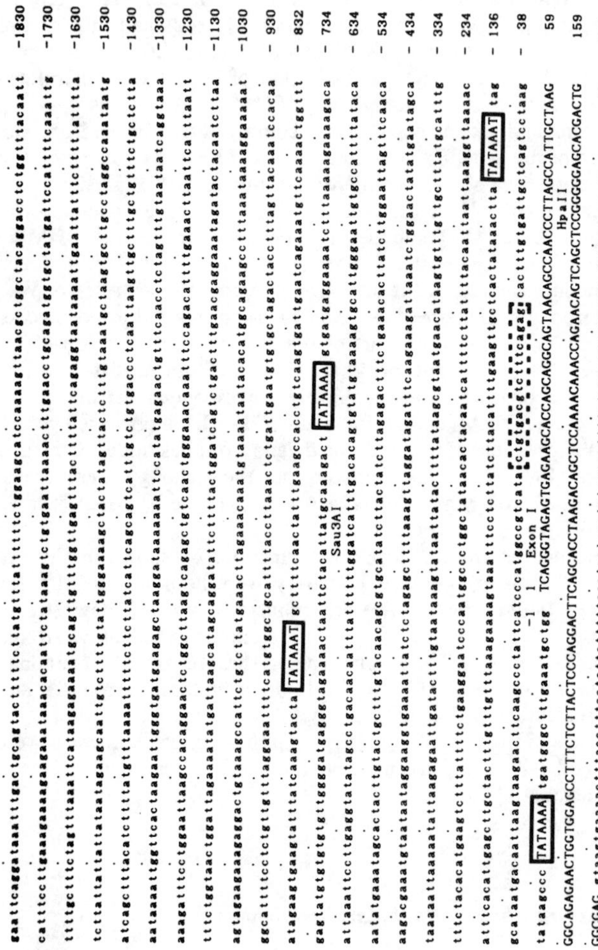

FIGURE 3. (Part 1)

gtacatcctgtatgaaagaattgtcccaggttattccagcactatagagatgtgcattcaacatagtatcggccaacatgtgccagacagt 1158

aggtgaaaagaattctaattttattcaagcacctgtcactgaagaaaatactgattttgaatgtatcatcttgcaattaactcttctacaaatga 1258

aaattactcttacaaactctgcagaggccattgaaaattacctgcaatcagaattacctgctggacatcttgctggaggaactgagtga 1358

    Exon II Met Asp Thr Arg Asn Lys Ala Gln Leu Leu Val Leu Leu Ser Val Le
ttctctctttag AGGCACAGA ATG GAC ACC AGA AAT AAG GCC CAG CTC CTG GTG CTC CTG ACT CTT CTC AGT GTG CT 1438

                Signal Peptide
u Phe Gln Thr Ser Ala Trp Pro Leu Tyr Arg Ala Pro Ser Ala Leu Ar
C TTC TCA ACT TCG GCA TGG CCT CTT TAC AGG GCA CCT TCT GCT CTC AG gtaagttcccttcaattcaaacatctgaac 1520

attcctcctcatctaaatgggaattctatacatttgttggacaactaaattatgtattatttaaattttcctgatgtgttg 1620

agtgagagtgttgtcaaatcaggtcatctgagtcctggaattcacttcaggcatgagagacactctcagttagttttatggctgagtgga 1720

tcacattcccaacatggtgaaaggaggctttcacttcacttttcttttttattcaaaacatcttagataaacatcttatccattgttatctcaagtca 1820

gttcaatttctggtggaaaaaagctgtttagttagttggccaacaccacattgagtttattttcaagttattcattttcaatttccttgatggttgattag 1920

tgaaacatgtataaaatcatgttgcacagaaatctatctaggccagagtcaattgccaattaaaatatggggtaaattgatctattgagataacactcccc 2020

caataggaaaatttgatatacttttgtttggaccataaatccttagtttattattgtctatatgttatatttatatattccaatccaaaagtataacaca 2120

actctattttaaaacttattaatgtatgcaaagaagtaaacaatataagaaactatatagctgaattttccttcaggttttgcttaaggtagacttacgccacctgta 2220

tctccaaaggaaaatataataatgggttggtttcctttcttttgcattattaggtcatcttgattttgtctctaaggtagacttatgctcaacagagaaat 2320

aacctcttagctattagtgttctctgtgaaatctgttttaatacagctcctgcgtgcttaagctgcttgataacctaaacaaaatggtctatcgaatagttctacc 2420

acagcagaatgaacaatcacaagagtgtcccagactgacacctctggcagtctgttgcctaagcttcagaacccacagaggacctagttgctctagtcgaaaatcgcacccaaatca 2520

ctgaaaagataaccaagtgtcccagactgcacacctcctggatgttgcctaacagtgaaaatcgcacacaaaattataagagttgccggtgatt 2620

gaaatatgcatccatcaaatatagtcatatccataaaacttattgaattcaaattcatctttagtctttcagtgtaacatccttattgctacatcccttattcttgaac 2720

ttaatacataagattagaaaaagaaaggcccataaaactatttgaagcaaactggggtcgagacgagaagaggcagttaatactctgttcttcagaga 2820

tcgtcaatacagagagaaatatataaatgccaaagtaaatattttgaaagctaacagttctcatccaaattgtcattgttatttctctatttgttccataaaatat 2920

tgtttggaacagcgtaatactgaactgcttgcaaatgaaaatatctttgccatagtaaattacaccaaagaagtatagtttgcttaatgctctgtaagaattgaat 3020

ttctacatacgaaatttgacttgctgtatattcacctataaaagtacatatggccatctactttatatctctattaactacta 3120

taaatagtcctctgtttgtttgtatatccatattatagagggctaataactcccagagtctaagtatctctatttaaggtcgttgccggaccacatacaca 3220

tgagccattaagtcaaattatgctatttcatattatgactggtaatacttccccatac g TTG GGT GAC AGA ATA CCC TTT GAC GGA GCA AAT GAA 3320
                    Exon III
        g Leu Gly Asp Arg Ile Pro Phe Glu Gly Ala Asn Glu

Pro Asp Gln Val Ser Leu Lys Glu Asp Ile Asp Met Leu Gln Asn Ala Glu Asn Asp Thr Pro Tyr Tyr
CCT GAT CAA GTT TCA TTA AAA GAA GAC ATT GAC ATG TTG CAA AAT GCA TTA GCT GAA AAT GAC ACA CCC TAT TAT 3407

Asp Val Ser Ar
GAT GTA TCC AG gtragtttattttataaaactatccaatagtttatttagaaaataatctaaaagtgctttattttatctcac 3482

catgaagctattccgatagcaaaacactagagtttctatgtcatgctcattactcagtcagaatctcagatttactgacgatctacagctactacagtctacataatttcat 3578

FIGURE 3. (Part 2)

```
actgaaaggttgtaacaagccaggatgaacacaccattcacttccattctgttgcacataattccaacatcacagattgtaccaattctgataaaagtac   3778
agcatttagcattccaatgatggaagagttgccaaggagttttgtctctatataaagaaaagatacctgatagagctgttcattcatagagctgtttgtc   3878
tagagcatcatttcaagtacagaccaagtagctctatagtacttggtacagacaaagtataaaaggtgcttcatttgaaagagaaaaggtgggatgatag   3978
gccttaatgccttctctatcttaagagattttgtttccaaatatttggaaaaagaaaaaaaaaggtgtactggggtttatgaactttccaaaatcagaa   4078
tattttcccattgtgaatgtctttattcagtggggcagacacaaagcaccatgtacaaatagcagctaatttaaatagatcatatttttacaccaatatt   4178
tcttagaaagaaatagttataaagattcaaccatggaggaatattgaaatgtgctcctagaaatgcctgtttctttaatttttcagtgtcttgggctaga   4278
aatatagggtatatcttgatataagtgactagaagatctcttttgttagggtgttaagaaatctccttttgaactttagttttaatgagaagctttcata   4378
                                                                                                g As
ataagcccataatttttttgttatttaataagccataataatattctagaaagccatttacaaaataatagctatttttttcttccttgttttag A AA   4476
 Exon IV  ┌──────────────────────────── PHM-27 ──────────────────────────────────────┐
n Ala Arg His Ala Asp Gly Val Phe Thr Ser Asp Phe Ser Lys Leu Leu Gly Gln Leu Ser Ala Lys Lys Thr Le
T GCC AGG CAT GCT GAT GGA GTT TTC ACC AGT GAC TTC AGT AAA CTC TTG GGT CAA CTT TCT GCC AAA AAG TAC CT   4551
────────────────────┐
u Glu Ser Leu Met Gly Lys Arg Val Se
T GAG TCT CTT ATG GGA AAA CGT GTT AG gtaaagagaatttattatttttataaaatatgttatcattattcaatctgaatattgtatttt   4641
cactcttaacaagttatttactttgtttgaaattgaaaactcgttgataatgtttaatttagttaaatgaaataacttgtattcttcaataacatctatc   4741
aagcccatggactaagactttttcataatatcatattcattgactccagacacacatttttctcaagtagcaatcatttagcaatctgcaatcaaattga   4841
acaagactcagtaaaacaatcaaaaagagatagtacagactgaggtaaatttaaggtcaaacagaatattctttttacttcctgctcaaattaaatgga   4941
gaattccaaatggccaacagtcaaatatttagatgacgttgctcagggtagcatagcttctaaagaagtaattatgtttttttaaaaaaaaaaaaaatt   5041
tctcccaatggcagagcacaacttcagctattcccaaatttttatttttggatgaattatttgctcagctgtacagaatgtgtcataaaacagtcccagg   5141
ccatgccaaaatatggcagatgattccttgctttccttcatccttaggtttagttgtatttttcttttagtctttttatgatagaaaattagttgggtgg   5241
                                                                                                   r
gaattgctttttatgtggctccaagaaacctggaacatgtgtgtatttatcatttcttgtgaaaactctttgatttccttttcctcatgttccttag C   5339
 Exon V                                      ┌──────────────────── VIP ──────────────────────┐
Ser Asn Ile Ser Glu Asp Pro Val Pro Val Lys Arg His Ser Asp Ala Val Phe Thr Asp Asn Tyr Tyr Arg Leu
AGT AAC ATC TCA GAA GAC CCT GTA CCA GTC AAA CGT CAC TCA GAT GCA GTC TTC ACT GAC AAC TAT ACC CGC CTT   5414
──────────────────────────────────────────────────────────┐
Arg Lys Gln Met Ala Val Lys Lys Tyr Leu Asn Ser Ile Leu Asn Gly Lys Arg Se
AGA AAA CAA ATG GCT GTA AAG AAA TAT TTG AAC TCA ATT CTG AAT GGA AAG AGG AG gtaaagaaaaagagaacttgctaaa   5495
atgaggaatcatgactgactttcaaaatagaagctgcacatggagacctctctatctcacttatctagctatactacatgaagcagtgattttcaacctt   5595
ggctgacattagactaccccgcagaactttaaaaatacagatgtctgggccttctcccaaaccaattgccaggaaatcggtgtcttcggtggtgtggccc   5695
tagacatacatttcttttaagagttccccagttgactttactatgctgccagtgttaaaaatgatgactatacagacatctagtctgaatctaagagcaa   5795
gtttcatcaaaagtgatgatttttaaaacatgtaaagcatagtcaattgcaatttggtaacacatggaactcacttcgtgtgcatattcactactgttat   5895
ttaatcaaattaaaccattaggtattttgtatatttagattctgtaaaatctatatctctctatggtgtgtaaatattggacacaatacataaacagtgt   5995
agtgttctgtctttttattccaattgtttttgtttaagtgatgagtattaaggataattctgtttgggtgtgatcagacaagatgacctctttgcccact   6095
agatgataattctgtgagaataatttagaaactctaagattgatgaataattcataggtactaacaaacctcaaagataattgtttagcctccccatac   6195
actttcagagcacagagaacagcacattcattatgtcataatagtttctttagaccctttctcatctgagagccttaatatgtacaatgtttttctggtc   6295
```

FIGURE 3. (Part 3)

```
       Exon VI
 . r Ser Glu Gly Glu Ser Pro Asp Phe Pro Glu Glu Leu Glu Lys End End
tgcag C AGT GAG GGA GAA TCT CCC GAC TTT CCA GAA GAG TTA GAA AAA TGA TGA AAAAGACCTTTGGAGCAAAGCTGATGAC    6377

AACTTCCCAGTG gtgggtatattcgtgcattccttctgtattcttatggctgtctctgattatataagtagctaagagtcacttagtaagaaacatctt    6476

agggttaaatagtttctcatcatgagacctcatccaagacagacacttctacaacagtggaccccaacccagtaaacagcttagaatgattcatgaaatt    6576

ttttgatcttgtaaaagagagcactcacaataagcaaacgttttgagatctgaatagtgttcctggcttacttggggttatttctacctttgtatcaag    6676

ataaaaaaacagaggaggctgactcacactgacaagaaaaatgggctttcctttt gaggatcgacccatgctgcttttattaattgaaggtttagtctca    6776

caattgactgttagctcctcaattaagtatagggaaatagcaccaaattagagcatggcccattactatgaaaatatcaaggcattctgggtctaactat    6876

attccttgaaacatggcaaacttcatagagcaaaagttaaatttagcttgttttacctgtaagtttgttttacctatatgactctaatagcattctctgc    6976

caacatttttttgagcagaaaaaacatggatagactttttttctttgtgaagtaataagcttgctatcaaaattgattttatataaatgtgggttcaag    7076

acatatttctttcctgagttacattacattaatattcacattcgctcataaaaaatctataatactgggcaagtgcttaaagaaatttcatgctgtcacc    7176

atatcaaaggttagcagatttaaagggctatggagtaaaatatgtttggctttgtgagccatctattttctgttagagtgacttaactctgctatggta    7276

gcacaaaagcagccacagttagatgtaaaacgaataggagtgactgtgttccaataaaactttattcataaaacctgaaggtgagccagattccaatccc    7376

taactaggttaaggagattaaattcacccatgctcaaactaaaggcaattcatggccttacctcagttcctgatggggttatctaaggttttcaacagtc    7476

atcaagagtggacatggtgtctgggaagatacctgcttaattgactgcttttgtccactaattacccttagacctctaagagaaagcagaggcaggagtg    7576

tggcccacatcaactctttatcttttatagacatctcagagaaacaagtccctttgctcaaagaagaaagttaattacatatagcttttctaagagtgtt    7676

tataagaaggcttctccatcaaattaagaaacacggtaggcactaaaatataaaggagaattgattaatcacactgtgctttgtaaatggtaagatcact    7776

tatgagattccatcctccattcttttctttttaaatgggtggctttggacaaattctttgaagaggaaatcatgtgggtcatccattagtgaaaattac    7876

aagtgaatcattaataatggttagttagacgtcttttcacattccagttcctctctgataatcagtcctctagaagctgctctcttggtatgtcccagga    7976

catgatcccccgacaggctgttaacaagggacaaagagaaataagtgtttatcagataagtaaatcagtgaatgaaactaagatgctagaaataaaatat    8076
                                    Exon VII                                ***
atttatgcctaaagcaacaatttttcttttcag AATTCTTGAAGGAAAATGATACGCAACATAATTAAATTTTGAGTTCTACATAAGTAATTCAAG    8175

AAAACAACTTCAATATCCAAACCA [AATAAA] AATATTCGTGTTGTGAATGTTGTGATGTATTCTAGCTAATGTAATAACTGTGAAGTTTACATTGTAAA    8273
                                                                                      * ↓
TAGTATTTGAGAGTTCTAAATTTTGTCTTTAACTCATAAAAAGCCTGCAATTTCATATGCTGTATATCCTTTCTAACAAAAAAATATATGTAATGATAAG    8373
   -         -
TAAATGCTAGGTTAATTCCAATTATATGAGACGTTTTTGGAAGAGTAGTAATAGAGCAAAATTGATGTGTTTATTTATAGAGTGTACTTAACTATTCAGG    8473

AGAGTAGAACAGATAATCAGTGTGTCTAAATTTGAATGTTAAGCAGATGGAATGCTGTGTTA [AATAAA] CCTCAAAATGTCTAAGATAGTAACAATGAA    8571

GATAAAAAGACATTCTTCCAAAAAGATTTTCAGAAAATATTATGTGTTTCCATATTTTATAGGCAACCTTTATTTTTAATGGTGTTTTAAAAAATCTCAA    8671

ATTTGGATTGCTAATCACCAAAGGCTCTCTCCTGATAGTCTTTCAGTTAAGGAGAACGACCCCTGCTTCTGACACTGAAACTTCCCTTTCTGCTTGTGTT    8771

AAGTATGTGTAAAATGTGAAGTGAATGAAACACTCAGTTGTTCAAT [AATAAA] TATTTTTGCCATAA tgactcagaatattgctttggtcatatgagc    8868

ttccttctgtgaaagtacatttggagacacaactatttttccaaaataatttaagaaatcaaagagagaaaataaagacctttgcttatgattgcagat    8968

aatttttttgtttgattattttatatgattcagcagtaactcattttagctctaaagttctaggcac    9035
```

FIGURE 3. (Part 4) Nucleotide sequence of the human VIP/PHM-27 gene. Exons are presented in capital letters, introns and flanking sequences in lower case letters. The numbering begins at 1, which is the transcription initiation site; negative values indicate 5′ flanking sequences. Four TATA-box sequences and three polyadenylation signals are boxed. The sequence that is supposed to be related to induction by cAMP is boxed by broken lines. Seven differences in nucleotide sequence between the human VIP/PHM-27 gene and the human preproVIP/PHM-27 cDNA[3] are indicated by asterisks (nucleotide change), top bars (addition) or an arrow (deletion).

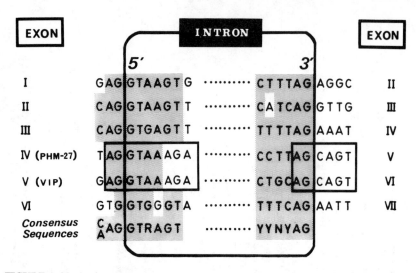

FIGURE 4. Nucleotide sequence conservation around splice junctions. Ten nucleotides around each exon-intron boundary are presented. Shaded regions indicate nucleotides identical to those of the consensus sequences.[16] Boxed nucleotides are identical stretches in introns IV and V. R, Purine; Y, pyrimidine; N, any nucleotide.

were hardly detectable with RNA from untreated cells (lane 1). The 220-base and 140-base transcripts were isolated from the gel and their sequences were determined by the method of Maxam and Gilbert.[17] The sequence of the 140-base transcript was identical to that of the 5′ portion of the 220-base transcript, suggesting the former was an incomplete product of the latter. In both the 220-base and 140-base transcripts, the primer extension was found to start from the cytosine residue corresponding to the guanine residue at 165 in FIGURE 3. Since the 50-base primer contained ten nucleotides complementary to the 3′-terminal portion of the 5′ untranslated region, it was indicated that the synthesis of the prepro-VIP/PHM-27 mRNA, which had a *ca.* 180-base 5′ untranslated region, was induced by Bt_2cAMP and TPA.

Exon mapping was done using the anti-sense RNA synthesized from the *Eco*RI fragment spanning −1,929 to 356. As shown in FIGURE 6, only one RNase-resistant fragment of about 170 bases was detected with RNA from TPA- or Bt_2cAMP-treated NB-1 cells (lanes 2 and 3). The amount of the fragment was also significantly increased with RNA from NB-1 cells that had been treated with both Bt_2cAMP and TPA (lane 4). The 170-base fragment was not detected with RNA from untreated cells (lane 1). The result of exon mapping indicated again that the synthesis of the prepro-VIP/ PHM-27 mRNA that had the same 5′ end was induced by either Bt_2cAMP or TPA and suggested that in the region upstream from exon II, there were no exons, other than 170 bp exon I, that were transcribed in the neuroblastoma cells.

We next determined the precise location of the 5′ end of exon 1 by mung bean nuclease mapping. A *Sau*3AI-*Hpa*II fragment (−689 to 143) containing the 5′ portion of exon I was hybridized with RNA from NB-1 cells treated with Bt_2cAMP and TPA and single-stranded regions were digested with mung bean nuclease. The resultant nuclease-resistant fragments were analyzed on a polyacrylamide-urea gel with a sequencing ladder of the labeled fragment. Only one distinctive band was detected, in agreement with the cytosine residue in the DNA template (FIG. 7). Since

Maxam-Gilbert DNA sequence reaction products have been shown to migrate 1-1.5 bp faster than the corresponding nuclease-resistant products,[18,19] it was indicated that the thymidine residue labeled 1 in FIGURE 3 was the 5′ end of exon I.

The results obtained from the primer extension, exon mapping, and mung bean nuclease mapping analyses suggest that among the four TATA-box sequences found in the 5′ flanking region, only the TATA-box sequence 28 bp upstream from the cap site is the promotor inducible by Bt$_2$cAMP and TPA.

DISCUSSION

In this paper, the complete nucleotide sequence of the human VIP/PHM-27 gene has been described for the first time. Bodner *et al.,*[20] Tsukada *et al.,*[21] and Linder *et*

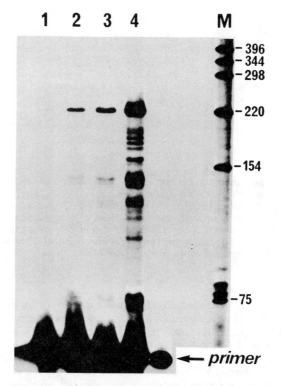

FIGURE 5. Analysis of the 5′ terminal region of the preproVIP/PHM-27 mRNA by primer extension. A synthetic oligodeoxyribonucleotide complementary to the first 50 nucleotides of the exon II was used as primer. The labeled primer was hybridized to total RNA from NB-1 cells and extended with avian myeloblastosis virus reverse transcriptase. RNA from untreated NB-1 cells (lane 1), RNA from NB-1 cells treated with TPA (lane 2), RNA from NB-1 cells treated with Bt$_2$cAMP (lane 3), RNA from NB-1 cells treated with TPA and Bt$_2$cAMP (lane 4). Labeled *Hinf*I fragments of pBR322 were used as size markers (lane M).

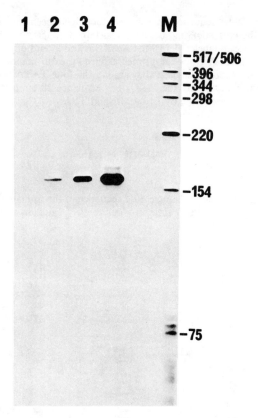

FIGURE 6. Characterization of the first exon of the human VIP/PHM-27 gene by exon mapping. ^{32}P-labeled anti-sense RNA spanning −1,929 to 356 was hybridized to total RNA from NB-1 cells and digested with RNase A and RNase T1. Nuclease-resistant fragments were analyzed on a 5% polyacrylamide/8 *M* urea gel. RNA from untreated NB-1 cells (lane 1), RNA from NB-1 cells treated with TPA (lane 2), RNA from NB-1 cells treated with Bt$_2$cAMP (lane 3), RNA from NB-1 cells treated with TPA and Bt$_2$cAMP (lane 4). Labeled *Hinf*I fragments of pBR322 were used as size markers (lane M).

al. [22] have recently reported the nucleotide sequence of a part of this gene. The sequence presented here is in good agreement with those reported by them.

VIP and PHM-27 are structurally related peptides having 44% homology in amino acid sequence and 52% homology in nucleotide sequence.[3] This study showed that PHM-27 was encoded in exon IV and VIP in the adjacent exon V. This suggests that the PHM-27-encoding and VIP-encoding exons have been duplicated from an ancestral exon as in the case of the glucagon/glucagon-like peptide gene[23] and the calcitonin/calcitonin-gene related peptide gene.[24] In addition, the sequence around boundaries between the PHM-27-encoding and VIP-encoding exons and their adjacent introns were highly conserved, suggesting that the duplication had occurred over a broad area containing the ancestral exon and its adjacent introns.

Another characteristic feature of the human VIP/PHM-27 gene is that it has four

TATA-box sequences (TATAAA$^T/_A$) at 28, 145, 772, and 900 bp upstream of the cap site. The presence and the differential usage of the plural number of TATA-box sequences have been reported in several genes such as mouse salivary and liver α-amylase gene,[25] mouse myosin light chain gene,[26] and rat insulin-like growth factor II gene.[27] In the human VIP/PHM-27 gene, only the TATA-box sequence 28 bp upstream of the cap site was found to be the promotor that is inducible by either cAMP or TPA in NB-1 cells (FIG. 5-7). The possibility, however, that the other three TATA-box sequences upstream of the inducible promotor may function in some circumstances or in other types of cells cannot be excluded.

Fifty-two bp upstream from the inducible TATA-box sequence of the human VIP/PHM-27 gene, there was found an 18-bp sequence that exhibited a high degree of

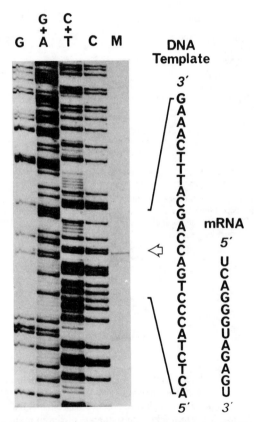

FIGURE 7. Determination of the cap site by mung bean nuclease mapping. The 830-bp *Sau*3AI-*Hpa*II fragment containing exon I and its 5' upstream region was labeled at the *Hpa*II 5' end. The labeled DNA fragment was hybridized to total RNA from NB-1 cells treated with TPA and Bt$_2$cAMP, digested with mung bean nuclease and run on a 6% polyacrylamide/8.3 M urea gel (lane M). In order to align the protected fragments with the genomic DNA sequence, a sequence ladder of the probe produced by chemical degradation[17] was run on the same gel (lanes G, G+A, C+T, and C).

homology with the consensus sequence of *E. coli* cAMP-inducible genes[28] and with the "cAMP-responsive element" of the rat phosphoenolpyruvate carboxykinase gene[29] and of the rat somatostatin gene[30] (TABLE 1). This 18-bp region may be related to the cAMP induction of the human VIP/PHM-27 gene. The 18-bp region may also be related to the induction by TPA, since Comb *et al.* have recently shown that the DNA sequences required for regulation by both cAMP and TPA mapped to the same 37-bp region located 107 to 71 bp 5' to the cap site of the human proenkephalin gene.[31] In fact, we have found through chloramphenicol acetyl transferase assay that a 50-bp region containing the 18-bp sequence is required for the induction by both cAMP and TPA of the human VIP/PHM-27 gene in the human neuroblastoma cells.[32]

TABLE 1. Nucleotide Sequence Homology in the 5' Flanking Region of Several cAMP-Inducible Genes[a]

Gene	Beginning Nucleotide	Sequence	Ending Nucleotide	Reference
VIP/PHM-27	−80	C T G T G A C G T C T T T C A G A G	−63	This paper
E. coli cAMP-inducible genes	−34--−86	* * * * * N N * N N N N * * N *	−33--−101	33–37
PEPCK	−91	* T * A C G * * * * * *	−80	29
Somatostatin	−48	* * * * * * * A G A G * * * *	−34	30

[a] Nucleotide identity with the 18-bp sequence found in the human VIP/PHM-27 gene is represented by asterisks. Negative numbers indicate nucleotide positions upstream from the cap site. *E. coli* cAMP-inducible genes include *lac*,[33] *gal*,[34] *araBAD*,[35] *malT*,[36] and *tna*;[37] PEPCK, the rat phosphoenol pyruvate carboxykinase gene; N, any nucleotide.

SUMMARY

We have previously shown that the VIP precursor contains a novel PHI-27-like peptide, PHM-27,[3] and that the synthesis of the prepro-VIP/PHM-27 mRNA is induced with cAMP and TPA in human neuroblastoma cells.[4-6] In this study, we have determined the complete nucleotide sequence of the human VIP/PHM-27 gene. The gene spans 8,837 bp and consists of seven exons and six introns. Exon I of 165 bp consists of the 5' untranslated region of the gene, exon II of 117 bp encodes the signal peptide of prepro-VIP/PHM-27, exon III of 123 bp encodes the amino-terminal region, exon IV of 105 bp encodes PHM-27, exon V of 132 bp encodes VIP, exon VI of 89 bp contains the termination codon of the prepro-VIP/PHM-27 mRNA, and exon VII of 724 bp consists of the 3' untranslated region of the gene. VIP and its structurally related peptide, PHM-27, were encoded in different exons V and IV, and the sequences around the splice junctions between these exons and their adjacent introns were highly conserved, suggesting that the VIP-encoding and PHM-27-encoding exons have been duplicated from an ancestral exon over a broad area containing its adjacent introns. We also determined the 1,929-bp sequence of the 5' flanking region of the human VIP/PHM-27 gene and found that four TATA-box sequences were present at 28 bp, 145 bp, 772 bp, and 900 bp upstream of the cap site. Primer extension, exon mapping, and mung bean nuclease mapping analyses revealed that only the TATA-box sequence 28 bp upstream of the cap site was the promoter that is inducible by cAMP and TPA in the human neuroblastoma cells. An 18-bp sequence 52 bp upstream from the TATA-box sequence was suggested to be a cAMP/phorbol esters-responsive element of the human VIP/PHM-27 gene.

REFERENCES

1. MUTT, V. & S. I. SAID. 1974. Eur. J. Biochem. **42:** 581-589.
2. SAID, S. I., ED. 1982. Vasoactive Intestinal Peptide, Advances in Peptide Hormone Research Series. Raven Press. New York.
3. ITOH, N., K. OBATA, N. YANAIHARA & H. OKAMOTO. 1983. Nature **304:** 547-549.
4. OBATA, K., N. ITOH, H. OKAMOTO, C. YANAIHARA, N. YANAIHARA & T. SUZUKI. 1981. FEBS Lett. **136:** 123-126.
5. HAYAKAWA, Y., K. OBATA, N. ITOH, N. YANAIHARA & H. OKAMOTO. 1984. J. Biol. Chem. **259:** 9207-9211.
6. OHSAWA, K., Y. HAYAKAWA, M. NISHIZAWA, T. YAMAGAMI, H.YAMAMOTO, N. YANAIHARA & H. OKAMOTO. 1985. Biochem. Biophys. Res. Commun. **132:** 885-891.
7. LAWN, R. M., E. F. FRITSCH, R. C. PARKER, G. BLAKE & T. MANIATIS. 1978. Cell **15:** 1157-1174.
8. BENTON, W. D. & R. W. DAVIS. 1977. Science **196:** 180-182.
9. WAHL, G. M., M. STERN & G. R. STARK. 1979. Proc. Natl. Acad. Sci. USA **76:** 3683-3687.
10. MESSING, J. 1983. Methods Enzymol. **101:** 20-78.
11. MIYAKE, S., T. SHIMO, T. KITAMURA, Y. NOJYO, T. NAKAMURA, S. IMASHUKU & T. ABE. 1973. Jiritsushinkei (The Autonomic Nervous System) **10:** 115-120. (In Japanese.)
12. CHIRGWIN, J. M., A. E. PRZYBYLA, R. J. MACDONALD & W. J. RUTTER. 1979. Biochemistry **18:** 5294-5299.
13. LEONALD, W. J., J. M. DEPPER, M. KANEHISA, M. KRÖNKE, N. J. PEFFER, P. B. SVETLIK, M. SULLIVAN & W. C. GREENE. 1985. Science **230:** 633-639.
14. MELTON, D. A., P. A. KRIEG, M. R. REBAGLIATI, T. MANIATIS, K. ZINN & M. R. GREEN. 1984. Nucleic Acids Res. **12:** 7035-7056.
15. GREEN, M. R. & R. G. ROEDER. 1980. Cell **22:** 231-242.
16. BREATHNACH, R. & P. CHAMBON. 1981. Ann. Rev. Biochem. **50:** 349-383.
17. MAXAM, A. M. & W. GILBERT. 1980. Methods Enzymol. **65:** 499-560.
18. HENTSCHEL, C., J-C. IRMINGER, P. BUCHER & M. L. BIRNSTIEL. 1980. Nature **285:** 147-151.
19. SOLLNER-WEBB, B. & R. H. REEDER. 1979. Cell **18:** 485-499.
20. BODNER, M., M. FRIDKIN & I. GOZES. 1985. Proc. Natl. Acad. Sci. USA **82:** 3548-3551.
21. TSUKADA, T., S. J. HOROVITCH, M. R. MONTMINY, G. MANDEL & R. H. GOODMAN. 1985. DNA **4:** 293-300.
22. LINDER, S., T. BARKHEM, A. NORBERG, H. PERSSON, M. SCHALLING, T. HÖKFELT & G. MAGNUSSON. 1987. Proc. Natl. Acad. Sci. USA **84:** 605-609.
23. BELL, G. I., R.SANCHEZ-PESCADOR, P. J. LAYBOURN & R. C. NAJARIAN. 1983. Nature **304:** 368-371.
24. JONAS, V., C. R. LIN, E. KAWASHIMA, D. SEMON, L. W. SWANSON, J-J. MERMOD, R. M. EVANS & M. G. ROSENFELD. 1985. Proc. Natl. Acad. Sci. USA **82:** 1994-1998.

25. YOUNG, R. A., O. HAGENBÜCHLE & U. SCHIBLER. 1981. Cell **23:** 451-458.
26. ROBERT, B., P. DAUBAS, M-A. AKIMENKO, A. COHEN, I. GARNER, J-L. GUENET & M. BUCKINGHAM. 1984. Cell **39:** 129-140.
27. FRUNZIO, R., L. CHIARIOTTI, A. L. BROWN, D. E. GRAHAM, M. M. RECHLER & C. B. BRUNI. 1986. J. Biol. Chem. **261:** 17138-17149.
28. CROMBRUGGHE, B., S. BUSBY & H. BUC. 1984. Science **224:** 831-838.
29. SHORT, J. M., A. WYNSHAW-BORIS, H. P. SHORT & R. W. HANSON. 1986. J. Biol. Chem. **261: 9721-9726.**
30. MONTMINY, M. R., K. A. SEVARINO, J. A. WAGNER, G. MANDEL & R. H. GOODMAN. 1986. Proc. Natl. Acad. Sci. USA **83:** 6682-6686.
31. COMB, M., N. C. BIRNBERG, A. SEASHOLTZ, E. HERBERT & H. M. GOODMAN. 1986. Nature **323:** 353-356.
32. OHSAWA, K., T. YAMAGAMI, M. NISHIZAWA, C. INOUE, E. GOTOH, H. YAMAMOTO & H. OKAMOTO. 1987. *In* Hormonal Regulation of Gene Expression. Gunma Symposia on Endocrinology. Vol. **24:** 169-181. Center for Academic Publications. Tokyo, Japan. VNU Science Press, BV. Utrecht, the Netherlands.
33. SCHMITZ, A. 1981. Nucleic Acids Res. **9:** 277-292.
34. SHANBLATT, S. H. & A. REVZIN. 1983. Proc Natl. Acad. Sci. USA **80:** 1594-1598.
35. OGDEN, S., D. HAGGERTY, C. M. STONER, D. KOLODRUBETZ & R. SCHLEIF. 1980. Proc. Natl. Acad. Sci. USA **77:** 3346-3350.
36. CHAPON, C. & A. KOLB. 1983. J. Bacteriol. **156:** 1135-1143.
37. DEELEY, M. C. & C. YANOFSKY. 1982. J. Bacteriol. **151:** 942-951.

Colocalization of VIP with Other Neuropeptides and Neurotransmitters in the Autonomic Nervous System[a]

M. COSTA,[b] J. B. FURNESS, I. L. GIBBINS, J. L.
MORRIS, J. C. BORNSTEIN, I. J. LLEWELLYN-SMITH,
AND R. MURPHY

Department of Physiology
Department of Anatomy and Histology and
Center for Neurosciences
Flinders University
Bedford Park, S.A., Australia

Since the first histochemical demonstration of VIP immunoreactivity in autonomic neurons,[1,2] numerous reports have appeared showing VIP-immunoreactive fibers in almost every organ of those species studied.[3] The widespread distribution of nerve fibers containing VIP immunoreactivity together with its potent biological actions on autonomic effectors had led to the proposal that VIP acts as a neurotransmitter in some autonomic nerves.[4,5] The use of immunoneutralization of endogenously released VIP in pharmacological studies has lent support to the role of VIP and related peptides as neurotransmitter.[6–10] The idea that VIP acts as a neurotransmitter fell on fertile ground because at the time of its discovery by Said and Mutt[11] it was known that substances other than acetylcholine and norepinephrine mediate autonomic neurotransmission in a variety of tissues.[12]

Over the last twelve years, in parallel with the discovery of VIP, numerous other peptides were found to be contained in autonomic neurons. Also, for some of them, evidence exists that they can act as neurotransmitters. The suggestion that neurons may utilize a cotransmitter in addition to the main neurotransmitter[13] led to research that compiled functional and morphological evidence confirming this possibility in the salivary glands. Lundberg[14] showed that both VIP and acetylcholine are contained in and released from the same postganglionic parasympathetic neurons. Thus the concept of cotransmission gave a new perspective to the increasing number of reports on the presence of peptides in autonomic neurons.[15]

[a] This work was supported by grants from the National Health and Medical Research Council of Australia, the National Heart Foundation of Australia, and the Flinders Medical Centre Research Foundation. The manuscript was written when Marcello Costa was a visiting scientist at the Institute for Advanced Biomedical Research, Oregon Health Sciences University, Portland, Oregon.

[b] Address for correspondence: M. Costa, Department of Physiology, Flinders University, Bedford Park 5042, S.A., Australia.

Our and other investigations on the coexistence of peptides in autonomic and visceral sensory neurons have shown that every neuron may, and indeed most of them do, contain several peptides.[16,17] These findings have led us to propose that neurons are chemically coded by a particular combination of peptide and nonpeptide transmitters and that the process of neurotransmission is likely to occur by a plurichemical process dependent upon the release and actions of several different transmitters.[18] In this context VIP-containing neurons are no exception, and in this article we will briefly describe some examples of coexistence of VIP with other transmitter substances and discuss some of the potential functional consequences. A full discussion of the role of each of the peptide and nonpeptide molecules is beyond the scope of this article, and because in most cases these molecules have biological actions and are likely to be released, we will regard all of them as potential transmitter substances. The evidence that this occurs in each case is still scanty and further investigation is necessary.

METHODS

Much of the evidence that VIP (and other peptides) coexists with other transmitters relies mainly on histochemical techniques for the simultaneous localization of the substances. The availability of antisera against peptides and against transmitter-specific enzymes raised in different species has allowed the use of double-labeling immunofluorescence for the simultaneous localization of two transmitters. The coexistence of any two such substances is directly deduced by the colocalization of two labels in the same neuron while the coexistence of three or more transmitters can only be deduced by a combination of experiments.[16,19] The details of double-labeling immunofluorescence techniques have been described in detail elsewhere.[16]

COEXISTENCE OF VIP WITH OTHER TRANSMITTERS

The observation of VIP immunoreactivity in nerve fiber and cell bodies in peripheral organs first raises the question whether the nerve fibers are viscerosensory or autonomic. Secondly, within the autonomic nervous system, they can be preganglionic, postganglionic sympathetic or parasympathetic, or enteric neurons. Only in a few cases the nature, origin, and connections of VIP neurons and the identity of their coexisting transmitters have been determined.

Blood Vessels

VIP immunoreactivity is present in nerve fibers around many blood vessels in different species.[3,20–23] Using the double-labeling immunofluorescence technique, Morris et al.[19] found that in the guinea pig uterine artery, nearly all perivascular axons with VIP immunoreactivity also contained neuropeptide Y (NPY) immunoreactivity. Since very few of the VIP immunoreactive axons contained dopamine β-hydroxylase (DBH) immunoreactivity, the authors deduced that the NPY-VIP axons are not noradrenergic. These axons also contain dynorphin (DYN) immunoreactivity. It is likely that this population of non-noradrenergic perivascular fibers is responsible for the neurogenic vasodilatation found in the guinea pig uterine artery.[24]

Autonomic Ganglia

VIP immunoreactive nerve terminals have been described in guinea pig prevertebral ganglia[25-27] and in human paravertebral ganglia.[28] In the guinea pig celiac ganglion, VIP coexists with cholecystokinin (CCK), DYN, enkephalin (ENK), and gastrin-releasing peptide (GRP) in neurons originating within the intestinal wall in the myenteric plexus.[16] This neuronal projection from the intestine to a prevertebral ganglion is likely to represent the afferent limb of the peripheral intestino-intestinal inhibitory reflex[29,30] and therefore these CCK/DYN/ENK/GRP/VIP neurons are likely also to contain acetylcholine.

In human sympathetic ganglia, VIP coexists with GRP in nerve terminals of preganglionic fiber and therefore these also contain acetylcholine.[17,28]

Enteric Nervous System

VIP is present in numerous different populations of enteric neurons with different projections and is colocalized with different combinations of transmitters. Most of the studies of coexistence have been performed in the guinea pig enteric nervous system.[16,31,32] Besides the CCK/DYN/ENK/GRP/VIP neurons that project to the celiac ganglion, there are at least two other populations of VIP-immunoreactive myenteric neurons and these project to the circular muscle. One is a short, anal projection of DYN/ENK/NPY/VIP neurons and the other is a longer anal projection of DYN/GRP/VIP neurons. Since there is only one other class of nerve fibers in the circular muscle and this is coded by substance P, which has been shown to mediate excitatory transmission to the muscle,[33,34] it is likely that both these populations of VIP neurons represent the enteric inhibitory motor neurons responsible for the relaxation of intestinal muscle. VIP is a good candidate for mediating transmission from such enteric inhibitory motor neurons.[35] However, on the basis of the action of apamin, two types of relaxation of intestinal muscle mediated by the enteric inhibitory motor neuron can be distinguished in the guinea pig gastrointestinal tract.[36] Only the apamin-insensitive component of the inhibitory transmission could be mediated by VIP or a related peptide. This implies that if VIP participates in the inhibitory transmission, other substances mediating the apamin-sensitive component are likely to be contained and released from these neurons.

In the submucous plexus of the guinea pig's small intestine, a significant proportion (45%) of the nerve cell bodies contain VIP. These neurons project to the mucosa and also contain DYN and galanin (GAL). These neurons are likely to mediate the powerful noncholinergic neuronal secretion of water and electrolytes. This conclusion is based on the powerful action of VIP and on the histochemical observation that the remaining 55% of submucous neurons contain the immunoreactivity for the acetylcholine-synthesizing enzyme choline-acetyltransferase (CHAT).[32,37] Some of these DYN/GAL/VIP neurons also supply small submucosal and mucosal arterioles and are likely to mediate the vasodilatation from intrinsic intestinal neurons.[37] Although no systematic studies of the coexistence of VIP with other substances have been done in enteric neurons of other species, Ekblat et al.[38] reported that in the rat VIP coexists with its related peptide PHI and with NPY.

PATTERNS OF COEXISTENCE OF TRANSMITTERS

The finding that VIP is often found with a multiplicity of other transmitters raises the question as to whether there is any specific and predictable association of transmitters in the same neurons. Following the discovery that VIP and acetylcholine coexist in parasympathetic neurons to the salivary glands,[14] the expectation that VIP and acetylcholine would be often associated could not be confirmed. Although VIP is present in some preganglionic, presumably cholinergic, fibers in human sympathetic ganglia[17,28] and in the enteric projections to prevertebral ganglia (see above), it is also found in noncholinergic neurons such as the enteric inhibitory motor neurons and in noncholinergic secretomotor neurons in the intestine. Furthermore VIP is present in vasodilatory nerve fibers, in some cases with a vasoconstrictor peptide NPY.[19] There is nevertheless a correlation between the combination of transmitters in a neuron and its location and connectivity. This chemical coding of autonomic neurons is only beginning to be unraveled. For example, the VIP vasodilatory fibers to pelvic viscera also contains DYN and NPY, but no such peptides are present in the VIP vasodilatory fibers to cranial blood vessels.[17] In sympathetic ganglia the VIP-containing terminals have specific connections with subgroups of postganglionic neurons. In human sympathetic ganglia the GRP/VIP axons terminate only around nonnoradrenergic neurons. Conversely preganglionic axons containing NPY are associated only with postganglionic noradrenergic neurons.[28] In the guinea pig celiac ganglion, there are three main subgroups of postganglionic noradrenergic neurons; that is, those with somatostatin (SOM) that project to submucous ganglia in the intestine, those with NPY that project to intestinal blood vessels, and those with no other peptides yet detected that project to myenteric ganglia.[16,25,39] The enteric neurons coded by CCK/DYN/ENK/GRP/VIP that project from the intestine to this ganglion end specifically around the two classes of sympathetic neurons that supply the myenteric and submucous ganglia but not those supplying blood vessels.[16,39] In the intestine the enteric inhibitory motor neurons that contain VIP are coded differently from the VIP secretomotor neurons (see above).

There is also a correlation between the chemical coding of a neuron and its functional inputs. For example, all the VIP-containing myenteric neurons have the morphology of Dogiel type I neuron, and all receive cholinergic synaptic inputs and thus are classified as S cells.[40] Of the two main classes of secretomotor submucous neurons, only the noncholinergic ones that are coded by DYN/GAL/VIP receive inhibitory synaptic inputs.[41,42]

CONCLUSIONS

This brief summary shows that VIP is present in a variety of functionally different autonomic neurons. This implies that no single function can be attributed to this potent peptide. Since VIP, like all the other transmitters, is most commonly found in combination with other transmitters in the same neuron, it is likely that the process of neurotransmission involves a multiplicity of chemicals. VIP is found in different combinations of transmitters, and there appear to be no specific association between them. However, a remarkable correlation exists between any given combination of transmitters and the location of a population of autonomic neurons, their projections, connections, and functions. Further, systematic work to establish the coding of all populations of autonomic neurons in different organs and species is required before the significance of the chemical coding can be understood.

ACKNOWLEDGMENTS

We would like to thank Gloria Ellis for the typing of this manuscript.

REFERENCES

1. BRYANT, M. G., J. M. POLAK, I. MODLIN, S. R. BLOOM, R. H. ALBUQUERQUE & A. G. E. PEARSE. 1976. Possible dual role for vasoactive intestinal peptide as gastrointestinal hormone and neurotransmitter substance. Lancet **1:** 991-993.
2. LARSSON, L. I., J. FAHRENKRUG, O. SCHAFFALITZKY DE MUKADELL, F. SUNDLER, R. HAKANSON & J. F. REHFELD. 1976. Localization of vasoactive intestinal polypeptide (VIP) to central and peripheral neurons. Proc. Natl. Acad. Sci. USA **73:** 3197-3200.
3. HAKANSON, R., F. SUNDLER & R. UDDMAN. 1982. Distribution and topography of peripheral VIP nerve fibers: Functional implications. *In* Vasoactive Intestinal Peptide. S. I. Said, Ed.: 121-144. Raven Press. New York.
4. FAHRENKRUG, J. 1982. VIP as a neurotransmitter in the peripheral nervous system. *In* Vasoactive Intestinal Peptide. S. I. Said, Ed.: 361-372. Raven Press. New York.
5. FURNESS, J. B. & M. COSTA. 1982. Enteric inhibitory nerves and VIP. *In* Vasoactive Intestinal Peptide. S. I. Said, Ed.: 391-406. Raven Press. New York.
6. GOYAL, R. K., S. RATTAN & S. I. SAID. 1980. Vasoactive intestinal polypeptide as a possible neurotransmitter of non-cholinergic, nonadrenergic neurons. Nature **288:** 378-380.
7. ANGEL, F., V. L. K. GO, P. F. SCHMALZ & J. H. SZURSZEWSKI. 1983. Vasoactive intestinal polypeptide: A putative transmitter in the canine gastric muscular is muscosa. J. Physiol. (London) **341:** 641-654.
8. BIANCANI, P., J. H. WALSH & J. BEHAR. 1984. Vasoactive intestinal polypeptide, a neurotransmitter for lower esophageal sphincter relaxation. J. Clin. Invest. **73:** 963-967.
9. GRIDER, J. R., M. B. CABLE, K. N. BITAR, S. I. SAID & G. M. MAKHLOUF. 1985. Vasoactive intestinal peptide, relaxant neurotransmitter in taenia coli of the guinea-pig. Gastroenterology **89:** 36-42.
10. GRIDER, J. R., M. B. CABLE, S. I. SAID & G. M. MAKHLOUF. 1985. Vasoactive intestinal peptide as a neural mediator of gastric relaxation. Am. J. Physiol. **248:** G73-G78.
11. SAID, S. I. & V. MUTT. 1970. Potent peripheral and splanchnic vasodilator peptide from normal gut. Nature **225:** 863-864.
12. CAMPBELL, G. 1970. Autonomic nervous supply to effector tissues. *In* Smooth Muscle. E. Bulbring, A. Brading, A. Jones & T. Tomita, Eds.: 451-495. Edward Arnold. London, England.
13. BURNSTOCK, G. 1980. Do some nerve cells release more than one transmitter? *In* Commentaries in the Neurosciences. A. D. Smith, R. Llinas & P. G. Kostyuk, Eds.: 151-160. Pergamon Press. Oxford, England.

14. LUNDBERG, J. M. 1981. Evidence for coexistence of vasoactive intestinal polypeptide (VIP) and acetylcholine in neurons of cat exocrine glands. Acta. Physiol. Scand. Suppl. **496:** 1-57.
15. LUNDBERG, J. M. & T. HÖKFELT. 1983. Co-existence of peptides and classical neurotransmitters. Trends Neurosci. **6:** 325-383.
16. COSTA, M., J. B. FURNESS & T. L. GIBBINS. 1986. Chemical coding of enteric neurons. *In* Progress in Brain Research. T. Hökfelt, K. Fuxe & B. Pernow, Eds. **68:** 217-239. Elsevier Science Publishers. Amsterdam, the Netherlands.
17. GIBBINS, T. L., J. L. MORRIS, J. B. FURNESS & M. COSTA. 1987. Chemical coding of autonomic neurons. Exp. Brain Res. Ser. **16:** 23-27.
18. FURNESS, J. B., M. COSTA, J. L. MORRIS & I. L. GIBBINS. 1987. Novel neurotransmitters and the chemical coding of neurons. Adv. Physiol. Res.: 143-165.
19. MORRIS, J. L., I. L. GIBBINS, J. B. FURNESS, M. COSTA & R. MURPHY. 1985. Co-localization of NPY, VIP and dynorphin in non-noradrenergic axons of the guinea-pig uterine artery. Neurosci. Lett. **67:** 31-37.
20. UDDMAN, R., J. ALUMETS, L. EDVINSSON, R. HAKANSON & R. SUNDLER. 1981. VIP fibres around peripheral blood vessels. Acta. Physiol. Scand. **112:** 65-70.
21. DELLA, N. G., R. E. PAPKA, J. B. FURNESS & M. COSTA. 1983. Vasoactive intestinal peptide-like immunoreactivity in nerves associated with the cardiovascular system of guinea-pigs. Neuroscience **9:** 605-619.
22. GIBBINS, I. L., J. E. BRAYDEN & J. A. BEVAN. 1984. Perivascular nerves with immunoreactivity to vasoactive intestinal polypeptide in cephalic arteries of the cat: Distribution, possible origins and functional implications: Neuroscience **13:** 1327-1346.
23. GIBBINS, I. L., J. L. MORRIS, J. B. FURNESS & M. COSTA. 1988. Innervation of systemic blood vessels. *In* Non-adrenergic Innervation of Blood Vessels. G. Burnstock & S. Griffith, Eds. C.R.C. Press. Boca Raton, FL. In press.
24. BELL, C. 1968. Dual vasoconstrictor and vasodilator innervation of the uterine arterial supply in the guinea-pig. Circ. Res. **23:** 279-289.
25. LUNDBERG, J. M., T. HOKFELT, A. ANGGARD, L. TERENIUS, R. ELDE, K. MARKEY, M. GOLDSTEIN & J. KIMMEL. 1982. Organizational principles in the peripheral sympathetic nervous system: Subdivision by coexisting peptides (somatostatin-, ovian pancreatic polypeptide-, and vasoactive intestinal polypeptide-like immunoreactive material. Proc. Natl. Acad. Sci. USA **79:** 1303-1307.
26. COSTA, M. & J. B. FURNESS. 1983. The origin, pathways and terminations of neurons with VIP-like immunoreactivity in the guinea-pig small intestine. Neuroscience **8:** 665-676.
27. DALSGAARD, C.-J., T. HOKFELT, M. SCHULTZBERG, J. M. LUNDBERG, L. TERENIUS, G. J. DOCKREY & M. GOLDSTEIN. 1983. Origin of peptide-containing fibers in the inferior mesenteric ganglion of the guinea-pig: Immunohistochemical studies with antisera to substance P, enkephalin, vasoactive intestinal polypeptide, cholecystokinin and bombesin. Neuroscience **9:** 191-211.
28. GIBBINS, I. L., D. WATTCHOW, J. WALSH, P. DUPONT, M. COSTA & J. B. FURNESS. 1986. Specific connections between immunohistochemically identified clones of preganglionic and postganglionic neurons in human lumbar sympathetic chain ganglia. Neurosci. Lett. Suppl. **23:** S49.
29. FURNESS, J. B. & M. COSTA. 1974. The adrenergic innervation of the gastrointestinal tract. Ergeb. Physiol. **69:** 1-51.
30. SZURSZEWSKI, J. H. 1976. Towards a new view of prevertebral ganglion. *In* Nerves and the Gut. F. P. Brooks & P. W. Evers, Eds.: 244-260. C. B. Black. Thorofare, NJ.
31. COSTA, M., J. B. FURNESS & I. J. LLEWELLYN-SMITH. 1986. Histochemistry of the enteric nervous system. *In* Physiology of the Gastrointestinal Tract, 2nd Edition. L. R. Jonnson, Ed. Vol. **1:** 1-41. Raven Press. New York.
32. FURNESS, J. B. & M. COSTA. 1986. The enteric nervous system. Churchill Livingstone. Edinburgh, U.K.
33. BARTHO, L. & P. HOLZER. 1985. Search for a physiological role of substance P in gastrointestinal motility. Neuroscience **16:** 1-32.
34. COSTA, M., J. B. FURNESS, C. O. PULLIN & J. BORNSTEIN. 1985. Substance P enteric neuron mediate non-cholinergic transmission to the circular muscle of the guinea-pig intestine. Naunyn-Schmied. Arch. Pharmacol. **328:** 446-453.

35. MARKHLOUF, G. M. 1985. Enteric neuropeptides: Role in neuromuscular activity of the gut. Trends Pharmacol. Sci. **6:** 214-218.
36. COSTA, M., J. B. FURNESS & C. M. S. HUMPHREYS. 1986. Apamin distinguishes two types of relaxation mediated by enteric nerves in the guinea-pig gastrointestinal tract. Naunyn-Schmied. Arch. Pharmacol. **332:** 79-88.
37. FURNESS, J. B. & M. COSTA. 1988. Identification of transmitters of functionally defined enteric neurons. *In* Handbook of Physiology. J. Wood, Ed. American Physiological Society. In press.
38. EKBLAT, E., R. HAKANSON & F. SUNDLER. 1984. VIP and PHI coexist with an NPY-like peptide in intramural neurones of the small intestine. Regul. Peptides **10:** 47-55.
39. MACRAE, I. M., J. B. FURNESS & M. COSTA. 1986. Distribution of subgroups of noradrenaline neurons in the coeliac ganglion of the guinea-pig. Cell Tissue Res. **244:** 173-180.
40. KATAYAMA, Y., G. M. LEES & G. T. PEARSON. 1985. Electrophysiological and morphology of vasoactive intestinal peptide immunoreactive neurones in the guinea-pig ileum. J. Physiol. (London) **378:** 1-11.
41. NORTH, R. A. & A. SURPRENANT. 1985. Inhibitory synaptic potentials resulting from α_2-adrenoceptor activation in guinea-pig submucuous plexus neurones. J. Physiol. (London) **358:** 17-33.
42. BORNSTEIN, J. C., M. COSTA & J. B. FURNESS. 1986. Synaptic inputs to immunohistochemically identified neurones in the submucous plexus of the guinea-pig small intestine. J. Physiol. (London) **381:** 465-488.

Vasoactive Intestinal Peptide as a Mediator of Intercellular Communication in the Cerebral Cortex

Release, Receptors, Actions, and Interactions with Norepinephrine[a]

PIERRE J. MAGISTRETTI,[b,c] MONIKA M. DIETL,[d]
PATRICK R. HOF,[b] JEAN-LUC MARTIN,[b] JOSÉ M.
PALACIOS,[d] NICOLAS SCHAAD,[b] AND MICHEL
SCHORDERET[b,e]

[b]Département de Pharmacologie
Centre Médical Universitaire
Geneva, Switzerland

[d]Preclinical Research
Sandoz, Ltd.
Basle, Switzerland

[e]Ecole de Pharmacie
Lausanne, Switzerland

INTRODUCTION

Investigations in the last decade have delineated an indisputable role for vasoactive intestinal peptide (VIP) in central neurotransmission. In particular, the commonly agreed criteria for establishing a neurotransmitter function for a substance identified

[a]This research is supported by Fonds National Suisse de la Recherche Scientifique Grants N° 3.357-0.86 and 3.969-0.84. PJM is the recipient of a Research Career Development Award (START) from Fonds National Suisse de la Recherche Scientifique. PRH is supported by the Fondation Centre de Recherches Médicales Carlos et Elsie de Reuter. NS is supported by Fellowships from the Fondation Suisse de Recherche sur l'Alcool and the Fondation Pierre Mercier.

[c]Address for correspondence: Pierre J. Magistretti, M.D., Ph.D., Department of Pharmacology, Centre Medical Universitaire, 1, rue Michel Servet, 1211 - Geneva 4, Switzerland.

in the nervous system have been fulfilled.[1,2] Thus, discrete populations of VIP-immunoreactive neurons have been described throughout the entire neuraxis,[3,4] the Ca^{2+}-dependent release of immunoreactive VIP has been demonstrated,[5,6] the kinetic properties of specific VIP recognition sites have been characterized,[7-9] and various cellular actions of VIP have been observed. These actions include alterations of neuronal excitability [10,11] and stimulation of various enzymatic activities, including activation of adenylate cyclase,[12-14] of choline acetyltransferase,[15] and of the cascade of reactions leading to the hydrolysis of glycogen.[16,17] Our interest has been focused in recent years on the VIP-containing neuronal system in the cerebral cortex (see Magistretti[1,18] for review), a CNS region where VIP is highly concentrated.

In the cerebral cortex VIP is contained in a homogeneous population of bipolar, radially oriented (i.e., oriented in a plane perpendicular to the pial surface) neurons, with minimal branching in the horizontal plane except in layers I and IV-V where the arborization spans for 60-100 μm[19,20] (see FIG. 1). These morphological characteristics imply that VIP released from VIP-containing neurons will act locally within radially restricted cortical volumes.[1,18] A quantitative analysis has revealed that the density of VIP-containing neurons is such that the cortical columns defined by the arborization pattern of each individual VIP cell partially overlap.[19] The functional implication of this arrangement is that, upon activation, a group of VIP-containing neurons has the capacity to "cover" a given region of the cerebral cortex. VIP neurons also contain acetylcholine, as revealed by indirect immunohistochemistry for choline acetyltransferase.[21] Recently, a functional interaction between VIP and acetylcholine has been demonstrated in the cerebral cortex whereby the stimulation of phosphoinositide turnover elicited by acetylcholine via muscarinic receptors is potentiated by VIP.[22] To summarize, it can be said that VIP neurons are capable of exerting input-output functions locally, within partially overlapping cortical columns.[1,18,23]

CELLULAR ACTIONS OF VIP IN THE CEREBRAL CORTEX

Role of Prostanoids in the Synergism between VIP and Norepinephrine

One of the actions of VIP in the CNS consists of the stimulation of cyclic-AMP formation.[12-14] In mouse cerebral cortex, a CNS region where norepinephrine (NE) stimulates cyclic-AMP formation predominantly via adrenergic receptors of the beta type,[24,25] Magistretti and Schorderet have described a synergistic interaction between VIP and NE in stimulating cyclic-AMP formation.[14] A pharmacological analysis of this synergism has revealed that NE, by acting at adrenergic receptors of the α_1-type, potentiates the increases in cyclic-AMP elicited by VIP.[26] The noradrenergic innervation of the neocortex is provided by fibers originating in the nucleus locus ceruleus in the brainstem.[27] Within the neocortex noradrenergic axons adopt a predominantly tangential trajectory (i.e., in a plane parallel to the pial surface) proceeding from the frontal to the occipital poles.[28,29] Thus, in contrast to the locally acting intracortical VIP-containing system, noradrenergic fibers are endowed with the capacity to exert their actions globally throughout the neocortex, simultaneously influencing functionally distinct regions. In view of the morphological characteristics of the VIP and NA-containing cortical neuronal systems, the synergistic interaction between VIP and NA, mediated by α_1-adrenergic receptors, should generate marked increases in cyclic-AMP

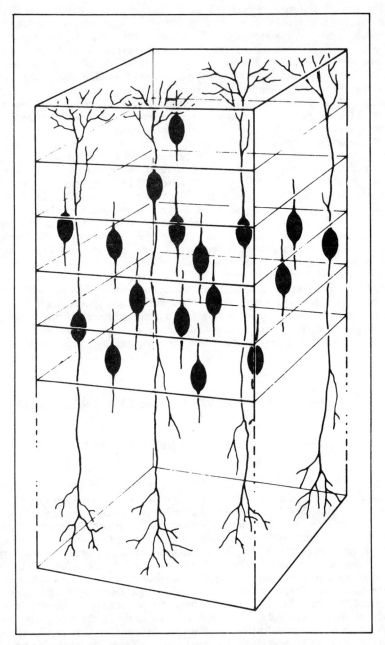

FIGURE 1. Schematic representation of VIP-immunoreactive neurons in rodent cerebral cortex. Note the bipolar and radial nature of these neurons that arborize only minimally in the superficial and deep cortical layers.

levels within discrete cortical volumes ("hot spots").[14] The spatial coordinates of such "hot spots" would be delineated by the intersection of the tangentially organized noradrenergic fibers and a group of activated, radially oriented VIP-containing neurons[14,26] (see FIG. 2).

Recently, the molecular mechanisms underlying the synergistic interaction between

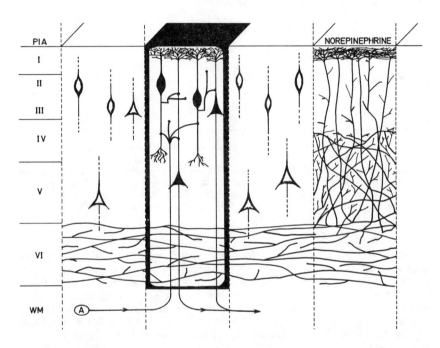

FIGURE 2. Diagrammatic representation of a "cortical hot spot" resulting from the concomitant activation of noradrenergic cortical afferents and a group of VIP-containing neurons. Bottom (layer VI), tangentially organized noradrenergic fibers. Right, detail of the arborization pattern of noradrenergic fibers within the cortex.[28,29] Ovoid-shaped cells, VIP-intracortical neurons; triangular-shaped cells, pyramidal neurons. Solid symbols refer to activated neurons. Far left, cortical layers. WM, white matter. The concomitant activation of noradrenergic fibers and of a group of VIP-containing intracortical neurons (by specific thalamic or cortico-cortical inputs, A, bottom left) would determine a drastic increase in cyclic-AMP levels within a discrete volume of cortex (delineated in this drawing by solid, thick lines). For graphic clarity, only the VIP-containing and the pyramidal cells have been represented here. In particular, the principal target cells of the thalamocortical afferents, that is, the small stellate cells in layer IV, have been omitted. However, any cell with the capacity of dendritic reception in layer IV may receive thalamic inputs[50] (taken from Magistretti and Schorderet[26]).

VIP and NE have been examined. Thus, we have observed that the α_1-adrenergic potentiation by NE of the increases in cyclic-AMP elicited by VIP was antagonized by indomethacin, a nonsteroidal antiinflammatory drug (TABLE 1). The degree of inhibition of the synergism by indomethacin was comparable to that observed in the presence of the selective α_1-adrenergic antagonist prazosin (TABLE 1). Indomethacin

TABLE 1. Effect of Indomethacin and Prazosin on the Synergism between VIP and NE in Increasing Cyclic-AMP Levels[a]

Agent Added	Concentration (μM)	cyclic-AMP (% of VIP 1 μM alone)
VIP	1	100 ± 7
VIP plus NE	1 10	282 ± 13
VIP plus NE plus Indomethacin	1 10 100	154 ± 6[b]
VIP plus NE plus Prazosin	1 10 10	146 ± 3[b,c]

[a] Results represent the mean $\pm$ SEM of four to seven separate determinations.
[b] Significantly different from cyclic-AMP levels in the presence of VIP and NE ($p < 0.005$).
[c] Not significantly different from cyclic-AMP levels in the presence of VIP and NE plus indomethacin. Basal cyclic-AMP levels were 18.2 ± 3.7 (pmol/mg prot), and were not statistically different in the presence of indomethacin 100 μM. Cyclic-AMP levels $\pm$ SEM observed in the presence of 1 μM VIP were 144.2 ± 9.4 (pmol/mg prot) and were not influenced by indomethacin μM 100 (data not shown).

is a rather selective inhibitor of cyclooxygenase, the enzyme regulating the synthesis of prostaglandins from arachidonic acid.[30] The inhibition of the synergism by indomethacin indicated, therefore, that a metabolite of arachidonic acid could be formed following α_1-adrenergic stimulation and mediate the potentiating effect of NE on cyclic-AMP increases elicited by VIP. We have tested various prostanoids for their potential ability to mimic the effects of NE, and we have observed that prostaglandins $F_{2\alpha}$ and E_2 selectively potentiate the stimulatory action of VIP on cyclic-AMP formation (TABLE 2).

This set of observations on the interaction between VIP and NE suggest that VIP- and NE-containing neuronal systems in the neocortex may converge, at least in part, on the same target cells, where the activation by NE of α_1-adrenergic receptors triggers the formation of arachidonic acid metabolites, possibly $PGF_{2\alpha}$ and PGE_2, which in turn potentiate the effect of VIP in stimulating cyclic-AMP formation. However, since prostanoids can be released in the extracellular fluid, it is conceivable that they are formed, following α_1-adrenergic receptor activation by NE, in a given cell type from where they would be released and potentiate the effect of VIP on another cell type. In fact, the molecular mechanism(s) through which prostanoids facilitate the formation of cyclic-AMP triggered by VIP still remain to be elucidated.

Differential Effect of Ouabain on the Stimulation of cyclic-AMP Formation and of Glycogenolysis Elicited by VIP

The cardiac glycoside ouabain, an inhibitor of the Na^+/K^+-ATPase,[31] has been previously shown to stimulate the formation of cyclic-AMP in rodent cerebral cortical slices and to potentiate the increases in the cyclic nucleotide elicited by NE and adenosine.[25,32,33] We have therefore examined whether a similar interaction was operative between VIP and ouabain. As shown in FIGURE 3A, ouabain potentiates the effect of VIP on cyclic-AMP formation. Interestingly, this effect of ouabain is observed at concentrations of the cardiac glycoside affecting only minimally basal cyclic-AMP levels.

VIP has been previously shown to promote the hydrolysis of glycogen newly synthesized by mouse cerebral cortical slices.[16,17] This action, when viewed in relation to the morphological characteristics of VIP-containing intracortical neurons (see FIG. 1), indicates that these neurons are in a position to regulate the availability of energy substrates locally, within cortical columnar ensembles.[16,17] One of the likely intracellular messengers that can trigger the cascade of enzymatic events leading to the hydrolysis of glycogen is cyclic-AMP.[34] In view of the synergistic interaction between VIP and ouabain in stimulating cyclic-AMP formation (FIG. 3A), we have examined the effect of the cardiac glycoside on the hydrolysis of glycogen promoted by VIP. As shown in FIGURE 3B, in contrast to its effect on cyclic-AMP levels, ouabain antagonized the glycogenolytic effect of VIP. This inhibition raises several points for discussion. A first possibility would be that ouabain could antagonize the stimulatory effect of VIP on cyclic-AMP formation and hence prevent the cyclic-AMP-activated glycogenolysis. However, the interaction observed between ouabain and VIP on cyclic-AMP levels is of a synergistic nature, rather than of an inhibitory one (FIG. 3A). This first hypothesis appears, therefore, unlikely.

A second possibility is that ouabain, by inhibiting the activity of the Na^+/K^+-ATPase and hence by modifying ionic gradients across the cell membrane, inhibits the activation of cyclic-AMP-dependent enzymes distal to cyclic-AMP formation, thus preventing the expression of the glycogenolytic action of VIP. This mechanism is supported by the observation indicating that ouabain inhibits hormone-stimulated glycogenolysis in adipocytes.[34] Furthermore, in the presence of ouabain or in K^+-free media, glycogen synthesis is stimulated in adipocytes[34] and in skeletal muscle.[35] The observation that ouabain antagonizes the glycogenolytic action of adenosine and NE[36] (TABLE 3), further supports the notion of a general inhibitory effect of the cardiac glycoside on the enzymatic process that leads to the breakdown of glycogen.

TABLE 2. Effect of $PGF_{2\alpha}$ and PGE_2 on Cyclic-AMP Increase Elicited by 1 μM VIP[a]

Agent Added	% Increase Elicited by I μM VIP[b]	(n)
VIP (1 μM)	100.0 ± 5.5	(18)
VIP (1 μM) + (PGF$_{2\alpha}$ (0.1 μM)	$173.0^c \pm 6.4$	(10)
VIP (1 μM) + PGE$_2$ (100 μM)	$154.5^c \pm 8.7$	(4)

[a] Results are the mean $\pm$ SEM of the number of determinations shown in parentheses. Absolute cyclic-AMP level observed in the presence of 1 μM VIP were 142.9 $\pm$ 13 (pmoles/mg prot).

[b] Basal cyclic-AMP levels $\pm$ SEM were 10.9 $\pm$ 1.1 pmoles/mg prot. In the presence of PGF$_{2\alpha}$ 1.0 μM and PGE$_2$ 100 μM, the levels were 15.7 $\pm$ 0.6 and 9.2 $\pm$ 1.2 pmoles/mg prot, respectively.

[c] $p < 0.001$.

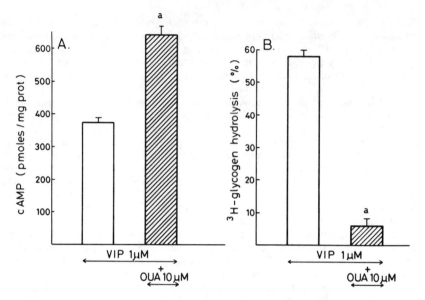

FIGURE 3. Differential effect of 10 μM ouabain on the increases in cyclic-AMP (**A**) and on the hydrolysis of glycogen (**B**) elicited by 1 μM VIP in mouse cerebral cortical slices. Results are the mean ± SEM of six different determinations. Basal cyclic-AMP levels were 14.6 ± 1.4 pmoles/mg protein. In the presence of 10 μM ouabain, cyclic-AMP levels were 38.4 ± 5.3 pmoles/mg prot. Basal [^{3}H]glycogen levels ± SEM (cpm/mg prot) were: 44,909 ± 2234.
  ^{a} Significantly different from VIP alone, $p < 0.001$.

It is also conceivable that VIP could activate a ouabain-sensitive, energy-consuming cellular process such as a Na^+/K^+-ATPase; this would in turn stimulate the mobilization of glycosyl units from glycogen, by causing a decrease in the energy charge of the cell.[37] However, this view seems unlikely, since no evidence exists for a direct activation of the Na^+/K^+-ATPase by VIP.

In summary this set of observations would indicate that one of the actions of ouabain in the CNS may be to impair neurotransmitter-mediated mobilization of energy stores.

RELEASE OF VIP

A sensitive radioimmunoassay (RIA) for the detection of small quantities of VIP (lower limit of detection 3 pg/tube, i.e. 1 fmol/ml) has been used to examine the regulation of VIP release from mouse cerebral cortical slices. For such a RIA a highly purified and characterized molecular form of [^{125}I]VIP, monoiodinated on Tyr[10] and oxidized to Met-sulfoxide on Met[17] was used.[38] This [mono[^{125}I]iodo-Tyr[10], MetO[17]]-VIP displays the following characteristics. (1) It constitutes quantitatively the major product of the iodination procedure (62.5%); (2) it is well resolved from other labeled and unlabeled products; (3) it is stable (two months at $-20°C$); (4) it possesses a high specific activity (2050 Ci/mmol); (5) it maintains the biological activity of native VIP; and (6) it binds to antibody and membrane recognition sites in a specific, saturable, and reversible manner. Two types of experimental paradigms have been used to assess VIP release: static and superfusion conditions. For the release under static conditions, mouse cerebral cortical slices (250 $\times$ 250 μm $\times$ ~ 1 mm, i.e., cortical thickness, 1-2 mg protein) are incubated for two minutes at 37°C in 450 μl of previously oxygenated Krebs-Ringer bicarbonate buffer (KRG) pH 7.4 containing (mM):NaCl, 120; KCl, 3; CaCl$_2$, 2.6; MgSO$_4$, 0.67; KH$_2$PO$_4$, 1.2; NaHCO$_3$, 27.5; and glucose, 3. Drugs are added as 50 μl. At the end of incubation, tubes are centrifuged and VIP released is assayed by RIA in the supernatant. VIP tissue content is assayed in the pellet after extraction with 1 M CH$_3$COOH. The effect of preincubation (P) time on basal and K$^+$-evoked VIP release has been examined. As shown in FIGURE 4A, basal and K$^+$-evoked release of VIP decrease as a function of P time up to 30 minutes. This decrease is not due to a decrease in VIP tissue content, which is remarkably stable up to 90 minutes of P time. After 90 minutes of preincubation, VIP is released, in a Ca^{2+}-dependent manner, by relatively small increases in extra-cellular K$^+$ concentration (range 12 to 25 mM K$^+$). At 25 mM K$^+$, VIP release increases 6.5 times over basal level (FIG. 4B). For the release under superfusion conditions mouse cerebral cortical slices (250 μm, 1.5 mg prot.) are distributed into four individual chambers and superfused with KRG buffer containing 30 μg/ml of bacitracin and 0.05% of BSA at a rate of 400 μl/min. The slices are equilibrated for one hour before the stimulation. Aliquots of 400 μl/min are collected, lyophilized and VIP release is measured by RIA. Under these conditions basal VIP release is 4.49 $\pm$ 0.31 pg/mg prot ($n = 9$) and is increased by 334.96% in the presence of 25 mM K$^+$ for two minutes. This K$^+$-evoked release is markedly decreased in the absence of Ca^{2+} in the medium.

TABLE 3. Inhibitory Effect of Ouabain on the Glycogenolytic Action of Adenosine and NE[a]

Agent(s) Added	Concentration (μM)	[³H]Glycogen Hydrolysis (%)
None	—	3.9 $\pm$ 1.3
Ouabain	10	5.7 $\pm$ 1.5[b]
Adenosine	100	46.2 $\pm$ 2.2
Adenosine + Ouabain	100 10	21 $\pm$ 2.5[c]
NE	1	50.6 $\pm$ 2
NE + Ouabain	1 10	9 $\pm$ 2.7[d]

[a] Results are the mean $\pm$ SEM of 12-24 determinations from four separate experiments and are expressed as percentages of basal [³H]glycogen hydrolyzed. Basal [³H]glycogen levels (cpm/mg prot): 44,427 $\pm$ 1192.
[b] Not significantly different from [³H]glycogen hydrolysis in the absence of added agents ($p > 0.05$).
[c] Significantly different from 100 μM adenosine alone ($p < 0.05$).
[d] Significantly different from 1 μM NE alone ($p < 0.05$).

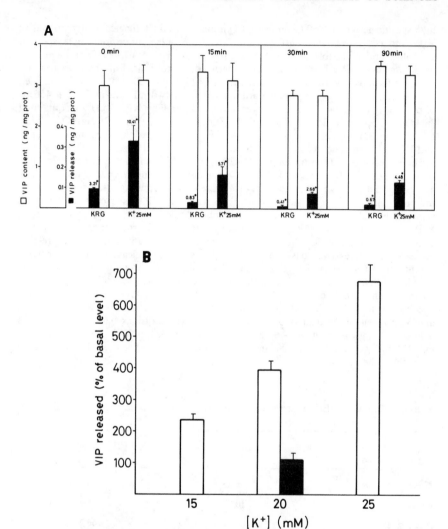

FIGURE 4. (A) Basal and K^+-stimulated release of VIP under static conditions, at various times after preparation of the slices (i.e., preincubation time in oxygenated KRG). Solid bars represent VIP release (ng/mg prot) under basal or stimulated conditions. Open bars represent VIP content (ng/mg prot). Numbers marked with an asterisk indicate the percentage of VIP tissue content that is released. Results are the mean ± SEM of triplicate determinations (except for 90-minute incubation time where $n = 8$).

(B) Effect of increasing concentrations of K^+ on basal VIP release under static conditions. The results are expressed in percent of basal VIP release. These results are the mean ± SEM of eight determinations in two separate experiments. The concentration of extracellular K^+ under basal conditions is 3 mM. The percentage of VIP release under basal conditions corresponds to 0.555% ± 0.027 ($n = 142$) of the VIP content. Open circle corresponds to the effect of 20 mM K^+ on VIP release in the absence of Ca^{2+}.

Open triangle corresponds to the effect of 25 mM K^+ on VIP release in a medium where the concentration of extracellular Cl^- has been adjusted in relation to KCl concentration.

AUTORADIOGRAPHIC MAPPING OF VIP RECEPTORS

Mammalian Brain

To further analyze the distribution of VIP binding sites in the nervous system and in peripheral tissues we have used *in vitro* receptor autoradiographic techniques. In these experiments we have examined tissues from lower vertebrates, laboratory rodents and other higher species, including man.

The distribution of VIP binding sites in the rat brain was examined by *in vitro* autoradiography on slide-mounted sections. A fully characterized monoiodinated form of VIP (M-^{125}I-VIP) was used for this study.[38,39] In initial kinetic and pharamacological experiments the binding of M-^{125}I-VIP to slide-mounted sections was shown to be time-dependent, saturable, and reversible. Association of M-^{125}I-VIP specific binding was maximal within 90 to 120 minutes. Specific binding, corresponding to approximately 50% of total binding, was saturable, of high affinity (Kd of 76.6 pM) and low capacity (fmol/mg prot range). Dissociation of M-^{125}I-VIP was maximal at 10 minutes. Unlabeled VIP and the two structurally related peptides PHI and secretin competed in a concentration-dependent manner for sites labeled by M-^{125}I-VIP with the following rank-order of potencies: VIP > PHI > secretin. VIP receptors, as revealed by quantitative autoradiography, are present at various levels of the neuraxis. High densities were observed in olfactory bulb, cerebral cortex (highest in layers I, II, IV), dentate gyrus, subiculum, various thalamic and hypothalamic nuclei, superior colliculus, locus ceruleus, area postrema, and pineal gland. Intermediate densities were found in the amygdala, nucleus accumbens, caudate-putamen, septum, bed nucleus of the stria terminalis, CA1 to CA4 fields of the hippocampus and central grey (see FIG. 5 and 6). No specific binding of M-^{125}I-VIP was observed in white-matter tracts such as corpus callosum, anterior commissure, medial forebrain bundle, and fornix.

These results are generally in good agreement with other studies;[40,41] when they are considered in reference to the previously described distribution of VIP immunoreactivity, a remarkable matching between VIP content and receptor density appears to exist, an observation that contrasts with what has been described for several other neurotransmitters.[42,43] A possible reason for such a matching may be the fact that the vast majority of VIP-containing cells are locally projecting neurons.[3,4,44] Nevertheless, even in the case of the long VIP-containing pathways, a good correlation exists between receptor density and VIP presence in the terminal areas of these pathways such as the bed nucleus of the stria terminalis and the anterior and preoptic areas of the hypothalamus.[45-48] A notable mismatch between receptor density and VIP content occurs in the dorsal cochlear nucleus, where the moderate density of autoradiographic grains observed is not accompanied by the presence in high amounts of immunoreactive VIP.[49]

It is also worth noting that these results indicate an association, although not exclusive, of VIP receptors with brain regions involved in the processing of specific sensory inputs. For example, the olfactory bulb, various thalamic nuclei including lateral and medial geniculate and lateral and medial ventroposterior, the habenular nuclei, the superior colliculus, the dorsal cochlear and the medial vestibular nucleus, as well as the central grey are all enriched in VIP receptors.

The distribution of VIP recognition sites in mouse and guinea pig brain is comparable, although not identical, to that observed in the rat brain (FIGS. 7-9). Some differences are worth noting. In mouse neocortex, the superficial layers (I-III) present

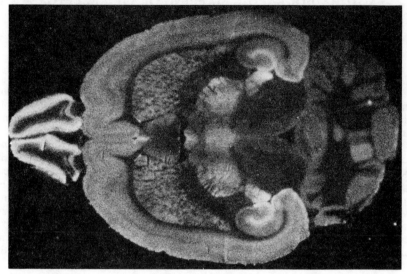

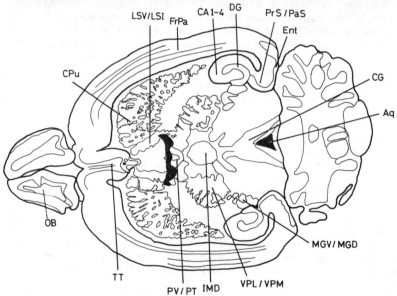

FIGURE 5. Autoradiographic localization of M-[^{125}I]VIP in the rat brain. Horizontal section at the level of the ventroposterior thalamic nuclei. White regions correspond to high receptor densities. Aq: acqueduct; CA1-4: fields CA1 to CA4 of Ammon's horn; CG: Central grey; CPu: caudate putamen; DG: dentate gyrus. Ent.: entorhinal cortex; FrPa: frontoparietal cortex; IMD: intermediodorsal thalamic nucleus; LSI/LSV: lateral septal nucleus; MGV/MGD: medial geniculate nucleus; OB: olfactory bulb; PrS/PaS: Pre- and parasubiculum; PV/PT: paraventricular and paratenial thalamic nuclei. Th: thalamic nuclei; TT: taenia tecta; VPL/VPM: ventroposterior thalamic nucleus.

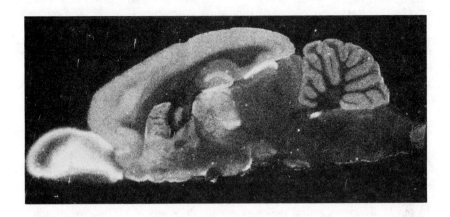

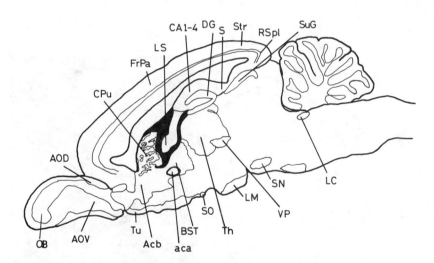

FIGURE 6. Autoradiographic localization of M-[^{125}I]VIP in rat brain. Sagittal section at the level of the locus ceruleus. aca: anterior commissure; Acb: nucleus accumbens; AM/AD/AV: anterior thalamic nuclei; AOD/AOV: olfactory nucleus; BST: bed nucleus of the stria terminalis; LC: locus coeruleus; LM: lateral mammillary nucleus; LP/LD: lateral thalamic nuclei; LS: lateral septum; RSpl: retrospenial cortex; S: subiculum; SN: substantia nigra; SO: supraoptic nucleus; Str: striate cortex; SuG: colliculus superior; Tu: olfactory tubercle; VM/VL: ventral thalamic nuclei. For other abbreviations, see legend for FIGURE 5.

a higher density of VIP receptors than deeper layers; this is particularly apparent in somatosensory cortex (see FIG. 7). In guinea pig neocortex the distribution of VIP binding sites appears rather homogeneous across layers and regions, except in the entorhinal cortex where a marked lamination is observed (FIG. 9). The cerebellar cortex of guinea pig and mouse presents a considerably higher density of VIP recognition sites than that observed in the rat; furthermore a marked lamination, confined to the granular layer, is apparent in the guinea pig cerebellar cortex (FIG. 9) but not in the mouse.

Lower densities of VIP binding sites were observed in cat brain.

Avian Brain

VIP binding sites as labeled by M-^{125}I-VIP were also present in lower vertebrate species such as frog, snake, and pigeon. For example, two coronal sections of the autoradiographic distribution of VIP receptors in pigeon brain are shown in FIGURES 10 and 11. The more rostral section shows a high density of VIP binding sites in the accessory hyperstriatum, dorsal and ventral hyperstriata, neostriatum, lateral septum,

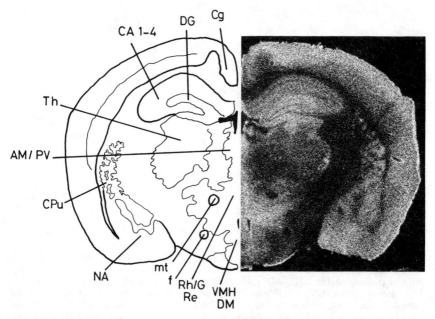

FIGURE 7. Autoradiographic localization of M-[^{125}I]VIP in mouse brain. Frontal section through the amygdaloid complex.

Cg: cingulate cortex; DM: dorsomedial hypothalamic nucleus; f: fornix; G: gelatinosus nucleus; mt: mammillothalamic tract; NA: amygdaloid nuclei; Re/Rh: reuniens and rhomboid nuclei; Rt: reticular thalamic nucleus; VHM: ventromedial hypothalamic nucleus. For other abbreviations see legends for FIGURES 5 and 6.

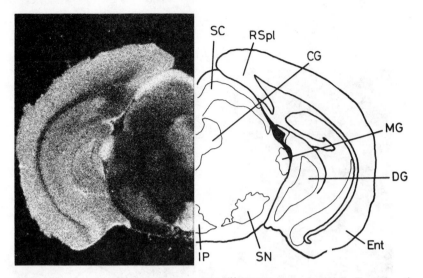

FIGURE 8. Autoradiographic localization of M-[^{125}I]VIP in the mouse brain. Frontal section at the level of the superior colliculus. IP: interpedoncular nucleus; MG: medial geniculate nucleus; SC: superior colliculus. For other abbreviations see legends for previous figures.

and intrapedoncular nucleus. A moderate density of VIP recognition sites is observed in the nucleus accumbens whereas a low density is present in the ectostriatum, paleostriatum, and in the parolfactory lobe. More caudally (FIG. 11), a very high density of VIP binding sites is observed in the tectum, particularly in the stratum griseum et fibrosum superficiale. At the same level the nucleus semilunaris is enriched with VIP receptors.

Rat Kidney

In the course of this autoradiographic study, we have examined various tissues in the rat and have made a surprising observation in the kidney. Here, two populations of VIP binding sites appear to exist (FIG. 12). Thus, a high-affinity site whose binding is selectively inhibited in the presence of 10 nM unlabeled VIP (FIG. 12B) is localized to the outer zone of the medullary pyramid as well as to punctate profiles in the renal cortex, which could correspond to glomerular structures (FIG. 12A). It is interesting to note that VIP has been shown to stimulate renin secretion, possibly by acting directly on the juxtaglomerular cells.[50] The remaining specific binding in the renal cortex is inhibited by 1 μM VIP (FIG. 12C). No specific binding is observed in the deeper medullary zone.

These autoradiographic studies have shown that VIP binding sites are present in most of the vertebrate brains examined and are particularly enriched in rodent brain. However, important species differences exist in the distribution and densities of these sites.

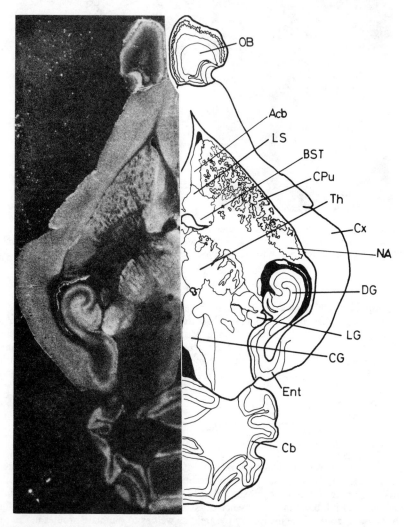

FIGURE 9. Autoradiographic localization of M-[¹²⁵I]VIP in the guinea pig brain. Horizontal section at the level of the lateral geniculate nucleus. Cb: cerebellar cortex; Cx: neocortex; LG: lateral geniculate nucleus; OB: olfactory bulb. For other abbreviations see legends for previous figures.

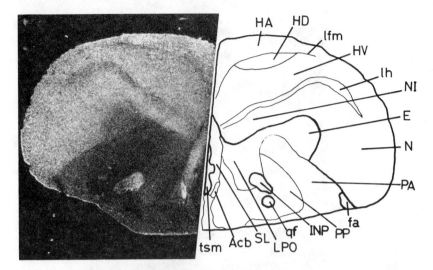

FIGURE 10. Autoradiographic localization of M-[^{125}I]VIP in pigeon brain. Frontal section at the level of the intrapedoncular nucleus. E: ectostriatum; fa: frontoarchistriatal tract; HA: accessory hyperstriatum; HV/HD: ventral and dorsal hyperstriata; INP: intrapedoncular nucleus; lfm: lamina frontalis suprema; lh: lamina hyperstriatica; LPO: parolfactory lobe; N: neostriatum; NI: neostriatum intermedium; PA: paleostriatum augmentatum; PP: paleostriatum primitivum; qf: quintofrontal tract; tsm: septomesencephalic tract. For other abbreviations see legends for previous figures.

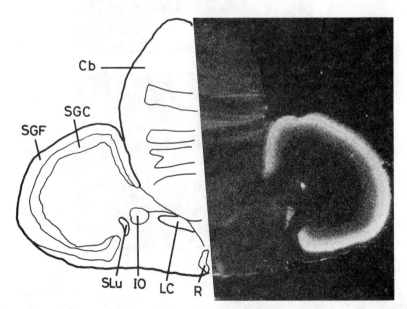

FIGURE 11. Autoradiographic localization of M-[^{125}I]VIP in pigeon brain. Frontal section through the tectum. IO: isthmooptic nucleus; R: nucleus raphes; SGC/SGF: central and superficial grey layer of the tectum; SLu: semilunate nucleus. For other abbreviations see legends for previous figures.

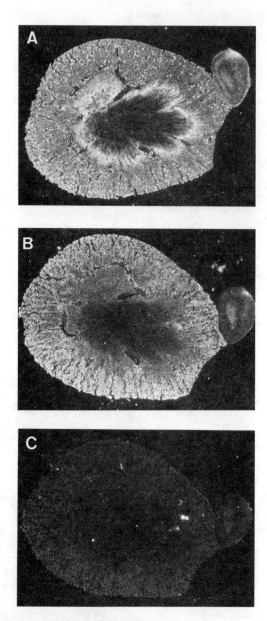

FIGURE 12. Autoradiographic localization of M-[^{125}I]VIP in rat kidney.

(A) Total binding. (B) Binding in the presence of 10 nM unlabeled VIP. Note that auto-radiographic grains in the outer zone of the medullary pyramid and in punctate structures in the renal cortex have disappeared. (C) Binding in the presence of 1 μM unlabeled VIP, cor-responding to nonspecific binding.

Note that M-[^{125}I]VIP-specific binding is also present in the adrenal gland.

ACKNOWLEDGMENTS

The authors wish to thank Ms. Sylvianne Bonnet for excellent secretarial work, Mr. Fred Pillonel for the graphs, and Ms. Nathalie Pellegrinelli and Gisèle Gilliéron for technical help.

REFERENCES

1. MAGISTRETTI, P. J. 1986. Intercellular communication mediated by VIP in the cerebral cortex. Peptides **7 (Suppl. 1):** 169-173.
2. ROSTENE, W. H. 1984. Neurobiological and neuroendocrine functions of the vasoactive intestinal peptide (VIP). Prog. Neurobiol. **22:** 103-129.
3. FUXE, K., T. HOKFELT, S. I. SAID & V. MUTT. 1977. Vasoactive intestinal polypeptide and the nervous system: Immunohistochemical evidence for localization in central and peripheral neurons, particularly intracortical neurons in the cerebral cortex. Neurosci. Lett. **5:** 241-246.
4. LOREN, I., P. C. EMSON, J. FAHRENKRUG, A. BJORKLUND, J. ALUMETS, R. HAKANSON & F. SUNDLER. 1979. Distribution of vasoactive intestinal polypeptide in the rat and mouse brain. Neuroscience **4:** 1953-1976.
5. GIACHETTI, A., S. I. SAID, R. C. REYNOLDS & F. C. KONIGES. 1977. Vasoactive intestinal polypeptide in brain: Localization in and release from isolated nerve terminals. Proc. Natl. Acad. Sci. USA **74:** 3424-3428.
6. BESSON, J., W. ROTSZTEJN, B. POUSSIN, A. M. LHIAUBET & G. ROSSELIN. 1982. Release of vasoactive intestinal peptide from rat brain slices by various depolarizing agents. Neurosci. Lett. **28:** 281-285.
7. TAYLOR, D. P. & C. B. PERT. 1979. Vasoactive intestinal polypeptide: Specific binding to rat brain membranes. Proc. Natl. Acad. Sci. USA **76:** 660-664.
8. STAUN-OLSEN, P., B. OTTESEN, P. D. BARTELS, M. H. NIELSEN, S. GAMMELTOFT & J. FAHRENKRUG. 1982. Receptors for vasoactive intestinal polypeptide on isolated synaptosomes from rat cerebral cortex. Heterogeneity of binding and desensitization of receptors. J. Neurochem. **39:** 1242-1251.
9. ROBBERECHT, P., P. DE NEEF, M. LAMMENS, M. DESCHODT-LANCKMAN & J.-P. CHRISTOPHE. 1978. Specific binding of vasoactive intestinal peptide to brain membranes from the guinea pig. Eur. J. Biochem. **90:** 147-154.
10. PHILLIS, J. W., J. R. KIRKPATRICK & S. I. SAID. 1978. Vasoactive intestinal polypeptide excitation of central neurons. Can. J. Physiol. Pharmacol. **56:** 337-340.
11. FERRON, A., G. R. SIGGINS & F. E. BLOOM. 1985. Vasoactive intestinal polypeptide acts synergistically with norepinephrine to depress spontaneous discharge rate in cerebral cortical neurons. Proc. Natl. Acad. Sci. USA **82:** 8810-8812.
12. QUIK, M., L. L. IVERSEN & S. R. BLOOM. 1978. Effect of vasoactive intestinal peptide (VIP) and other peptides on cAMP accumulation in rat brain. Biochem. Pharmacol. **27:** 2209-2213.
13. DESCHODT-LANCKMAN, M., P. ROBBERECHT & J. CHRISTOPHE. 1977. Characterization of VIP-sensitive adenylate cyclase in guinea pig brain. FEBS Lett. **83:** 76-80.
14. MAGISTRETTI, P. J. & M. SCHORDERET. 1984. VIP and noradrenaline act synergistically to increase cyclic AMP in cerebral cortex. Nature **308:** 280-282.
15. LUINE, V. N., W. ROSTENE, J. RHODES & B. S. MCEWEN. 1984. Activation of choline acetyltransferase by vasoactive intestinal peptide. J. Neurochem. **42:** 1131-1134.
16. MAGISTRETTI, P. J., J. H. MORRISON, W. J. SHOEMAKER, V. SAPIN & F. E. BLOOM. 1981. Vasoactive intestinal polypeptide induces glycogenolysis in mouse cortical slices: A possible regulatory mechanism for the local control of energy metabolism. Proc. Natl. Acad. Sci. USA **78:** 6535-6539.

17. MAGISTRETTI, P. J., J. H. MORRISON, W. J. SHOEMAKER & F. E. BLOOM. 1984. Morphological and functional correlates of VIP neurons in cerebral cortex. Peptides **5:** 213-218.
18. MAGISTRETTI, P. J. 1986. VIP-containing neurons in the cerebral cortex: Cellular actions and interactions with the noradrenergic system *In* Ionic Channels in Neural Membranes. J. M. Ritchie, R. D. Keynes & C. L. Bolis, Eds.: 323-331. Alan R. Liss. Inc. New York.
19. MORRISON, J. H., P. J. MAGISTRETTI, R. BENOIT & F. E. BLOOM. 1984. The distribution and morphological characteristics of the intracortical VIP-positive cell: An immunohistochemical analysis. Brain Res. **292:** 269-282.
20. CONNOR, J. R. & A. PETERS. 1984. Vasoactive intestinal polypeptide-immunoreactive neurons in rat visual cortex. Neuroscience **12:** 1027-1044.
21. ECKENSTEIN, F. & R. W. BAUGHMAN. 1984. Two types of cholinergic innervation in cortex, one co-localized with vasoactive intestinal polypeptide. Nature **309:** 153-155.
22. RAITERI, M., M. MARCHI & P. PAUDICE. 1987. Vasoactive intestinal polypeptide (VIP) potentiates the muscarinic stimulation of phosphoinositide turnover in rat cerebral cortex. Eur. J. Pharmacol. **133:** 127-128.
23. MAGISTRETTI, P. J. & J. H. MORRISON. 1985. VIP neurons in the neocortex. TINS **8:** 7-8.
24. BLOOM, F. E. 1975. The role of cyclic nucleotides in central synaptic transmission. Rev. Physiol. Biochem. Pharamacol. **74:** 1-103.
25. DALY, J. 1975. Role of cyclic nucleotides in the nervous system. *In* Handbook of Psychopharmacology. L. L. Iversen, S. D. Iversen & S. H. Snyder, Eds.: 47-129. Plenum Press. New York.
26. MAGISTRETTI, P. J. & M. SCHORDERET. 1985. Norepinephrine and histamine potentiate the increases in cAMP elicited by vasoactive intestinal polypeptide in mouse cerebral cortical slices: Mediation by α_1-adrenergic and H1-histaminergic receptors. J. Neurosci. **5:** 362-368.
27. DAHLSTROM, A. & K. FUXE. 1964. Evidence for the existence of monoamine-containing neurons in the central nervous system. I. Demonstration of monoamines in the cell bodies of brain stem neurons. Acta Physiol. Scand. **62(Suppl. 232):** 1-55.
28. MORRISON, J. H., R. GRZANNA, M. MOLLIVER & J. T. COYLE. 1978. The distribution and orientation of noradrenergic fibers in neocortex of the rat: An immunofluorescence study. J. Comp. Neurol. **181:** 17-40.
29. MORRISON, J. H., M. E. MOLLIVER, R. GRZANNA & J. T. COYLE. 1981. The intra-cortical trajectory of the coeruleo-cortical projection in the rat: A tangentially organized cortical afferent. Neuroscience **6:** 139-158.
30. VANE, J. R. 1971. Inhibition of prostaglandin synthesis as a mechanism of action for aspirin-like drugs. Nature **231:** 232-235.
31. SKOU, J. C. 1965. Enzymatic basis for active transport of Na$^+$ and K$^+$ across cell membrane. Physiol. Rev. **45:** 596-617.
32. SHIMIZU, H. & J. W. DALY. 1972. Effect of depolarizing agents on accumulation of cyclic adenosine 3',5'-monophosphate in cerebral cortical slices. Eur. J. Pharmacol. **17:** 240-252.
33. SHIMIZU, H., C. R. CREVELING & J. W. DALY. 1970. Cyclic adenosine 3',5'-monophosphate formation in brain slices: Stimulation by batrachotoxin, ouabain, veratridine, and potassium ions. Mol. Pharmacol. **6:** 184-188.
34. HO, R. J. & B. JEANRENAUD. 1967. Insulin-like action of ouabain. I. Effect on carbohydrate metabolism. Biochim. Biophys. Acta **144:** 61-73.
35. CLAUSEN, T. 1966. The relationship between the transport of glucose and cations across cell membranes in isolated tissues. II. Effects of K$^+$-free medium, ouabain and insulin upon the fate of glucose in rat diaphragm. Biochim. Biophys. Acta **120:** 361-368.
36. MAGISTRETTI, P. J., P. R. HOF & J.-L. MARTIN. 1986. Adenosine stimulates glycogenolysis in mouse cerebral cortex: A possible coupling mechanism between neuronal activity and energy metabolism. J. Neurosci. **6:** 2558-2562.
37. SIESJO, B. K., ED. 1978. Brain Energy Metabolism. Wiley. New York.
38. MARTIN, J.-L., K. ROSE, G. H. HUGHES & P. J. MAGISTRETTI. 1986. [mono[^{125}I]iodo-Tyr^{10},MetO^{17}]-Vasoactive intestinal polypeptide: Preparation, characterization, and use for radioimmunoassay and receptor binding. J. Biol. Chem. **261:** 5320-5327.

39. MARTIN, J.-L., M. M. DIETL, P. R. HOF, J. M. PALACIOS & P. J. MAGISTRETTI. 1987. Autoradiographic mapping of [mono-(^{125}I)iodo-Tyr^{10}, MetO^{17} vasoactive intestinal peptide binding sites in the rat brain. Neuroscience **23**: 539-565.
40. SHAFFER, M. M. & T. W. MOODY. 1986. Autoradiographic visualization of CNS receptors for vasoactive intestinal peptide. Peptides **7**: 283-288.
41. BESSON, J., A. SARRIEAU, M. VIAL, J.-C. MARIE, G. ROSSELIN & W. ROSTENE. 1986. Characterization and autoradiographic distribution of vasoactive intestinal peptide binding sties in the rat central nervous system. Brain Res. **398**: 329-336.
42. HERKENHAM, M. & S. MCLEAN. 1986. Mismatches between receptor and transmitter localizations in the brain. In Quantitative Receptor Autoradiography. A. C. Boast, E. W. Snowhill & A. C. Altar, Eds.: 137-171. Alan R. Liss, Inc. New York.
43. KUHAR, M. J. Quantitative receptor autoradiography: An overview. In Quantitative Receptor Autoradiography. A. C. Boast, E. W. Snowhill & A. C. Altar, Eds.: 1-12. Alan R. Liss, Inc. New York.
44. ABRAMS, G. M., G. NILAVER & E. A. ZIMMERMAN. 1985. VIP-containing neurons. In Handbook of Chemical Neuroanatomy, Vol. 4: GABA and Neuropeptides in the CNS, Part I. A. Björklund & T. Hökfelt, Eds.: 335-354. Elsevier Science Publishers B.V.
45. EIDEN, L. E., T. HOKFELT, M. J. BROWNSTEIN & M. PALKOVITS. 1985. Vasoactive intestinal polypeptide afferents to the bed nucleus of the stria terminalis in the rat: An immunohistochemical and biochemical study. Neuroscience **15**: 999-1013.
46. MARLEY, P. D., P. C. EMSON, S. P. HUNT & J. FAHRENKRUG. 1981. A long ascending projection in the rat brain containing vasoactive intestinal polypeptide. Neurosci. Lett. **27**: 261-266.
47. ROBERTS, G. W., P. L. WOODHAMS, M. G. BRYANT, T. J. CROW, S. R. BLOOM & J. M. POLAK. 1980. VIP in the rat brain: Evidence for a major pathway linking the amygdala and hypothalamus via the stria terminalis. Histochemistry **65**: 103-119.
48. ROBERTS, G. W., P. L. WOODHAMS, T. J. CROW & J. M. POLAK. 1980. Loss of immunoreactive VIP in the bed nucleus following lesions of the stria terminalis. Brain Res. **195**: 471-475.
49. EIDEN, L. E., G. NILAVER & M. PALKOVITS. 1982. Distribution of vasoactive intestinal polypeptide (VIP) in the rat brain stem nuclei. Brain Res. **231**: 472-477.
50. WHITE, E. L. 1981. Thalamocortical synaptic relations. In The Organization of the Cerebral Cortex. F. O. Schmitt, F. G. Worden, G. Adelman & S. G. Dennis, Eds.: 153-161. MIT Press. Cambridge, MA.

Functional Implications of the Radial Organization of VIP-Containing Neurons in the Neocortex

JOHN H. MORRISON[a]

Scripps Clinic and Research Foundation
La Jolla, California 92037

INTRODUCTION

The pioneering anatomic studies of Lorento de No[1] led to the proposal that the neocortex consisted of adjacent overlapping radial units, capable of information processing at the most basic local level. He termed this collection of radially interconnected afferents and intrinsic neurons an "elementary unit," which was the conceptual forerunner of the cortical column, initially described by Mountcastle[2] as "a vertically oriented column or cylinder of cells capable of input-output functions of considerable complexity, independent of horizontal intragriseal spread of activity." Extensive electrophysiological and anatomic analyses have elaborated on and extended our knowledge of the columnar organization of neocortex in numerous cortical sensory and motor regions.[3-10] In addition, we now understand the laminar pattern of termination of the afferents in great detail[11-15] and realize that the cortical efferents exhibit laminar segregation based on their target tissue[16] (layer VI pyramids to thalamus, layer V to brain stem, etc.) and that the afferents terminate discontinuously.[17] Furthermore, interconnections of neurons within the cortex have been defined extensively by combined Golgi-electronic microscopic studies[12,18] and by anatomic reconstruction of physiologically characterized cells identified by intracellular marker injections.[19] Thus, the "elementary unit" has grown in complexity, to become a more dynamic module whose boundaries float with the activity patterns of their afferents. Also, it is clear that until recently, the capacity for horizontal interactions in neocortex was greatly underestimated. Not only do pyramidal and nonpyramidal cell axons extend for several millimeters in the plane tangential to the pial surface[20] but the monoamine-containing afferents such as the ceruleo-cortical projection sweep across vast expanses of neocortex modulating activity in several functionally discrete regions simultaneously.[21,22]

As we obtain more information on neurotransmitter distributions and functions in neocortex, we will be able to attach additional functional and biochemical relevance to the radial and horizontal morphologic characteristics of specific elements of cortical

[a] Address for correspondence: John H. Morrison, Ph.D., Scripps Clinic and Research Foundation, BCR-1, 10666 North Torrey Pines Road, La Jolla, CA 92037.

circuitry. One problem in this regard is that the same neurotransmitter may be utilized by different cell types with different anatomic characteristics. This is clearly the case for GABA[23] and somatostatin.[24-26] However, as described below, vasoactive intestinal peptide (VIP) can be correlated with one particular cell type in rat neocortex, namely, the bipolar cell. In addition, extensive information has been obtained on the cellular effects of VIP in rodent cortex (see Magistretti, this volume) and interactions between VIP and norepinephrine, the neurotransmitter utilized by one of the major horizontal (or tangential) systems in neocortex.[27,28] Thus, by considering the cellular effects of these two neurotransmitters in relation to their morphologic constraints, a model for radial-tangential interactions in neocortex emerges.

MORPHOLOGY OF VIP-CONTAINING CORTICAL NEURONS

VIP-positive neurons can be visualized in all areas of rat cortex. The laminar distribution of VIP-positive cells is consistent throughout the cortex; labeled cells are most numerous in layers II and III, but are present in all layers (see FIG. 1 and 2). Laminar analysis of the distribution of labeled cells in primary visual cortex is presented in FIGURE 1. In the visual cortex, approximately 50% of the labeled cells are in layers II and III, and 80% of the labeled cell bodies are contained within layers I-IV (superficial 600 μm of cortex), whereas in somatosensory cortex approximately 48% are in layers II and III and 65% are present in layers I-IV. A fine plexus of highly varicose axonal fibers is present in layers I-V, with the highest density in layers II-IV. Presynaptic VIP-positive profiles engaging in conventional axodendritic synaptic complexes with small dendritic profiles are present in layers I-V.

In coronal and sagittal sections, the vast majority of VIP-positive profiles appears as bipolar, radially oriented neurons (see FIG. 2). The cell body is ovoid in shape, with one main process emanating from both the superficial and deep poles. These two processes proceed radially toward the pial surface and white matter, respectively, with minimal horizontal branching (FIG. 2). The same process can be followed for long distances, in some cases as far as 1 mm, in a 40-μm coronal section, indicating the extreme radial nature of the trajectory through the cortical thickness. In layer I, the radial processes often branch in a Y-shaped fashion, where a single branch may extend for 100 μm obliquely with no further branching. These processes often extend up to the pial surface and occasionally appear to extend to the apparent limits of the cortical neuropil. The ascending and descending dendrites often proceed through layers II, III, and superficial IV as single processes with a very low degree of arborization.

The branching pattern of the descending dendrite is usually more variable than the ascending dendrite and may terminate in a few oblique branches or in a fairly tight and spherical "burst" of relatively short but more highly arborized processes (see FIG. 3). The descending process rarely extends as deep as mid-layer V. The branches from an individual cell generally extend within a sphere of 60-120 μm diameter in layer I and 50-100 μm in deep layer IV and superficial V (see FIG. 3).

In some instances, a very fine axonal process emanates from one of the two main radial processes (see FIGS. 2 and 3). This fine process generally egresses horizontally or obliquely for a short distance (30-50 μm) and leaves the plane of section; however, occasionally we have observed a bifurcation of this process into two radial branches that proceed obliquely, or parallel to the main radial dendritic process. The shape and dimensions of an idealized VIP-positive bipolar cell, based on observations in the coronal and sagittal planes, are represented in FIGURE 3.

The nonbipolar cells are more likely to occur in layers I and VI than in the intervening layers. Labeled cells in I and VI that are not bipolar are usually round rather than ovoid. In addition, the orientation of the labeled bipolar cells in layers I and VI is more variable, in that they are more likely to be oriented obliquely or horizontally than are the labeled cells in layers II-V.

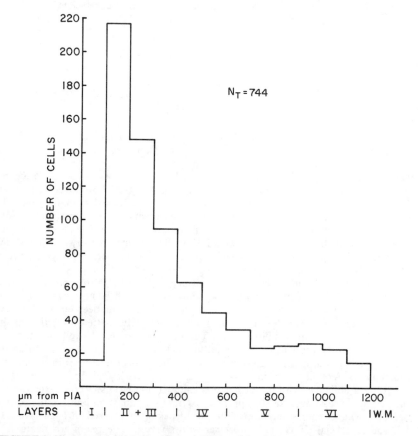

FIGURE 1. Histogram showing distribution of VIP-positive cell bodies in primary visual cortex. Cell counts were derived from photomontages of 550-μm-wide strips of 50-μm-thick coronal sections. Total cells = 744. (Taken from Morrison *et al.;*[29] used with permission.)

The predominant radial orientation of the VIP-positive cell also is apparent in tangential sections through the neocortex. In tangential sections through layers II-IV, the labeled profiles are restricted to cell bodies and processes cut in cross section; there are no processes that run more than 25-50 μm in the tangential plane of section. Tangential sections through layers I and deep IV through superficial V contain unique, coarse "fusilli-like" profiles that correspond to the oblique, varicose dendritic processes seen in sagittally or coronal sections.

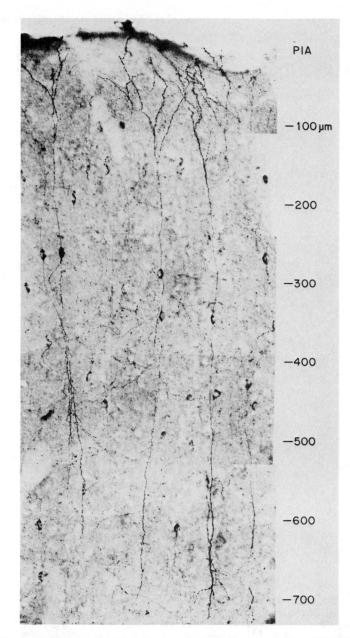

PIA

−100 μm

−200

−300

−400

−500

−600

−700

FIGURE 2. Photomontage of VIP-positive neurons in lateral neocortex (50-μm coronal section). Note the following features: (1) most cell bodies are ovoid, with a major ascending and descending process. (2) These processes extend radially for several hundred microns within the plane of section and do not arborize extensively, except within layers I (pia-100 μm) and superficial V (600-700 μm). (3) The distal branches are more heavily stained and of larger diameter than the segments closer to the cell bodies. (4) Processes that arise from proximal segments may be axons, as they are very fine, highly varicose and more variable in orientation. (Taken from Morrison *et al.*[29]; used with permission.)

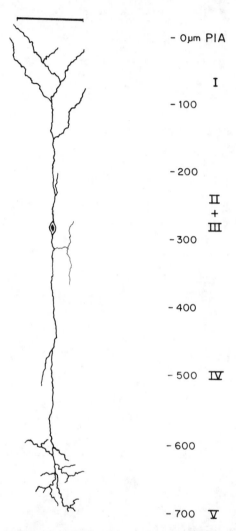

- 0µm PIA

I

- 100

- 200

II
+
III

- 300

- 400

- 500   IV

- 600

- 700   V

FIGURE 3. Diagram showing shape and dimensions of idealized VIP-positive bipolar cell, based on photographs of actual cells. The cell is accurately drawn to scale. Radial length is approximately 700 µm and tangential dendritic spread is approximately 100 µm. Note paucity of branching in layers II, III, and superficial IV. Also, note axon emanating from descending dendrite and bifurcating. The axon rarely is seen in continuity with the cell, and in those rare cases cannot be followed for any significant distance. Bar at top equals 100 µm. Radial depth shown on right. Roman numerals on far right refer to cortical layers. The dendritic patterns appear similar in both the coronal and sagittal planes. (Taken from Morrison *et al.*[29]; used with permission.)

In order to determine the density and three-dimensional distribution pattern of these cells, serial tangential sections (40 μm thick) were prepared from the primary visual cortex (see Fig. 4). Cell bodies were easily discriminated from dendritic profiles by their general appearance and far greater diameter; dendritic profiles were barely resolvable at the final magnification of the photomontages. Since virtually all of the

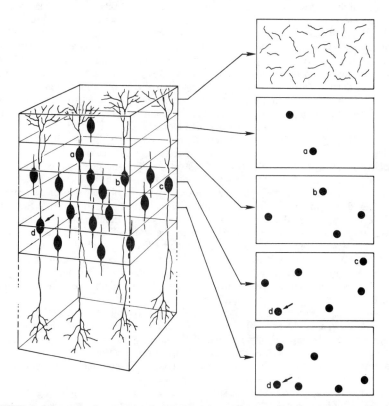

FIGURE 4. Schematic diagram showing design of tangential analysis. Cell plots of each 40-μm-thick tangential section are made through the superficial 600 μm of primary visual cortex. The assumption is made that each cell body represents a bipolar cell, and thus represents a radial volume. The individual cell plots are then superimposed to generate a two-dimensional depiction of the three-dimensional array of VIP-containing cells. If a cell is represented on two adjacent sections (such as cell d) then it is only counted on the more superficial section, to avoid counting any cell twice.

labeled cells are radially bipolar, with a limited dendritic and axonal arbor in the tangential plane, the position of the VIP-positive cell body in the tangential plane is an accurate reflection of the three-dimensional extension of that cell relative to that of the neighboring labeled cell.

The quantitative observations derived from this reconstruction are the following. The mean density of VIP-positive cells in a vertically compressed region of visual cortex is one cell per 737 μm;[2] this is equivalent to a density of approximately one cell per 27-μm square or circle of 30.6-μm diameter. The uniformity of this distribution is reflected by two measures: (1) the largest areas lacking a VIP-positive cell are generally 60-90 μm in diameter, (2) the average nearest neighbor (i.e., the mean minimum horizontal distance between VIP-positive cells in the horizontal plane) is approximately 15 μm. By relating the average nearest neighbor to the mean density, we conclude that the distribution of VIP cells is random, and not clustered.[29]

Finally, it should be recalled that, by absolute counts, approximately 80% of VIP-positive cell bodies are located within the superficial 600 μm of cortex. Thus, the figure for the density of VIP-positive neurons includes the great majority (80%) but not all immunoreactive cell bodies and, as such, is slightly underestimated. While the data were derived from the compressed tangential series, the strictly radial shape of the VIP-positive cells permits analysis with reference to the entire cortical depth. Thus, a circle of 30.6 μm diameter actually represents a vertical column that extends across the entire cortical mantle with a diameter of 30.6 μm.

The VIP-positive cells clearly represent a subclass of the bipolar cells as described by Peters and Kimerer;[30] their analysis suggests that the axonal arborization of a bipolar cell (as defined in Golgi studies) is strictly radial and does not extend outside of a narrow radial column that is largely within the domain of the dendritic arbor. Therefore, an individual VIP-positive neuron is presumably capable of synaptic reception and transmission within a narrow radial column that extends from the pia to layer V. If one makes the conventional assumption that dendrites receive and axon terminals transmit synaptic information, then the VIP cell is best suited to receive input in layers I, deep IV, and superficial V and synapse on other neurons predominantly in layers II through IV. However, given the high concentration of immunoreactive VIP in the distal dendrites, this conventional concept of polarity may not be valid. It is possible that, as with neurons in the substantia nigra,[31] release occurs from both the dendrites and axon terminals.

Thus, each VIP-containing cell is identified with a unique radial volume, which is generally between 15 and 60 μm in diameter, and overlaps with the contiguous domains of neighboring VIP-positive cells.[29] The density is such that any given location in neocortex is included within the radial domain of at least one VIP-containing cell. The emergence of an approximate density of one VIP-containing cell per 30-μm diameter column is of interest for two reasons. First, Powell and his colleagues have shown that across several different species and cortical regions, including rat visual cortex, a cylinder of cortex 25 μm by 30 μm consistently contains approximately 70 pyramidal cells, 30 stellate cells, and 5 large stellate cells.[32,33] On the average, this same region would contain one VIP-containing cell. Thus, approximately 1% of the neurons in rat visual cortex are VIP-positive (if shrinkage is taken into consideration, this figure would be closer to 1.5%). Second, a column of this size, the so-called "minicolumn," is viewed by some investigators as the smallest unit of resolution in the anatomic and functional organization of neocortex.[3,34] The concept of a hardwired minicolumn has been controversial and somewhat resistant to analysis. Given that the distribution of the VIP-containing cells is random, our data cannot be taken as evidence for the existence of anatomic or functional minicolumns of a specific diameter. However, should the concept of the minicolumns gain additional experimental verification, it is comforting to know that each minicolumn is likely to contain at least one VIP-positive neuron.

The morphological characteristics and distribution of the VIP-containing cell are ideally suited for a role in local, radial regulation of cortical activity.[27-29] The precise nature of this role is dependent upon the cellular effect of VIP (see Magistretti et al., this volume) and the anatomic constraints of the circuits involving VIP-containing cells.

MORPHOLOGY OF NORADRENERGIC INNERVATION OF NEOCORTEX

The noradrenergic innervation of the neocortex is organized according to strikingly different morphological principles.[27] Noradrenergic neurons originate in the nucleus locus ceruleus in the brain stem, from where they project to every level of the neuraxis including the neocortex (for reviews see Foote et al.[35] and Foote and Morrison[36]). The ascending noradrenergic fibers enter the cortex rostrally and proceed caudally through the cortical gray matter predominantly in a plane parallel to the pial surface.[21,22] The intracortical noradrenergic fibers branch widely and pass across cytoarchitectonic boundaries, thus furnishing the ceruleocortical system with the unique capacity to modulate neuronal activity synchronously and globally throughout a vast rostrocaudal expanse of neocortex (FIG. 5). Fibers branch from the tangentially oriented fibers and arborize with a specific laminar pattern.[37] Subtle regional differences in the density pattern of the noradrenergic innervation exist in the rat neocortex;[38] however, these regional differences are more pronounced in the primate.[39–41] Thus, the density is high in the primary somatosensory and motor, relative to primary visual and temporal cortices.[39–41] Furthermore, laminar specializations are more pronounced in the primate.[42] Thus, there are preferred regional and laminar targets within this highly divergent neurotransmitter specified afferent system; however, in contrast to the locally restricted VIP neurons, the spatial domain of noradrenergic cortical fibers is quite expansive.

INTERACTIONS BETWEEN NOREPINEPHRINE AND VIP

As described above, the anatomic constraints of these two systems are quite divergent; norepinephrine is likely to exert a global effect on cortical activity, whereas VIP-containing neurons are positioned for local regulation. However, these two neurotransmitters share important cellular effects, suggesting that they may regulate similar processes in different domains, and in some cases synergistically interact (see Magistretti, this volume).

Both norepinephrine and VIP increase glycogenolysis.[43] The glycogenolytic actions of VIP and norepinephrine are independent.[44] The hydrolysis of glycogen, induced by VIP and NA, will result at the cellular level in an increased availability of energy substrates. This action, when viewed in relation to the morphological characteristics of the VIP- and NA-containing neurons, indicates the existence of two complementary neuronal systems that participate in the regulation of energy metabolism within the neocortex: (1) the intracortical VIP-containing system endowed with the capacity to regulate glycogenolysis locally, within individual cortical columns of 60-100 μm diameter, and (2) the tangentially organized monoaminergic fibers exerting their metabolic effect globally and synchronously, intersecting a longitudinal array of columns (FIG. 6).

NA and VIP both increase cAMP synthesis when applied separately, and furthermore, when both are present they act synergistically to increase cAMP in rodent cerebral cortex.[45,46] Within the cerebral cortex, this synergism reveals that VIP and NA-containing neurons, when simultaneously active, may act in a functionally coordinated manner to generate a "cortical hot-spot" where cAMP levels are drastically

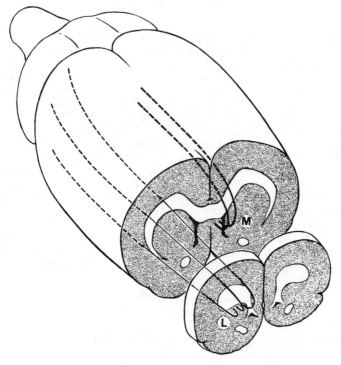

FIGURE 5. Intracortical trajectory of noradrenaline fibers in the rat. The majority of the corticopetal NA fibers in the medial forebrain bundle follow one of two routes to the neocortex: a medial group (M) ascends through the septal area, and a lateral group (L) continues rostrally through the ventral telencephalon. Once they enter neocortex, these fibers form a continuous sheet of axons, largely within layer VI, that proceeds caudally throughout the longitudinal extent of the medial and dorsolateral cortex, supplying the cortical NA innervation throughout their trajectory. (Taken from Morrison et al.[21]; used with permission.)

increased in comparison to surrounding regions to activate those intracellular processes that are regulated by cAMP-dependent phosphorylations.[28,46] The spatial coordinates of such a cortical domain are delineated by the intersection of the tangentially organized NA fibers and a group of activated, radially oriented VIP-containing neurons (FIG. 6).

Certain behavioral situations would be likely to bring about the simultaneous activity of VIP- and NA-containing neurons. Electrophysiological recordings in be-

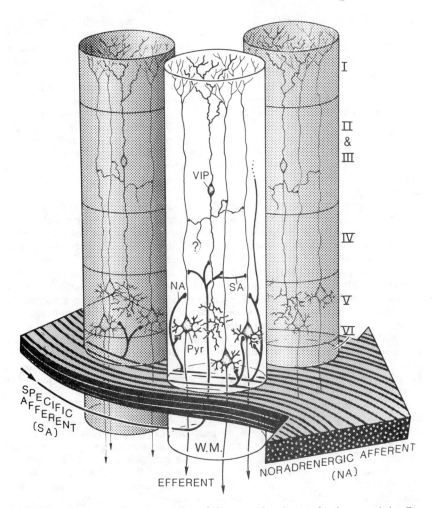

FIGURE 6. Diagrammatic representation of the anatomic substrate for the synergistic effects of NA and VIP following the concomitant activation of noradrenergic cortical afferents and a group of VIP-containing neurons. Such an arrangement would allow for the establishment of temporary columnar "hot spots." VIP: VIP-containing bipolar cell. NA: noradrenergic afferent. S.A.: specific afferent (i.e. from thalamus). PYR: pyramidal cell furnishing major efferent projections. W.M.: subcortical white matter. Cortical layers denoted by Roman numerals. Note tangential orientation of NA fibers, and radially restricted domain of VIP-containing neuron. The concomitant activation of noradrenergic fibers (large arrow bottom) by unexpected sensory stimuli and of a group of VIP-containing intracortical neurons by specific thalamic inputs would lead to a drastic increase in cAMP level within a discrete volume of somatosensory cortex, delineated here by the cylinder with dark background. Adjoining gray-background cylinders represent nonactivated cortical volumes. For graphic clarity, only the VIP-containing and the pyramidal cells have been represented here. In particular the principal target cells of the thalamocortical afferents, that is, the small stellate cells in layer IV, have been omitted. Furthermore, also for graphic clarity, only one VIP neuron per cylinder has been drawn, in representation of a group of VIP neurons. (Taken from Magistretti and Morrison;[28] used with permission.)

having rats have demonstrated that NA-containing neurons exhibit pronounced responses to nonnoxious, unexpected auditory, visual, and somatosensory stimuli.[47,48] The firing pattern and activating inputs to VIP intracortical neurons are not known. However, at the light microscopic level, the overall morphological characteristics and pattern of dendritic arborization of VIP-immunoreactive neurons resemble those of the "biopolar cell" described in Golgi-impregnated material by Peters and Kimerer.[30] These authors, by using a combined Golgi-electron microscopy technique, have demonstrated that in rat visual cortex "bipolar cells" receive direct thalamocortical inputs and synapse on pyramidal cells.[30] These observations would therefore suggest that VIP-bipolar neurons could also be activated by sensory inputs relayed by specific thalamocortical afferents and hence, that sensory stimulation could constitute a behavioral event whereby the synergistic interaction between VIP and NA would become operative within the terminal field of thalamocortical afferents in primary sensory cortex.[28]

A synergistic interaction has recently been described electrophysiologically as well.[49] NA has been described as having an "enabling" effect on cortical neuron responsivity.[35] Ferron et al.[49] have demonstrated that VIP iontophoretically applied to cortical neurons has both excitatory and inhibitory effects, but when applied with NE, a substantial augmentation of the VIP-mediated inhibition occurs. The synergistic effects of VIP and NE in both stimulating cAMP formation and depressing the firing rate of cortical neurons suggest that VIP- and NA-containing terminals converge on the same target cells; however, this has yet to be definitively demonstrated anatomically. The anatomic and electrophysiological evidence both suggest a common neuronal target, which is likely to be the pyramidal cell. However, evidence also exists for NA and VIP effects on glial cells and the vasculature (see Magistretti, this volume and Edvinsson, this volume). These latter two interactions may be nonsynaptic and in fact, may occur largely in layer I.[28] If the glial and vascular interactions occur largely in layer I and are nonsynaptic, they may be dependent on dendritic release of VIP from the VIP-rich dendrites that arborize in layer I.

Thus, as a working hypothesis we would suggest the following:[28] (1) VIP and NA neurons have contrasting geometric designs that define different domains of action, local for VIP and global for NA. This independent regulatory role may be most clearly reflected in their effect on metabolism. (2) Both neurotransmitter systems may act on three cell types: neurons, glia, and cells of the vasculature. Actions on the latter two cells may be mediated nonsynaptically, suggesting that a given cortical system may be capable of both synaptic and nonsynaptic release, each being related to a specific target. In addition each mode of release, and thus each physiologic effect, may exhibit a certain degree of laminar specificity with the synaptic-neuronal mode in the intermediate layers and the nonsynaptic glial and vascular regulation occurring largely in layer I.

REFERENCES

1. LORENTO DE NO, R. 1938. In Physiology of the Nervous System. J. F. Fulton, Ed.: 291-339. Oxford University Press. New York.
2. MOUNTCASTLE, V. B. 1957. J. Neurophysiol. 20: 408-434.
3. MOUNTCASTLE, V. B. 1979. In The Neurosciences Fourth Study Program. F. O. Schmitt & F. G. Worden, Eds.: 21-42. MIT Press. Cambridge, MA.
4. ASANUMA, H. 1975. Physiol. Rev. 55: 143-156.
5. ABELES, M. & M. H. GOLDSTEIN. 1970. J. Neurophysiol. 33: 172-187.

6. HUBEL, D. H. & T. N. WIESEL. 1970. Proc. R. Soc. B. **196:** 1-59.
7. COLONNIER, M. 1981. *In* The Organization of the Cerebral Cortex, Proceedings of a Neurosciences Research Program Colloquium. F. O. Schmitt, F. G. Worden, G. Adelman & S. G. Dennis, Eds.: 125-152. MIT Press. Cambridge, MA.
8. JONES, E. G. 1981. *In* The Organization of the Cerebral Cortex. F. O. SCHMITT, F. G. WORDEN, G. ADELMAN & S. G. DENNIS, Eds.: 199-236. MIT Press. Cambridge, MA.
9. POWELL, T. P. S. 1981. *In* Brain Mechanisms and Perceptual Awareness. O. Pompeiano & C. Marsan Ajmone, Eds.: 1-19. Raven Press. New York.
10. SZENTAGOTHAI, J. 1975. Brain Res. **95:** 475-496.
11. FISKEN, R. A., L. J. GAREY & T. P. S. POWELL. 1925. Phil. Trans. R. Soc. Lond. **272:** 487-536.
12. WHITE, E. L. 1978. J. Comp. Neurol. **181:** 627-662.
13. PETERS, A. 1979. Trends Neurosci. **2:** 183-185.
14. WINFIELD, D. A., M. RIVERA-DOMINGUEZ & T. P. S. POWELL. 1982. Brain Res. **231:** 19-32.
15. BLASDEL, G. G. & J. S. LUND. 1983. J. Neurosci. **3:** 1389-1413.
16. JONES, E. G. *In* Cerebral Cortex. A. Peters & E. G. Jones, Eds. **1:** 521-548. Plenum Press. New York.
17. GOLDMAN, P. S. & W. J. H. NAUTA. 1977. Brain Res. **122:** 393-413.
18. PETERS, A. & A. FAIREN. 1978. J. Comp. Neurol. **181:** 129-172.
19. GILBERT, C. D. & T. N. WIESEL. 1981. *In* The Organization of the Cerebral Cortex. F. O. Schmitt, F. G. Worden, G. Adelman & S. G. Dennis, Eds.: 163-191. MIT Press. Cambridge, MA.
20. VALVERDE, F. 1986. Neuroscience **18:** 1-24.
21. MORRISON, J. H., M. E. MOLLIVER & R. GRZANNA. 1979. Science **205:** 313-316.
22. MORRISON, J. H., M. E. MOLLIVER, R. GRZANNA & J. T. COYLE. 1981. Neuroscience **6:** 139-158.
23. SOMOGYI, P. 1986. Soc. Neurosci. Abstr. **12:** 583.
24. MORRISON, J. H., S. SCHERR, M. J. CAMPBELL & D. A. LEWIS. 1985. Soc. Neurosci. Abstr. **11:** 679.
25. LEWIS, D. A., M. J. CAMPBELL & J. H. MORRISON. 1986. J. Comp. Neurol. **248:** 1-18.
26. CAMPBELL, M. J., D. A. LEWIS, R. BENOIT & J. H. MORRISON. 1987. J. Neurosci. **7:** 1133-1144.
27. MORRISON, J. H. & P. J. MAGISTRETTI. 1983. TINS **6:** 146-151.
28. MAGISTRETTI, P. J. & J. H. MORRISON. 1987. Neuroscience, in press.
29. MORRISON, J. H., P. J. MAGISTRETTI, R. BENOIT & F. E. BLOOM. 1984. Brain Res. **292:** 269-282.
30. PETERS, A. & L. M. KIMERER. 1981. J. Neurocytol. **9:** 163-183.
31. GLOWINSKI, J. 1979. *In* The Neurosciences, 4th Study Program. F. O. Schmitt & F. G. Worden, Eds.: 1069-1084. MIT Press. Cambridge, MA.
32. POWELL, T. P. S. 1981. *In* Brain Mechanisms and Perceptual Awareness. O. Pompeiano & C. Ajmone Marsan, Eds.: 1-19 Raven Press. New York.
33. ROCKEL, A. J., R. W. HIORNS & T. P. S. POWELL. 1980. Brain **103:** 221-244.
34. D. H. HUBEL & T. N. WIESEL. 1974. J. Comp. Neurol. **158:** 267-294.
35. FOOTE, S. L., F. E. BLOOM & G. ASTON-JONES. 1983. Physiol. Rev. **63:** 844-914.
36. FOOTE, S. L. & J. H. MORRISON. 1987. Annu. Rev. Neurosci. **10:** 67-95.
37. MORRISON, J. H., R. GRAZANNA, M. MOLLIVER & J. T. COYLE. 1978. J. Comp. Neurol. **181:** 17-40.
38. MORRISON, J. H., M. E. MOLLIVER, R. GRZANNA & J. T. COYLE. 1979. Brain Res. Bull. **4:** 849-857.
39. LEVITT, P., P. RAKIC & P. GOLDMAN-RAKIC. 1984. J. Comp. Neurol. **227:** 23-36.
40. MORRISON, J. H., S. L. FOOTE, D. O'CONNOR & F. E. BLOOM. 1982. Brain Res. Bull **9:** 309-319.
41. MORRISON, J. H. & S. L. FOOTE. 1986. J. Comp. Neurol. **243:** 117-138.
42. MORRISON, J. H., S. L. FOOTE, M. E. MOLLIVER, F. E. BLOOM & H. G. W. LIDOV. 1982. Proc. Natl. Acad. Sci. USA **79:** 2401-2405.
43. MAGISTRETTI, P. J., J. H. MORRISON, W. J. SHOEMAKER, V. SAPIN & F. E. BLOOM. 1981. Proc. Natl. Acad. Sci. USA **78:** 6535-6539.

44. MAGISTRETTI, P. J., J. H. MORRISON, W. J. SHOEMAKER & F. E. BLOOM. 1983. Brain Res. **261:** 159-162.
45. MAGISTRETTI, P. J. & M. SCHORDERET. 1984. Nature **308:** 280-282.
46. MAGISTRETTI, P. J. & M. SCHORDERET. 1985. J. Neurosci. **5:** 362-368.
47. ASTON-JONES, G. & F. E. BLOOM. 1981. J. Neurosci. **1:** 876-886.
48. ASTON-JONES, G. & F. E. BLOOM. 1981. J. Neurosci. **1:** 887-900.
49. FERRON, A., G. R. SIGGINS & F. E. BLOOM. 1985. Proc. Natl. Acad. Sci. USA **82:** 8810-8812.

Vasoactive Intestinal Peptide in the Peripheral Nervous System[a]

F. SUNDLER,[b,c] E. EKBLAD,[c] T. GRUNDITZ,[e]
R. HÅKANSON,[d] AND R. UDDMAN[e]

[c]Department of Medical Cell Research and
[d]Department of Pharmacology
University of Lund
Lund, Sweden
and
[e]Department of Otolaryngology
Malmö General Hospital
Malmö, Sweden

About ten years ago the first reports appeared on the immunocytochemical localization of vasoactive intestinal peptide (VIP) in the central and peripheral nervous systems.[1-9] Already from these initial observations, it was apparent that VIP was a major neuropeptide in both the brain and the periphery, and that VIP-containing fibers were widely distributed, particularly in the cardiovascular system and in the respiratory, gastrointestinal, and genitourinary tracts where they innervated smooth muscle and glands. During the years that followed, an extensive literature emerged describing the occurrence and distribution of VIP-containing neuronal elements in peripheral organs and tissues.[10-13]

Although originally identified, as its name implies, on the basis of its strong vasodilator effect,[14] VIP possesses a wide spectrum of pharmacological actions on a number of target organs. These effects include stimulation of intestinal secretion,[15,16] inhibition of histamine- and pentagastrin- stimulated gastric acid secretion,[14,17] stimulation of pancreatic flow and bicarbonate secretion,[18,19] bronchodilatation,[20] gastric relaxation,[21] and induction of choleresis[22] and glycogenolysis.[23] In addition VIP stimulates lipolysis in fat cells[24] and releases thyroid hormones,[25,26] insulin, and glucagon (cf. Fahrenkrug et al.[27]). Clinically, VIP has attracted much interest because of its possible role in pancreatic cholera.[28]

A few years ago the amino acid sequence of the VIP precursor was elucidated.[29] The precursor was found to contain not only VIP but also peptide histidine isoleucine amide (PHI), a VIP-like peptide originally isolated from porcine intestine by Tatemoto and Mutt.[30] A common origin of VIP and PHI explained the observation that the two peptides coexisted in the same neurons in several peripheral organs.[31-33]

Below we review the distribution of VIP-containing nerve fibers in the periphery and discuss their possible functional roles. Also the origin of the VIP-containing fibers and the coexistence of VIP with other neuronal messenger compounds will be dealt with.

[a]Grant support was provided by the Swedish MRC (projects No. 4499, 6859, and 1007), from Albert Påhlsson's Foundation, and from the Swedish Diabetes Association.

[b]Address for correspondence: Dr. Frank Sundler, Department of Medical Cell Research, University of Lund, Biskopsgatan 5, S-223 62 Lund, Sweden.

CARDIOVASCULAR SYSTEM

Most peripheral blood vessels are supplied with VIP-containing nerve fibers (FIG. 1a and b). Comprehensive studies of the vascular innervation have been performed in the cat[34] and the guinea pig.[35] On the whole, VIP-containing fibers are numerous around arteries, while veins and venules are supplied with fewer VIP-containing fibers. Characteristic regional differences have been noted in the distribution of perivascular VIP-containing fibers. Pial vessels,[3,34,36–38] intestinal vessels (cf. Håkanson et al.[10] and Hökfelt et al.[11]), and vessels supplying the genitourinary tract[4–6] are notably rich in VIP-containing nerve fibers. At the other extreme are blood vessels in skeletal muscle,[39] liver, and kidney[34] that receive a comparatively scarce supply of VIP-containing nerve fibers. It is generally assumed that perivascular VIP-containing fibers arise mainly from ganglia situated close to or within the tissue (cf. Håkanson et al.[10]). In blood vessels supplying the head and neck, a contribution from major parasympathetic ganglia (e.g., the sphenopalatine and otic ganglia) is likely (cf. Gibbins et al.[38]).

There are several lines of evidence supporting the view that VIP-containing neurons of presumed parasympathetic nature are cholinergic (cf. Lundberg et al.[40] and Lundberg[41]). Thus, VIP is present in virtually all nerve cell bodies in cholinergic ganglia such as the sphenopalatine and otic ganglia.[42–44] This does not necessarily imply that acetylcholine and VIP occur in the same neurovesicles. Peptide-containing vesicles are transported via axonal transport from the cell body to the terminals. Once such a vesicle has released its content, it cannot be refilled with peptide. The terminals manufacture classical transmitters only. Thus, retrieval of a vesicle that previously contained peptides means that it can now be loaded to become a classical neurotransmitter-containing vesicle. Accordingly, VIP-containing nerve fibers (wherever they are found) seem to harbor two vesicle populations[43]: one consisting of fairly large (100 nm) dense-cored vesicles (peptide vesicles) and another consisting of small (40 nm) electron-lucent vesicles (retrieval vesicles?). VIP has been demonstrated immunocytochemically in the large dense-cored vesicles,[43,45–47] whereas acetylcholine seems to be associated mainly with small neurovesicles.[48] The vasodilation evoked by stimulation of VIP- and acetylcholine-containing nerves is biphasic. A differential storage of the two transmitter candidates within the neuron could explain the observation made in several tissues that continuous low-frequency stimulation gives rise to responses that are predominantly atropine-sensitive, whereas high-frequency stimulation, particularly when applied in bursts, induces predominantly atropine-resistant responses.[4,49–51] Under these latter conditions, the release of VIP is greatly enhanced.[41,49–52] The release of acetylcholine from the acetylcholine/VIP-containing nerves seems to be feedback regulated via a muscarinic autoreceptor. Consequently, disinhibition may explain why atropine treatment leads to enhanced release of acetylcholine.[53–55] Acetylcholine inhibits the release of VIP via muscarinic autoreceptors,[41] and VIP acting at VIP receptors inhibits the release of acetylcholine.[41,56]

Several studies have dealt with the VIP innervation of the portal vein showing that VIP is released in response to electrical field stimulation.[57] VIP effectively inhibits the mechanical activity of the rat portal vein.[58,59] Most of the neurogenic dilatation of the portal vein of the rabbit persists in the presence of adrenergic and cholinergic antagonists.[60]

It is conceivable that VIP plays an important physiological role in cardiovascular physiology and pathology. Nilsson and Bill[61] studied the effect of VIP on regional blood flow in rabbits. The doses used did not affect the arterial blood pressure. The most pronounced vasodilation was observed in the pancreas, the thyroid gland, and the parotid gland. In these tissues local blood flow increased by more than 100%. VIP also produced marked vasodilation in the stomach but had no effect on the blood flow in the small intestine (the dose used was too low). Interestingly, there was no correlation between the density of innervation and the vasodilatory response to VIP; blood vessels in the small intestine, which have a rich VIP nerve supply, did not respond, while vasodilation was observed in the less densely innervated heart muscle.[35]

In the heart VIP-containing fibers are present in close contact not only with the vasculature, but also with nodal cells, juxtanodal intracardiac ganglia, and single intranodal ganglionic cells.[62,63] VIP exerts a positive inotropic effect in dog.[64] De Neef *et al.*[65] studied monkey heart and reported that VIP increased the rate of beating of the isolated right atrium as well as the contractility of both atria. VIP also stimulated the contractility of papillary muscle and the authors concluded that VIP exerts a direct chronotropic and inotropic effect. In man it acts as a coronary vasodilator[66] and as a positive chronotropic agent,[67] the latter effect possibly being attributable to the hypotensive effect of the peptide. Recently, an inotropic effect of VIP has also been demonstrated in the human heart.[68]

RESPIRATORY TRACT

VIP-containing fibers are numerous in the mammalian nasal mucosa where they occur beneath the surface epithelium and around blood vessels; a moderate supply of such fibers is also seen around seromucous glands (FIG. 1c).[69] The fibers derive from the sphenopalatine ganglion (FIG. 1d).[44] Electrical stimulation of the Vidian nerve results in an atropine-sensitive nasal secretion and an atropine-resistant vasodilatation.[70,71] Electrical stimulation of chronically sympathectomized cats induced a frequency-dependent increase in the VIP concentration in nasal venous blood.[31,33] After atropine treatment, the VIP output was somewhat reduced following electrical stimulation of the Vidian nerve while hexamethonium pretreatment almost totally abolished the rise in VIP.[72] This effect may be due to blockade of preganglionic cholinergic fibers terminating on VIP-containing nerve cell bodies in the sphenopalatine ganglion.[73] VIP given intraarterially close to the nose induced an atropine-resistant dilatation of both resistance and capacitance vessels.[74] Methacholine promotes mucoglycoprotein secretion from the lateral nasal gland of the dog. VIP, on the other hand, was without effect in concentrations that have powerful vasodilator effects.[75] This seems to be compatible with the view that the postganglionic parasympathetic mediation of nasal secretion is mainly cholinergic, whereas vasodilatation is mediated predominantly by noncholinergic mechanisms. VIP (and PHI) have emerged as strong candidates for mediating the latter response.

In the tracheobronchial region VIP-containing fibers are numerous around vascular and nonvascular smooth muscle bundles and close to seromucous glands. The fibers probably originate from the nodose ganglion, from nerve cell bodies in small ganglia scattered along laryngeal branches of the vagus nerve and from small ganglionic formations in the tracheal wall.[33,69,76-78] Isolated precontracted tracheobronchial smooth muscle and pulmonary and bronchial arteries relaxed upon exposure to VIP.[79-82] In addition, VIP may regulate fluid secretion over the surface epithelium in the respiratory tract.[83] Mapping of VIP receptors by autoradiography revealed binding sites on blood vessels, smooth muscle bundles, seromucous glands, and surface epithelium.[84] Immunocytochemical studies have suggested the existence of several distinct VIP-con-

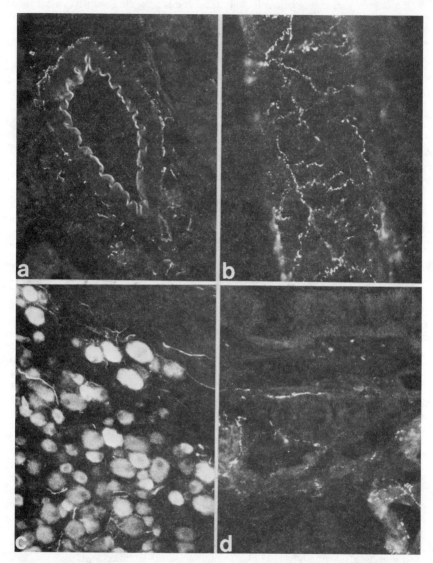

FIGURE 1. Numerous perivascular VIP-containing nerve fibers in (a) artery of rat tongue (cryostat section) and (b) guinea pig pial artery (whole mount preparation). (c) Cat sphenopalatine ganglion (cryostat section). Virtually all nerve cell bodies are VIP-immunoreactive. (d) Cat nasal mucosa (cryostat section). VIP-containing nerve fibers surround seromucous glands and blood vessels. Original magnifications: (a) ×180, (b) ×200, (c) ×175, (d) ×175; all reduced by 10%.

taining nerve fiber populations in the respiratory tract of the rat. In one subpopulation VIP coexists with neuropeptide Y (NPY) (Uddman *et al.,* unpublished observations) and in another VIP coexists with galanin.[85]

THE GASTROINTESTINAL TRACT

VIP has a widespread distribution in the digestive tract of both mammals and nonmammals. It occurs in large amounts in the gut of man, pig, dog, cat, rat (*cf.* Fahrenkrug[86]), and guinea pig (*cf.* Furness *et al.*[87]), as well as of birds[88] and fish.[89,90] In the cat the highest VIP concentrations were found in sphincteric regions.[91]

It is generally agreed that in the gut of mammals VIP is confined to neuronal elements,[92] with the possible exception of the cat where immunoreactive VIP occurs in a population of endocrine cells in the antrum.[2,93] In lower vertebrates there is evidence for the existence of VIP or VIP-like peptides in endocrine cells in the gut.[89,94–96]

Distribution and Topography of Enteric VIP-Containing Nerves

VIP-containing nerve fibers are numerous in all layers throughout the mammalian gastrointestinal tract (FIG. 2; *cf.* Håkanson *et al.*[10] and Furness & Costa[97]). The submucous ganglia harbor many more VIP-immunoreactive cell bodies (45% of all submucous neurons) than the myenteric ganglia (2.5% of all myenteric neurons) as studied in the guinea pig small intestine.[98] Also in the avian gastrointestinal tract, VIP-containing nerve fibers occur in all layers,[88,94,95] and VIP-containing nerve cell bodies are numerous in the submucous ganglia (27%) but few in the myenteric ganglia (2%).[88,95]

In reptiles and amphibians VIP-immunoreactive nerve fibers are numerous in all layers throughout the gut, particularly in the stomach and duodenum.[95,99] Immunoreactive nerve cells occur in both submucous and myenteric ganglia, however, less frequently than in mammals.

VIP immunoreactive nerve fibers have been reported to occur in many species of bony and cartilaginous fish.[89,95,96,100–103] The fibers are mainly myenteric; only a few fibers have been observed in the mucosa and submucosa, mainly associated with blood vessels. Scattered VIP-immunoreactive nerve cell bodies have been reported in both submucous ganglia[95] and myenteric ganglia.[100] In some bony fish[95] VIP-immunoreactive endocrine cells have been observed, predominantly in the upper part of the gut. In two species of cartilaginous fish, the ray[89,96] and the shark,[95] VIP-immunoreactive endocrine cells occur in all parts of the intestine. They are particularly numerous in the colon where they form an almost continuous layer basally in the epithelium. Finally, VIP-immunoreactive nerve fibers have been demonstrated in the gut wall of an insect, the cockroach.[104]

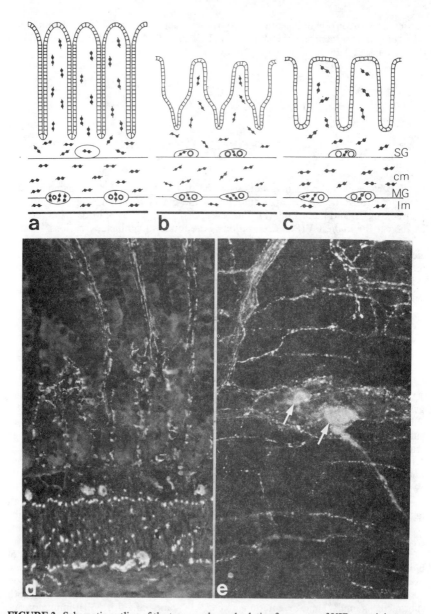

FIGURE 2. Schematic outline of the topography and relative frequency of VIP-containing nerve
fibers -•-•- and nerve cell bodies (○) in the rat stomach (**a**), small intestine (**b**), and large
intestine (**c**). SG, submucous ganglia; cm, circular muscle; MG, myenteric ganglia; lm, longitudinal muscle. (**d**) Rat jejunum, cryostat section. Numerous VIP-containing nerve fibers in the
mucosa, submucosa, smooth muscle, and intramural ganglia. (**e**) Rat jejunum, whole-mount
preparation of the outer longitudinal smooth muscle with adherent myenteric ganglia. Numerous
VIP-containing nerve fibers and two VIP-containing nerve cell bodies (arrows) can be seen.
Original magnifications: (d) ×150, (e) ×175; both reduced by 10%.

Origin and Projections of VIP-Containing Enteric Nerve Fibers

The great majority of VIP-containing nerves in the gastrointestinal tract are intrinsic in origin. This conclusion is based on the finding of numerous VIP nerve cell bodies in both the submucous and myenteric ganglia (see above), and the fact that extrinsic denervation fails to affect the VIP nerve supply of the gut.[97,105-108]

Within the rat intestine, VIP-containing fibers originating in the submucous ganglia seem to terminate mainly in other submucous ganglia and in the mucosa with ascending projections up to 4 mm long in the small intestine[108] and up to 2 mm long in the large intestine.[109] Myenteric VIP-containing neurons send descending projections to other myenteric ganglia and to the smooth muscle layer; these fibers are approximately 6 mm long in guinea pig small intestine,[106] approximately 2 mm long in the rat small intestine (FIG. 3),[108] approximately 4 mm long in the rat large intestine,[109] and up to 20 mm in the dog ileum.[110]

Enteric VIP-containing fibers have also been shown to terminate in ganglia located outside the intestines such as the celiac and the inferior mesenteric ganglia.[106,111]

VIP Release from Enteric Neurons

The gastrointestinal tract is a major source of endogenous VIP released into the portal circulation. Several investigators have demonstrated VIP release following vagal stimulation[112,113] and various intramural stimuli including gastric distension,[114] intraduodenal administration of HC1, ethanol, and fats,[115] and jejunal administration of hypertonic saline.[116] Reid *et al.*[117] proposed that VIP is released from inhibitory neurons involved in relaxation of the stomach and that the entry of food in the small intestine causes release of VIP. VIP seems to increase in portal but not in peripheral blood after a test meal.[114,115,118,119] For VIP to exert a systemic effect, it must first traverse the liver and the efficiency of the liver in extracting VIP from portal blood is therefore an important factor in determining its physiological role as a circulating agent. There is abundant evidence that VIP is cleared as it passes through the liver (cf. Brook *et al.*[120]). Misbin *et al.*[121] demonstrated that VIP binds to specific, high-affinity hepatocyte receptors and is internalized and degraded by lysosomes. Hepatic clearance of VIP[122] may therefore account for the lack of detectable increases in peripheral blood in situations when portal plasma VIP is elevated.[118] On the whole therefore, it seems likely that under normal circumstances the actions of VIP are exerted locally, close to the terminals from which it is released.

Coexistence with Other Neurotransmitters

Our knowledge of the coexistence of VIP with "classical" transmitters is very limited as far as the gut is concerned. VIP-containing neurons have been found to be identical with acetylcholinesterase-positive ones in the rat duodenum and have therefore been interpreted as cholinergic.[123] This observation is in contrast to findings in

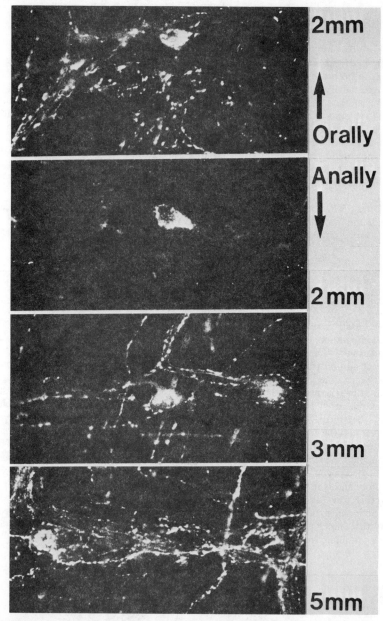

FIGURE 3. VIP-containing nerve fibers and cell bodies in rat jejunum, 10 days after myectomy. Whole mounts of longitudinal smooth muscle with adherent myenteric ganglia. No loss of VIP-immunoreactive fibers orally to the lesion. Up to 2 mm anally to the lesion the number of VIP-containing nerve fibers was markedly reduced. More distally, the nerve fiber frequency gradually normalized. The occurrence and distribution of VIP-containing nerve cell bodies were not affected by the lesion. Original magnification ×225; reduced by 10%.

the guinea pig small intestine where VIP-immunoreactive nerve fibers seem to be distinct from those that contain immunoreactive choline acetyltransferase.[124]

More information is available with respect to the coexistence of VIP and other neuropeptides. The coexistence of VIP and PHI[31–33,125] could be predicted since the two peptides share the same precursor. In pig stomach, VIP fibers have been reported to be more numerous than PHI fibers.[126] This discrepancy could not be confirmed in studies of the stomach of rat and mouse[107] and is most probably related to the specificity of the PHI antisera used. Recent studies have revealed relatively large amounts of COOH-terminally extended forms of PHI in stomach extracts.[127] Such forms will not be recognized by all PHI antibodies.

VIP is also reported to coexist with neuropeptides that have no relation to the VIP precursor. Thus, subpopulations of myenteric VIP-containing neurons in the guinea pig small intestine have been found to contain immunoreactive cholecystokinin, enkephalin, dynorphin, gastrin-releasing peptide (GRP), and NPY in various combinations (cf. Costa *et al.*[98]). Immunoreactive NPY has been demonstrated in the entire population of myenteric VIP-containing neurons in the rat stomach and in both myenteric and submucous VIP-containing neurons of the mouse stomach.[107] Submucous VIP-containing neurons in the rat stomach seem to harbor GRP rather than NPY (Ekblad *et al.*, unpublished). In the small intestine of rat, mouse, and pig, all VIP-containing neurons seem to store NPY (FIG. 4).[32] In the rat colon a few VIP-containing neurons store NPY.[109] Further, in the rat colon some intrinsic perivascular VIP-containing nerve fibers also harbor calcitonin gene-related peptide (CGRP).[109] Galanin has also been reported to coexist with VIP in intramural neurons in the guinea pig and pig small intestine.[128]

VIP-Containing Nerves in Pathophysiological Conditions

Achalasia of the esophagus and gastro-esophageal reflux are both associated with failure to regulate the lower esophageal sphincter properly. Achalasia is characterized by an increased tone in the lower esophageal sphincter and a reduced number of nerve cells in the myenteric ganglia. Patients with hiatus hernia and gastro-esophageal reflux have reduced pressure in the lower sphincter region. Specimens taken from the lower esophageal sphincter region of patients suffering from achalasia had a reduced content of immunoreactive VIP and a lower number of VIP-containing nerve fibers than control specimens. In contrast, specimens taken from patients with hiatus hernia and severe gastro-esophageal reflux had an elevated concentration of immunoreactive VIP and an increased number of VIP fibers.[129] Hirschsprung's disease (aganglionic megacolon) is characterized by a lack of nerve cell bodies in a segment of the distal colon. This deficiency is associated with local constriction and a consequent proximal enlargement of the gut. VIP nerve fibers are greatly reduced in number or absent in the muscle layers of the aganglionic (constricted) segment (FIG. 4).[130–133] The supply of mucosal VIP-containing fibers in the aganglionic segment is much less affected.[134]

Crohn's disease, a segmental inflammatory bowel disease, is accompanied by an increase in the number of intramural ganglion cells and in the number and thickness of enteric nerve fibers.[135] This includes the VIP-containing nerve fibers in the afflicted segment of the bowel, which are thickened, coarse, and intensely immunostained.[136,137]

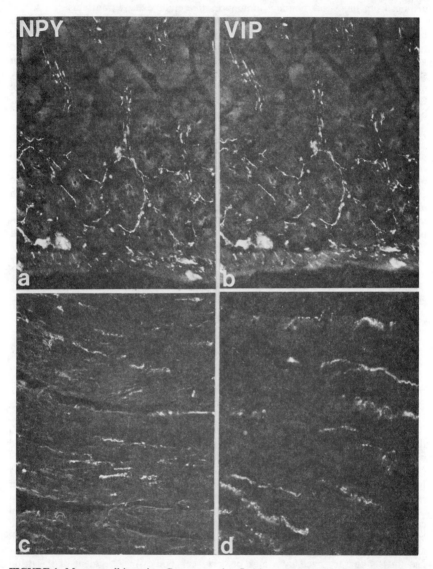

FIGURE 4. Mouse small intestine: Cryostat section first immunostained for NPY (**a**) and then for VIP (**b**) after removal of the NPY antibodies. Note coexistence of NPY and VIP immunoreactivity in the same nerve cell bodies and nerve fibers. Human colon: VIP-immunoreactive nerve fibers in smooth muscle from a control patient (**c**) and a patient with Crohn's disease (**d**). VIP-containing fibers in afflicted smooth muscle are more coarse than in the control. Original magnification (a–d): ×150; all reduced by 10%.

Functional Aspects

VIP relaxes intestinal smooth muscle[138] and has been proposed to be a relaxatory neurotransmitter.[139] VIP neurons may play a part in mediating the atropine-resistant receptive relaxation of the stomach following swallowing and also the hyperemia of the intestinal mucosa that occurs during digestive activity. Evidence for VIP as a causal agent in both these phenomena has been provided by observations of the effects of exogenous VIP.[140,141] Also, when receptive relaxation and intestinal hyperemia were stimulated by nervous reflexes, VIP increased in the gastric and intestinal venous effluents.[113]

Three nerve-mediated vasodilator mechanisms in the feline intestines are accompanied by release of VIP.[113,142] The three mechanisms are: (1) vasodilation in the small intestine evoked by mechanical mucosal stimulation, (2) increase in intestinal blood flow occurring upon intraarterial infusion of 5-HT, and (3) colonic vasodilation evoked by pelvic nerve stimulation. Jodal *et al.*[143] showed that these vasodilator responses were diminished or totally abolished by the bee venom peptide, apamin. Concomitantly, the release of VIP was also markedly reduced.[144]

It has been suggested that VIP might play a role in the neural control of intestinal and gallbladder mucosal fluid transport. Cassuto *et al.*[145,146] demonstrated the involvement of cholinergic nicotinic receptors in the nervous reflexes that are important in cholera toxin induced intestinal secretion and the release of VIP from intestines exposed to cholera toxin. These observations might suggest that VIP neurons play a role in cholera and that they are supplied with nicotinic receptors.[146] VIP nerves are numerous close to the feline and human gallbladder epithelium[9] and specific VIP receptors occur in gallbladder epithelial cells.[147] Intravenous infusion of VIP stimulates gallbladder mucosal fluid secretion by a direct action on the epithelial cells.[148,149]

GENITOURINARY TRACT

VIP-containing nerve fibers occur in the smooth muscle all along the genitourinary tract as studied in several mammals (FIG. 5).[4-6,150,151] The fibers are particularly numerous in regions having a sphincter function, such as the uterine cervix, the neck region of the bladder, and the distal portion of the ureters at their entrance into the bladder wall. VIP-containing fibers are also fairly numerous in the mucosa of the uterine cervix, the vas deferens, the urinary bladder, and the urethra. VIP nerves are found in the oviducts and ovaries of some mammals and in the vaginal wall of all species (*cf.* Ottesen *et al.*[151]). In the female genital tract the highest concentrations of VIP were found in the uterus, particularly in the cervix region. Pregnancy induced approximately 50% reduction in the content of VIP in the rat uterine horns (changes were less marked in the cervix). The change was associated with a reduced number of visible VIP-containing nerve fibers. The innervation was back to normal 25 days following delivery.[152] In the male genital tract the prostate gland was found to receive a rich supply of VIP-containing fibers distributed around the glandular acini and the blood vessels. VIP nerve fibers were fairly numerous in penile tissues of rat, rabbit, cat, monkey, and man, particularly in the erectile tissue, including blood vessels and intrinsic smooth muscle.[4,153-156]

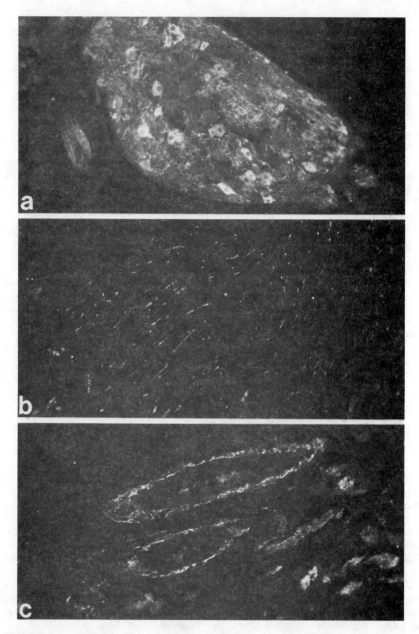

FIGURE 5. Cat, cryostat sections: (a) Paraurethral ganglion with numerous VIP-containing nerve cell bodies and nerve fibers. (b) Vas deferens with a moderate number of VIP-containing nerve fibers in the smooth muscle. (c) Prostate gland with numerous VIP-containing nerve fibers surrounding blood vessels and running in nerve bundles in the stroma. Magnification: a, ×100; b and c, ×125.

The vascular smooth muscle and intrinsic smooth muscle of penile erectile tissue are under the control of the autonomic nervous system. An essential mechanism in penile erection is dilation of the vessels supplying the corpus cavernosum whereby the organ is filled with blood. The most important nervous pathway, mediating the relaxation, is the sacral parasympathetic nerves that constitute the "nervii erigentes." Acetylcholine has been put forward as one of the vasodilator compounds responsible. It is unlikely to be of major significance, however, since local infusion of acetylcholine does not induce erection and since atropine does not prevent erection evoked by stimulation of the pelvic nerve.[157] A noncholinergic mechanism seems more likely. VIP reduces spontaneous contractile activity of isolated corpus cavernosum smooth muscle from several species.[153–155] Upon infusion, it causes erection. Hence, VIP is the only known putative neurotransmitter that is found in nerves associated with the corpus cavernosum and that is capable of causing noncholinergic, nonadrenergic relaxation of penile smooth muscle and penile erection upon local infusion.

VIP was found to inhibit smooth muscle activity in the feline vas deferens[158] and the electrically induced twitch in the mouse[159] but had no direct or indirect effects on the smooth muscle of the guinea pig vas deferens and seminal vesicle.[160] VIP inhibited the spontaneous motor activity of the uterine smooth muscle.[151,161] This effect was more pronounced in the cervix than in the corpus uteri.[161] VIP reduced the spontaneous rhythmic activity of the rat uterine cervix and caused a dose-dependent inhibition of contractions evoked by electrical field stimulation. Stjernquist and Owman[162] suggested that VIP affects not only the smooth muscle cells but also the cholinergic nerves of the rat uterine cervix. VIP is a potent inhibitor of spontaneous and nerve-induced tubal motor activity,[163,164] and it has been suggested that VIP may be the neurotransmitter that mediates the relaxation of the isthmic sphincter.[163] VIP-containing fibers in the genitourinary tract seem to have a local origin in paraurethral and paracervical ganglia, which harbor numerous VIP-containing nerve cell bodies (cf. Alm *et al.:*[150] and Mattiasson *et al.*[165]).

The kidney seems also to be a target of VIP. The effects of VIP on renal function appear to be complex, involving hemodynamic, secretory, and excretory actions.[166–170] Some evidence exists that VIP acts predominantly on the tubular system rather than on the vascular or glomerular compartments.[170,171]

ENDOCRINE GLANDS

Many endocrine glands harbor VIP-containing nerve fibers. In the adenohypophysis such fibers are few and scattered (Sundler, unpublished), whereas they are numerous in the thyroid gland (FIG. 6a and b)[25,172,173] and the adrenal cortex (FIG. 6c).[10,174,175] In the thyroid the VIP-containing fibers occur around blood vessels and follicles (FIG. 6a). The origin of the VIP-containing fibers in the thyroid has been studied in the rat and mouse. Most of the fibers originate in the so-called thyroid ganglion, which is situated outside the thyroid capsule at the dorsomedial aspect (FIG. 6b).[172,173] VIP stimulated thyroid hormone secretion *in vivo* (mice)[25,172] and *in vitro* (dog)[26] and enhanced TSH-induced hormone secretion.[25,176] VIP was found to stimulate cyclic AMP production in the mouse thyroid[25] and to enhance thyroid blood flow.[61,177]

In the adrenal cortex VIP-containing fibers form a dense plexus beneath the capsule. From this plexus single fibers penetrate radially into the cortical tissue (FIG. 6c).[10,174,175] Many of these fibers run close to the cortical cells. VIP-containing fibers occur in

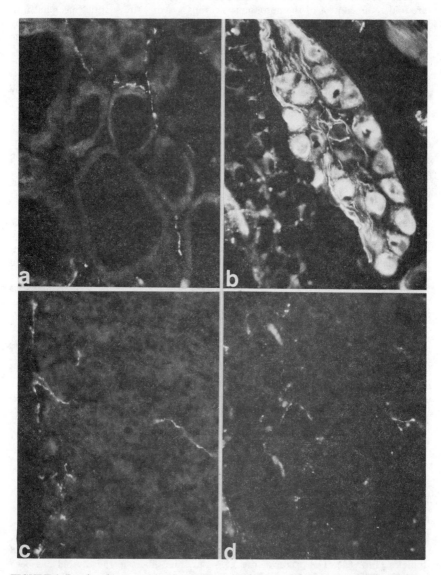

FIGURE 6. Rat thyroid, cryostat sections: VIP-containing nerve fibers ramify among the follicles (a). VIP immunoreactive nerve cell bodies and nerve fibers are numerous in the thyroid ganglion (b). (c) Rat adrenal cortex, cryostat section. VIP-containing nerve fibers form a plexus beneath the capsule (left in fig) with single fibers penetrating into the cortical tissue. (d) Cat pineal gland: VIP-containing nerve fibers occur scattered in the parenchyma. Original magnifications: a and b ×200, c and d ×175; all reduced by 10%.

moderate numbers in the testes and the ovaries, both around blood vessels and in the stroma.[4,5,150] It has been suggested from studies on isolated cells[178,179] and from animal experiments that VIP participates in the regulation of steroid hormone synthesis and secretion. Thus, VIP-stimulated progesterone secretion in the female rabbit,[180,181] and Ahmed *et al.*[182] reported that the rat ovary responds to VIP with steroid secretion. Ottesen *et al.*[183] recently reported that VIP raised serum estradiol and testosterone concentrations in normal women. There was no effect on progesterone or cortisol. They concluded that the stimulatory effect of VIP might reflect a direct action on the ovary or the adrenal gland. This conclusion is supported by the observation that VIP stimulates steroidogenesis in cultured granulosa cells.[184]

Also the pancreatic islets receive VIP-containing nerve fibers; they often form a loose plexus in the peripheral parts of the islet. Both VIP and PHI stimulate pancreatic endocrine secretion in experimental animals.[185–187] Intravenous infusion of VIP evoked a moderate increase in basal insulin secretion in mice. In addition, VIP potentiated glucose- and isoprenaline-evoked insulin secretion.[188] Intravenous infusion of fairly large amounts of VIP to healthy volunteers stimulated secretion of insulin, C-peptide and glucagon. The human variety of PHI, PHM, did not have this effect. Fahrenkrug *et al.*[27] concluded that VIP is a likely neurotransmitter in control of the endocrine pancreas while PHM is not. The pineal gland, finally, receives numerous VIP-containing fibers as studied in several mammals (FIG. 6d).[189]

EXOCRINE GLANDS

Several studies have dealt with the occurrence, distribution, and functional role of VIP-containing nerve fibers in exocrine glands, notably the salivary glands[41,190,191] and the pancreas.[192,193] In all these glands VIP-containing nerve fibers are numerous around blood vessels and glandular acini (FIG. 7a and c).

It is generally assumed that VIP-containing fibers in exocrine glands are parasympathetic. This assumption is supported by the presence of numerous VIP-storing nerve cell bodies in parasympathetic ganglia supplying exocrine glands and in small local ganglia of presumed parasympathetic nature located close to or within the glandular parenchyma (FIG. 7b and d).[33,40,41,44,191–193]

Several reports indicated that VIP has no or only a weak sialogogic effect.[40,194] However, VIP was found to induce a flow of saliva from both the parotid and the submaxillary gland in the rat,[195] and parotid glands in the rat responded to VIP with amylase secretion.[196,197] The effect of VIP was direct; it occurred after removal of the adrenals, after degeneration of intraglandular nerves, and in the presence of autonomic blockers. Local infusions of acetylcholine induced both vasodilation and salivary secretion in the submandibular gland of the cat. Although VIP in the cat caused vasodilation but no secretion per se, it enhanced the secretory response to acetylcholine.[49,198] The VIP-induced potentiation of cholinergic salivary secretion may be in part due to the additional increase in blood flow and in part to a direct effect of VIP on secretory elements.[199–201] VIP was found to potentiate the salivary secretion induced by acetylcholine from the cat submandibular gland.[201] VIP increased muscarinic ligand binding in this tissue suggesting that the peptide, which is costored and coreleased with acetylcholine, could increase the affinity of muscarinic receptors for the primary transmitter.[198]

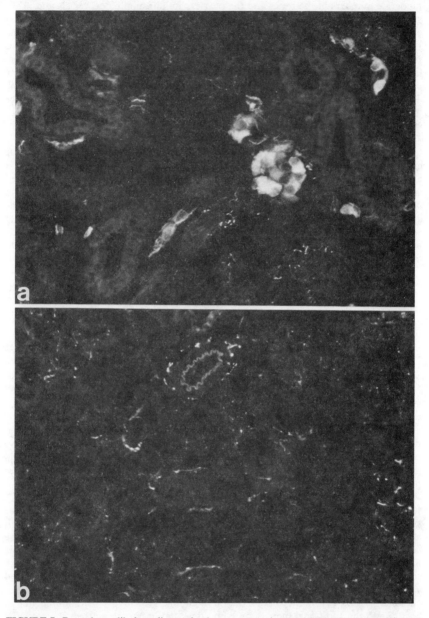

FIGURE 7. Rat submandibular salivary gland, cryostat sections. (a) VIP-containing nerve cell bodies in ganglionic formations located close to the salivary ducts. (b) Numerous VIP-containing nerve fibers around blood vessels and penetrating in between the glandular acini. Magnification: both a and b ×140.

Electrical stimulation of the vagus caused an atropine-resistant profuse secretion of fluid and bicarbonate from the pancreas[202,203] that cannot be accounted for by the release of secretin.[203] Under these conditions a splanchnic release of VIP could be demonstrated[204] and part of the VIP output was from the pancreas.[205] VIP, like secretin, stimulates pancreatic flow and bicarbonate output, but its efficacy in this respect appears to be species dependent[206] and to depend on the mode of administration.[207] In an elegant series of experiments using the isolated perfused pig pancreas with intact vagal nerve supply, Holst and coworkers[208] provided evidence for the view that VIP is responsible for at least part of the neurally controlled fluid and bicarbonate secretion.

SENSORY AND SYMPATHETIC NEURONS

There are several reports suggesting the presence of VIP in sensory neurons. Thus, VIP has been demonstrated in nerve fibers in the dorsal horn of the spinal cord[209,210] and in a minor population of nerve cell bodies in the dorsal root ganglia at the lumbar and sacral levels (about 5% of the cell bodies in the feline dorsal root ganglia at the levels L7 and S2).[211–213] The number of VIP-immunoreactive nerve cell bodies increased markedly after exposure to colchicine (*cf.* de Groat[214]). Leah *et al.*[213] in addition described complex patterns of coexistence of VIP and other neuropeptides in these ganglia. Thus, some of the VIP-containing cell bodies were found to harbor SP and/ or somatostatin (see also de Groat[214]). Interestingly, the level of VIP (and PHI) increased markedly after peripheral nerve injury both in dorsal root ganglia and in the dorsal horn of the spinal cord.[215–218] Whether VIP is present also in the peripheral ramifications of sensory neurons has yet to be established. The function of VIP in sensory neurons is unclear.

Immunocytochemistry has provided evidence for the presence of a few VIP-containing nerve cell bodies in various sympathetic ganglia, such as the superior cervical ganglion,[44,173] the stellate and lumbar sympathetic ganglia of the rat,[219] and thoracic sympathetic ganglia of the pig.[220] It has been suggested that VIP-containing fibers arising from cell bodies in sympathetic ganglia may innervate certain blood vessels,[41] sweat glands,[219] and bone tissue.[220]

VIP-RECEPTOR INTERACTIONS

VIP appears to be highly conserved among mammals since identical sequences have been reported in rat,[221] dog,[222] pig,[223] cow,[224] and man.[29] Guinea pig VIP, however, differs in positions 5, 9, 19, and 26.[225] Interestingly, guinea pig VIP is equipotent with the more common type of VIP in binding to pancreatic acini from the guinea pig and in stimulating amylase release from these acini.[226] Marie *et al.*[227] recently reported that modification of positions 10 and 17 does not interfere with the biological activity and that iodination of tyrosine in position 22 actually increased the effectiveness of VIP interaction with its receptors.

The VIP fragments VIP_{1-6}, VIP_{1-10}, VIP_{18-28}, VIP_{15-28}, and VIP_{7-28} have been compared with authentic VIP in different test systems. The fragments showed no or weak bioactivity.[228–230] The results of these studies suggested that both the NH_2-

terminal and the COOH-terminal portions of VIP were essential. Two peptides were synthesized where VIP_{1-6} or VIP_{1-9} were joined with VIP_{20-28} or VIP_{21-28}, respectively, with the consequent omission of the midportion of VIP. These peptides had no detectable bioactivity.[231] Also Gly^{17-19} VIP was tested; it had very weak VIP-like bioactivity in high concentrations. The results suggest that not only the NH_2-terminal and COOH-terminal parts but also the midportion of VIP is important for full bioactivity.

The first step in VIP's action on its target cell is its binding to specific cell surface receptors that are usually coupled to adenylate cyclase.[171,232-239] Raiteri et al.[240] recently suggested another second messenger coupling by showing that VIP potentiated the stimulation by acetylcholine of phosphoinositide turnover in rat brain.

It should perhaps be mentioned that binding sites for VIP may not always represent functionally important receptors and that they may interact with other peptides of the secretin-glucagon-VIP family. Recently, helodermin, a novel peptide with VIP-like properties, has been demonstrated in mammalian tissues, notably thyroid C cells.[241] The ability of helodermin to act on VIP receptors[242] and the possibility that VIP acts on helodermin receptors illustrates the difficulty in discriminating between receptors to related peptides.

REFERENCES

1. BRYANT, M. G., S. R. BLOOM, J. M. POLAK, R. H. ALBUQUERQUE, I. MODLIN & A. G. E. PEARSE. 1976. Lancet I: 991-993.
2. LARSSON, L.-I., J. FAHRENKRUG, O. SCHAFFALITZKY DE MUCKADELL, F. SUNDLER, R. HÅKANSON & J. F. REHFELD. 1976. Proc. Natl. Acad. Sci. USA 73: 3197-3200.
3. LARSSON, L.-I., L. EDVINSSON, J. FAHRENKRUG, R. HÅKANSON, CH. OWMAN, O. B. SCHAFFALITZKY DE MUCKADELL & F. SUNDLER. 1976. Brain Res. 113: 400-404.
4. LARSSON, L.-I., J. FAHRENKRUG & O. B. SCHAFFALITZKY DE MUCKADELL. 1977. Life Sci. 21: 503-508.
5. LARSSON, L.-I., J. FAHRENKRUG & O. B. SCHAFFALITZKY DE MUCKADELL. 1977. Science 197: 1374-1375.
6. ALM, P., J. ALUMETS, R. HÅKANSON & F. SUNDLER. 1977. Neuroscience 2: 751-754.
7. FUXE, K., T. HÖKFELT, S. I. SAID & V. MUTT. 1977. Neurosci. Lett. 5: 241-246.
8. HÖKFELT, T., L.-G. ELFVIN, M. SCHULTZBERG, K. FUXE, S. I. SAID, V. MUTT & M. GOLDSTEIN. 1977. Neuroscience 2: 885-896.
9. SUNDLER, F., J. ALUMETS, R. HÅKANSON, S. INGEMANSSON, J. FAHRENKRUG & O. B. SCHAFFALITZKY DE MUCKADELL. 1977. Gastroenterology 72: 1375-1377.
10. HÅKANSON, R., F. SUNDLER, & R. UDDMAN. 1982. In Vasoactive Intestinal Peptide. S. I. Said, Ed.: 121-144. Raven Press. New York.
11. HÖKFELT, T., M. SCHULTZBERG, J. M. LUNDBERG, K. FUXE, J. FAHRENKRUG & S. I. SAID. 1982. In Vasoactive Intestinal Peptide. S. I. Said, Ed.: 65-90. Raven Press. New York.
12. LARSSON, L.-I. 1982. In Vasoactive Intestinal Peptide. S. I. Said, Ed.: 51-63. Raven Press. New York.
13. POLAK, J. M. & S. R. BLOOM. 1982 In Vasoactive Intestinal Peptide, S. I. Said, Ed.: 107-120. Raven Press. New York.
14. SAID, S. I. & V. MUTT. 1970. Science 169: 1217-1218.
15. PEARSE, A. G. E., J. M. POLAK & S. R. BLOOM. 1977. Gastroenterology 72: 746-761.
16. KREJS, G., R. M. BARKELY, N. W. READ & J. S. FORDTRAN. 1978. J. Clin. Invest. 61: 1337-1345.
17. EL MUNSHID, H. A., R. HÅKANSON, G. LIEDBERG & F. SUNDLER. 1980. J. Physiol. 305: 249-265.

18. KONTUREK, S. J., A. PUCHER & R. RADECKI. 1976. J. Physiol. **255:** 497-509.
19. DOMSCHKE, S., W. DOMSCHKE, W. ROSCH, S. J. KONTUREK, W. SPRUGEL, P. MITZNEGG, E. WUNSCH & L. DEMLING. 1977. Gastroenterology **73:** 478-480.
20. MORICE, A., R. J. UNWIN & P. S. SEVES. 1983. Lancet **II:** 1225-1227.
21. BITAR, K. N. & G. M. MAKHLOUF. 1982. Science **216:** 531-535.
22. THULIN, L. & M. HELLGREN. 1976. Acta Chir. Scand. **142:** 235-237.
23. MATSUMARA, M., H. AKIYOSHI & S. FUJI. 1977. J. Biochem. (Tokyo) **82:** 1073-1076.
24. FRANDSEN, E. K. & A. J. MOODY. 1973. Horm. Metab. Res. **5:** 196-199.
25. AHRÉN, B., J. ALUMETS, M. ERICSSON, J. FAHRENKRUG, R. HÅKANSON, P. HEDNER, I. LORÉN, A. MELANDER, C. RERUP & F. SUNDLER. 1980. Nature **287:** 343-345.
26. LAURBERG, P. 1986. Horm. Metab. Res. **18:** 230-233.
27. FAHRENKRUG, J., J. HOLST PEDERSEN, Y. YAMASHITA, B. OTTESEN, T. HÖKFELT & J. M. LUNDBERG. 1987. Regul. Peptides **18:** 51-61.
28. MODLIN, I. M., S. R. BLOOM & S. J. MITCHELL. 1978. Gastroenterology **75:** 1051-1054.
29. ITOH, N., K. I. OBATA, N. YANAIHARA & H. OKAMOTA. 1983. Nature **304:** 547-549.
30. TATEMOTO, K. & V. MUTT. 1981. Proc. Natl. Acad. Sci. USA **78:** 6603-6607.
31. YANAIHARA, N., K. NOKIHARA, C. YANAIHARA, T. IWANAGA & T. FUJITA. 1983. Arch. Histol. Jpn. **46:** 575-581.
32. EKBLAD, E., R. HÅKANSON & F. SUNDLER. 1984. Regul. Peptides **10:** 47-55.
33. LUNDBERG, J., J. FAHRENKRUG, T. HÖKFELT, C.-R. MARTLING, O. LARSSON, K. TATEMOTO & A. ÄNGGÅRD. 1984. Peptides **5:** 593-606.
34. UDDMAN, R., J. ALUMETS, L. EDVINSSON, R. HÅKANSON & F. SUNDLER. 1981. Acta Physiol. Scand. **112:** 65-70.
35. DELLA, N. G., R. E. PAPKA, J. B. FURNESS & M. COSTA. 1983. Neuroscience **9:** 605-619.
36. DUCKLES, S. P. & S. I. SAID. 1982. Eur. J. Pharmacol. **78:** 371-374.
37. EDVINSSON, L., J. FAHRENKRUG, J. HANKO, C. OWMAN, F. SUNDLER & R. UDDMAN. 1980. Cell Tissue Res. **208:** 135-142.
38. GIBBINS, I. L., J. E. BRAYDEN & J. A. BEVAN. 1984. Neuroscience **13:** 1327-1346.
39. JÄRHULT, J., P. HELLSTRAND & F. SUNDLER. 1980. Cell Tissue Res. **207:** 55-64.
40. LUNDBERG, J. M., A. ÄNGGÅRD, J. FAHRENKRUG, T. HÖKFELT & V. MUTT. 1980. Proc. Natl. Acad. Sci. USA **77:** 1651-1665.
41. LUNDBERG, J. M. 1981. Acta Physiol. Scand. 112(Suppl. 496): 1-57.
42. LUNDBERG, J. M., T. HÖKFELT, M. SCHULTZBERG, K. UVNÄS-WALLENSTEN, C. KÖHLER & S. I. SAID. 1979. Neuroscience **4:** 1539-1559.
43. JOHANSSON, O. & J. M. LUNDBERG. 1981. Neuroscience **6:** 847-862.
44. UDDMAN, R., L. MALM & F. SUNDLER. 1980. Acta Otolaryngol. **89:** 152-156.
45. LARSSON, L.-I. 1977. Histochemistry **54:** 153-176.
46. POLAK, J. M. & S. R. BLOOM. 1978. Invest. Cell. Pathol. **1:** 301-326.
47. SUNDLER, F., R. HÅKANSON, S. LEANDER & R. UDDMAN. 1982. *In* Cytochemical Methods in Neuroanatomy.: 341-356. Alan R. Liss, Inc. New York.
48. LUNDBERG, J. M., G. FRIED, J. FAHRENKRUG, B. HOLMSTEDT, T. HÖKFELT, H. LAGERCRANTZ, G. LUNDGREN & A. ÄNGGÅRD. 1981. Neuroscience **6:** 1001-1010.
49. LUNDBERG, J. M., A. ÄNGGÅRD & J. FAHRENKRUG. 1982. Acta Physiol. Scand. **116:** 387-392.
50. BLOOM, S. R. & A. V. EDWARDS. 1980. J. Physiol. **300:** 41-53.
51. EDWARDS, A. V., J. JÄRHULT, P.-O. ANDERSSON & S. R. BLOOM. 1982. *In* Systemic Role of Regulatory Peptides. S. R. Bloom, J. M. Polak & E. Lindenlaub, Eds.: 145-168. F. K. Schattauer Verlag. Stuttgart-New York.
52. UDDMAN, R., L. MALM, J. FAHRENKRUG & F. SUNDLER. 1981. Acta Otolaryngol. **91:** 135-138.
53. POLAK, R. L. & M. M. MEEUWS. 1966. Biochem. Pharmacol. **15:** 989-992.
54. VIZI, E. S. 1979. Prog. Neurobiol. **12:** 181-290.
55. ALBERTS, P., T. BARTFAI & L. STJÄRNE. 1982. J. Physiol. (London) **322:** 93-112.
56. BARTFAI, T., A. WESTLIND, J. ABENS, C. ENGSTRÖM & P. ALBERTS. 1984. *In* Regulation of Transmitter Function. E. S. Vizi & K. Magyar, Eds.: 497-500. European Society of Neurochemists.
57. JÄRHULT, J., J. FAHRENKRUG, P. HELLSTRAND & R. UDDMAN. 1982. Cell Tissue Res. **221:** 617-624.

58. HELLSTRAND, P. & J. JÄRHULT. 1980. Acta Physiol. Scand. **110:** 89-94.
59. ISHII, T. & R. SHIMO. 1983. Arch. Int. Pharmacodyn. **261:** 291-301.
60. HUGHES, J. & J. R. VANE. 1970. Br. J. Pharmacol. **39:** 476-489.
61. NILSSON, S. F. E. & A. BILL. 1984. Acta Physiol. Scand. **121:** 385-392.
62. FORSSMANN, W. G., M. REINECKE & E. WEIHE. 1982. *In* Systemic Role of Regulatory Peptides. S. R. Bloom, J. M. Polak & E. Lindenlaub, Eds.: 329-349. Schattauer Verlag. Stuttgart-New York.
63. WEIHE, E. & M. REINECKE. 1981. Neurosci. Lett. **26:** 283-288.
64. SAID, S. I. 1980. *In* Gastrointestinal Hormones. G. B. J. Glass, Ed.: 246-273. Raven Press. New York.
65. DE NEEF, P., P. ROBBERECHT, P. CHATELAIN, M. WAELBROECK. & J. CHRISTOPHE. 1984. Regul. Peptides **8:** 237-244.
66. SMITHERMAN, T. C., H. SAKIO, A. M. GEUMEI, T. YOSHIDA, M. OYAMADA & S. I. SAID. 1982. *In* Vasoactive Intestinal Peptide. S. I. Said, Ed.: 169-176. Raven Press. New York.
67. DOMSCHKE, S. & W. DOMSCHKE. 1982. *In* Vasoactive Intestinal Peptide. S. I. Said, Ed.: 201-209. Raven Press. New York.
68. FRANCO-CERECEDA, A., L. BENGTSSON & J. M. LUNDBERG. 1987. Eur. J. Pharmacol. **134:** 69-76.
69. UDDMAN, R., J. ALUMETS, O. DENSERT, R. HÅKANSON & F. SUNDLER. 1978. Acta Otolaryngol. **86:** 443-448.
70. ECCLES, R. & H. WILSON. 1973. J. Physiol. **23:** 213-223.
71. ÄNGGÅRD, A. 1974. Acta Otolaryngol. **78:** 98-195.
72. LUNDBLAD, L., A. ÄNGGÅRD & J. LUNDBERG. 1983. Acta Physiol. Scand. **119:** 7-13.
73. LUNDBERG, J., A. ÄNGGÅRD, P. EMSON, J. FAHRENKRUG & T. HÖKFELT. 1981. Proc. Natl. Acad. Sci. USA **78:** 5255-5259.
74. MALM, L., F. SUNDLER & R. UDDMAN. 1980. Acta Otolaryngol. **90:** 304-308.
75. WELLS, U. M. & J. G. WIDDICOMBE. 1986. J. Physiol. **374:** 359-374.
76. DEY, R. D., A. SHANNON, JR. & S. I. SAID. 1981. Cell Tissue Res. **220:** 231-238.
77. GHATEI, M. A., M. N. SHEPPARD, D. J. O'SHAUGHNESSY, T. E. ADRIAN, G. P. MCGREGOR, J. M. POLAK & S. R. BLOOM. 1982. Endocrinology **111:** 1248-1254.
78. POLAK, J. M. & S. R. BLOOM. 1985. Recent Results Cancer Res. **99:** 1-16.
79. ALTIERE, R. J. & L. DIAMOND. 1983. Eur. J. Pharmacol. **93:** 121-124.
80. ALTIERE, R. J. & L. DIAMOND. 1984. Br. J. Pharmacol. **82:** 321-328.
81. HAND, J. M., R. B. LARAVUSO & J. A. WILL. 1984. Eur. J. Pharmacol. **98:** 279-284.
82. HAMASAKI, Y., M. MOJARAD & S. I. SAID. 1983. J. Appl. Physiol. **54:** 1607-1611.
83. NATHANSON, I., J. H. WIDDICOMBE & P. BARNES. 1983. J. Appl. Physiol. **55:** 1844-1848.
84. CARSTAIRS, J. R. & P. BARNES. 1986. J. Pharmacol. Exptl. Exp. Ther. **239:** 249-255.
85. CHEUNG, A., J. M. POLAK, F. E. BAUER, A. CADIEUX, N. D. CHRISTOFIDES, D. R. SPRINGALL & S. R. BLOOM. 1985. Thorax **40:** 889-896.
86. FAHRENKRUG, J. 1979. Digestion **19:** 149-169.
87. FURNESS, J. B., M. COSTA, R. MURPHY, A. M. BEARDSLEY, J. R. OLIVER, I. J. LLEWELLYN-SMITH, R. L. ESKAY, A. A. SHULKES, T. W. MOODY & D. K. MEYER. 1982. Scand. J. Gastroenterol. **17(71):** 61-70.
88. VAILLANT, C., R. DIMALINE & G. J. DOCKRAY. 1980. Cell Tissue Res. **211:** 511-523.
89. FALKMER, S., J. FAHRENKRUG, J. ALUMETS, R. HÅKANSON & F. SUNDLER. 1980. Endocrinol. Jpn. **27:** 31-35.
90. FOUCHEREAU-PERON, M., M. LABURTHE, J. BESSON, G. ROSSELIN & Y. LEBAL. 1980. Comp. Biochem. Physiol. **65A:** 489-492.
91. ALUMETS, J., J. FAHRENKRUG, R. HÅKANSON, O. SCHAFFALITZKY DE MUCKADELL, F. SUNDLER & R. UDDMAN. 1979. Nature **280:** 155-156.
92. LARSSON, L.-I., J. M. POLAK, R. BUFFA, F. SUNDLER & E. SOLCIA. 1979. J. Histochem. Cytochem. **27:** 936-938.
93. YAMADA, J., N. KITAMURA, T. YAMASHITA, M. MISU & N. YANAIHARA. 1982. Cell Tissue Res. **226:** 113-120.
94. SUNDLER, F., J. ALUMETS, J. FAHRENKRUG, R. HÅKANSON & O. B. SCHAFFALITZKY DE MUCKADELL. 1979. Cell Tissue Res. **196:** 193-201.

95. REINECKE, M., P. SCHLUTER, N. YANAIHARA & W. G. FORSSMANN. 1981. Peptides 2(2): 149-156.
96. EKBLAD, E., J. ALUMETS, R. EKMAN, S. FALKMER, R. HÅKANSON & F. SUNDLER. 1985. Peptides 6(3): 383-388.
97. FURNESS, J. B. & M. COSTA. 1980. Neuroscience 5: 1-20.
98. COSTA, M., J. B. FURNESS & I. L. GIBBINS. 1986. *In* Progress in Brain Research. T. Hökfelt, K. Fuxe & B. Pernow, Eds. 68: 217-239.
99. JUNQUERA, C., M. J. AZANZA, B. PARRA, M. T. PEG & P. GARIN. 1986. Gen. Pharmacol. 17(5): 597-605.
100. LANGER, M., S. VAN NOORDEN, J. M. POLAK & A. G. E. PEARSE. 1979. Cell Tissue Res. 199: 493-508.
101. HOLMGREN, S., C. VAILLANT & R. DIMALINE. 1982. Cell Tissue Res. 223: 141-153.
102. HOLMGREN, S. & S. NILSSON. 1983. Acta Zool. (Stockholm) 64: 25-32.
103. JENSEN, J. & S. HOLMGREN. 1985. Comp. Biochem. Physiol. 82C(1): 81-89.
104. FUJITA, T., R. YUI, T. IWANAGA, J. NISHIITSUTSUJI-UWO, Y. ENDO & N. YANAIHARA. 1981. Peptides 2(2): 123-131.
105. MALMFORS, G., S. LEANDER, E. BRODIN, R. HÅKANSON, T. HOLMIN & F. SUNDLER. 1981. Cell Tissue Res. 214: 225-238.
106. COSTA, M. & J. B. FURNESS. 1983. Neuroscience 8: 665-676.
107. EKBLAD, E., M. EKELUND, H. GRAFFNER, R. HÅKANSON & F. SUNDLER. 1985. Gastroenterology 89: 73-85.
108. EKBLAD, E., C. WINTHER, R. EKMAN, R. HÅKANSON & F. SUNDLER. 1987. Neurosci. 20: 169-188.
109. EKBLAD, E., R. EKMAN, R. HÅKANSON & F. SUNDLER. 1988. Neuroscience. Submitted.
110. DANIEL, E. E., J. B. FURNESS, M. COSTA & L. BELBECK. 1987. Cell Tissue Res. 247: 377-384.
111. DALSGAARD, C.-J., T. HÖKFELT, M. SCHULTZBERG, J. M. LUNDBERG, L. TERENIUS, G. J. DOCKRAY & M. GOLDSTEIN. 1983. Neuroscience 9: 191-211.
112. BLOOM, S. R. & A. V. EDWARDS. 1980. J. Physiol. 299: 437-452.
113. FAHRENKRUG, J., U. HAGLUND, M. JODAL, O. LUNDGREN, L. OLBE & O. B. SCHAFFALITZKY DE MUCKADELL. 1978. J. Physiol. (London) 284: 291-305.
114. CHAYVIALLE, J.-A., M. MIYATA, P. L. RAYFORD & J. C. THOMPSON. 1980. Gut 21: 745-749.
115. SCHAFFALITZKY DE MUCKADELL, O. B., J. FAHRENKRUG, J. J. HOLST & J. B. LAURITSEN. 1977. Scand. J. Gastroent. 12: 793-799.
116. EBEID, A. M., P. MURRAY, P. B. SOETERS, P. MURRAY & J. E. FISCHER. 1977. J. Surg. Res. 23: 25-30.
117. REID, A. M., A. SHULKES & D. A. TITCHEN. 1985. Regul. Peptides 12: 43-50.
118. WOLFE, M. M., R. I. MISBIN, D. F. GARDNER & J. E. McGUIGAN. 1983. Regul. Peptides 5: 103-109.
119. MITCHELL, S. J. & S. R. BLOOM. 1978. Gut 19: 1043-1048.
120. BROOK, C. W., R. B. SEWELL, A. SHULKES & R. A. SMALLWOOD. 1987. Regul. Peptides, in press.
121. MISBIN, R. I., M. M. WOLFE, P. MORRIS, S. J. BUYNITZKY & J. E. McGUIGAN. 1982. Am. J. Physiol. 243: G103-G111.
122. EBEID, A. M., J. ESCOURROU, P. B. SOETERS, P. MURRAY & J. E. FISHER. 1978. Ann. Surg. 188: 28-33.
123. IWANAGA, T., T. FUJITA & N. YANAIHARA. 1983. Biomed. Res. 4: 167-172.
124. FURNESS, J. B., M. COSTA & J. R. KEAST. 1984. Cell Tissue Res. 237: 329-336.
125. FAHRENKRUG, J., T. BEK, J. M. LUNDBERG & T. HÖKFELT. 1985. Regul. Peptides 12: 21-34.
126. BISHOP, A. E., J. M. POLAK, Y. YIANGOU, N. D. CHRISTOFIDES & S. R. BLOOM. 1984. Peptides 5: 255-259.
127. YIANGOU, Y., F. REQUEJO, J. M. POLAK & S. R. BLOOM. 1986. Biochem. Biophys. Res. Commun. 139: 1142-1149.
128. MELANDER, T., T. HÖKFELT, Å. RÖKAEUS, J. FAHRENKRUG, K. TATEMOTO & V. MUTT. 1985. Cell Tissue Res. 239: 253-270.

129. AGGESTRUP, S., R. UDDMAN, F. SUNDLER, J. FAHRENKRUG & R. HÅKANSON. 1983. Gastroenterology **84:** 924-927.
130. BISHOP, A. E., J. M. POLAK, B. D. LAKE, M. G. BRYANT & S. R. BLOOM. 1981. Histopathology **5:** 679-688.
131. TSUTO, T., H. OKAMURA, K. FUKUI, H. OBATA, T. HIROFUMI, N. IWAI, S. MAJIMA, N. YANAIHARA & Y. IBATA. 1982. Neurosci. Lett. **34:** 57-62.
132. TAGUCHI, T., K. TANAKA, K. IKEDA, F. MATSUBAYASHI & N. YANAIHARA. 1983. Virchows Arch. A Pathol. Anat. **401:** 223-235.
133. LARSSON, L. T., G. MALMFORS & F. SUNDLER. 1983. Z. Kinderchir. **38:** 301-304.
134. LARSSON, L. T., G. MALMFORS & F. SUNDLER. 1988. Pediatr. Surg. Int. In press.
135. DAVIS, D. R., M. B. DOCKERTY & C. W. MAYO. 1955. Surg. Gynecol. Obstet. **101:** 208-216.
136. BISHOP, A. E., J. M. POLAK, M. G. BRYANT, S. R. BLOOM & S. HAMILTON. 1980. Gastroenterology **79:** 853-860.
137. SJÖLUND, K., O. B. SCHAFFALITZKY DE MUCKADELL, J. FAHRENKRUG, R. HÅKANSON, B. G. PETERSSON & F. SUNDLER. 1983. Gut **24:** 724-733.
138. LEANDER, S., R. HÅKANSON & F. SUNDLER. 1981. Cell Tissue Res. **215:** 21-39.
139. FURNESS, J. B. & M. COSTA. 1982. *In* Vasoactive Intestinal Peptide. S. I. Said, Ed.: 391-406. Raven Press. New York.
140. MORGAN, K. G., P. F. SCHMALZ & J. H. SZURSZEWSKI. 1978. J. Physiol. **282:** 437-450.
141. EKLUND, S., M. JODAL, O. LUNDGREN & A. SJÖQVIST. 1979. Acta Physiol. Scand. **105:** 461-468.
142. EKLUND, S., J. FAHRENKRUG, M. JODAL, O. LUNDGREN, SCHAFFALITZKY DE MUCKADELL & A. SJÖQVIST. 1980. J. Physiol. **302:** 549-557.
143. JODAL, M., O. LUNDGREN & A. SJÖQVIST. 1983. J. Physiol. **338:** 207-219.
144. SJÖQVIST, A., J. FAHRENKRUG, M. JODAL & O. LUNDGREN. 1983. Acta Physiol. Scand. **119:** 69-76.
145. CASSUTO, J., J. FAHRENKRUG, M. JODAL, R. TUTLE & O. LUNDGREN. 1981. Gut **22:** 958-963.
146. CASSUTO, J., M. JODAL & O. LUNDGREN. 1982. Acta Physiol. Scand. **114:** 573-577.
147. BJÖRCK, S. 1982. Ph.D. thesis, University of Göteborg, Sweden.
148. JANSSON, R. & J. SVANVIK. 1978. Gastroenterology **75:** 47-49.
149. JIVEGÅRD, L., J. FAHRENKRUG & J. SVANVIK. 1988. Regul. Peptides, submitted.
150. ALM, P., J. ALUMETS, R. HÅKANSON, CH. OWMAN, N.-O. SJÖBERG, F. SUNDLER & B. WALLES. 1980. Cell Tissue Res. **205:** 337-347.
151. OTTESEN, B., J. J. LARSEN, J. FAHRENKRUG, M. STJERNQUIST & F. SUNDLER. 1981. Am. J. Physiol. **240:** E32-E36.
152. STJERNQUIST, M., P. ALM, R. EKMAN, CH. OWMAN, N.-O. SJÖBERG & F. SUNDLER. 1985. Biol. Reprod. **33:** 157-163.
153. WILLIS, E., B. OTTESEN, G. WAGNER, F. SUNDLER & J. FAHRENKRUG. 1981. Acta Physiol. Scand. **113:** 545-547.
154. WILLIS, E. A., B. OTTESEN, G. WAGNER, F. SUNDLER & J. FAHRENKRUG. 1983. Life Sci. **33:** 383-391.
155. ANDERSSON, K. E., H. HEDLUND, A. MATTIASSON, C. SJÖGREN & F. SUNDLER. 1983. World J. Urol. **1:** 203-208.
156. DAIL, W. G., M. A. MOLL & K. WEBER. 1983. Neuroscience **10:** 1379-1386.
157. SJÖSTRAND, N. O. & E. KLINGE. 1979. Acta Physiol. Scand. **106:** 199-214.
158. LARSEN, J. J., B. OTTESEN, J. FAHRENKRUG & L. FAHRENKRUG. 1981. Invest. Urol. **19:** 211-213.
159. KASTIN, A. J., D. H. COY, A. V. SCHALLY & CH. A MEYERS. 1978. Pharamacol. Biochem. Behav. **9:** 673-676.
160. STJERNQUIST, M., R. HÅKANSON, S. LEANDER, CH. OWMAN, F. SUNDLER & R. UDDMAN. 1983. Regul. Peptides **7:** 67-86.
161. HELM, G., B. OTTESEN, J. FAHRENKRUG, J.-J. LARSEN, CH. OWMAN, N.-O. SJÖBERG, B. STOLBERG, F. SUNDLER & B. WALLES. 1981. Biol. Reprod. **25:** 227-234.
162. STJERNQUIST, M. & C. OWMAN. 1984. Regul. Peptides **8:** 161-167.
163. WALLES, B., R. HÅKANSON, G. HELM, CH. OWMAN, N.-O. SJÖBERG & F. SUNDLER. 1980. Am. J. Obstet. Gynecol. **138:** 337-338.

164. HELM, G., R. HÅKANSON, S. LEANDER, CH. OWMAN, N.-O. SJÖBERG & B. SPORRONG. 1982. Regul Peptides **3:** 145-153.
165. MATTIASSON, A., E. EKBLAD, F. SUNDLER & B. UVELIUS. 1985. Cell Tissue Res. **239:** 141-146.
166. CALAM, J., R. DIMALINE, W. S. PEART, J. SINGH & R. J. UNWIN. 1983. J. Physiol. **345:** 469-475.
167. DIMALINE, R., W. S. PEART & R. J. UNWIN. 1983. J. Physiol. **344:** 379-388.
168. PORTER, J. P., I. A. REID, S. I. SAID & W. F. GANONG. 1982. Am. J. Physiol. **243:** F306-F310.
169. PORTER, J. P., S. I. SAID & W. F. GANONG. 1983. Neuroendocrinology **36:** 404-408.
170. ROSA, R. M., P. SILVA, J. S. STOFF & F. EPSTEIN. 1985. Am. J. Physiol. **249:** E494-E497.
171. AMENTA, F., E. BROZETTI & W. L. COLLIER. 1987. Regul. Peptides **17:** 295-299.
172. GRUNDITZ, T., R. HÅKANSON, G. HEDGE, C. RERUP, F. SUNDLER & R. UDDMAN. 1986. Endocrinology **118:** 783-790.
173. GRUNDITZ, T., R. HÅKANSON, F. SUNDLER & R. UDDMAN. 1988. Neuroscience, in press.
174. HÖKFELT, T., J. M. LUNDBERG, M. SCHULTZBERG & J. FAHRENKRUG. 1981. Acta Physiol. Scand. **113:** 575-576.
175. HOLZWARTH, M. A. 1984. J. Auton. Nerv. System **11:** 269-283.
176. AHRÉN, B., R. HÅKANSON & C. RERUP. 1982. Acta Physiol. Scand. **114:** 471-473.
177. HUFFMAN, L. & G. A. HEDGE. 1986. Endocrinology **118:** 550-557.
178. KOWAL, J. 1982. *In* Vasoactive Intestinal Peptides. S. I. Said, Ed.: 277-284. Raven Press. New York.
179. MORERA, A. M., A. M. CATHIARD, M. LABURTHE & J. M. SAEZ. 1979. Biochem. Biophys. Res. Commun. **90:** 78-85.
180. FREDERICKS, C. M., L. E. LUNDQUIST, R. S. MATHUR, S. H. ASHTON & S. LANDGREBE. 1983. Biol. Reprod. **28:** 1052-1060.
181. FREDERICKS, C. M., S. H. ASHTON, W. F. ANDERSON, R. S. MATHUR, L. E. LUNDQUIST & S. C. LANDGREBE. 1985. Peptides **6:** 205-210.
182. AHMED, C. E., W. L. DEEDS & S. R. OJEDA. 1986. Endocrinology **118:** 1682-1689.
183. OTTESEN, B., B. PEDERSEN, J. NIELSEN, D. DALGAARD & J. FAHGRENKRUG. 1986. Regul. Peptides **16:** 299-304.
184. DAVOREN, J. B. & J. W. A. HSUEH. 1985. Biol. Reprod. **33:** 37-52.
185. SCHEBALIN, M., S. I. SAID & G. M. MAKHLOUF. 1977. Am. J. Physiol. **232:** E197-E200.
186. SZECOWKA, J., P. E. LINS, K. TATEMOTO & S. EFENDIC. 1983. Endocrinology **112:** 1469-1473.
187. SZECOWKA, J., D. TENDLER & S. EFENDIC. 1983. Am. J. Physiol. **245:** E313-E317.
188. AHRÉN, B. & I. LUNDQUIST. 1981. Diabetologia **20:** 1-6.
189. UDDMAN, R., J. ALUMETS, R. HÅKANSON, I. LORÉN & F. SUNDLER. 1980. Experientia **36:** 1119-1120.
190. WHARTON, J., J. M. POLAK, M. G. BRYANT, S. VAN NOORDEN, S. R. BLOOM & A. G. E. PEARSE. 1979. Life Sci. **25:** 273-280.
191. UDDMAN, R., J. FAHRENKRUG, L. MALM, J. ALUMETS, R. HÅKANSON & F. SUNDLER. 1980. Acta Physiol. Scand. **110:** 31-38.
192. LARSSON, L.-I., J. FAHRENKRUG, J. J. HOLST & O. B. SCHAFFALITZKY DE MUCKADELL. 1978. Life Sci. **22:** 773-780.
193. SUNDLER, F., J. ALUMETS, R. HÅKANSON, J. FAHRENKRUG & O. B. SCHAFFALITZKY DE MUCKADELL. 1978. Histochemistry **55:** 173-176.
194. SHIMIZU, T. & N. TAIRA. 1979. Br. J. Pharmacol. **65:** 683-687.
195. EKSTRÖM, J., B. MÅNSSON & G. TOBIN. 1983. Acta Physiol. Scand. **119:** 169-175.
196. INOUE, Y. & T. KANNO. 1982. Biomed. Res. **3:** 384-389.
197. DEHAYE, J.-P., J. CHRISTOPHE, F. ERNST, P. POLOCZEK & P. VAN BOGAERT. 1985. Arch. Oral Biol. **30:** 827-832.
198. LUNDBERG, J. M., B. HEDLUND & T. BARTFAI. 1982. Nature **295:** 147-149.
199. LUNDBERG, J. M., A. ÄNGGÅRD & J. FAHRENKRUG. 1981. Acta Physiol. Scand. **113:** 317-327.
200. LUNDBERG, J. M., A. ÄNGGÅRD & J. FAHRENKRUG. 1981. Acta Physiol. Scand. **113:** 329-336.

201. LUNDBERG, J. M., A. ÄNGGÅRD & J. FAHRENKRUG. 1982. Acta Physiol. Scand. 114: 329-337.
202. HICKSON, J. C. D. 1970. J. Physiol. 206: 257-297.
203. HOLST, J. J., O. B. SCHAFFALITZKY DE MUCKADELL & J. FAHRENKRUG. 1979. Acta Physiol. Scand. 105: 33-51.
204. FAHRENKRUG, J., H. GALBO, J. J. HOLST & O. B. SCHAFFALITZKY DE MUCKADELL. 1978. J. Physiol. 280: 405-422.
205. FAHRENKRUG, J., O. B. SCHAFFALITZKY DE MUCKADELL & S. L. JENSEN. 1979. Am. J. Physiol. 237: E535-E540.
206. CHRISTOPHE, J. & P. ROBBERECHT. 1982. In Vasoactive Intestinal Peptide. S. I. Said, Ed.: 235-252. Raven Press. New York.
207. ROCHE, C., M. VAGNE, C. SCARPIGNATO & V. MUTT. 1985. Regul. Peptides 12: 125-132.
208. HOLST, J. J., J. FAHRENKRUG, S. KNUHTSEN, S. L. JENSEN, S. SEIER POULSEN & O. VAGN NIELSEN. 1984. Regul. Peptides 8: 245-259.
209. EMSON, P. C., R. F. T. GILBERT, I. LORÉN, J. FAHRENKRUG, F. SUNDLER & O. B. SCHAFFALITZKY DE MUCKADELL. 1979. Brain Res. 177: 437-444.
210. GIBSON, S. J., J. M. POLAK, S. R. BLOOM & P. D. WALL. 1981. J. Comp. Neurol. 201: 65-79.
211. KAWATANI, M., I. P. LOWE, I. NADELHAFT, C. MORGAN & W. C. DE GROAT. 1983. Neurosci. Lett. 42: 311-316.
212. OTTEN, U. & H. P. LOREZ. 1983. Neurosci. Lett. 34: 153-158.
213. LEAH, J. D., A. A. CAMERON, W. L. KELLY & P. J. SNOW. 1985. Neuroscience 16: 683-690.
214. DE GROAT, W. C. 1986. Progr. Brain Res. 67: 165-187.
215. MCGREGOR, G. P., S. J. GIBSON, I. M. SABATE, M. A. BLANK, M. D. CHRISTOFIDES, P. D. WALL, J. M. POLAK & S. R. BLOOM. 1984. Neuroscience 13: 207-216.
216. SHEHAB, S. A. S. & M. E. ATKINSON. 1984. J. Anat. (London) 13: 725.
217. SHEHAB, S. A. S. & M. E. ATKINSON. 1986. Exp. Brain Res. 62: 422-430.
218. JU, G., T. HÖKFELT, E. BRODIN, J. FAHRENKRUG, J. A. FISCHER, P. FREY, R. P. ELDE & J. C. BROWN. 1987. Cell Tissue Res. 24: 417-431.
219. LANDIS, S. & J. R. FREDIEU. 1986. Brain Res. 377: 177-181.
220. HOHMANN, E. L., R. P. ELDE, J. A. RYSAVY, S. EINZIG & R. L. GEBHARD. 1986. Science 232: 868-871.
221. DIMALINE, R., J. R. REEVE, JR., J. E. SHIVELY & D. HAWKE. Peptides 5: 183-187.
222. WANG, S. C., B.-H. DU, J. ENG, M. CHANG, J. D. HULMES, Y.-C. E. & R. S. YALOW. 1985. Life Sci. 37: 979-983.
223. MUTT, V. & S. I. SAID. 1974. Eur. J. Biochem. 42: 581-589.
224. CARLQUIST, M., V. MUTT & H. JÖRNVALL. 1979. FEBS Lett. 108: 457-460.
225. DU, B.-H., J. ENG, J. D. HULMES, M. CHANG, Y.-C. E. PAN & R. S. YALOW. 1985. Biochem. Biophys. Res. Commun. 128: 1093-1098.
226. KAUFMAN, J.-P., J. ENG, B.-H. DU, E. STRAUS & R. S. YALOW. 1986. Regul. Peptides 14: 93-97.
227. MARIE, J.-C., D. HUI BEN HOA, R. JACKSON, G. HEJBLUM & G. ROSSELIN. 1985. Regul. Peptides 12: 113-123.
228. BODANZKY, M. 1977. In First International Symposium on Hormonal Receptors in Digestive Tract Physiology. INSERM Symposium No. 3. S. Bonfils, P. Fromageot & G. Rosselin, Eds.: 13-18. Elsevier. Amsterdam; New York.
229. BODANZKY, M., Y. S. KLAUSNER & S. I. SAID. 1973. Proc. Natl. Acad. Sci. USA 70: 382-384.
230. BODANZKY, M., I. B. HENES, A. E. YIOTAKIS & S. I. SAID. 1977. J. Med. Chem. 20: 1461-1464.
231. PIPKORN, R. & R. HÅKANSON. 1984. Peptides 5: 267-269.
232. SCHWARTZ, C. J., D. V. KIMBERG, H. E. SHEERIN, M. FIELD & S. I. SAID. 1974. J. Clin. Invest. 54: 536-544.
233. SIMON, B. & H. KATHER. 1978. Gastroenterology 74: 722-725.
234. CHATELAIN, P., P. ROBBERECHT, P. DE NEEF, J. C. CAMUS, D. HEUSE & J. CHRISTOPHE. 1980. Pflugers Arch. 389: 29-35.

235. KITAMURA, S., Y. ISHIHARA & S. I. SAID. 1980. Eur. J. Pharmacol. **67:** 219-223.
236. INOUE, Y., K. KAKU, T. KANERO, N. YANAIHARA & T. KANNO. 1985. Endocrinology **116:** 686-692.
237. SCHOEFFTER, P. & J. C. STOCLET. 1985. Eur. J. Pharmacol. **109:** 275-279.
238. HUANG, M. & O. P. RORSTAD. 1983. J. Neurochem. **40:** 719-726.
239. VAN BOGAERT, P., Y. SOUKIAS, J.-P. DEHAYE, M. LAMBERT, P. POLOCZEK, J. WINAND, R. MAYER & J. CHRISTOPHE. 1987. Regul. Peptides **17:** 339-348.
240. RAITERI, M., M. MARCHI & P. PAUDICE. 1987. Eur. J. Pharmacol. **133:** 127-128.
241. SUNDLER, F., J. CHRISTOPHE, P. ROBBERECHT, N. YANAIHARA, C. YANAIHARA, T. GRUNDITZ & R. HÅKANSON. 1988. Regul. Peptides **20:** 83-89.
242. VANDERMEERS, A., P. GOURLET, M.-C. VANDERMEERS-PIRET, A. CAUVIN, P. DE NEEF, J. RATHE, M. SVOBODA, P. ROBBERECHT & J. CHRISTOPHE. 1987. Eur. J. Biochem. **164:** 321-327.

Glucagon and Related Peptides

Molecular Structure and Biological Specificity[a]

D. BATAILLE, P. BLACHE, F. MERCIER,
C. JARROUSSE, A. KERVRAN, M. DUFOUR,
AND P. MANGEAT

Centre CNRS-INSERM de Pharmacologie-Endocrinologie
CCIPE
34094, Montpellier Cédex, France

M. DUBRASQUET

INSERM U. 10
Hôpital Bichat 75877
Paris Cédex 18, France

A. MALLAT, S. LOTERSZTAJN, C. PAVOINE,
AND F. PECKER

INSERM U. 99
94010 Créteil, France

INTRODUCTION

The family of peptides[1] comprising glucagon and the structurally related molecules derives from an ancestral gene which, by duplication followed by mutations, has given the preproglucagon gene and the genes producing vasoactive intestinal peptide (VIP) and its related peptides (see the other contributions in this volume).

[a]The work of the authors included in this review was supported by INSERM (CRL 79 5 449 7 and 82 7 009), CNRS, Swedish MRC (MFR K75 60F 4896 and B81 13F 60044 01), European Economic Community (85 1000001 BE02 PUJU 1), and the Fonds pour la Recherche Médicale.

[b]This peptide terminology uses the one-letter code[42] of the first and last amino acids followed by the number of amino acids. In this terminology, glucagon would be HT-29, oxyntomodulin HA-37, and so forth.

As for the VIP family, the members of the glucagon family are synthesized at different levels of the digestive tract, the pancreas, and the central nervous system. However, in spite of these similarities in terms of structure and localization, the glucagon-related peptides display original biological features that are triggered by receptors that VIP and its parent molecules do not share. This cleavage between the receptor-effector systems of the two families was discovered fourteen years ago[2-4] and has since been a developing subject of research. Glucagon and related peptides, as well as the biological pathways by which they act, appear to be an ensemble of regulatory systems that have evolved in parallel to that represented by the peptides described in the contributions by our colleagues.

In this paper we shall present what is known about this family of regulatory peptides, with a special reference to the molecular structure and the consequent biological specificity of the different fragments produced from preproglucagon. Other aspects of this peptide family have been the subject of recent reviews.[5-12]

MOLECULAR STRUCTURE OF THE PEPTIDES PRODUCED FROM PREPROGLUCAGON

The structure of preproglucagon was determined by cloning the mRNA-deriving cDNA corresponding to the preproglucagon gene from five animal species: anglerfish,[13] ox,[14] hamster,[15] human,[16] and rat.[17] If we focus on the mammalian species, it may be seen that the general structure is conserved in all the different preproglucagons (see FIG. 1). After elimination of the hydrophobic 20 amino acid signal peptide, the translated protein is 160 amino acids long. There are two distinct domains:

(1) The left part codes for a 69 amino acid peptide, initially isolated from the porcine intestine[18,19] and referred to as glicentin,[19] proglucagon,[19] or glucagon-69.[20] Inside this structure are found the 37 amino acid oxyntomodulin or glucagon-37 isolated from intestinal[20,21] and pancreatic[22] origins, and glucagon, also referred to as glucagon-29, historically the first in the series, that was isolated from the pancreas.[23] These three peptides contain the whole glucagon sequence justifying the terms "glucagon-xx" or "G-xx" (G-69, G-37, and G-29) for peptides containing glucagon, with 69, 37, and 29 amino acids, respectively.[20]

The right part codes for two peptides arranged in tandem, with structures resembling those of glucagon and accordingly named "glucagon-like peptide 1" (GLP-1) and "glucagon-like peptide 2" (GLP-2).

As relatively little is known about these latter peptides, except some biological activities[24,25] and their probable presence in tissues,[26-29] we shall focus here on the glucagon-containing peptides and their derivatives.

Dibasic peptides (Arg-Lys, Lys-Arg, Arg-Arg, or Lys-Lys) are the most commonly encountered sites for processing enzymes (see Rholam *et al.*[30] for a recent paper on this topic). Ten different fragments may theoretically be produced from the first 69 amino acids of preproglucagon by classical processing, with elimination of the two basic amino acids (see FIGS. 1 and 2). Among them, five fragments have already been isolated and sequenced (see FIGS. 1 and 2). Fragment 1-30 corresponds to the glicentin-related pancreatic peptide (GRPP), isolated from porcine pancreas.[31] It has been shown to be released at the same rate as glucagon from a preparation of isolated pancreas.[8] It corresponds to a fragment generated from preproglucagon during the pancreatic processing of the precursor leading to glucagon production. No data are

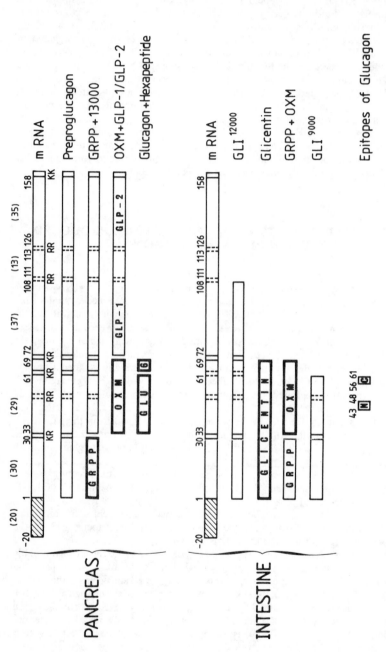

FIGURE 1. Schematic representation of mammalian preproglucagon and preproglucagon messenger RNA (taken from Refs. 14-17). The processing of preproglucagon in pancreas and intestine are the ones that are the most likely to exist, according to available data.[28,43-49] GRPP: Glicentin-related pancreatic peptide[31]; OXM: Oxyntomodulin, or glucagon-37[20,21]; GLP-1 and GLP-2: Glucagon-like peptide-1 and -2[43-49]; GLI[12000]: 12,000-dalton, glucagon-like immunoreactive peptide[52]; Glicentin (or proglucagon)[19]; GLI[9000]: 9,000-dalton glucagon-like immunoreactive peptide[36]; Epitopes of glucagon: NH₂-terminal and COOH-terminal glucagon epitopes.[37-40]

available concerning a potential biological regulatory role (such as an endocrine function). It must be noticed that GRPP is rather variable in its structure depending on the animal species,[14-17] unlike oxyntomodulin, which is very stable from an evolutionary point of view, despite a very small change (arginine in hamster, human, and rat or lysine in ox and pig) at position 33 (position 65 of preproglucagon). Glucagon is identical in all mammals studied so far,[32] except in the guinea pig.[33] This evolutionary stability is obtained despite some mutations in the genetic code (silent mutations, see sequences in References 14-17).

Fragments 1-69, 33-61, and 33-69 are glicentin (proglucagon or G-69), glucagon (G-29), and oxyntomodulin (G-37), respectively. Their implication in the succession of events occurring during the preproglucagon processing as well as their possible biological roles will be discussed.

Fragment 64-69 (oxyntomodulin 32-37 or NA-6[b]) has a very similar story to that of GRPP: It has been isolated and sequenced from pancreas[34] and shown to be released

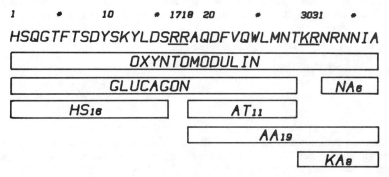

FIGURE 2. Peptides certainly or possibly produced from oxyntomodulin with a classical processing at dibasic peptides (Arg-Arg). The fragments are named according to the one-letter code[42] of the first and the last amino acid, followed by the number of amino acids. KA$_8$ is unlikely to exist *in vivo*, but has a great deal of pharmacological interest (see text).

from perfused pancreas at the same rate as glucagon[35]; like GRPP it is a side product of glucagon production. No data are available concerning its potential regulatory role.

Five other peptides may exist, but the proof of their occurrence in tissue or plasma is still debatable: Fragment 1-48 is purely hypothetical. However, fragment 1-61 may be the 9,000 MW peptide with both NH$_2$-terminal and COOH-terminal glucagon-like immunoreactivities (see below) that are observed in pathological states (such as chronic renal failure.[36] Its exact role, if any, has still to be established. Fragment 33-48 (called HS-16[b]) as well as fragment 51-61 (called AT-11[b]) may be produced from glucagon (glucagon 1-16 and 19-29, respectively). A possible role for these peptides will be discussed below. The same holds true for fragment 51-69 (AA-19[b] or oxyntomodulin 19-37).

Obviously, these peptides are, or may be, those that are produced after a "classical" processing at dibasic peptides. Other sites of processing exist in other series of regulatory peptides and, if the same happens for preproglucagon, more fragments may indeed be produced; this would further complicate the research on preproglucagon processing.

From an immunological point of view, four different epitopes appear within the first 69 amino acids of preproglucagon. The so-called "NH$_2$-terminal" and "COOH-terminal" glucagon epitopes[37-39]) are shown in FIGURE 3, as well as one borne by the COOH-terminal octapeptide of oxyntomodulin or glicentin.[40,41] Another epitope is borne by GRPP.[8]

BIOSYNTHESIS CONSIDERATIONS

According to the present knowledge on the biosynthesis of glucagon-containing peptides,[28,43-49] it may be assumed that, whatever the tissue considered, the same preproglucagon is produced from the same mRNA. The different peptides therefore appear to be the result of differential tissue-specific processing (see FIG. 1).

Pancreas

In contrast to what was initially believed, Glicentin does not appear to be the pancreatic proglucagon. Indeed, the first cleavage of preproglucagon in this tissue appears to be at site 31-32, releasing GRPP and a 13,000-dalton glucagon-containing peptide. At this point, a cleavage at site 70-71 leads to oxyntomodulin, which is further processed at site 62-63, leading to glucagon and NA-6. The existence of this process is supported by direct studies on glucagon biosynthesis[28,43-49] and on the pancreatic content in the different peptides. Glicentin content is very low if not nil, whereas the predominent peptides are glucagon, GRPP,[31] NA-6,[35] and oxyntomodulin (ca. 30% of the glucagon content in the rat).[50,51]

Intestine

In contrast to what is observed in pancreas, glicentin appears to be a biosynthetic intermediate in intestine. Indeed, this peptide is released from preproglucagon by a cleavage at site 70-71, following a possible first cut at site 109-110, leading to "GLI^{12000}" (see FIG. 1).[52] Thus, in this tissue, the separation between glucagon-containing peptides and glucagon-like peptides (GLP-1 and -2) appears early. A further processing at site 31-32 leads to the release of oxyntomodulin. This last processing seems to be quantitatively different from one animal species to another; whereas in pig intestine, the glicentin : oxyntomodulin ratio is about one order of magnitude in favor of the former, a roughly 1 : 1 ratio is observed in man[53] and rat.[50,51] This holds true in the systemic circulation.[50,51]

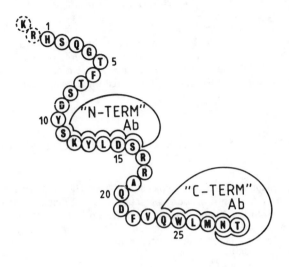

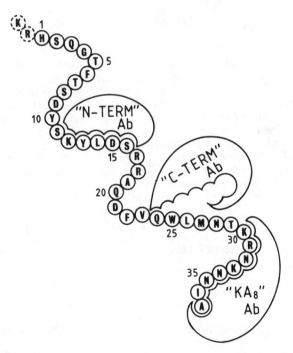

FIGURE 3. "NH$_2$-terminal" and "COOH-terminal" epitopes of glucagon.[37–40] "KA$_8$" antiserum may be produced by immunization with KA$_8$ (Bataille *et al.*, unpublished) or with longer fragments.[41]

Central Nervous System

Glucagon-like material has also been found at this level.[54-58] However, much less is known about the precise molecular forms existing there, although it is likely to be essentially the COOH-terminally extended forms (glicentin, oxyntomodulin,...), as they react poorly with COOH-terminally directed antiglucagon antisera.[56]

BIOLOGICAL ACTIVITIES AND BIOLOGICAL SPECIFICITY

Among glucagon's numerous biological activities (for a review, see Lefebvre[6]), some are certainly the result of a cross-reaction with biological systems that are not primarily adapted to the 29 amino acid molecule. Since the discovery, five years ago, of an original tissue specificity of oxyntomodulin,[59] two categories may be distinguished within the targets for glucagon and related peptides.

The "Classical" Glucagon Targets

The classical glucagon targets are usually linked to the control of metabolism.[6,10] The hepatic glycogenolysis and gluconeogenesis are among them, with the addition of fat cell lipolysis, ketogenesis, and so forth. Still in the field of metabolism is the stimulation of insulin secretion by the pancreatic B cells.[60] All these examples have at least two points in common. (1) The second messenger appears to be cyclic AMP. (2) Oxyntomodulin, which contains an additional COOH-terminal octapeptide, is one order of magnitude less potent than glucagon in these systems[5,20,60] (see FIG. 4). This indicates that these biological actions are linked to a receptor type that is, at most, adapted to the 29 amino acid glucagon molecule, the COOH-terminal octapeptide introducing a steric hindrance within the peptide-receptor interaction. It must be noted that the NH_2-terminally extended glicentin molecule does not display any significant effect on these glucagon-sensitive targets,[8] as expected from other data[61]; this allowed us to use the glucagon radioreceptor assay in liver membranes to specifically assay oxyntomodulin and glucagon in tissue extracts and plasma after HPLC separation.[50,51,53] This receptor, linked to adenylate cyclase, is the one initially described by Rodbell *et al.* in 1971[62] (see also Rodbell[10]) and ever since largely studied (see Herberg *et al.*[63]).

A New Type of Target for the Peptides of the Glucagon Family

This new type of target is exemplified by the gastric mucosa, which display very different reactivities toward the nonelongated compared with the elongated peptides (see FIG. 5). In 1981, we showed[59] that oxyntomodulin (glucagon plus the COOH-terminal octapeptide) is one order of magnitude *more* potent than glucagon in stimulating cyclic AMP production in isolated acid-secreting gastric glands (oxyntic glands) from the rat, or in membranes prepared from these glands. The two log difference between the tissue-specificities of the two peptides (hepatic versus gastric target) gave to the 37 amino acid peptide the status of a new biological entity.[5,59]

This was confirmed by *in vivo* data. Indeed, when oxyntomodulin and glucagon were compared for their effects on acid secretion in anesthetized rats,[64] both peptides were found to be inhibitory, with the same efficacy. As for the *in vitro* experiments (cyclic AMP), oxyntomodulin was one order of magnitude more potent than glucagon in its effect on acid secretion, indicating that a relationship between the two phenomena exists. A relationship was found in the gastric glands where an original receptor, different from the glucagon receptor present in liver, fat cell, and so forth was discovered.[65] This new type of receptor displays pharmacological characteristics (see FIG. 6) that explain both the *in vitro* data (cyclic AMP) and the *in vivo* data (inhibition

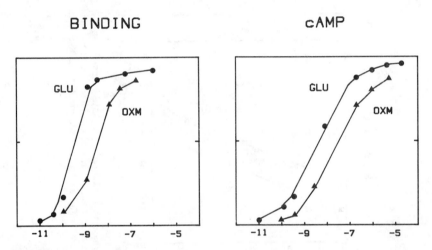

FIGURE 4. Effects of glucagon (GLU) and oxyntomodulin (OXM) on mono-[^{125}I]glucagon binding (left) and activation of adenylate cyclase (right) in rat liver membranes. Data from Bataille *et al.*[20]

of gastric acid secretion). This receptor is indeed more adapted to oxyntomodulin than to glucagon, with a 10 times higher affinity for the former peptide than for the latter. Accordingly, it may be called "oxyntomodulin receptor."[65] No direct data are available concerning a possible interaction of the 69 amino acid peptide glicentin with this receptor-effector system. However, this peptide has been shown to be able to inhibit *in vivo* gastric acid secretion at a dosage where glucagon was ineffective.[66] This suggests either that glicentin interacts with the gastric oxyntomodulin receptor-effector system, or that oxyntomodulin is released *in vivo* from glicentin. At present, we have no clear picture of the relationship between the oxyntomodulin receptor, cyclic AMP, and inhibition of acid secretion, inasmuch as peptides deriving from oxyntomodulin, incapable of modifying the cyclic nucleotide levels, are able to mimic oxyntomodulin's effect *in vivo*. This is clear with the COOH-terminal octapeptide, differentiating oxyntomodulin from glucagon. Indeed, this peptide, named KA-8 according to the

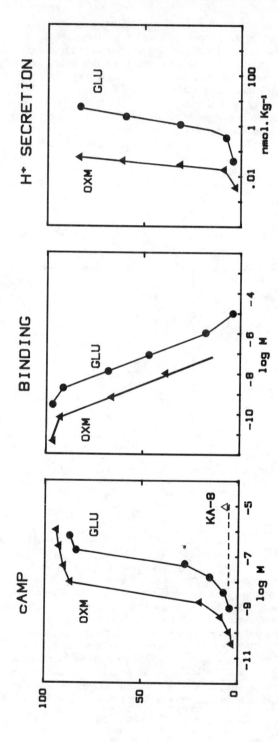

FIGURE 5. Effects of oxyntomodulin (OXM) and glucagon (GLU) on cyclic AMP accumulation in rat oxyntic glands (left), binding of mono-[125I]OXM in the same glands (middle) and inhibition of pentagastrin-induced gastric acid secretion in anesthetized rats (right). Data from Bataille *et al.*,[59] left, Depigny *et al.*,[65] middle, and Dubrasquet *et al.*,[64] right; used with permission. KA_8: COOH-terminal octapeptide of oxyntomodulin (see FIG. 2).

terminology described above (see FIG. 2), is unable to modulate the cyclic AMP of the gastric mucosa (see FIG. 5), but displays oxyntomodulin's features through its capacity to inhibit gastric acid secretion both in the anesthetized[67,68] and conscious rat[67,69,70] (see FIG. 7), although it is 100-150-fold less potent than the entire 37 amino acid molecule (see FIG. 8). This clearly indicates that the molecular signal triggering the inhibition of acid secretion is mainly, if not completely, borne by the octapeptide. The rest of the molecule is likely to increase the number of molecular interactions with the recognition system(s) and thus to decrease the peptide concentrations necessary to allow the occurrence of biological effects at physiological concentrations.

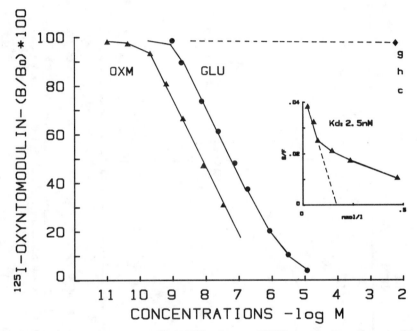

FIGURE 6. Effects of oxyntomodulin (OXM), glucagon (GLU), gastrin or pentagastrin (g), histamine (h) and carbachol (c) on mono-[^{125}I]oxyntomodulin binding to isolated rat oxyntic glands. Inset: Scatchard transformation of the data obtained with unlabeled OXM. Data from Depigny *et al.*[65]

The *in vivo* effectiveness of KA-8 in the absence of any modulation of cyclic AMP raises the question of the second messenger implicated in the inhibitory effect of oxyntomodulin and their derivatives on acid secretion. At the present time, there is no data indicating that calcium ions could be this messenger. However, recent data on *in vitro* biological effectiveness of glucagon and related peptides shed new light on two important questions:

  1. What are the effects of glucagon and related peptides that are transmitted by cyclic AMP?

  2. Are there other effects that may be transmitted by other messengers, such as Ca^{2+}?

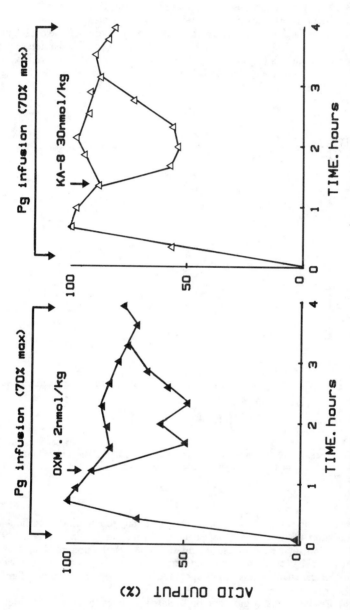

FIGURE 7. Effects of oxyntomodulin (OXM) and COOH-terminal octapeptide of oxyntomodulin (KA-8) on pentagastrin (Pg) stimulated (70% of the maximal response) gastric acid secretion in the conscious rat bearing a gastric fistula. OXM and KA-8 were bolus-injected. Upper curves: control in the absence of injected peptides (plateau level); lower curves: inhibition observed with 200 pmol·Kg⁻¹ OXM (left) or 30 nmol·Kg⁻¹ KA-8 (right). Data from Jarrousse et al.[69]

GLUCAGON-CONTAINING PEPTIDES AND CELLULAR CALCIUM

Until recently, all glucagon's effects appeared to be transduced by cyclic AMP (for a review, see Rodbell[10]). In 1984, glucagon was observed to lower the enzymatic activity and pumping rate of the hepatic membrane Ca^{2+}-ATPase,[71] in a cyclic AMP-independent manner. This was the first clue showing that an effect of glucagon is not mediated by cyclic AMP. However, this was observed only at a high peptide concentration suggesting that a glucagon-like peptide, rather than glucagon itself was implicated. The suppression of the effect by performing the incubation in the presence

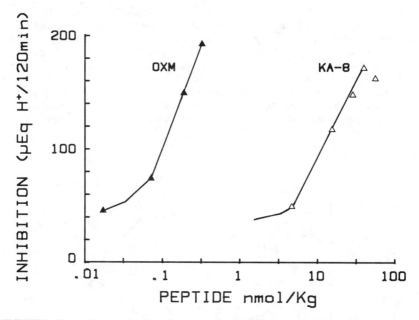

FIGURE 8. Dose-effect relationship of oxyntomodulin (OXM) and COOH-terminal octapeptide of oxyntomodulin (KA-8) in inhibiting the pentagastrin-induced gastric acid secretion in the conscious rat. Data from Jarrousse *et al.*[69]; used with permission.

of inhibitors of proteolysis suggested that the mechanism was brought into action by a fragment produced during incubation.[71] A candidate molecule was the COOH-terminal moiety of glucagon (glucagon$_{19-29}$ or AT-11) because of the presence of a dibasic peptide (Arg- Arg), a possible processing site, in the glucagon molecule and because the NH_2-terminal moiety of glucagon is required to modulate cyclic AMP. The peptide produced from natural glucagon by tryptic digestion[72] and HPLC-purified was compared to glucagon in its actions on the liver membrane Ca^{2+} pump and was found to be 1,000 times more potent than the entire molecule[72] (see FIG. 9). This opened up a new era for research on glucagon and related peptides both in terms of molecular structure (a fragment of a hormone is a "hormone" itself) and in terms of second messenger (calcium versus cyclic AMP).

The existence of a link between the effects of glucagon-containing peptides and calcium ion as a second messenger was confirmed and extended to another system: indeed, glucagon, at physiological concentrations, was shown to increase inositol phosphate breakdown, independently of cyclic AMP.[73] These authors proposed the separation of glucagon receptors into two categories: "GR-1" linked to calcium (via the inositol phosphates pathway) and "GR-2" linked to adenylate cyclase.[73] A third receptor, recognizing glucagon fragments, in particular AT-11 (coupled to the calcium pathway via the calcium pump?), might also exist.[72] FIGURE 10 summarizes the present hypothesis on the action of glucagon and glucagon fragments. The existence of the three receptors are for the moment hypothetical, and further studies using direct approaches such as using binding of labeled probes are necessary to confirm these hypotheses.

Regarding the regulation system(s) controlled by the COOH-terminally extended glucagon molecules (in particular oxyntomodulin) a similar, although probably different, heterogeneity in the recognition and the second messenger pathways is likely to exist. Indeed, oxyntomodulin negatively controls gastric acid secretion. At the same time, this glucagon-containing peptide induces a sharp rise in gastric glands' cyclic AMP, as does histamine, a major stimulator of acid secretion. Although the cell type(s) from the gastric mucosa responding to histamine and/or oxyntomodulin when cyclic AMP is concerned are not yet precisely established, it seems contradictory that a stimulator and an inhibitor of the same biological event act through the same second

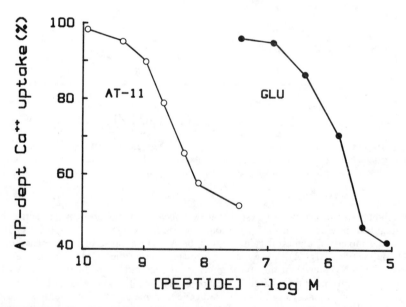

FIGURE 9. Effects of glucagon (GLU) and glucagon$_{19-29}$ (AT-11) on the pumping rate of liver membrane calcium ATPase *in vitro*. Data from Lotersztajn *et al.*,[71] glucagon and Mallat *et al.*,[72] AT-11; used with permission.

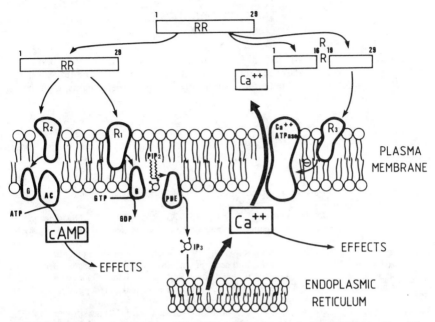

FIGURE 10. Present hypothesis on the action of glucagon and glucagon fragments on the hepatocyte. R2: "Classical" glucagon receptor[10,62] linked to adenylate cyclase (AC) through a GTP-binding protein (G). R1: suspected glucagon receptor[73] linked to a phospholipase C (PDE) through a GTP-binding protein (G). The consecutive production of inositol triphosphate (IP$_3$) induces a Ca^{2+} release from intracellular stores (endoplasmic reticulum), leading to an increase in cytosolic Ca^{2+}. R3: Suspected receptor[72] for the COOH-terminal fragment of glucagon (19-29 or AT-11), negatively linked to the plasma membrane-calcium pump (Ca^{2+}-ATPase), leading to an increase in cytosolic Ca^{2+}.

messenger. Part of this question is solved by the observation that COOH-terminal fragments of oxyntomodulin (e.g., the COOH-terminal octapeptide KA-8) display the inhibitory effect of oxyntomodulin on acid secretion without interacting with the cyclic AMP system (see FIGS. 5, 7, and 8). Further investigation is required to establish whether calcium (via any of the calcium pathways) is implicated in the inhibitory effect of oxyntomodulin and peptides deriving from it.

Whatever the case, the two parallel regulatory systems displayed by glucagon and derived peptides on one hand, and oxyntomodulin and derived peptides on the other, all produced from the same biosynthetic precursor, appear to be more complicated than initially supposed. Tissue specific processing, *in vivo* secretory pathways (endocrine, neurocrine, paracrine . . .), subclasses of receptors coupled to different second messengers are presently the subject of an increasing number of studies. The data already obtained on the family of glucagon-containing peptides strongly support the concept of "one hormone-inside another hormone." It is a good example of evolutionary phenomena that match the increasing demands of more complex organisms requiring more sophisticated regulatory systems.

ACKNOWLEDGMENTS

The authors thank C. Bunoust, M. Passama, and A. Sahuquet for their invaluable help in graphic work. Thanks are due to Mrs. B. Hurson for her helpful secretarial assistance. Mrs. A. Turner-Madeuf is acknowledged for her expert linguistic guidance.

REFERENCES

1. MUTT, V. 1976. Further investigation on intestinal hormonal polypeptides. Clin. Endocrinol. Suppl. **5:** 175s-183s.
2. BATAILLE, D. P., P. FREYCHET, P. E. KITABGI & G. ROSSELIN. 1973. Gut glucagon: A common receptor site with pancreatic glucagon in liver cell plasma membranes. FEBS Lett. **30:** 215-218.
3. BATAILLE, D., P. FREYCHET & G. ROSSELIN. 1974. Interactions of glucagon, gut glucagon, vasoactive intestinal polypeptide and secretin with liver and fat cell plasma membranes: Binding to specific sites and stimulation of adenylate cyclase. Endocrinology **95:** 713-721.
4. DESBUQUOIS, B. 1974. The interaction of vasoactive intestinal polypeptide and secretin with liver-cell membranes. Eur. J. Biochem. **46:** 439-450.
5. BATAILLE, D., C. JARROUSSE, A. KERVRAN, C. DEPIGNY & M. DUBRASQUET. 1986. The biological significance of "Enteroglucagon." Present status. Peptides 7(Suppl. 1): 37-42.
6. LEFEBVRE, P. J. Ed. 1983. Glucagon, Handbook of Experimental Pharmacology. Vol. 66, I and II. Springer Verlag. Heidelberg, West Germany.
7. HOLST, J. J. 1983. Gut glucagon, enteroglucagon, gut glucagon-like immunoreactivity, glicentin—current status. Gastroenterology **84:** 1602-1613.
8. MOODY, A. J. & L. THIM. 1983. Glucagon, glicentin and related peptides. *In* Glucagon. P. J. Lefebvre, Ed. Vol. I: 139-174. Springer Verlag. Berlin, West Germany.
9. ORCI, L., C. BORDI, R. H. UNGER & A. PERRELET. 1983. Glucagon- and glicentin-producing cells. *In* Glucagon. P. J. Lefebvre, Ed. Vol I: 57-79. Springer Verlag. Berlin, West Germany.
10. RODBELL, M. 1983. The actions of glucagon at its receptor: Regulation of adenylate cyclase. *In* Glucagon. P. J. Lefebvre, Ed. Vol. I: 263-290. Springer Verlag. Berlin, West Germany.
11. TAGER, H. S. 1984. Glucagon-containing and glucagon-related peptides: Evolutionary, structural and biosynthetic considerations. *In* Evolution and tumor pathology of the neuroendocrine system. S. Falkmer, R. Hakanson, and F. Sundler, Eds.: 285-311. Elsevier. Amsterdam, Oxford, New York.
12. VALVERDE, I. 1983. Heterogeneity of circulating glucagon and glucagon-like immunoreactivity. *In* Glucagon. P. J. Lefebvre, Ed. Vol. I: 223-244. Verlag-Springer. Berlin, West Germany.
13. LUND, P. K., R. H. GOODMAN, P. C. DEE & J. F. HABENER. 1982. Pancreatic preproglucagon cDNA contains two glucagon-related coding sequences arranged in tandem. Proc. Natl. Acad. Sci. USA **79:** 345-349.
14. LOPEZ, L. C., M. L. FRAZIER, C.-J. SU, A. KUMAN & G. F. SAUNDERS. 1983. Mammalian Preproglucagon contains three Glucagon-related peptides. Proc. Natl. Acad. Sci. USA **80:** 5485-5489.
15. BELL, G. I., R. F. SANTERRE & G. T. MULLENBACH. 1983. Hamster preproglucagon contains the sequence of glucagon and two related peptides. Nature **302:** 716-718.
16. BELL, G. I., R. SANCHEZ-PESCADOR, P. J. LAYBOURN & R. C. NAJARIAN. 1983. Exon duplication and divergence in the human preproglucagon gene. Nature **304:** 368-371.
17. HEINRICH, G., P. GROS & J. F. HABENER. 1984. Glucagon gene sequence. Four of six exons encode separate functional domains of rat preproglucagon. J. Biol. Chem. **259:** 14082-14087.

18. SUNDBY, F., H. JACOBSEN & A. J. MOODY. 1976. Purification and characterization of a protein from porcine gut with glucagon-like immunoreactivity. Horm. Metab. Res. **8:** 366-371.
19. THIM, L. & A. J. MOODY. 1981. The primary structure of porcine glicentin (proglucagon). Regul. Pept. **2:** 139-150.
20. BATAILLE, D., K. TATEMOTO, C. GESPACH, H. JORNVALL, G. ROSSELIN & V. MUTT. 1982. Isolation of glucagon-37 (bioactive Enteroglucagon/Oxyntomodulin) from porcine jejuno-ileum. Characterization of the peptide. FEBS Lett. **146:** 79-86.
21. BATAILLE, D., A. M. COUDRAY, M. CARLQVIST, G. ROSSELIN & V. MUTT. 1982. Isolation of glucagon-37 (bioactive Enteroglucagon/Oxyntomodulin) from porcine jejuno-ileum. Isolation of the peptide. FEBS Lett. **146:** 73-78.
22. TAGER, H. S. & D. F. STEINER. 1973. Isolation of a glucagon-containing peptide: Primary structure of a possible fragment of proglucagon. Proc. Natl. Acad. Sci. USA **80:** 2321-2325.
23. BROMER, W. W., L. G. SINN & O. K. BEHRENS. 1957. The amino acid sequence of glucagon. V. Location of amide groups, acid degradation studies and summary of sequential evidence. J. Am. Chem. Soc. **79:** 2807-2810.
24. HOOSEIN, N. M & R. S. GURG. 1984. Human glucagon-like peptides 1 and 2 activate rat brain adenylate cyclase. FEBS Lett. **178:** 83-86.
25. SCHMIDT, W. E., E. G. SIEGEL & W. CREUTZFELDT. 1985. Glucagon-like peptide-1 but not glucagon-like peptide-2 stimulates insulin release from isolated rat pancreatic islets. Diabetologia **28:** 704-707.
26. GEORGE, S. K., L. O. UTTENTHAL, M. GHIGLIONE & S. R. BLOOM. 1985. Molecular forms of glucagon-like peptides in man. FEBS Lett. **192:** 275-278.
27. ORSKOV, C., J. J. HOLST, S. KNUHTSEN, F. G. A. BALDISSERA, S. S. POULSEN & V. NIELSEN. 1986. Glucagon-like peptides GLP-1 and GLP-2, predicted products of the glucagon gene, are secreted separately from pig small intestine but not pancreas. Endocrinology **119:** 1467-1475.
28. PHILIPPE, J., S. MOJSOV, D. J. DRUCKER & J. F. HABENER. 1986. Proglucagon processing in a rat islet cell line resembles phenotype of intestine rather than pancreas. Endocrinology **119:** 2833-2839.
29. UTTENTHAL, L. O., M. GHIGLIONE, S. K. GEORGE, A. E. BISHOP, J. M. POLAK & S. R. BLOOM. 1985. Molecular forms of glucagon-like peptide-1 in human pancreas and glucagonomas. J. Clin. Endocr. Metabol. **61:** 472-479.
30. RHOLAM, M., P. NICOLAS & P. COHEN. 1986. Precursors for peptide hormones share common secondary structures forming features at the proteolytic processing sites. FEBS Lett. **207:** 1-6.
31. THIM, L. & A. J. MOODY. 1982. Purification and chemical characterization of a glicentin-related pancreatic peptide (proglucagon fragment) from porcine pancreas. Biochem. Biophys. Acta **703:** 134-141.
32. THOMSEN, J., K. CHRISTIANSEN & K. BRUNFELDT. 1972. The amino acid sequence of human glucagon. FEBS Lett. **21:** 315-319.
33. CONLON, J. M., H. F. HANSEN & T. W. SCHWARTZ. 1985. Primary structure of glucagon and a partial sequence of oxyntomodulin (glucagon-37) from the guinea pig. Regul. Peptides **11:** 309-320.
34. YANAIHARA, C., T. MATSUMOTO, Y.-M. HONG & N. YANAIHARA. 1985. Isolation and chemical characterization of glicentin C-terminal hexapeptide in porcine pancreas. FEBS Lett. **189:** 50-56.
35. YANAIHARA, C., T. MATSUMOTO, M. KADOWAKI, K. IGUCHI & N. YANAIHARA. 1985. Rat pancreas contains the proglucagon (64-69) fragment and arginine stimulates its release. FEBS Lett. **187:** 307-310.
36. ENSICK, J. W. 1983. Immunoassays for glucagon. *In* Glucagon. P. J. Lefebvre, Ed. Vol **1:** 203-221. Springer Verlag. Berlin, West Germany.
37. ASSAN, R. & N. SLUSHER. 1972. Structure/function and structure/immunoreactivity relationships of the glucagon molecule and related synthetic peptides. Diabetes **21:** 843-855.
38. HEDING, L., E. K. FRANDSEN & H. JACOBSEN. 1976. Glucagon. Structure-function relationship: Immunologic. Metabolism **25:** 1327-1329.

39. UNGER, R. H., A. M. EISENTRAUT, M. S. MCCALL & L. L. MADISON. 1961. Glucagon antibodies and an immunoassay for glucagon. J. Clin. Invest. **40:** 1280-1289.
40. YANAIHARA, C., T. MATSUMOTO, T. NISHIDA, T. UCHIDA, S. KOBAYASHI, A. J. MOODY, L. ORCI & N. YANAIHARA. 1984. Chemical approach to develop glicentin COOH-terminal specific radioimmunoassay. Biomed. Res. **5**(Supp.): 19-32.
41. BLACHE, P., A. KERVRAN & D. BATAILLE. 1987. Oxyntomodulin and glicentin: Brain-gut peptides. Regul. Peptides **18:** 349.
42. IUPAC-IUB COMMISSION ON BIOCHEMICAL NOMENCLATURE. 1968. Eur. J. Biochem. **246:** 2833-2827.
43. HATTON, T. W., C. C. YIP & M. VRANIC. 1985. Biosynthesis of Glucagon (IRG 3500) in canine gastric mucosa. Diabetes **34:** 38-46.
44. NOE, B. D. & G. E. BAUER. 1975. Evidence for sequential metabolic cleavage of proglucagon to glucagon in glucagon biosynthesis. Endocrinology **97:** 868-877.
45. NOE, B. D., C. A. BASTE & G. E. BAUER. 1977. Studies on proinsulin and proglucagon biosynthesis at the cellular level. J. Cell. Biol. **74:** 589-604.
46. PATZELT, C. & E. SCHILTZ. 1984. Conversion of proglucagon in pancreatic alpha cells: The major endproducts are glucagon and a single peptide, the major proglucagon fragment, that contains two glucagon-like sequences. Proc. Natl. Acad. Sci. USA **81:** 5007-5011.
47. PATZELT, C., H. S. TAGER, R. J. CARROLL & D. F. STEINER. 1979. Identification and processing of proglucagon in pancreatic islets. Nature **282:** 260-266.
48. SHIELDS, D., T. G. WARREN, S. E. ROTH & M. J. BRENNER. 1981. Cell-free synthesis and processing of multiple precursors to glucagon. Nature **289:** 511-514.
49. TAGER, H. S. & J. MARKESE. 1979. Intestinal and pancreatic glucagon-like peptides: Evidence for identity of higher molecular weight forms. J. Biol. Chem. **254:** 2229-2233.
50. KERVRAN, A., C. JARROUSSE & D. BATAILLE. 1984. Oxyntomodulin (G-37) and glucagon (G-29): Distribution in the gastrointestinal tract of the rat. Diabetologia **27:** 295-296.
51. KERVRAN, A., P. BLACHE & D. BATAILLE. 1987. Distribution of oxyntomodulin and glucagon in the gastro-intestinal tract and the plasma of the rat. Endocrinology **121:** 704-713.
52. WIDER, M. D. 1985. Characterization of a heat stable 12,000 Da, glucagon-like immunoreactivity (GLI) peptide from porcine ileum that stimulates hepatic glucose production *in vivo* and *in vitro*. Proc. Soc. Exp. Biol. Med. **179:** 356-364.
53. MUNCK, A., A. KERVRAN, J. C. MARIE, D. BATAILLE & G. ROSSELIN. 1984. Glucagon-37 (Oxyntomodulin) and glucagon-29 (pancreatic glucagon) in human bowel: Analysis by HPLC and radioreceptorassay. Peptides **5:** 553-561.
54. CONLON, J. M., W. K. SAMSON, R. E. DOBBS, L. ORCI & R. H. UNGER. 1979. Glucagon-like polypeptides in canine brain. Diabetes **28:** 700-702.
55. HATTON, T. W., N. KOVACEVIC, M. DUTCZAK & M. VRANIC. 1982. Glucagon-like im-munoreactants in extracts of the rat hypothalamus. Endocrinology **111:** 572-577.
56. LOREN, I., J. ALUMETS, R. HAKANSON, F. SUNDLER & J. THORELL. 1979. Gut-type glucagon immunoreactivity in nerves of the rat brain. Histochemistry **61:** 335-341.
57. TAGER, H., M. HOHENBOKEN, J. MARKESE & R. J. DINERSTEIN. 1980. Identification and localization of glucagon-related peptides in rat brain. Proc. Natl. Acad. Sci. USA **77:** 6229-6233.
58. TOMINAGA, M., H. KANEDA, S. MARUBASHI, T. KAMIMURA, T. KATAGIRI & H. SASAKI. 1984. Synaptosomal localization and release of glucagon-like materials in the rat brain. Brain Res. Bull. **12:** 373-375.
59. BATAILLE, D., C. GESPACH, A. M. COUDRAY & G. ROSSELIN. 1981. "Enteroglucagon": A specific effect on gastric glands isolated from the rat fundus. Evidence for an oxyntomodulin action. Biosci. Rep. **1:** 151-155.
60. JARROUSSE, C., D. BATAILLE & B. JEANRENAUD. 1984. A pure enteroglucagon, oxyntomodulin (glucagon-37), stimulates insulin release in perfused rat pancreas. Endocrinology **115:** 102-105.
61. EPAND, R. M., G. ROSSELIN, D. HUI BON HOA, T. E. COTE & M. LABURTHE. 1981. Structural requirements for glucagon receptor binding and activation of adenylate cyclase in liver. J. Biol. Chem. **255:** 653-658.

62. RODBELL, M., H. M. J. KRANS, S. L. POHL & L. BIRNBAUMER. 1971. The glucagon sensitive adenyl cyclase system in plasma membranes of rat liver. III. Binding of glucagon: Method of assay and specificity. J. Biol. Chem. **246:** 1861-1871.

63. HERBERG, J. T., J. CODINA, K. A. RICH, F. J. ROJAS & R. IYENGAR. 1984. The hepatic glucagon receptor. Solubilization, characterization and development of an affinity adsorption assay for the soluble receptor. J. Biol. Chem. **259:** 9285-9294.

64. DUBRASQUET, J. M., D. BATAILLE & C. GESPACH. 1982. Oxyntomodulin (glucagon-37 or bioactive Enteroglucagon): A potent inhibitor of pentagastrin-stimulated acid secretion in rats. Biosci. Rep. **2:** 391-395.

65. DEPIGNY, C., B. LUPO, A. KERVRAN & D. BATAILLE. 1984. Evidence for a specific binding site for glucagon-37 (Oxyntomodulin/ Bioactive enteroglucagon) in the rat oxyntic glands. C.R. Acad. Sci. Paris III **299:** 677-680.

66. KIRKEGAARD, P., A. J. MOODY, J. J. HOLST, F. B. LOUD, P. S. OLSEN & J. CHRISTIANSEN. 1982. Glicentin inhibits gastric acid secretion in the rat. Nature **297:** 156-157.

67. AUDOUSSET-PUECH, M. P., C. JARROUSSE, M. DUBRASQUET, A. AUMELAS, B. CASTRO, D. BATAILLE & J. MARTINEZ. 1985. Synthesis of the C-terminal octapeptide of pig oxyntomodulin: Lys-Arg-Asn-Lys-Asn-Asn-Ile-Ala: A potent inhibitor of pentagastrin-induced acid secretion. J. Med. Chem. **28:** 1529-1533.

68. DUBRASQUET, J. M., M. P. AUDOUSSET-PUECH, J. MARTINEZ & D. BATAILLE. 1986. Somatostatin enhances the inhibitory effect of oxyntomodulin and its C-terminal octapeptide on acid secretion. Peptides 7(Suppl. 1): 257-259.

69. JARROUSSE, C., M. P. AUDOUSSET-PUECH, M. DUBRASQUET, H. NIEL, J. MARTINEZ & D. BATAILLE. 1985. Oxyntomodulin (glucagon-37) and its C-terminal octapeptide inhibit gastric acid secretion. FEBS Lett. **188:** 81-84.

70. JARROUSSE, C., H. NIEL, M. P. AUDOUSSET-PUECH. J. MARTINEZ & D. BATAILLE. 1986. Oxyntomodulin and its C-terminal octapeptide inhibit liquid meal-stimulated acid secretion. Peptides 7(Supp. 1): 253-256.

71. LOTERSZTAJN, S., R. M. EPAND, A. MALLAT & F. PECKER. 1984. Inhibition by glucagon of the calcium pump in liver plasma membranes. J. Biol. Chem. **259:** 8195-8201.

72. MALLAT, A., C. PAVOINE, M. DUFOUR, S. LOTERSZTAJN, D. BATAILLE & F. PECKER. 1987. Glucagon-(19-29), a proteolytic fragment of glucagon, is responsible for the inhibition of the liver Ca^{2+} pump by glucagon. Nature **325:** 620-622.

73. WAKELAM, M. J. O., G. J. MURPHY, V. J. HRUBY & M. D. HOUSLAY. 1986. Activation of two signal-transduction systems in hepatocytes by glucagon. Nature **323:** 68-71.

Helodermin-like Peptides

PATRICK ROBBERECHT, ANDRÉ VANDERMEERS,
MARIE-CLAIRE VANDERMEERS-PIRET, PHILIPPE
GOURLET, ANNICK CAUVIN, PHILIPPE DE NEEF,
AND JEAN CHRISTOPHE

Department of Biochemistry and Nutrition
School of Medicine
Université Libre de Bruxelles
Brussels, Belgium

DISCOVERY OF HELODERMIN-LIKE PEPTIDES

In 1982, Raufman et al.[1] showed that the venom of the venomous lizards *Heloderma suspectum* and *Heloderma horridum* caused an increase in amylase secretion from dispersed acini of guinea pig pancreas. This effect was attributed to a thermostable peptide structurally related but distinct from VIP on the basis of the following arguments: As for VIP, the venom efficacy on amylase secretion and cyclic AMP production was increased by theophylline; the venom did not alter calcium outflux but potentiated the enzyme secretion caused by secretagogues that mobilized calcium; the venom totally inhibited [^{125}I]VIP binding; the venom effects were inhibited by (Gln^9)-secretin$_{5-27}$, an inhibitor of both secretin and VIP receptors. At variance with VIP, the venom was unable to interact with a VIP-specific antiserum. The presence in the venom of both lizards of a VIP-like peptide was further substantiated by Amiranoff et al.[2] who demonstrated an inhibition of the binding of [^{125}I]VIP to human and rat intestinal epithelial cell membranes and an activation, in the presence of GTP, of the adenylate cyclase system. In 1984, Gillet et al.[3] in our laboratory described the activation of adenylate cyclase in rat pancreatic plasma membranes by the two venoms and obtained evidence, based on the use of competitive inhibitors of secretin action, that this effect could be mediated through interaction with secretin-preferring receptors.

The purification of the VIP-secretin-like material present in the venom of *Heloderma suspectum* was undertaken independently by Pisano's group at the National Institutes of Health (USA) and by our group in Brussels.

The purification of the active material was monitored by the capability of the material to stimulate amylase production by isolated guinea pig pancreatic acini (Pisano's group) or to activate adenylate cyclase in rat pancreatic plasma membranes (our group). In January 1984, we published[4] the isolation and purification to homogeneity of a 5.9-kDa peptide that interacted with VIP and secretin receptors in several mammalian tissues[5] and was called helodermin.

A sample of this essentially pure peptide was sent to Dr. N. Yanaihara (Shizuoka, Japan) who published the complete amino acid sequence of helodermin in December

1984,[6] demonstrating clearly that this new peptide exhibited strong homologies with VIP, PHI, and secretin.

In October 1984, Pisano's group had published[7] the isolation and amino acid sequence of two peptides that were called helospectins I and II and were also clearly related to the VIP family of peptides. Helodermin and helospectins I and II (TABLE 1) differed not only on the total number of amino acids (respectively, 35 and 37/38 amino acids) but also on the identity of amino acids in positions 5, 8, 24, 30, and 34. Furthermore, the number of peptides obtained after tryptic digestion was unequal. Despite the fact that such disparities between helodermin and helospectin were unlikely to reflect errors in sequence analysis we tried, in collaboration with Dr. Yanaihara who synthesized helodermin analogues and fragments, to prove that both peptides were indeed present in the lizard venoms. The experiments performed (see below) led us to conclude that:

1. helodermin and helospectin coexist as distinct molecular entities;
2. helodermin is the major component of *Heloderma suspectum* venom whereas helospectin is predominant in *Heloderma horridum* venom;
3. multiple variants of helodermin and helospectin coexist in each venom;
4. the amino acid sequence of the major form of helodermin differs from that previously reported, glutamic acid being present in positions 8 and 9 instead of glutamine.

In parallel with these studies conducted on lizard peptides, rabbits were immunized against natural helodermin (our group) or against the synthetic fragment helodermin$_{7-35}$ (Yanaihara's group). The development of highly specific radioimmunoassays allowed us to discover, in 1985, the presence of helodermin-immunoreactive material in rat and human tissues[8,9] while Yanaihara's group established in 1986 the regional distribution of helodermin-immunoreactive material in porcine brain and gut.[10] We observed recently the presence of enough helodermin-immunoreactive material in human endocrine tumors to hope to elucidate the structure of mammalian helodermin.

IDENTIFICATION OF HELODERMIN-LIKE PEPTIDES

As soon as sufficient amounts of pure helodermin were available, polyclonal antibodies were produced by injecting rabbits with the peptide coupled to bovine serum albumin by carbodiimide. The production of specific antiserums as well as the easy iodination of helodermin[11] allowed the design of a sensitive radioimmunoassay.[8,9] Our antibody 15/3[9] detected 2.5 to 5.0 pg helodermin; was NH$_2$-terminally directed; and did not recognize the parent peptides VIP, PHI, PHM, GRF, glucagon, and secretin but cross-reacted fully with synthetic helospectin I and helospectin II (FIG. 1A). We also looked for a possible cross-reactivity of helodermin and helospectin in specific radioimmunoassays of VIP, PHI, and secretin and found to our surprise (FIG. 1B) that both helospectins—but not helodermin—cross-reacted in a PHI radioimmunoassay using the NH$_2$-terminal specific antiserum R8403 from Professor Yanaihara.[12] By combining the two radioimmunoassays, we were thus easily able to distinguish helodermin-like peptides from helospectin-like peptides.

A systematic analysis of the chromatographic profiles of several batches of *Heloderma suspectum* and *Heloderma horridum* venoms purchased from Sigma Chemical Co. (St. Louis, MO) revealed a much higher heterogeneity than that previously

TABLE 1. Comparison of the Amino Acid Sequence of Helodermin and Helospectins with Those of VIP, PHI, Secretin, and GRF[a]

Species	Peptide	1	5	10	15	20	25	30	35	40	45
ls	Helodermin[b]	H-S-D-A-I-F-T-Q-Q-Y-S-K-L-L-A-K-L-A-L-Q-K-Y-L-A-S-I-L-G-S-R-T-S-P-P-P-*									
lh	Helospectin(s)[c]	H-S-D-A-T-F-T-A-E-Y-S-K-L-L-A-K-L-A-L-Q-K-Y-L-E-S-I-L-G-S-S-T-S-P-R-P-P-S-(S)									
p/h	VIP	H-S-D-A-V-F-T-D-N-Y-T-R-L-R-K-Q-M-A-V-K-K-Y-L-N-S-I-L-N-*									
p	PHI	H-A-D-G-V-F-T-S-D-F-S-R-L-L-G-Q-L-S-A-K-K-Y-L-E-S-L-I-*									
p	Secretin	H-S-D-G-T-F-T-S-E-L-S-R-L-R-D-S-A-R-L-Q-R-L-L-Q-G-L-V-*									
h	GRF$_{1-44}$	Y-A-D-A-I-F-T-N-S-Y-R-K-V-L-G-Q-L-S-A-R-K-L-L-Q-D-I-M-S-R-Q-Q-G-E-S-N-Q-E-R-G-A-R-A-R-L-*									

[a] Identities are represented by bold letters and bars. * = α-carboxyamide group. Species: b: bovine; c: chicken; h: human; ls: lizard *Heloderma suspectum*; lh: lizard *Heloderma horridum*; p: porcine. Underlined: identifies with helodermin.
ALA A; ARG R; ASN N; ASP D; CYS C; GLN Q; GLU E; GLY G; HIS H; ILE I; LEU L; LYS K; MET M; NH$_2$*; PHE F; PRO P; SER S; THR T; TRP W; TYR Y; VAL V.
[b] According to Hoshino et al.[6] The batches of helodermin used here contain E-E in positions 8 and 9 (Vandermeers et al.[13]).
[c] According to Parker et al.[7]

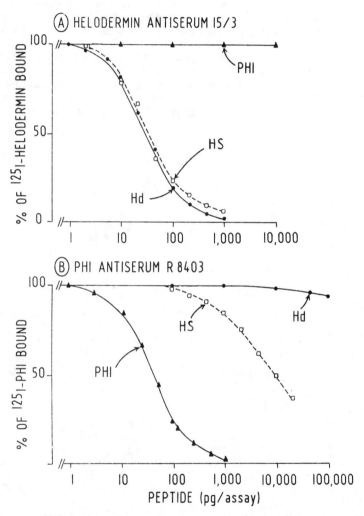

FIGURE 1. Displacement of [^{125}I]helodermin bound to helodermin antiserum 15/3 (upper panel A) and [^{125}I]PHI bound to antiserum R8403 (lower panel B) by increasing concentrations of PHI (▲), helodermin (●), and synthetic helospectin I from Peninsula (□). VIP, secretin, and GRF were ineffective in both assays.

reported by either Pisano's group or our group (FIGS. 2 and 3). On the basis of the immunological properties previously described, it appeared that six forms of helospectin-like peptides were present in *Heloderma horridum* venom, and that two minor forms of helospectin-like peptides and at least two forms of helodermin coexisted in *Heloderma suspectum* venom. These results were confirmed by the chemical analysis of the major forms of the pure peptides. Indeed, all helospectin-like variants exhibited a similar pattern of four peptide fragments after tryptic digestion (FIG. 4A), whereas all helodermin-like peptides generated five tryptic fragments (FIG. 4B). The main form among helodermin-like peptides (peak 4 in FIG. 2B) was reanalyzed; at variance with the sequence published by Hoshino *et al.*,[6] we found that: (a) the peptide was more acidic than helodermin synthesized according to Hoshino; (b) a treatment with the endoproteinase Glu-C from *Staphylococcus aureus* under conditions restricting the enzyme specificity to glutamoyl bonds generated two fragments, the first being iden-

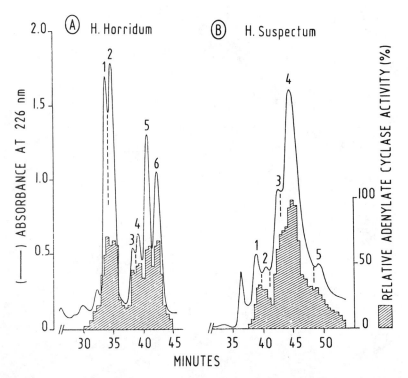

FIGURE 2. High-performance liquid chromatography elution profile of bioactive fractions isolated from *Heloderma horridum* venom (panel A) and *Heloderma suspectum* (panel B). After a first purification on a Supelcosil LC8 DB8 column (1 × 25 cm) eluted with a linear gradient (25 to 75%) of acetonitrile, the active fractions were further chromatographed on the Supelcosil LC308 column (0.46 × 25 cm) that was eluted with solvent A (0.25 M H_3PO_4 adjusted to pH 3 with triethylamine) and solvent B (CH_3CN- H_2O, 4 : 1), using a linear gradient (30 to 32%) of B in 45 minutes at 30°C. Flow rate was 0.8 ml/min. Absorbance was recorded at 226 nm; the biological activity tested was the stimulation of adenylate cyclase activity in rat pancreatic plasma membranes measured on 1 μl aliquots of each fraction. The activity was expressed as percent of maximal activity.

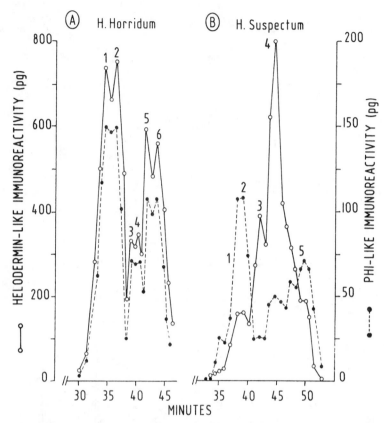

FIGURE 3. Elution profile of immunoreactive helodermin-like (O——O) and PHI-like (-•-) activities in the chromatograms illustrated in FIGURE 2. Radioimmunoassays were performed as described in Vandermeers *et al.*[13] The data were expressed in µg equivalents of each reference peptide.

tified as fragment 1-9, whereas synthetic helodermin was unaffected under similar conditions; and (c) 10 cycles of Edman's degradation revealed glutamic acid in positions 8 and 9.[13]

A direct comparison of the first batch of helodermin analyzed by Hoshino and the subsequent batches could not be performed and a careful analysis of Hoshino's data did not reveal any ambiguity *a posteriori.* Possible explanations for the discrepancy are that: (a) the first batch of venom was rich in a component that was underrepresented in the next batches; and (b) a change in the processing of the crude venom (by the manufacturer) had occurred leading to the deamidation of glutamine 8 and glutamine 9. The final proof of the sequence of natural helodermin will require a direct analysis of the lizard glands and/or the determination of the DNA sequence coding for the peptide.

Peaks 5 and 6 of the chromatographic profile of *Heloderma horridum* venom were found to be identical to helospectins I and II of Pisano's group. For both venoms the other forms were not yet completely sequenced but the differences appeared to be

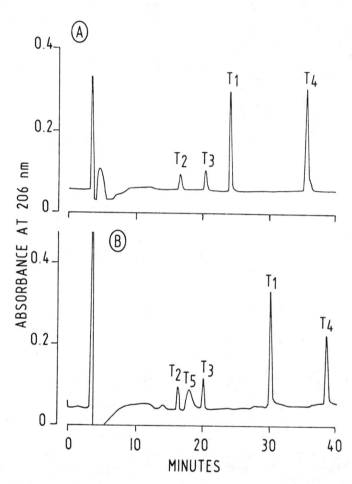

FIGURE 4. Comparative high-performance liquid chromatography elution profiles on Vydac 10-C18 of tryptic peptides from helospectin I (panel A) and helodermin (panel B). Each sample contained 12 nmol of tryptic digest. Solvent A was 0.1% CF_3COOH in water. Solvent B was 0.1% CF_3COOH in acetonitrile/H_2O in a 4 : 1 ratio. A linear gradient (0-10%) of solvent B was applied from 0 to 5 minutes and a second linear gradient (10-40%) of B applied from 5 to 50 minutes. Column temperature was 30°C and the flow rate 1 ml/min. The rank number of the tryptic fragments (T_1, T_2 ...) corresponds to their position in the peptide of origin.

located in the COOH-terminal part of the molecule (see Vandermeers *et al.*, this volume): Deamidation of the terminal prolineamide, glycosylation and/or phosphorylation of the multiple serine residues and/or the addition of a COOH-terminal glycine residue are at present under investigation.

PRESENCE OF HELODERMIN-LIKE PEPTIDES IN MAMMALIAN TISSUES

Immunoreactive helodermin was found in various mammalian tissues of rat,[8] dog,[9] human,[9] and pig.[10] Precise quantification of the material was difficult in crude total tissue extracts due to the lack of parallelism between inhibition curves of serial extract dilutions and the standard helodermin curve in the radioimmunoassays performed with different antisera.[8,9] A more accurate (although not yet precise) quantification was obtained after a partial purification of the immunoreactive material, either on a TSK-G2000-SW column (performing gel permeation chromatography) or a reverse-phase column (performing hydrophic chromatography). In most tissues, the amount of helodermin-like material recovered was 25- to 200-fold lower than that of VIP or PHI/PHM. Due to the low level of immunoreactive material present, we have not yet succeeded in purifying peptide(s) in sufficient amounts to obtain their amino acid composition and sequence. Collecting material is further complicated by the presence of multiple immunoreactive forms separated by ion-exchange chromatography.

FIGURES 5 to 8 summarize our efforts to purify helodermin-like peptides from dog saliva that was chosen as starting material considering its relatively high concentration of helodermin-like material[9] and the low level of other peptides of the same family. Two liters of saliva were collected on ice from anesthetized dogs stimulated with pilocarpine (i.m. injections of 10 mg). The saliva was boiled in 1.0 N acetic acid. After centrifugation the supernatant was lyophilized, redissolved in 1.0 N acetic acid and chromatographed on a Lichroprep column (porosity, 25-50 μ) eluted with an acetonitrile gradient (FIG. 5). The material eluting between 30 and 45% acetonitrile (pool of two chromatographic products) was rechromatographed (after evaporation of the organic solvent) on a RP8 Lichrosorb column (porosity, 10 μ) and eluted with a propanol gradient (FIG. 6). The fractions containing the immunoreactive material were pooled, lyophilized, and further chromatographed on a RP8 Lichrosorb column (porosity, 5 μ) eluted again with an acetonitrile gradient (FIG. 7). The immunoreactive material was pooled, lyophilized, resuspended in 20 mM ammonium acetate-3% propanol (pH 4.2), and chromatographed on an ion-exchange Mono S HR 5/5 column eluted with an ammonium acetate gradient (FIG. 8). At least six peaks of immunoreactive material were identified. Peak IV eluted in the same position as the standard of natural helodermin. The total amount of material recovered before the Mono S step was 1.5 μg of helodermin equivalent. The quantities of material found in each chromatographic peak were too small to justify further purification. VIP and PHI (assayed with, respectively, antibody R502 and R8403[12,14]) were not present in the chromatogram represented in FIGURE 8.

Human endocrine tumors are likely to represent an adequate starting material for the purification of helodermin-like peptides. We have so far examined three specimens: one pancreatic tumor containing VIP and PHM but no gastrin that provoked an unusual clinical history of severe diarrhea and duodenal ulcers; one hepatic metastasis of a medullary thyroïd carcinoma responsible for severe diarrhea; and one endocrine

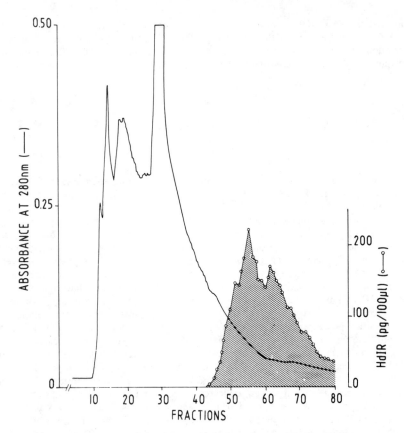

FIGURE 5. High-performance liquid chromatography profile on Lichroprep RP-8 Lobar column of a concentrated boiled acidic extract of dog saliva. The sample (10 ml) was equivalent to 100 ml of dog saliva. The column was eluted with a linear gradient (20 to 70% acetonitrile) applied in 50 minutes. The flow rate was 2 ml/min and 30-second fractions were collected. The absorbance was recorded at 280 nm and the fractions containing immunoreactive helodermin were collected (O——O, hatched area).

pancreatic tumor in a five-year-old girl.[15] We have detected the presence of helodermin-like peptides in each tumor. Four grams of the tumor (and metastasis) of the five-year-old girl (her clinical history is reported in Santangelo et al.[15]) were extracted in boiling water, then acidified with 1.0 N acetic acid, and the supernatant was chromatographed on a RP8 Lichrosorb column (10 μ porosity) eluted with an acetonitrile gradient. The helodermin immunoreactive material was clearly separated from VIP and PHM immunoreactivities (FIG. 9). The levels of VIP, PHM, and helodermin-like material were of the same order of magnitude (± 1 μg per g tumor). Secretin-like material was not found.

BIOLOGICAL PROPERTIES OF HELODERMIN-LIKE PEPTIDES

In Vitro *Biological Properties*

In order to screen target tissues susceptible to be modulated by helodermin-like peptides, we looked for the presence of helodermin binding sites and/or for the presence of helodermin-sensitive adenylate cyclase in various membranes.

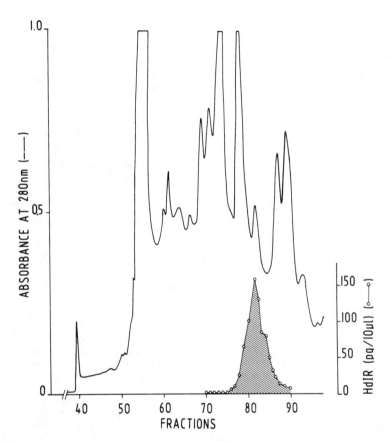

FIGURE 6. High-performance liquid chromatography profile on a Lichrosorb RP-8 column (porosity 10 μ) of the helodermin-immunoreactive material collected from 10 successive chromatograms described in FIGURE 5. Solvent A was 0.4 M ammonium acetate (pH 7) and solvent B was 0.4 M ammonium acetate pH 7, propanol 50%. The column was eluted with a linear gradient (0-80%) of solvent B in 50 minutes. The flow rate was 2 ml/min and 30 sec fractions were collected. The absorbance was recorded at 280 nm and the fractions containing immunoreactive helodermin were pooled (O——O, hatched area).

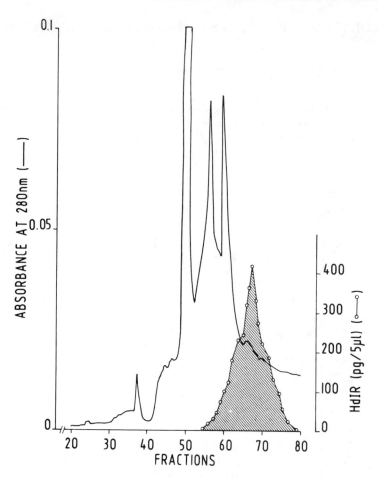

FIGURE 7. High-performance liquid chromatography profile on a Lichrosorb RP-8 column (porosity 5 μ) of the sample prepared in FIGURE 6, lyophilized and dissolved in 0.4 *M* ammonium acetate (pH 7.0). The column was eluted with a linear gradient of acetonitrile (0-50%) in ammonium acetate developed in 50 minutes. The flow rate was 2 ml/min and 30-second fractions were collected. The absorbance was recorded at 280 nm and the fractions containing immunoreactive helodermin were pooled (O——O, hatched area).

Presence of Helodermin Binding Sites

Helodermin receptors were identified by [^{125}I]helodermin binding and its inhibition by the unlabeled peptide. In most experiments, helodermin was radioiodinated by the chloramine T method[11] and separated from free iodine by adsorption on cellulose and elution by a high concentration of bovine serum albumin. In some experiments, the tracer was purified by reverse-phase chromatography: this last procedure (FIG. 10) allowed the separation of free iodine, unlabeled peptide, and six radioactive peaks that could be precipitated by 10% trichloroacetic acid. Peaks I and II were identified as, respectively, monoiodinated (Tyr[10])-helodermin and monoiodinated (Tyr[22])-helodermin (P. Gourlet *et al.*, to be published). The other peaks have not yet been precisely characterized. Although the use of peaks I and II as tracers improved the quality of binding studies, the results obtained were similar to those previously published with unpurified [^{125}I]helodermin. [^{125}I]helodermin binding sites were identified on liver membranes,[11] pulmonary membranes,[16] and pancreatic acini[17] from rat. We did not observe significant tracer binding on heart, pituitary, and synaptic membranes from rat as well as on human heart membranes. In rat liver and pulmonary membranes, [^{125}I]helodermin identified a single class of receptors that could be considered high-affinity VIP receptors.[11] We were unable to identify a specific helodermin receptor in these tissues. The use of [^{125}I]helodermin to identify and quantify the high-affinity subclass of VIP receptors allowed significant progress as compared to methods based on the decomposition of complex binding curves.

In rat pancreatic acini, [^{125}I]helodermin labeled two classes of receptors that were identified by Dehaye *et al.*[17] as a high-affinity receptor for secretin (S_2) and a receptor with low affinity for secretin and high affinity for VIP (S_3). In this tissue, [^{125}I]helodermin was a nonselective ligand occupying VIP and secretin receptors with the same affinity. In pancreatic acini we cannot find any selective helodermin receptor.

In the experiments performed on hepatic, pulmonary, and pancreatic preparations, a major advantage of using [^{125}I]helodermin as tracer was its remarkable stability even at 37°C.

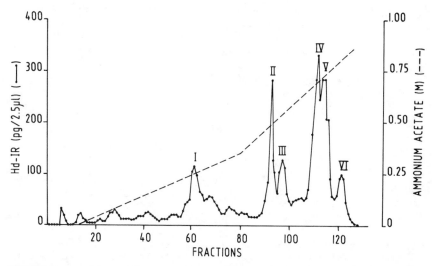

FIGURE 8. Ion-exchange chromatography on Mono S HR 5/5 column of the immunoreactive helodermin obtained in FIGURE 7. The pool of helodermin was lyophilized, dissolved in 20 m*M* ammonium acetate (pH 4.2), propanol 10% and eluted with a gradient of ammonium acetate (pH 4.2). A first linear gradient (20 m*M*-300 m*M*) was developed in 40 minutes and was followed by a second linear gradient (0.3 *M*-1.0 *M*) during 30 further minutes. The flow rate was 1 ml/min and 30-second fractions were collected. A radioimmunoassay of helodermin was performed on each fraction (●——●). Six peaks were separated and peak IV eluted in the same position as the helodermin standard.

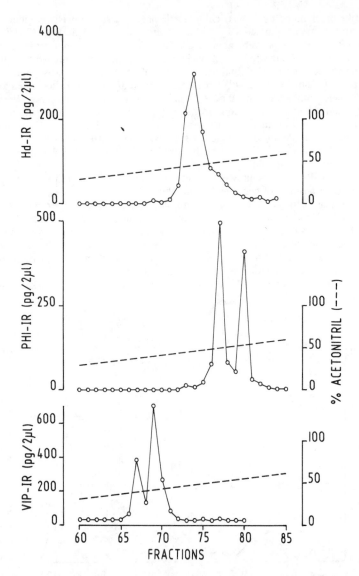

FIGURE 9. High-performance liquid chromatography profile of a 1.0 N acetic acid extract of two grams of an endocrine tumor.[15] The Lichrosorb RP-8 column (porosity 10 μ) was eluted with a linear gradient (0-60%) of acetonitrile in 50 minutes. The flow rate was 2 ml/min and 30-second fractions were collected. Helodermin, PHM, and VIP immunoreactivity were determined with, respectively, antiserum 15/3, AC24, and R502. Antiserums 15/3 and R502 were characterized in, respectively, Robberecht *et al.*[8] and Yanaihara *et al.*[14]; the rabbit anti-PHM serum AC24 was obtained after four injections of PHI coupled to BSA by carbodiimide and cross-reacted fully with human PHI(PHM).

Presence of Helodermin-Stimulated Adenylate Cyclase

As a member of the VIP/PHI/secretin/GRF/glucagon superfamily of peptides, helodermin was likely to act essentially by activation of membrane adenylate cyclase so that the stimulation of this enzyme could be a tool for the identification of helodermin receptors.

Helodermin stimulated adenylate cyclase activity in several rat tissue membranes, including synaptic, pituitary, heart, lung, liver, intestinal smooth muscle, intestinal epithelium, and pancreatic membranes (Refs. 5, 11, 16, 18, and unpublished data)

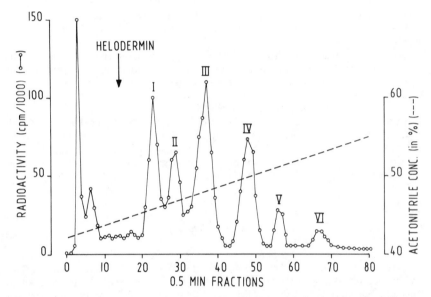

FIGURE 10. High-performance liquid chromatography profile of radioiodinated [^{125}I]helodermin. The C18 Microbondapak column was eluted with a linear gradient (43-55%) of acetonitrile, trifluoroacetic acid 0.1% that developed in 40 minutes; 0.5-minute fractions were collected. The flow rate was 1.0 ml/min. At least 90% of the radioactivity of peaks I to VI was precipitated by 10% trichloroacetic acid. The arrow indicates the elution position of unlabeled helodermin.

and on human tissue membranes including lung, heart, coronary vessel, and pancreatic membranes (unpublished data). In all these tissues helodermin probably acted through interaction with VIP and/or secretin receptors although direct proof is still lacking.

In rat pituitary membranes (in which helodermin could conceivably activate adenylate cyclase through interaction with VIP and/or GRF receptors) the peptide stimulated the enzyme with the same efficacy but a lower potency than VIP and its effect was not antagonized by the GRF antagonist[19] (N-Ac-Tyr^1,D-Arg^2)-GRF$_{1-29}$-NH$_2$ (unpublished results). In rat pancreatic membranes, helodermin activated adenylate cyclase through interaction with VIP and secretin receptors as the VIP antagonists (N-Ac-Tyr^1,D-Phe^2)-GRF$_{1-29}$-NH$_2$[20] and (D-Phe^2)-VIP,[21] as well as the secretin antagonist secretin$_{7-27}$ inhibited helodermin effects. Preliminary data obtained on human pancreatic membranes suggest that helodermin activates adenylate cyclase through interaction with secretin receptors only. In rat pancreatic, pituitary, and hepatic membranes, helodermin and helopectin(s) had the same efficacies and potencies on adenylate cyclase activation.

In Vitro *Effects on Intact Tissues*

To the best of our knowledge, pure helodermin and helospectin(s) have been tested on pancreatic preparations only. The relaxing effect of Gila monster venom on rabbit urethrea and anococcygeus muscle[23] cannot be definitely attributed to helodermin-like peptides as such crude preparations also contain active forms of phospholipases A_2.[24]

In rat pancreatic acini, helodermin increased in a dose-dependent manner the production of cyclic AMP, phosphorylation of three particulate proteins, and amylase secretion; it also potentiated the secretion of amylase induced by the COOH-terminal octapeptide of cholecystokinin.[17,25] As previously mentioned, helodermin recognized both secretin and VIP receptors in this model. In guinea pig acini, helospectins induced amylase hypersecretion, their maximal efficacy being 10-15% lower than that of VIP and their potency 100 times lower. Finally, synthetic helodermin, in the 10^{-9} M to 10^{-7} M concentration range, exhibited a marked potentiation of glucose-induced insulin release from the isolated perfused rat pancreas: the potency of helodermin in this system was 25% of that of VIP.[10]

In Vivo *Biological Effects*

Intra-arterial infusion of helodermin caused a dose-dependent increase in the femoral arterial blood flow in the anesthetized dog. Helodermin was 16 times less potent than VIP but more potent than PHM. The COOH-terminal fragment helodermin$_{7-35}$ was completely inactive while the NH_2-terminal fragment helodermin$_{1-27}$-NH_2 retained full biological activity. However, the mean half-life of the vascular effect of helodermin was 9.1 minutes while that of VIP and helodermin$_{1-27}$-NH_2 was 1.4 and 2.2 minutes, respectively.[26] An intravenous injection of helodermin (200 pmol/kg) induced a prolonged systemic hypotension and tachycardia and an increase in carotid arterial blood flow. The effect was lower than that of VIP but markedly longer.[26] Intravenous injection of helodermin to conscious dogs with chronic pancreatic fistula resulted in a dose-dependent increase in pancreatic water and bicarbonate secretion but not in protein secretion. In this respect helodermin was four times less potent than secretin but four times more potent than VIP.[10]

CONCLUSIONS

Helodermin and helospectin-like peptides represent clearly distinct chemical entities. Helodermin is the major peptide of *Heloderma suspectum* venom and helospectin is the major peptide of *Heloderma horridum* venom. The existence of these peptides, obviously related to the VIP/secretin/PHI/glucagon/GRF family of peptides, in an exocrine secretion supports the concept of an overlap of exocrine and (neuro)endocrine functions.[27] A detailed study of the structure and distribution of all parent peptides in lizard tissues would be of great interest.

Helodermin- and/or helospectin-like peptides are present in mammalian tissues on the basis of radioimmunoassays. Both types of peptides cannot be differentiated so far with the antiserums at hand. As helospectin cross-reacted with specific antibodies developed against porcine PHI, there is a possibility that some PHI variants could be in fact helospectin-like peptides. This might offer an explanation for the marked heterogeneity of mammalian PHI-immunoreactive material[28,29] that contrasts with the relatively limited number of VIP and secretin molecular forms.[30]

The spectrum of biological activities of helodermin is comparable to that of VIP, PHI, and secretin: Helodermin appears to interact with VIP and/or secretin receptors. The longer half-life of its biological action, due to the original COOH-terminal extension 28-35 (resistant to proteolytic cleavage by carboxypeptidase Y, for instance: A. Vandermeers *et al.*, unpublished data) is of major pharmacological interest.

ACKNOWLEDGMENTS

We thank the following colleagues who made this work possible: Drs. Chizuko and Noboru Yanaihara (Department of Bioorganic Chemistry, Shizuoka School of Pharmacy, Japan) for their active participation in this work and for their generous gift of synthetic peptides and specific antibodies, Dr. Jacques De Graef and Marie-Claire Woussen-Colle (Laboratory of Experimental Surgery, Université Libre de Bruxelles, Brussels, Belgium) for helping us in producing antisera and collecting dog saliva, and Dr. Guenter Krejs (Department of Internal Medicine, University of Texas at Dallas, Dallas, TX) for sending us a sample of a human endocrine tumor.

REFERENCES

1. RAUFMAN, J. P., R. T. JENSEN, V. E. SUTLIFF, J. J. PISANO & J. D. GARDNER. 1982. Actions of Gila monster venom on dispersed acini from guinea pig pancreas. Am. J. Physiol. **242:** 6470-6474.
2. AMIRANOFF, B., N. VAUCLIN-JACQUES, N. BOIGE, C. ROUYER-FESSARD & M. LABURTHE. 1983. Interaction of Gila monster venom with VIP receptors in intestinal epithelium of human. A comparison with rat. FEBS Lett. **164:** 299-302.
3. GILLET, L., P. ROBBERECHT, M. WAELBROECK, J. C. CAMUS, P. DE NEEF, W. KÖNIG & J. CHRISTOPHE. 1984. Interaction of Gila monster venom with secretin receptors in rat pancreatic membranes. Peptides **5:** 407-409.
4. VANDERMEERS, A., M. C. VANDERMEERS-PIRET, P. ROBBERECHT, M. WAELBROECK, J. P. DEHAYE, J. WINAND & J. CHRISTOPHE. 1984. Purification of a novel pancreatic secretory factor (PSF) and a novel peptide with VIP- and secretin-like properties (helodermin) from Gila monster venom. FEBS Lett. **166:** 273-276.
5. ROBBERECHT, P., M. WAELBROECK, J. P. DEHAYE, J. WINAND, A. VANDERMEERS, M. C. VANDERMEERS-PIRET & J. CHRISTOPHE. 1984. Evidence that helodermin, a newly extracted peptide from Gila monster venom, is a member of the secretin/VIP/PHI family of peptides with an original pattern of biological properties. FEBS Lett. **166:** 277-282.

6. HOSHINO, M., C. YANAIHARA, Y. M. HONG, S. KISHIDA, Y. KATSUMARU, A. VANDER-MEERS, M. C. VANDERMEERS-PIRET, P. ROBBERECHT, J. CHRISTOPHE & N. YANAI-HARA. 1984. Primary structure of helodermin, a VIP-secretin-like peptide isolated from Gila monster venom. FEBS Lett. **178:** 233-239.
7. PARKER, D. S., J. P. RAUFMAN, T. O'DONOHUE, M. BLEDSOE, H. YOSHIDA & J. J. PISANO. 1984. Amino acid sequences of helospectins, new members of the glucagon superfamily, found in Gila monster venom. J. Biol. Chem. **259:** 11751-11755.
8. ROBBERECHT, P., J. DE GRAEF, M. C. WOUSSEN, M. C. VANDERMEERS-PIRET, A. VAN-DERMEERS, P. DE NEEF, A. CAUVIN, C. YANAIHARA, N. YANAIHARA & J. CHRISTOPHE. 1985. Immunoreactive helodermin-like peptides in rat: A new class of mammalian neu-ropeptides related to secretin and VIP. Biochem. Biophys. Res. Commun. **130:** 333-342.
9. ROBBERECHT, P., P. DE NEEF, A. VANDERMEERS, M. C. VANDERMEERS-PIRET, M. SVOBODA, S. MEURIS, J. DE GRAEF, M. C. WOUSSEN-COLLE, C. YANAIHARA, N. YANAIHARA & J. CHRISTOPHE. 1985. Presence of helodermin-like peptides of the VIP-secretin family in mammalian salivary glands and saliva. FEBS Lett. **190:** 142-146.
10. NARUSE, S., A. YASUI, S. KISHIDA, C. YANAIHARA, P. ROBBERECHT, J. CHRISTOPHE & N. YANAIHARA. 1986. Helodermin: Synthesis, existence and biological actions in mam-mals. Can. J. Physiol. Pharmacol. (Gastrointestinal Hormones) July: 23.
11. ROBBERECHT, P., M. WAELBROECK, P. DE NEEF, J. C. CAMUS, A. VANDERMEERS, M. C. VANDERMEERS-PIRET & J. CHRISTOPHE. 1984. Specific labelling by ^{125}I-helodermin of high-affinity VIP receptors in rat liver membranes. FEBS Lett. **172:** 55-58.
12. YANAIHARA, N., C. YANAIHARA, R. NOKIHORA, K. IGUCHI, S. FUKATA, M. TANAKA, Y. YAMAMOTO & T. MOCHIZUKI. 1984. Immunochemical study on PHI/PHM with use of synthetic peptides. Peptides **5:** 247-254.
13. VANDERMEERS, A., P. GOURLET, M. C. VANDERMEERS-PIRET, A. CAUVIN, P. DE NEEF, J. RATHE, M. SVOBODA, P. ROBBERECHT & J. CHRISTOPHE. 1987. Chemical, immu-nological and biological properties of vasoactive intestinal peptide-peptide histidine is-oleucinamide (VIP-PHI)-like peptides extracted from the venom of two lizards (*Heloderma horridum* and *Heloderma suspectum*). Eur. J. Biochem. In press.
14. YANAIHARA, N., M. SAKAGONI, H. SATO, K. YAMAMOTO, T. HOSHIMOTO, C. YANAI-HARA, Z. ITO, K. YAMAGUCHI & K. ABE. 1977. Immunological aspects of secretin, substance P, and VIP. Gastroenterology **72:** 803-810.
15. SANTANGELO, W. C., A. J. STRICKLAND, J. M., DUCORE & G. J. KREJS. 1986. Long-term treatment of a child with pancreatic cholera syndrome with somatostatin analog (SMS 201-995). Can. J. Physiol. Pharmacol. (Gastrointestinal Hormones) July: 66-67.
16. ROBBERECHT, P., A. VANDERMEERS, M. C. VANDERMEERS-PIRET, P. DE NEEF, J. C. CAMUS, M. WAELBROECK, D. H. COY & J. CHRISTOPHE. 1985. Specific labelling of high affinity VIP receptors in rat liver and lung membranes by [^{125}I]helodermin. *In* Regulatory Peptides in Digestive, Nervous and Endocrine Systems. INSERM Symposium n° 25. M. J. M. Lewin & S. Bonfils, Eds.: 149-152. Amsterdam, the Netherlands.
17. DEHAYE, J. P., J. WINAND, C. DAMIEN, F. GOMEZ, P. POLOCZEK, P. ROBBERECHT, A. VANDERMEERS, M. C. VANDERMEERS-PIRET, M. STIEVENART & J. CHRISTOPHE. 1986. Receptors involved in helodermin action on rat pancreatic acini. Am. J. Physiol. **251:** G602-G610.
18. ROBBERECHT, P., N. YANAIHARA, C. YANAIHARA, P. DE NEEF, J. C. CAMUS, A. VAN-DERMEERS, M. C. VANDERMEERS-PIRET & J. CHRISTOPHE. 1986. Interaction of syn-thetic NH$_2$- and COOH-terminal fragments of helodermin with rat liver VIP receptors. Peptides 7(Suppl. 1): 79-82.
19. ROBBERECHT, P., D. H. COY, M. WAELBROECK, M. L. HEIMAN, P. DE NEEF, J. C. CAMUS & J. CHRISTOPHE. 1985. Structural requirements for the activation of rat anterior pituitary adenylate cyclase by growth hormone-releasing factor (GRF): Discovery of (N-AC-TYR^1, D-ARG^2)-GRF(1-29)-NH$_2$ as a GRF antagonist on membranes. En-docrinology **117:** 1759-1764.
20. WAELBROECK, M., P. ROBBERECHT, D. H. COY, J. C. CAMUS, P. DE NEEF & J. CHRIS-TOPHE. 1985. Interaction of growth hormone-releasing factor (GRF) and 14 GRF analogs with rat pancreatic VIP receptors. Discovery of (N-AC-TYR^1, D-PHE^2)-GRF(1-29)-NH$_2$ as a vasoactive intestinal peptide (VIP) antagonist. Endocrinology **116:** 2643-2649.

21. ROBBERECHT, P., D. H. COY, P. DE NEEF, J. C. CAMUS, A. CAUVIN, M. WAELBROECK & J. CHRISTOPHE. 1986. Interaction of vasoactive intestinal peptide (VIP) and N-terminally modified VIP analogs with rat pancreatic, hepatic and pituitary membranes. Eur. J. Biochem. **159:** 45-49.

22. ROBBERECHT, P., P. CHATELAIN, M. WAELBROECK & J. CHRISTOPHE. 1982. Heterogeneity of VIP-recognizing binding sites in rat tissues. *In* Vasoactive Intestinal Peptide. S. I. Said, Ed.: 323-332. (In the series, Advances in Peptide Hormone Research.) Raven Press. New York.

23. BLANK, M. A., J. R. BROWN, J. C. HUNTER, S. R. BLOOM & M. B. TYERS. 1986. Effects of VIP and related peptides and Gila monster venom on genitourinary smooth muscle. Eur. J. Pharmacol. **132:** 155-161.

24. DEHAYE, J. P., J. WINAND, P. MICHEL, P. POLOCZEK, C. DAMIEN, M. C. VANDERMEERS-PIRET, A. VANDERMEERS & J. CHRISTOPHE. 1984. Phospholipase A2 activity of pancreatic secretory factor, a new secretagogue isolated from the venom of *Heloderma suspectum.* FEBS Lett. **172:** 284-288.

25. CHRISTOPHE, J., M. C. VANDERMEERS-PIRET, J. RATHE, J. P. DEHAYE, N. D. BUI-NGUYEN, J. WINAND & A. VANDERMEERS. 1984. A comparison of the phosphorylation of M_r = 33k, 21k, and 25k membrane-bound proteins in the rat pancreas, submitted to various secretagogues. W. Paton, J. Mitchell, P. Turner, Eds. Vol. **2:** 147-156. Macmillan Press Ltd. London.

26. NARUSE, S., A. YASUI, S. KISHIDA, M. KADOWAKI, M. OSHINO, T. OZAKI, P. ROBBER-ECHT, J. CHRISTOPHE, C. YANAIHARA & N. YANAIHARA. 1986. Helodermin has a VIP-like effect upon canine blood flow. Peptides 7(Suppl. 1): 237-240.

27. ROTH, J., D. LEROITH, J. SHILOACK, J. L. ROZENZWEIG, M. LESNIAK & J. HAVRANKOVE. 1982. The evolutionary origins of hormones, neurotransmitters and other extracellular chemical messengers. Implications for mammalian biology. New Engl. J. Med. **306:** 523-527.

28. YIANGOU, Y., N. D. CHRISTOFIDES, M. A. BLANK, N. YANAIHARA, K. TATEMOTO, A. E. BISHOP, J. M. POLAK & S. R. BLOOM. 1985. Molecular forms of peptide histidine isoleucine-like immunoreactivity in the gastrointestinal tract. Gastroenterology **89:** 516-524.

29. CAUVIN, A., A. VANDERMEERS, M. C. VANDERMEERS-PIRET, P. DE NEEF, C. YANAI-HARA, N. YANAIHARA, P. ROBBERECHT & J. CHRISTOPHE. 1986. Multiple variants of the PHI/VIP/Helodermin family in rat brain. Arch. Int. Physiol. Biochem. **94:** B69.

30. DIMALINE, R. & G. J. DOCKRAY. 1982. Molecular forms of VIP in normal tissue. *In* Vasoactive Intestinal Peptide. S. I. Said, Ed.: 23-33. Raven Press. New York.

Distribution and Pharmacology of Vasoactive Intestinal Peptide Receptors in the Brain and Pituitary

JACQUELINE BESSON[a]

INSERM U. 55
Unité de Recherches sur les Peptides Neurodigestifs et le Diabète
Hôpital St. Antoine
75571 Paris Cedex 12, France

In spite of the fact that extensive studies have been published on putative neurobiological, behavioral, and neuroendocrine roles of the vasoactive intestinal peptide (VIP),[1] only a few investigations have been carried out in the last decade on the localization and characterization of VIP binding sites in the central nervous system (CNS) and in the pituitary gland. However, binding to specific recognition sites represents the first step of any physiological action of VIP in those structures.

This lack of information was mainly due, on the one hand, to the difficulty of working properly on a highly heterogeneous tissue such as the brain, and on the other hand, to the fact that a highly purified radiolabeled ligand was absolutely necessary in order to study VIP binding sites due to the specific lipidic composition of the neural tissue. The problem was solved in part by the recent introduction of a mono-[^{125}I]VIP purified on HPLC,[2] now commercially available, and by autoradiographic studies that allow a precise localization of VIP binding sites.

Until recently, evidence of the presence of VIP binding sites has been found in guinea pig or rat brain membrane preparations[3-8] and in rat isolated cortical synaptosomes.[9-11] However, membranes obtained by dissecting brain regions cannot provide the same degree of resolution and anatomical localization of VIP binding sites within a given structure that can be obtained with autoradiographic methods.[12]

We described in 1984 the first *in vitro* autoradiographic localization of VIP binding sites in the rat brain,[13] a distribution that was recently confirmed and extended by several studies.[14-19]

The aim of this paper is to review the characterization and the anatomical distribution of [^{125}I]VIP binding sites in the brain and pituitary, in an attempt to correlate those binding data with the physiological effects of the peptide in brain and pituitary functions.

[a] In memorium. This manuscript is dedicated to Dr. Jacqueline Besson who suddenly died on January 16, 1987. This paper was written and prepared by Dr. Besson's close collaborators: Dr. William H. Rostene, Micheline Vial, and Monique Dussaillant who wish to thank all their colleagues of the INSERM U.55, Paris, France (Director, Dr. Gabriel Rosselin) for their help; Martine le Hein and Chantal Brunet for secretarial assistance; and Yves Issoulie for the illustrations. Correspondence should be sent to: Dr. William H. Rostene, INSERM U.55, Hôpital St. Antoine, 184, rue du Fg. St. Antoine, 75571 Paris Cedex 12, France.

PHARMACOLOGICAL CHARACTERIZATION OF BRAIN VIP BINDING SITES

The overall autoradiographic procedure used here has already been described in detail for several neuroactive substances.[12,20-22]

For VIP, briefly, Wistar male rats (200-250 g) from our breeding colony were sacrificed by decapitation. Brains were removed and frozen with dry ice on microtome chucks. Twenty-μm sections were cut on a cryostat, mounted onto gelatin-coated slides, stored overnight at $-20°C$, and then kept at $-70°C$ until assay. Sections identified with the atlas of Paxinos and Watson[23] were incubated in 300 μl of 50 mM Trizma buffer, pH 7.4, containing 2% bovine serum albumin, 0.1% bacitracin, 5 mM MgCl$_2$ in the presence of 100 pM mono-[^{125}I]VIP (3-iodotyrosyl-[^{125}I]VIP)[2] with or without unlabeled VIP, various VIP fragments or related peptides. At the end of incubation, sections were washed twice for 15 minutes in 40 mM Trizma buffer at 4°C since steady state conditions were obtained under those experimental conditions (FIG. 1). This procedure gave the highest ratio of specific versus nonspecific binding, nonspecific binding being defined as that obtained with 1 μM unlabeled VIP. For biochemical determinations, tissues were wiped off of the slides with Schleicher and Schüll filters and the radioactivity was measured in a gamma Packard Multiprias counter.

For autoradiography, the sections were washed twice after incubation as described above, dipped in cold distilled water to remove salts and dried with a cold stream of air. Film autoradiographs were produced by the apposition of [^{3}H]Ultrofilm (LKB, France) or [^{3}H]Hyperfilm (Amersham) on the radiolabeled sections in Kodak X-O Matic film holders. Following three to four weeks of exposure at room temperature in darkness, according to the amount of radioactivity recovered on the sections, films were developed for three minutes in Kodak D19, rinsed in water and fixed with Kodak fixer. After development, the optical density of the autoradiograms was measured with a densitometer that converts the amount of light into millivolts.[12,22] Using iodinated standards prepared from brain homogenates incubated with increasing concentrations of mono-[^{125}I]TiTx γ toxin, the optical density of each structure was referred to a standard curve computed on a Hewlett Packard (HP 85) so that the results were expressed as femtomoles [^{125}I]VIP bound per milligram of protein.[24] Protein concentrations were measured by the method of Bradford using bovine serum albumin as the standard.[25] Under our experimental conditions, nonspecific binding obtained with 1 μM unlabeled VIP was subtracted from the total binding to obtain specific concentrations of VIP binding sites.

Before proceeding to autoradiographic studies, optimal binding conditions of [^{125}I]VIP to rat brain sections incubated in vitro were carried out to determine VIP binding parameters using sections at the level of the dorsal hippocampus, Bregma -2.3 mm to -8.8 mm, according to the atlas of Paxinos and Watson.[23]

The kinetic of specific [^{125}I]VIP association to slide mounted brain sections is shown in FIGURE 2. At 37°C, the specific binding increased and reached a steady state after 120 minutes that was stable up to four hours. The specific binding of [^{125}I]VIP obtained after four hours of incubation at 22°C was lower than that at 37°C, whereas no specific binding was observed at 4°C up to 24 hours (data not shown). Thus a two-hour incubation time was routinely used at 37°C. Under those conditions, VIP determination in the incubation medium by radioimmunoassay[26] showed that 50% of the peptide was degraded after two hours of incubation at 37°C in spite of the presence of 0.1% bacitracin. However, since the amount of VIP specifically bound

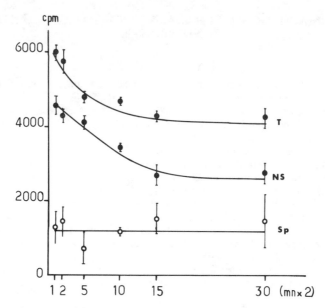

FIGURE 1. Effect of washing time in 40 m*M* Tris buffer at 4°C on total (T), nonspecific (NS), and specific (Sp) [^{125}I]VIP binding on rat brain hippocampal sections.

represented less than 10% of the total amount of the peptide incubated with the sections, and that none of the possible degrading product peptides were able to bind to VIP receptors (FIG. 5), this degradation of VIP does not seem to be an important factor in the characterization of VIP binding sites.

Using a 1,000-fold dilution of VIP in incubation buffer, 35 to 40% of the specific binding dissociated by two hours (data not shown). Thus, [^{125}I]VIP slowly binds to and dissociates from rat brain receptors in agreement with previous data on membranes[8,9] and recently on brain slices at the striatal level.[17]

FIGURE 3 shows the competition between [^{125}I]VIP and increasing concentrations of unlabeled VIP for binding to brain slices. The total binding represents around 6% of the added [^{125}I]VIP and the nonspecific around 2%. Maximal inhibition of [^{125}I]VIP binding that corresponds to 65-70% of the initial binding is obtained with 1 μ*M* of unlabeled peptide and half-maximum inhibition (IC$_{50}$) occurs with 3 n*M*. Scratchard analysis of the displacement curve illustrated in FIGURE 3 suggests the presence of two classes of [^{125}I]VIP binding sites obtained by regression lines computerized by means of the least-squares method. The apparent dissociation constant (Kd) and the maximal binding capacity (B$_{max}$) are estimated at 1.03 ± 0.11 (5) n*M* and 43.3 ± 5.1 (5) fmol/mg protein for the high-affinity and low-capacity binding sites and 68 ± 14 (5) n*M* and 713 ± 117 (5) fmol/mg protein for the low-affinity and high-capacity binding sites. These data are in agreement with those obtained on purified synaptosomes from rat cerebral cortex[9] and on membranes from various rat brain regions.[6] Furthermore, Hill representation of the data showed no cooperative interactions between VIP binding sites (FIG. 4).

The specificity of the [^{125}I]VIP binding to brain slices is shown in FIGURE 5. Natural peptides structurally related to VIP, such as peptide histidine isoleucine amide

(PHI), human and rat growth hormone releasing factors (hGRF and rGRF), secretin, insulin, and glucagon as well as synthetic fragments of VIP, were tested under our experimental conditions. PHI, rat GRF, secretin, VIP_{2-28}, and human GRF are able to compete with $[^{125}I]VIP$, whereas glucagon, insulin, VIP_{1-14}, VIP_{14-28}, and VIP_{20-28} do not modify $[^{125}I]VIP$ binding even at 1 μM concentration. The order of potency of the peptides able to inhibit $[^{125}I]VIP$ binding is VIP_{1-28} > PHI > rGRF > secretin > VIP_{2-28} > hGRF. A quite similar pharmacological pattern was recently obtained on the isolated 46,000 M_r protein involved in the specific high-affinity binding of VIP to synaptosomes from rat cerebral cortex.[27]

Among the different synthetic fragments of VIP tested, only VIP_{2-28} shows some activity (FIG. 5). This result confirms previous pharmacological studies in peripheral tissues showing that the whole sequence of VIP is necessary to bind to the receptor and to induce full physiological action.[28] The order of potency of the different peptides in inhibiting the binding of $[^{125}I]VIP$ to central VIP receptors is thus very similar to that observed in the periphery such as in the liver, gastric cells, epididymal fat cells, and intestinal epithelium.[29] PHI seems to have the most potent inhibitory effect (FIG. 5). PHI[30] was recently reported to be present in the brain with a distribution very similar to that of VIPergic neurons.[31] The fact that the two peptides are encoded by the same precursor molecule[32,33] and that PHI has a potent interaction with VIP binding sites suggests that PHI may have physiological effects in the CNS at least via VIP receptors since PHI-specific receptors have not yet been described. Rat GRF is more potent than human GRF in displacing $[^{125}I]VIP$ binding, but high concentrations are necessary to obtain this effect. Previous studies have reported that high concen-

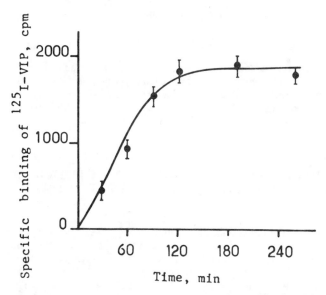

FIGURE 2. Kinetic of $[^{125}I]VIP$ binding: 100 pM $[^{125}I]VIP$ were incubated alone or in the presence of 1 μM unlabeled VIP at 37°C for indicated times and the specific binding was determined as the difference between total and nonspecific binding. Each point is the mean ± SEM of four determinations.

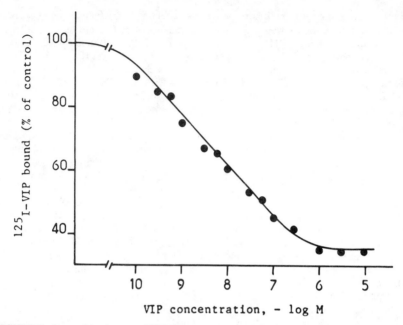

FIGURE 3. Competition between [^{125}I]VIP and unlabeled VIP for binding to rat brain sections: 100 pM [^{125}I]VIP were incubated alone or in the presence of increasing concentrations of unlabeled VIP at 37°C for two hours. [^{125}I]VIP binding is expressed as the percentage of initial binding. The curve represents the mean of five experiments.

trations of secretin and of some fragments of secretin are able to inhibit [^{125}I]VIP binding to brain membranes whereas glucagon has no effect,[3,4,9] and the results on brain sections corroborate those data. The presence of specific receptors for secretin and glucagon in rat brain[34,35] and in bovine pituitary for GRF[36] suggests possible biological effects of those peptides via their own binding sites.

AUTORADIOGRAPHIC DISTRIBUTION OF [^{125}I]VIP BINDING SITES IN THE RAT BRAIN AND PITUITARY

The rostrocaudal topographical distribution of [^{125}I]VIP binding sites is shown in TABLE 1 and illustrated in FIGURE 6. The densities of specific binding sites expressed as fmol [^{125}I]VIP/mg protein are estimated as follows: high from 6 to 8.5, moderate from 3 to 6, and low when values are below 3.

The external plexiform layer of the olfactory bulbs show a high density of binding sites whereas the internal granular layer has a moderate labeling (FIG. 6a).

A moderate level of binding sites is found in different parts of cortex mainly in the intermediate (IV) and deepest layers (VI) of the neocortex as shown in FIGURE 6b, d, and e.

The basal ganglia only shows moderate (accumbens nucleus and caudate putamen) (FIG 6b) or low (globus pallidus) (FIG. 6c) densities of binding sites.

In the hypothalamus, the suprachiasmatic (FIG. 6c) and dorsomedial nuclei (FIG. 6d) show a high concentration of VIP binding sites. Moderate densities are found in the arcuate (FIG. 6d), mammillary (except its dorsal part, FIG. 6e) para and periventricular nuclei, whereas in the other nuclei, the specific labeling is not significantly different from the nonspecific background.

In the amygdaloid complex, only the central nucleus (FIG. 6c, d) presents a high concentration of VIP binding sites.

In the hippocampal formation, a high to moderate labeling is observed in the dentate gyrus, in the subiculum and in the different subfields of Ammon's horn. In the dentate gyrus, the labeling is mainly located in the molecular layer of the fascia dentata but some labeling is also observed in the granular layer (FIG. 6d, e). In the thalamus, the highest densities of binding sites are found in the mediodorsal, the gelatinosus (FIG. 6d), the lateral posterior (FIG. 6e), the dorsolateral and medial geniculate nuclei (FIG. 6d, e). Caudally, the superficial grey layers of the superior colliculus are strongly labeled in contrast to the other regions of the midbrain, brainstem, and cerebellum, which show a low concentration of binding sites with the exception of the facial nucleus, the dorsal raphe (FIG. 6g) and the area postrema.[17] An intense labeling is observed in the pineal gland (FIG. 6f). In the pituitary gland, the anterior lobe is highly labeled in contrast to the neural and particularly the intermediate lobe (FIG. 6h).

The autoradiographic localization of [^{125}I]VIP binding sites reported in the present study gives a more detailed topographical distribution of these binding sites than that

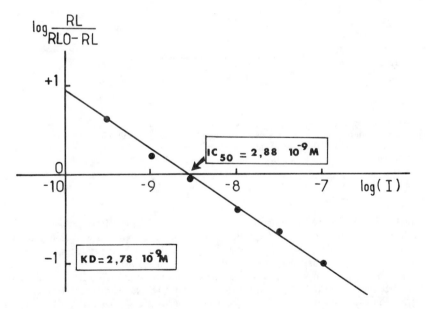

FIGURE 4. Hill representation of the data obtained from competition curves between [^{125}I]VIP and increasing concentrations of unlabeled VIP.

reported either on membranes prepared from various regions of rat brain[4,6] or in our previous preliminary[13] or recent autoradiographic studies.[14,17,18]

VIP binding sites are generally located in regions that also contain VIPergic neurons.[26,37-39] Moreover, VIP binding sites are often associated with a VIP-stimulated adenylate cyclase in several brain regions, such as the olfactory bulbs, hippocampus, cerebral cortex, thalamus, hypothalamus, and striatum,[40-42] and this may have relevant functional implications for the peptide in the CNS.

In the cerebral cortex, VIP promotes both cAMP accumulation[43] and enzymatic

SPECIFICITY OF ^{125}I-VIP BINDING

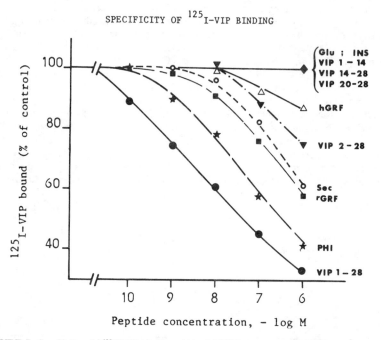

FIGURE 5. Specificity of [^{125}I]VIP binding: 100 pM [^{125}I]VIP were incubated alone or in the presence of increasing concentrations of unlabeled peptides at 37°C for two hours. [^{125}I]VIP binding is expressed as the percentage of initial binding. The curve represents the mean of three experiments. Glu = glucagon; Ins = insulin, h and rGRF = human and rat GRF; Sec = secretin.

breakdown of glycogen to glucose in mouse cortical slices.[44] VIP stimulates glucose utilization locally at the site of injection in the cingulate cortex as well as in anatomically related brain areas.[45,46] Iontophoretic application of VIP produces a potential excitatory effect on neurons of cerebral cortex.[47] This may be related to the well-documented effect of VIP as a vasodilatory neurotransmitter.[48] VIP-like immuno-reactivity was reported in cerebral arteries[48] and VIP was shown to stimulate the formation of cyclic AMP in cerebral cortical microvessels.[49] Recently, VIP binding sites have been localized in bovine cerebral arteries[19,50] and represent functional receptors on cerebrovascular functions.[19]

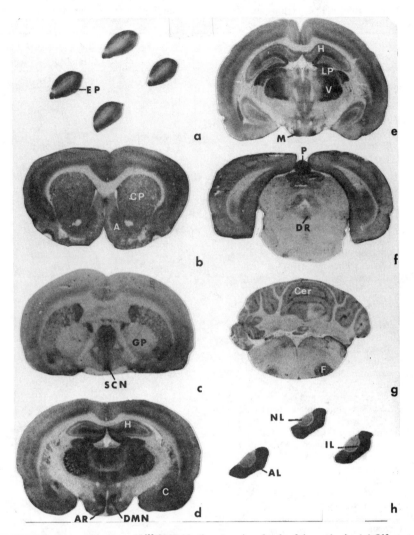

FIGURE 6. Autoradiograms of [^{125}I]VIP binding at various levels of the rat brain. (a) Olfactory bulbs; (b) caudate-putamen; (c) globus pallidus, anterior hypothalamus; (d) diencephalon; (e) hippocampal formation; (f) rostral midbrain; (g) cerebellum and brainstem; (h) pituitary gland. Sections were incubated two hours at 37°C with 100 pM [^{125}I]VIP.

Abbreviations: EP = external plexiform layer (olfactory bulbs); CP = caudate putamen; A = accumbens; GP = globus pallidus; SCN = suprachiasmatic nucleus; C = central amygdaloid nucleus; H = hippocampus; DMN = hypothalamic dorsomedial n.; AR = arcuate nucleus; M = mammillary bodies; LP = lateral postthalamic n.; V = ventral thalamic nucleus; P = pineal gland; DR = dorsal raphe; Cer = cerebellum; F = facial nucleus; AL = anterior lobe; NL = neural lobe; IL = intermediate lobe (pituitary).

Sections were exposed to [^{3}H]Ultrofilm for 25 days. Densitometric readings of the autoradiograms are tabulated in TABLE 1.

TABLE 1. Regional Distribution of [^{125}I]VIP Binding Sites in the Rat Brain and Pituitary[a]

Areas	Specific [^{125}I]VIP Bound fmol/mg Protein
Olfactory bulb	
External plexiform layer	High
Internal Granular Layer	Moderate
Cerebral Cortex	
Frontoparietal cortex ⎫	
Cingulate cortex ⎬	Moderate
Temporal cortex ⎪	
Entorhinal cortex ⎭	
Basal forebrain	
Septohippocampal nucleus	Moderate
Lateral septal dorsal nucleus	Low
Bed nucleus of the stria terminalis	Low
Basal ganglia	
Accumbens nucleus	Moderate
Caudate putamen	Moderate
Globus pallidus	Low
Hypothalamus	
Suprachiasmatic nucleus ⎫	High
Dorsomedial nucleus ⎬	
Arcuate nucleus	Moderate
Paraventricular nucleus ⎫	
Periventricular nucleus ⎬	
Mammillary nucleus ⎭	
Amygdala	
Central nucleus	High
Thalamus	
Lateral posterior nucleus ⎫	
Dorsolateral geniculate nucleus ⎪	
Medial geniculate nucleus ⎬	High
Mediodorsal nucleus ⎪	
Gelatinosus (submedius) nucleus ⎭	
Lateral dorsal nucleus ⎫	
Ventroposterior nucleus ⎪	
Ventromedial nucleus ⎬	Moderate
Reuniens nucleus ⎪	
Rhomboid nucleus ⎭	
Hippocampal formation	
Dentate gyrus	High
CA1	Moderate
CA2	Low
CA3 ⎫	
CA4 ⎬	Moderate
Subiculum ⎭	
Brainstem and cerebellum	
Substantia nigra	Low
Superior colliculus	High
Periaqueductal central grey ⎫	
Dorsal raphe ⎪	
Interfascicular nucleus ⎬	Low
Interpeduncular nucleus ⎪	
Cerebellum ⎭	

TABLE 1. *Continued*

Areas	Specific [^{125}I]VIP Bound fmol/mg Protein
Pineal Gland	High
Pituitary Gland	
Anterior lobe	High
Intermediate lobe	Low
Neural lobe	Low

[a] Results determined by densitometry on film autoradiograms represent the mean of six determinations and were obtained by transformation of optical densities in fmol/mg protein as described in the text. Nonspecific binding (1 μM unlabeled VIP) was subtracted from each total value so that data are expressed as specific binding.

The presence of VIP binding sites in the hippocampal formation correlates with the excitatory effect of the peptide on neurons of this brain structure.[51] Furthermore, the high density of VIP binding sites in the subiculum may be related to the specific effect of the peptide in the modulation of serotoninergic pathways and receptors in this hippocampal region,[52-54] an effect that is under the control of peripheral adrenal steroids[55] and that may serve as a neurobiological support for behavioral actions of the peptide.[56,57]

The discrete and specific localization of VIP binding sites in some hypothalamic nuclei is in close relation with the known neuroendocrine roles of VIP.[1] Functional interactions between VIP and serotoninergic innervation are also evidenced by anatomical observations in the hypothalamus.[58,59] In the suprachiasmatic nucleus, where a high density of both VIP cell bodies and neurons have been described,[58-61] VIP binding sites are highly concentrated, and the peptide was reported to stimulate the secretion of serotonin[62] and to decrease the number of serotoninergic receptors.[55] Besides, preliminary data (Besson and Beaudet, unpublished results) suggest that VIP receptors are probably located in the dorsomedial hypothalamic nucleus in the same region as the discrete group of serotoninergic perikarya found in this nucleus.[63] The presence of VIP binding sites in the paraventricular nucleus may be implicated in the physiological action of adrenal steroids in this target nucleus, since VIP and CRF neurons have been shown to coexist in the parvocellular portion of the nucleus[64] and that adrenalectomy resulted in the appearance of VIP-immunoreactive cell bodies.[64] Furthermore, corticosterone has been shown to increase hypothalamic VIP-mRNA levels, an effect that may be located in the paraventricular nucleus.[65] Finally, VIP has been reported to affect several neuroendocrine functions by acting directly at the hypothalamic level as shown for the inhibition of somatostatin release.[66,67] These data may be related to the presence of VIP binding sites in the arcuate region of the hypothalamus and have important physiological relevance in the regulation of anterior pituitary functions.[1] In that respect, it is interesting to note that high densities of [^{125}I]VIP binding sites are found in the anterior pituitary in contrast to both the neural and intermediate lobes (FIG. 6).

The high density of VIP binding sites found in the pineal gland is in agreement with previous reports showing the presence of such binding sites in rat dispersed pineal cells[68] and in the pineal gland of the gerbil[15] and gives a functional basis to the stimulation by VIP of serotonin-N-acetyltransferase, enzyme involved in the synthesis of melatonin.[69,70]

In the thalamus, the autoradiographic study demonstrates high densities of VIP binding sites in the dorsolateral and medial geniculate nuclei, in the ventrobasal

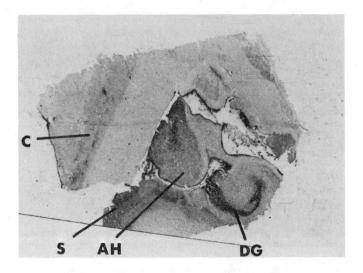

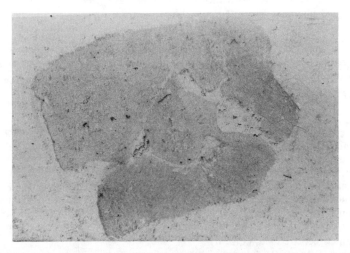

FIGURE 7. Autoradiograms of [^{125}I]VIP binding at the level of the hippocampal formation of the human postmortem brain. (A) Represents the total binding obtained with 100 pM [^{125}I]VIP; (B) represents the nonspecific binding observed in the presence of 1 μM unlabeled VIP. Abbreviations: DG = dentate gyrus; AH = Ammon's horn; S = subiculum; C = temporal cortex.

complex, in the posterior lateral nucleus, and in the submedius nucleus, which are all relay nuclei for various sensory pathways connected to the reticular nucleus.[71] The latter contains a majority of GABAergic neurons[72] and immunocytochemical data suggest that VIP and GABA may be colocalized in neurons in this nucleus.[73] Finally, the high concentration of [^{125}I]VIP binding sites in the geniculate nuclei of the thalamus, in the hypothalamic suprachiasmatic nucleus, and in the superior colliculus suggests that VIP may play a role in visual processes.

Some of the biological effects of VIP reported above may be related to human brain physiology since [^{125}I]VIP binding sites have been already described on human brain membranes.[74] Preliminary autoradiographic data (FIG. 7) show for the first time a high specifically distributed labeling in the human hippocampus mainly in the dentate gyrus and in the subiculum.

In conclusion, the localization of [^{125}I]VIP binding sites generally correlates with the immunocytochemical distribution of VIP neurons even if quantitatively the endogenous concentration of VIP does not always parallel that of its receptors. Nevertheless, as shown in this paper, the majority of the physiological actions of VIP in brain and pituitary functions may be easily related to the anatomical localization of its receptors.

Modulation of brain and pituitary VIP binding sites in various experimental of physiopathological conditions may represent in the near future a great challenge to enhance our knowledge on the possible involvement of the peptide in neurological and neuroendocrine disorders.

REFERENCES

1. ROSTENE, W. H. 1984. Neurobiological and neuroendocrine functions of the vasoactive intestinal peptide (VIP). Prog. Neurobiol. **22:** 103-129.
2. MARIE, J. C., D. HUI BON HOA, R. JACKSON, G. HEJBLUM & G. ROSSELIN. 1985. The biological relevance of HPLC-purified vasoactive intestinal polypeptide monoiodinated at tyrosine 10 or tyrosine 22. Regul. Pept. **12:** 113-123.
3. ROBBERECHT, P., P. DE NEEF, M. LAMMENS, M. DESCHODT-LANCKMAN & J. CHRISTOPHE. 1978. Specific binding of vasoactive intestinal peptide to brain membranes from the guinea pig. Eur. J. Biochem. **90:** 147-154.
4. TAYLOR, D. P. & C. B. PERT. 1979. Vasoactive intestinal polypeptide: Specific binding to rat brain membranes. Proc. Natl. Acad. Sci. USA **76:** 660-664.
5. ROBBERECHT, P., W. KONIG, M. DESCHODT-LANCKMAN, P. DE NEEF & J. CHRISTOPHE. 1979. Specificity of receptors to vasoactive intestinal peptide in guinea pig brain. Life Sci. **25:** 879-884.
6. STAUN-OLSEN, P., B. OTTESEN, S. GAMMELTOFT & J. FAHRENKRUG. 1985. The regional distribution of receptors for vasoactive intestinal polypeptide (VIP) in the rat central nervous system. Brain Res. **330:** 317-321.
7. OGAWA, N., S. MIZUNO, A. MORI, I. NUKINA & N. YANAIHARA. 1985. Properties and distribution of vasoactive intestinal polypeptide receptors in the rat brain. Peptides. **6:** 103-109.
8. MOODY, T. W., D. P. TAYLOR & C. B. PERT. 1981. Effects of guanine nucleotides on CNS neuropeptide receptors. J. Supramol. Str. Cell. Biochem. **15:** 153-159.
9. STAUN-OLSEN, P., B. OTTESEN, P. D. BARTELS, M. H. NIELSEN, S. GAMMELTOFT & J. FAHRENKRUG. 1982. Receptors for vasoactive intestinal polypeptide on isolated synaptosomes from rat cerebral cortex. Heterogeneity of binding and desensitization of receptors. J. Neurochem. **39:** 1242-1251.

10. FAHRENKRUG, J., S. GAMMELTOFT, P. STAUN-OLSEN, B. OTTESEN & A. SJOQUIST. 1983. Multiplicity of receptors for VIP: Differential effects of apamin on binding in brain, uterus and liver. Peptides **4:** 133-136.
11. STAUN-OLSEN, P., B. OTTESEN, S. GAMMELTOFT & J. FAHRENKRUG. 1986. VIP binding sites on synaptosomes from rat cerebral cortex: Structure-binding relationship. Peptides **7:** 181-186.
12. ROSTENE, W., J. BESSON, Y. BROER, M. DUSSAILLANT, D. GROUSELLE, P. KITABGI, A. M. LHIAUBET, J. L. MORGAT, A. SARRIEAU & M. VIAL. 1985. Localisation par radioautographie des récepteurs des neuropeptides dans le système nerveux central. Ann. Endocrinol. **46:** 27-33.
13. BESSON, J., M. DUSSAILLANT, J. C. MARIE, W. ROSTENE & G. ROSSELIN. 1984. In vitro autoradiographic localization of vasoactive intestinal peptide (VIP) binding sites in the rat central nervous system. Peptides **5:** 339-340.
14. DE SOUZA, E. B., H. SEIFERT& M. J. KUHAR. 1985. Vasoactive intestinal peptide receptor localization in rat forebrain by autoradiography. Neurosci. Lett. **56:** 113-120.
15. MOLLER, M., J. D. MIKKELSEN, J. FAHRENKRUG & H. W. KORF. 1985. The presence of VIP-like immunoreactive nerve fibres and VIP-receptors in the pineal gland of the Mongolian gerbil: An immunohistochemical and receptor-autoradiographic study. Cell Tissue Res. **241:** 333-340.
16. BESSON, J., A. SARRIEAU, M. VIAL, J. C. MARIE, G. ROSSELIN & W. ROSTENE. 1986. Characterization and autoradiographic distribution of vasoactive intestinal peptide binding sites in the rat central nervous system. Brain Res. **398:** 329-336.
17. SHAFFER, M. & T. W. MOODY. 1986. Autoradiographic visualization of CNS receptors for vasoactive intestinal peptide. Peptides **7:** 283-288.
18. MARTIN, J. L., M. R. DIETL, P. M. HOF, J. M. PALACIOS & P. J. MAGISTRETTI. 1987. Autoradiographic mapping of mono-[^{125}I]Tyr$_{10}$-Met 0$_{17}$-VIP binding sites in the rat brain. Neuroscience **23:** 539-566.
19. POULIN, P., Y. SUZUKI, K. LEDERIS & O. P. RORSTAD. 1986. Autoradiographic localization of binding sites for VIP in bovine cerebral arteries. Brain Res. **381:** 382-384.
20. KUHAR, M. J. 1983. Autoradiographic localization of drug and neurotransmitter receptors. In Handbook of Chemical Neuroanatomy. A. Björklund and T. Hökfelt, Eds. Vol. **1:** 398-415. Elsevier. Amsterdam, the Netherlands.
21. HERKENHAM, M. 1984. Autoradiographic demonstration of receptor distributions. In Brain Receptor Methodologies. P. J. Marangos, I. C. Campbell & R. M. Cohen, Eds. Part A: 127-152. Academic Press. New York.
22. ROSTENE, W. H., D. HERVE, P. KITABGI, J. MAGRE & A. SARRIEAU. 1986. Hormonal receptor plasticity in the brain as shown by in vitro quantitative autoradiography. In Neuroendocrine Molecular Biology. G. Fink, A. J. Harmar & K. W. McKerns, Eds.: 405-416. Plenum Press. New York.
23. PAXINOS, G. & C. WATSON. 1982. The Rat Brain in Stereotaxic Coordinates. Academic Press. New York.
24. ROSTÈNE, W. & C. MOURRE. 1985. Préparation de standards iodés pour radioautographie quantitative in vitro à l'aide d'un film sensible au tritium. C. R. Acad. Sci. Paris. **301:** 245-250.
25. BRADFORD, M. M. 1976. A rapid and sensitive method for the quantification of microgram quantities of protein utilizing the principle of protein-dye binding. Anal. Biochem. **72:** 248-254.
26. BESSON, J., W. ROTSZTEJN, M. LABURTHE, J. EPELBAUM, A. BEAUDET, C. KORDON & G. ROSSELIN. 1979. VIP: Brain distribution, subcellular localization and effect of deafferentation of the hypothalamus in male rats. Brain Res. **165:** 79-85.
27. COUVINEAU, A., S. GAMMELTOFT & M. LABURTHE. 1986. Molecular characteristics and peptide specificity of vasoactive intestinal peptide receptors from rat cerebral cortex. J. Neurochem. **47:** 1469-1475.
28. FOURNIER, A., J. K. SAUNDERS & S. ST PIERRE. 1984. Synthesis, conformational studies and biological activities of VIP and related fragments. Peptides **5:** 169-177.
29. ROSSELIN, G. 1986. The receptors of the VIP family peptides (VIP, secretin, GRF, PHI, PHM, GIP, glucagon and oxyntomodulin). Specificities and identity. Peptides **7:** 89-100.

30. TATEMOTO, K., M. CARLQUIST, T. J. McDONALD & V. MUTT. 1983. Isolation of a brain peptide identical to the intestinal PHI (peptide HI). FEBS Lett. **153**: 248-252.
31. HOKFELT, T., J. FAHRENKRUG, B. EVERITT, S. WERNER, A. L. HULTING, K. TATEMOTO & V. MUTT. 1983. Immunohistochemical studies on the CNS using antisera to VIP and PHI and some functional aspects. Regul. Peptides **6**: 308-314.
32. ITOH, N., K. OBATA, N. YANAIHARA & H. OKAMOTO. 1983. Human preprovasoactive intestinal polypeptide (VIP) mRNA contains the coding sequence for a novel PHI-27 like peptide, PHM-27. Nature (London) **304**: 547-549.
33. BODNER, M., M. FRIDKIN & I. GOZES. 1985. Coding sequences for vasoactive intestinal peptide and PHM-27 peptide are located on two adjacent exons in the human genome. Proc. Natl. Acad. Sci. USA **82**: 3548-3551.
34. FREMEAU, R. T., R. T. JENSEN, C. G. CHARLTON, R. L. MILLER, T. L. O'DONONUE & T. W. MOODY. 1983. Secretin: Specific binding to rat brain membranes. J. Neurosci. **3**: 1620-1625.
35. HOOSEIN, N. M. & R. S. GURD. 1984. Identification of glucagon receptors in rat brain. Proc. Natl. Acad. Sci. USA **81**: 4368-4372.
36. VELICELEBI, G., T. M. SANTACROCE & H. M. HARPOLD. 1985. Specific binding of synthetic human pancreatic growth hormone-releasing factor (1-40-OH) to bovine anterior pituitaries. Biochem. Biophys. Res. Commun. **126**: 33-39.
37. FUXE, K., T. HOKFELT, S. I. SAID & V. MUTT. 1977. Vasoactive intestinal polypeptide and the nervous system: Immunohistochemical evidence for localization in central and peripheral neurons, particularly intracortical neurons of the cerebral cortex. Neurosci. Lett. **5**: 241-246.
38. LOREN, I., P. C. EMSON, J. FAHRENKRUG, A. BJORKLUND, J. ALUMETS, R. HAKANSON & F. SUNDLER. 1979. Distribution of vasoactive intestinal polypeptide in the rat and mouse brain. Neuroscience **4**: 1953-1976.
39. SIMS, K. B., D. L. HOFFMAN, S. I. SAID & E. A. ZIMMERMAN. 1980. Vasoactive intestinal polypeptide (VIP) in mouse and rat brain: An immunocytochemical study. Brain Res. **186**: 165-183.
40. QUIK, M., L. L. IVERSEN & S. R. BLOOM. 1978. Effect of vasoactive intestinal peptide (VIP) and other peptides and cAMP accumulation in rat brain. Biochem. Pharmacol. **27**: 2209-2213.
41. BORGHI, C., S. NICOSIA, A. GIACHETTI & S. I. SAID. 1979. Vasoactive intestinal polypeptide (VIP) stimulates adenylate cyclase in selected areas of rat brain. Life Sci. **24**: 65-70.
42. KERWIN, R. W., S. PAY, K. D. BHOOLA & C. J. PYCOCK. 1980. Vasoactive intestinal polypeptide (VIP) sensitive adenylate cyclase in rat brain: Regional distribution and localization on hypothalamic neurons. J. Pharm. Pharmacol. **32**: 561-566.
43. MAGISTRETTI, P. J. & M. SCHORDERET. 1984. VIP and noradrenaline act synergistically to increase cyclic AMP in cerebral cortex. Nature (London) **308**: 280-282.
44. MAGISTRETTI, P. J., J. H. MORRISON, W. H. SHOEMAKER, V. SAPIN & F. E. BLOOM. Vasoactive intestinal polypeptide induces glycogenolysis in mouse cortical slices: A possible regulator mechanism for the local control of energy metabolism. Proc. Natl. Acad. Sci. USA **78**: 6535-6539.
45. McCULLOCH, J. & P. A. T. KELLY. 1983. A functional role for vasoactive intestinal polypeptide in anterior cingulate cortex. Nature (London) **304**: 438-440.
46. McCULLOCH, J., P. A. T. KELLY, R. UDDMAN & L. EDVINSSON. 1983. Functional role for vasoactive intestinal polypeptide in the caudate nucleus: A 2-deoxy-14C-glucose investigation. Proc. Natl. Acad. Sci. USA **80**: 1472-1476.
47. PHILLIS, J. W. & J. R. KIRKPATRICK. 1978. The actions of motilin, luteinizing hormone-releasing hormone, cholecystokinin, somatostatin, vasoactive intestinal peptide and other peptides on rat cerebral cortical neurons. Can. J. Pharmacol. **56**: 337-340.
48. EDVINSSON, L., J. FAHRENKRUG, J. HANKO, J. McCULLOCH, C. OWMAN & R. UDDMAN. 1981. Vasoactive intestinal polypeptide distribution and effects on cerebral blood flow and metabolism. *In* Cerebral Microcirculation and Metabolism. J. Cervos-Navarro & E. Fritschka, Eds.: 147-155. Raven Press. New York.
49. HUANG, M. & O. P. RORSTAD. 1984. Cerebral vascular adenylate cyclase: Evidence for coupling to receptors for vasoactive intestinal peptide and parathyroid hormone. J. Neurochem. **43**: 849-856.

50. SUZUKI, Y., D. MCMASTER, M. HUANG, K. LEDERIS & O. P. RORSTAD. 1985. Characterization of functional receptors for vasoactive intestinal peptide in bovine cerebral arteries. J. Neurochem. **45:** 890-899.

51. DODD, J., J. S. KELLY & S. I. SAID. 1979. Excitation of CA_1 neurons of the rat hippocampus by the octacosapeptide vasoactive intestinal peptide (VIP). Br. J. Pharmacol. **66:** 125.

52. STUCKEY, J., D. ALLEN & B. S. MCEWEN. 1985. Vasoactive intestinal peptide effects on serotonin turnover in the hippocampus. Soc. Neurosc. Abstract. N° 170-15: 571.

53. ROSTENE, W., C. T. FISCHETTE & B. S. MCEWEN. 1984. Modulation by vasoactive intestinal peptide (VIP) of serotonin$_1$ receptors in membranes from rat hippocampus. J. Neurosci. **3:** 2414-2419.

54. ROSTENE, W., C. T. FISCHETTE, T. C. RAINBOW & B. S. MCEWEN. 1983. Modulation by vasoactive intestinal peptide of serotonin$_1$ receptors in the dorsal hippocampus of the rat brain: An autoradiographic study. Neurosci. Lett. **37:** 143-148.

55. ROSTENE, W. H., C. T. FISCHETTE, M. DUSSAILLANT & B. S. MCEWEN. 1985. Adrenal steroid modulation of vasoactive intestinal peptide effect on serotonin$_1$ binding sites in the rat brain shown by *in vitro* quantitative autoradiography. Neuroendocrinology **40:** 129-134.

56. RIOU, F., R. CESPUGLIO & M. JOUVET. 1982. Endogenous peptides and sleep in the rat: The hypnogenic properties of vasoactive intestinal polypeptide. Neuropeptides **2:** 265-277.

57. COTTRELL, G. A., H. D. VELDHUIS, W. H. ROSTENE & E. R. DE KLOET. 1984. Behavioural actions of VIP. Neuropeptides. **4:** 331-341.

58. KISS, J. Z., CS. LERANTH & B. HALASZ. 1984. Serotoninergic ending on VIP-neurons in the suprachiasmatic nucleus and on ACTH-neurons in the arcuate nucleus of the rat hypothalamus. A combination of high-resolution autoradiography and electronmicroscopic immunocytochemistry. Neurosci. Lett. **44:** 119-124.

59. BOSLER, O. & A. BEAUDET. 1985. VIP neurons as prime synaptic targets for serotoninergic afferents in rat suprachiasmatic nucleus: A combinated radioimmunological and immunocytochemical study. J. Neurocytol. **14:** 749-763.

60. CARD, J. P., N. BRECHA, H. J. KARTEN & R. Y. MOORE. 1981. Immunocytochemical localization of vasoactive intestinal polypeptide-containing cells and processes in the suprachiasmatic nuleus of the rat: Light and electron microscopic analysis. J. Neurosci. **1:** 1289-1303.

61. ROSTENE, W. H., CS. LERANTH, M. MALETTI, E. MEZEY, J. BESSON, L. E. EIDEN, G. ROSSELIN & M. PALKOVITS. 1982. Distribution of VIP following various brain transections in the rat by radioimmunoassay and electron-microscopic immunocytochemistry. Neuropeptides **2:** 337-350.

62. HERY, M., M. FAUDON & F. HERY. 1984. Effect of vasoactive intestinal peptide on serotonin release in the suprachiasmatic area of the rat. Modulation by oestradiol. Peptides **5:** 313-317.

63. DESCARRIES, L. & A. BEAUDET. 1978. The serotonin innervation of adult rat hypothalamus. *In* Biologie Cellulaire des Processus Neurosécrétoires Hypothalamiques. J. D. Vincent & C. Kordon, Eds. Vol. **280:** 135-153. CNRS. Paris, France.

64. MEZEY, E. & J. Z. KISS. 1985. Vasoactive intestinal peptide-containing neurons in the paraventricular nucleus may participate in regulating prolactin secretion. Proc. Natl. Acad. Sci. USA **82:** 245-247.

65. GOZES, I. 1988. Biosynthesis and regulation of expression: The vasoactive intestinal peptide gene. Ann. N.Y. Acad. Sci. This volume.

66. EPELBAUM, J., L. TAPIA-ARANCIBIA, J. BESSON, W. ROTSZTEJN & C. KORDON. 1979. Vasoactive intestinal peptide inhibits release of somatostatin from hypothalamus *in vitro*. Eur. J. Pharmacol. **58:** 493-495.

67. SHIMATSU, A., Y. KATO, N. MATSUSHITA, H. KATAKAMI, N. YANAIHARA & H. IMURA. 1982. Effects of glucagon, neurotensin and vasoactive intestinal polypeptide on somatostatin release from perifused rat hypothalamus. Endocrinology **110:** 2113-2117.

68. KAKU, K., Y. INOUE, A. MATSUTANI, M. OKUBO, K. HATAO, T. KANEKO & N. YANAIHARA. 1983. Receptors for vasoactive intestinal polypeptide on rat dispersed pineal cells. Biomed. Res. **4:** 321-328.

69. KANEKO T., P. Y. CHENG, H. OKA, T. ODA, N. YANAIHARA & C. YANAIHARA. 1980. Vasoactive intestinal polypeptide stimulates adenylate cyclase and serotonin N-acetyl-transferase activities in rat pineal *in vitro.* Biomed. Res. **1:** 84-87.
70. YUWILER, A. 1983. Vasoactive intestinal peptide stimulation of pineal serotonin-N-ace-tyltransferase activity: General characteristics. J. Neurochem. **41:** 146-153.
71. JONES, E. G. 1985. The Thalamus. Plenum Press. New York.
72. KANEKO, T., K. TASHIRO, T. SUGIMOTO, A. KONISHI & N. MIZUNO. 1985. Identification of thalamic neurons with vasoactive intestinal polypeptide-like immunoreactivity in the rat. Brain Res. **347:** 390-393.
73. HOUSER, C. R., J. E. VAUGHN, R. P. BARBER & E. ROBERTS. 1980. GABA neurons are the major cell type of the nucleus reticularis thalami. Brain Res. **200:** 341-354.
74. FARMERY, S. M., F. OWEN, M. POULTER & T. J. CROW. 1984. Characterization and distribution of vasoactive intestinal polypeptide binding sites in human brain. Neuro-pharmacology **23:** 101-104.

Regulation of the Vasoactive Intestinal Peptide Receptor

G. ROSSELIN,[a] A. ANTEUNIS, A. ASTESANO, C.
BOISSARD, P. GALI, G. HEJBLUM, AND J. C. MARIE

Unité de Recherches sur les Peptides Neurodigestifs et le Diabète
INSERM U.55 de l'Institut National de la Santé et de la Recherche
Médicale
75012 Paris, France

Most of the data now available indicate that the biological action of vasoactive intestinal peptide or VIP[1] is mediated by the adenylyl cyclase system.[2,3] The stimulation of adenylyl cyclase by VIP involved at least three components: (a) the receptor binding proteins that bind the natural ligand or its agonist; (b) the stimulatory guanyl regulator protein that binds GTP or Ns, which is represented by a heterotrimer made of three units—alpha S, beta, and alpha; (c) the catalytic moiety of the adenylyl cyclase. The regulation of the VIP effect via the receptor as described up to now might be attributed to: (1) the modification of the conformation of binding site by VIP agonists or antagonists; (2) the modulation of the VIP-induced stimulation of adenylate cyclase through the activation of other receptors; or (3) the cellular regulation of the cell surface expression of the VIP binding site. We will briefly review (1) and (2) and emphasize (3), since few data exist on the cellular traffic of the VIP and the VIP receptor as compared to that collected for the catecholamine,[4] the insulin, and the EGF (review in Pastan & Willingham[5]) receptors.

REGULATION OF THE VIP RECEPTOR AT THE LEVEL OF THE BINDING SITES AND OF THE ADENYLYL CYCLASE

Specific binding of agonists or antagonists to the VIP binding site mimics or inhibits the VIP effect. This type of antagonist regulation of the VIP receptor is described for synthetic analogues,[6–9] such as modified growth hormone releasing factor, 4-Cl-D-Phe-6, leucine 17 VIP.[9] Such analogues are of interest in pharmacological study in the effort to characterize biological or physiological actions that are specifically transmitted to cells via VIP receptors. The antagonist effect of VIP fragments was also reported for VIP_{10-28}[10] showing that a fragment that might be physiologically produced acts as a competitive antagonist of VIP. The effect of VIP agonists or antagonists varies

[a] Address for correspondence: Dr. G. Rosselin, Unité de Recherches sur les Peptides Neu-rodigestifs et le Diabète, INSERM U.55 de l'Institut National de la Santé et de la Recherche Médicale, 184, rue du Faubourg Saint-Antoine, 75012 Paris Cedex 12, France.

according to species[11-13] and according to tissue.[3] The molecular basis of this heterogeneity might be due to the existence of different subtypes of VIP binding sites. It might be also related to tissue-specific changes in the membrane-induced secondary configuration of the ligand and/or the receptor that positions the specific interacting group.

The only well-documented mechanism by which other hormones or neurotransmitters act on the response to VIP is the adenylyl cyclase modulation. Somatostatin (SRIF) decreases the effect of VIP in many tissues.[14-22] The mechanism of the inhibitory effect of SRIF on VIP action is the suppression of VIP-stimulated adenylate cyclase as shown in most experiments by the somatostatin-induced decrease in the cyclic AMP generated by VIP. The inhibitory effect is determined by the SRIF activation of the guanyl nucleotide-binding protein Ni, since the SRIF effect is suppressed after treatment by the islet activator protein (IAP) contained in the pertussis toxin. IAP blocks the function by ATP-ribosylation of Ni.[23,24] The site(s) of the somatostatin regulation is still a subject of investigation. In cells such as ATT-20 that produce ACTH, the rise in cyclic AMP induced by a secretagogue such as VIP determines an increase of the cytosolic calcium.[25] It was therefore proposed that somatostatin blocks the increase of cytosolic calcium by inhibiting the stimulation of the adenylyl cyclase system. In HGH-4 Cl cells[23] the intracellular calcium was increased without altering intracellular cyclic AMP. This effect is also prevented by somatostatin, suggesting a new function for Ni[23] that could directly block the Ca^{2+} transfer.

Dopamine also directly inhibits cyclic AMP production through the interaction of the D-2-dopaminergic receptors with Ni. Thus VIPs have been shown to stimulate prolactin release by prolactinoma only after dopamine inhibition.[26,27] The IAP that inactivates Ni also uncouples the dopamine inhibition of the VIP action on striatal neurons in primary culture.[28] MET-enkephalin inhibits the VIP effect on those cells via the same mechanism. The regulation of VIP effect by dopamine has been also studied in the rabbit retina.[29] In that model, the effect of dopamine is partially synergic of that of VIP suggesting that part of the VIP-dependent adenylate cyclase pool is related to the dopamine receptor D1, which stimulates the cyclase activity.

The alpha-adrenergic agonists were shown to act synergistically with VIP in cerebral cortex.[30] In human colonic crypts[31] as in human cancerous colonic cells in culture, alpha-2 agonists partially (1/3) inhibit the VIP action at pharmacological doses. This inhibition is reversed by alpha-2 antagonists.[31,32] It was not observed, however, in intestinal epithelial cells isolated from rat when maximally stimulatory concentrations of VIP were added.[33]

The possibility of an inhibitory regulation of VIP receptor via the activation of receptors of the alpha-1 type, which are coupled to the phosphoinositide release and stimulation of kinase C, is now being investigated in several laboratories.[34] A phorbol ester, belonging to a family of toxic drug that stimulates the kinase C, was shown to inhibit the stimulating effect of VIP on cyclic AMP in GH3 cells.[34] This effect is similar to the inhibition by phorbol ester of the beta-adrenergic receptor stimulation of adenylyl cyclase. In these experiments, the inhibition was attributed to a phosphorylation of the beta-adrenergic receptor.[4] However, the thyroid releasing hormone that mimics the effect of phorbolester in GH3 cells did not inhibit the VIP stimulation.[34] To what extent the muscarinic agonists (which also activate the phosphoinositide turnover[35]) inhibit the VIP-induced stimulation of adenylyl cyclase and the VIP effect on prolactin secretion[36] through a phosphorylation of the VIP receptor is still unknown. Recently, it has been shown that VIP per se is able to provoke a large inositol phospholipid breakdown by acting directly on ganglionic cells.[37] The half-maximal response to VIP, however, was obtained at pharmacological concentration (1 μM)

and corresponds to the concentration of VIP that is necessary for the occupancy of the low-affinity sites.

Regulation of peptide action by proteolytic cleavage *in situ* has been suggested for glucagon[38]: Glucagon 19-29, which is totally ineffective in activating adenylate cyclase, inhibits the calcium Ca^{2+} transport in liver plasma membranes with an efficiency 1,000-fold higher than that of glucagon. Such a situation is not described for VIP and might be interesting to investigate since the VIP molecule also contains pairs of basic amino acids that represent potential cleavage sites in the cells.

The regulation of the VIP effect via the VIP receptor might also occur by an unknown mechanism, as for the steroid-induced inhibition of the prolactin release due to VIP.[39] On the other hand, the addition of insulin to VIP has also been shown to elicit a significant increase in gastrin release and bombesin-like immunoreactivity by the rat stomach.[40]

CELLULAR REGULATION OF VIP ACTION

The cellular traffic of VIP and VIP receptor is likely to represent a powerful system in the regulation of the VIP receptor. We have previously demonstrated that desensitization of VIP receptor activity was associated with a retroregulation of the VIP binding sites associated with a drop of the VIP-induced cyclic AMP generation.[41] This effect was obtained after a short-term exposure of cells in culture flasks and was also observed under different experimental conditions.[41-45] Chronic treatment by VIP might induce a biological refractoriness to a second acute challenge with VIP as shown in mouse calvaria[46] or in human gastric cell line HGT-1[47] and osteocarcinoma cells.[48] The data related to the desensitization of VIP effect are of general interest since suppression of VIP effect after VIP exposure was observed in different biological and physiological models. Besides the suppression of the VIP effect on glycogenolysis in gut cancerous cells[49,41] and on the resistance to the bone resorption,[46] the refractoriness to VIP was also noticed in cultured muscle of the rat mesenteric artery.[50] VIP treatment of T lymphocytes decreases their ability to localize in mesenteric lymph node and Peyer's patches of recipient animals soon after cell transfer.[51] This effect is associated with the loss of the ability of T cells to specifically bind radioiodinated VIP. In the initial pharmacological demonstration of an excitatory action of VIP on cerebral cortical neurons,[52] Phillis *et al.* indicated that when applications were repeated at relatively short intervals of a few minutes, the excitatory effects of VIP were frequently attenuated and could even fail to appear. Kinetic data were collected leading to the conclusion that VIP receptors in brain synaptosomes were desensitized.[53] In the rat pineal gland, VIP binding and cyclic AMP accumulation in response to VIP were significantly increased in animals kept exposed to constant light compared to those in animals that experienced a dark night before the experiments.[54] Prior treatment of pineal gland with VIP decreased [^{125}I]VIP binding by reducing the number of receptors and significantly inhibited subsequent VIP stimulation of cyclic AMP accumulation. In other systems the refractoriness to VIP is less obvious: in GH3 pituitary cell,[15] VIP is able to stimulate long-term PRL production (24 h in GH3-B6 cells). Similarly the effect of VIP perfusion on the intestinal hydroelectrolytic exchanges might be prolonged for several hours[55] although it has been noticed in cancerous human colonic cells in culture that after addition of 10^{-7} M VIP, ^{36}Cl accumulation reached a peak at about 10 minutes and declined thereafter.[56] It is therefore of interest to study in detail the characteristics of the cellular regulation of the VIP receptor associated with the desensitization and to see under what conditions and to what extent the VIP signal might be ended. To carry out this study, we have used the human colonic cancer cells in culture[45] because they are rich in VIP receptors and retain many regulatory sites similar to those observed in normal epithelial intestinal cells, such as the receptors of insulin,[57] EGF,[58] dopamine,[59] and alpha-2-catecholamines.[32]

The characteristics of the desensitization to VIP in those cells are the following: It requires a previous exposure to VIP; it is dependent on time and VIP concentration; and it retains the pharmacological specificity of the VIP receptor since, for example, the ID_{50} of secretin is more than 100-fold higher than that of VIP. The loss of response to VIP is temporally and quantitatively related to the disappearance of the cell surface receptor. It is partly reversible.[45] We have further studied the characteristics of this receptor regulation in order to find out what happens to VIP and to the VIP receptor after cell exposure to VIP.[43,45] The experimental conditions were chosen after experiments determined optimal time and temperature conditions of the internalization process (TABLE 1). In those experiments, [^{125}I]VIP was directly incubated with the cell layers in 9.6-cm^2 Petri dishes at a concentration of 4.10^{-11} M. The reaction is ended at the time indicated by washing the cells with ice-cold buffer. Thereafter, cells were acid treated and washed to suppress the surface-bound radioactivity without removing the internalized peptide. The internalization is rapid at 37°C with a half-time of three minutes. The rate of internalization slows down with decreasing temperature; At 10°C, the internalization is much lower. Notice that the accumulation of VIP inside the cells at 20°C is higher than at 10 or 37°C.. At this low concentration of VIP, even at 37°C, internalization of VIP reaches its maximum only after 60 minutes. In fact, when concentrations of VIP are increasing in the medium, the internalization is more rapidly achieved.[45] This is due to the fact that the binding at 37°C increases with the concentration of VIP in the external medium[45,44] indicating that the rate of receptor occupancy increases with VIP concentrations, whereas the rate of internalization of the occupied sites remains constant. Given those data, it is possible to choose conditions where most of the VIP is bound to the cell surface (for example 60 minutes' incubation at 10°C) or most of the VIP is internalized (for example 90 minutes at 37°C).

The fate of VIP after internalization was studied after exposure at 37°C for the times indicated (TABLE 2) using mono[^{125}I]Tyr^{10}-VIP.[43] The HPLC analysis of the intracellular VIP indicates that internalized VIP molecules have the same retention time as those of intact VIP. In the medium only few intact VIP molecules remain after an incubation time as short as 10 minutes (20%) and are likely to represent VIP molecules that are dissociated from the receptor directly in the medium after exposure of the cell at 37°C. After 20 minutes, there is no more intact VIP left indicating that all the VIP that has been recycled in the cell appears degraded in the medium. The persistence of [^{125}I]VIP as intact molecules into the cells during the internalization process is of interest because it gives the opportunity to further proceed in the determination of the molecular species of the VIP bound in the cells with an unaltered tracer and to directly characterize by autoradiography the specifically labeled organelles involved in the VIP processing.

The nature of the internalized VIP-bound receptor was studied after incubation at 20 and 37°C and suppression at 4°C of the cell-surface-bound radioactivity by acetic acid. The cells are thereafter collected, Dounce-broken at 4°C, and, after a series of centrifugations, the affinity labeling of the pellet containing the radioactivity is performed with different chemical cross-linkers. After solubilization, samples were run on an SDS polyacrylamide gel. The affinity labeling of the cell surface binding sites was performed as a control under similar conditions on cells incubated with [^{125}I]VIP

TABLE 1. Internalization of the [125I]VIP-Bound Receptor According to Time and Temperature[a]

Temperature °C		Time (minutes)									
		5	10	20	30	40	60	80	90	120	180
10	Qi[b]						0.05			0.1	0.2
	Fi[c]						6.3			10.3	15.8
15	Qi	0.008	0.02	0.05	0.1		0.5		0.6		
	Fi	3.5	6.6	8.8	13.7		30.8		34.3		
20	Qi		0.12	0.31			0.95		1.43	1.63	1.62
	Fi		33.1	45.3			48.3		66.8	73.1	77.4
37	Qi	0.25	0.7	0.82		1.13		1.16		1.1	1
	Fi	47.5	67	70.5		83.5		90.1		89.5	97.5

[a] Monoiodinated [125I][Tyr10]-VIP at the concentration of 4×10^{-11} M was incubated directly with confluent HT-29 cells for the time and the temperature indicated. Compartmental partition and measure of internalized VIP was performed as previously published.[43,45]

[b] Quantity internalized, [125I]VIP bound in fmol/10^6 cells.

[c] Fraction internalized, [125I]VIP internalized × 100/total [125I]VIP bound.

at 10°C. Under all conditions, the molecular mass on the internalized binding sites was identical to those of the cell surface receptors. The major protein species was 66.7 kDa indicating a binding site of 63.4 kDa. Those results are in agreement with the molecular mass found by Muller[42] on the cell surface receptor VIP cross-linked after incubation of cells at 15°C and with the data of Couvineau on the VIP receptor cross-linked on the HT-29 membranes.[60] In agreement with the data of Luis,[44] we also observed that the labeling of the major polypeptide was greatly reduced on the cell surface after incubation at 37°C. A major polypeptide of 63 and 62 kDa was also characterized after affinity labeling of the membranes of human normal colonic epithelial cells[61] and human lung,[62] respectively. The band obtained by the comigration of VIP with albumin (64 kDa) had a different molecular mass from that of the VIP receptor (66.7 kDa) under the conditions of our comparative experiments (molecular mass = 62 kDa). In intact human lymphoblasts,[63] the migration of the VIP receptor was also distinct from that of albumin and the major bands were found to be at 50 kDa. From our data, the affinity-labeled receptor of VIP remains unaltered during the internalization. The internalized VIP-bound binding site also retains its specificity

TABLE 2. HPLC Analysis of the Radioactivity Present inside the Cells (Intracellular) and Processing from the Cells into the Medium (Medium)[a]

Incubation Time (min)	$\dfrac{\text{Intracellular} \times 100}{\text{Total VIP Bound}}$	Intact VIP in Percent of	
		Total Intracellular Radioactivity	Total Medium Radioactivity
10	54	65	20
20	35	68	5
60	30	69	0
90	27	67	0

[a] Monoiodinated [^{125}I]Tyr^{10}-VIP at the concentration of 10^{-9} M was incubated with confluent HT-29 cells in 75-cm^2 flasks for 90 minutes at 10°C and then washed and reincubated at 37°C for the time indicated. VIP is extracted and analyzed by HPLC as previously described.[43]

as assessed by the inhibition of the bands in presence of native VIP, whereas no displacement is observed with unrelated peptide. Besides the major degraded band of 66 kDa, we occasionally found other bands of 31, 44, and 99 kDa. Those bands were also identical to those found after cross-linking of the VIP-bound cell surface. A detailed analysis of the major and the minor VIP-binding proteins was recently performed in reference to the glycoprotein nature of the VIP receptor in HT-29 cells,[64] as initially observed in liver cells by N'Guyen.[65] Our data indicated either that those different forms of bound VIP might be internalized, or that similar procedures in the affinity labeling experiments might induce the same type of alteration in the cell surface or internalized VIP receptor. We have, however, no indication of the relative proportion of the different VIP binding proteins inside the cell since in the conditions of our experiment we measure inside the cells only the labeled pool of VIP receptors that come from the cell surface and not the entire intracellular VIP receptor including the VIP receptor processed by biosynthesis from the Golgi and the putative intracellular pool of VIP receptors absent at the cell surface during the labeling period.

The functional ability of the internalized VIP-bound receptor to stimulate adenylyl cyclase inside the cell was tested by comparing the effects of forskolin on the VIP

TABLE 3. Effect of Delayed Application of Forskolin (Time Indicated) and of Temperature on the Potentiative Effect of Forskolin on the VIP-Induced Stimulation of Cyclic AMP[a]

Temperature (°C)	Time of Forskolin Application after VIP Binding (minutes)							
	0	3	10	20	60	90	120	180
10					705			
20	1330		623	358	363	332	282	223
37	1330	613	452	422	220		120	51.43

[a] Cell monolayers in 9.6-cm^2 dishes were directly incubated with VIP at the concentration of 10^{-8} M, then washed at 10°C. After the time indicated forskolin at the concentration of 3 μM is added with the new medium. At 0 time forskolin and VIP were directly added together at 10°C. Thereafter all the dishes are incubated for 90 minutes at 10°C. Results are given in picomoles of cAMP produced / 10^6 cells. cAMP generated by forskolin alone does not exceed 10 picomoles / 10^6 cells.

bound at the cell surface or on the internalized receptor (TABLE 3). Forskolin is a diterpen known to directly activate adenylyl cyclase in intact cells[66] and to potentiate the action of ligands by stabilizing the complex between the guanine nucleotide binding subunit and the catalytic moiety of adenylyl cyclase.[67] Forskolin was shown to potentiate the effect of VIP in generating cyclic AMP, and this effect is retained at 10°C when no internalization occurs.[45] Forskolin alone is efficient in cyclic AMP generation in the range of concentrations of 3 to 300 μM. In the presence of a 10 nM VIP concentration, this curve is shifted to the left by two orders of magnitude. Forskolin was used at a 3 μM concentration for the experiments shown in TABLE 3 since in this condition forskolin alone has practically no effect in comparison to the considerable cyclic AMP obtained when forskolin is added in combination with VIP. In TABLE 3 are indicated the results obtained when forskolin is added to the culture medium at different times following the internalization of VIP. At 10°C when no internalization occurs, the potentiative effect of a delayed application of forskolin (60 minutes) is largely retained as compared to that obtained in controls by simultaneous application of VIP and forskolin. At 37°C or 20°C, the potentiative effect of forskolin on the VIP-bound receptor decreases with the rate of internalization of VIP. The reduction of the forskolin effect is also quicker at 37°C than at 20°C, in agreement with the temperature dependence of the rate of internalization. These data indicate that the potentiative effect of forskolin is closely related to the presence of VIP-bound receptor at the cell surface. The lack of potentiative effect of forskolin on the internalized site is not due to the alteration of the VIP or of the VIP-bound receptor since we have seen by HPLC that VIP was intact (see TABLE 2) and that VIP-bound receptor has the same molecular mass as the VIP-bound receptor at 10°C. This loss of effect was also not associated with a loss of the adenylyl cyclase pool during the internalization since the effect of forskolin alone is identical in control and VIP-pretreated cells.[45] Those experiments substantiate the hypothesis that the internalized VIP-bound receptor is no longer coupled to the adenylyl cyclase.

The analysis of the fate of [^{125}I]VIP after internalization was performed by quantitative autoradiographic ultrastructural analysis. This technique gives interesting results, but is rarely used because the calculations are long and tedious. Those calculations are, however, necessary because the autoradiographic grains do not correspond exactly to the original source for geometric reasons. To facilitate this type of approach, we have created a system by which the image of the electron microscopy is transferred to a computer. Briefly, the analogical signal of the scanning obtained on the STEM screen is converted by a digitalizer from the electronic signal into a numerical input. The transferred image is analyzed on the computer screen by the ARGIA program.[68] Results of this analysis show, for example, that after a 60-minute incubation at 15°C with [^{125}I]VIP, nearly 70% of the disintegrations are on the plasma membrane and microvilli. After 10 minutes at 37°C, the pattern of the [^{125}I]VIP distribution in the cell organelles is completely different. Only 21% of the label remains at the cell surface and nearly half the activity if contained in endosomes. Most of the grains present in the vesicle remain bound to the endosome-limiting membrane, whereas some are found in the lumen, suggesting that VIP is detached from its receptor at some steps of the internalization process.[69] More detailed studies on the repartition of VIP in the endosomal compartment are shown in FIGURE 1.

The compartment termed "endosome" and multivesicular endosome includes both the grains of VIP that were attributed to the clear round or ovoid vesicles surrounded by smooth membrane as well as the tubular (FIG. 2a) and C-shaped endosome (FIG. 2b) components. The compartment termed "multivesicular bodies" includes the grains of VIP that are contained in larger vesicles containing small vesicles of medium density that might represent the association of several endosomal vesicles (FIG. 3). This pattern

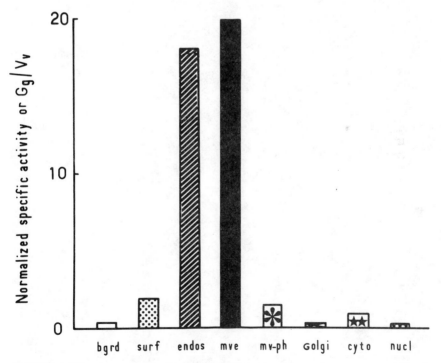

FIGURE 1. Ultrastructural repartition of [^{125}I]VIP in the endosomal compartment. Abbreviations are: bgrd, background; surf, cell surface and microvilli; endos, endosome (see FIG. 2a); mve, multivesicular endosome (see FIG. 2b); mv-ph, multivesicular bodies and phagosomes; cyto, cytoplasm; nucl, nucleus. The normalized specific activity represents the relative density of grain divided by the relative volume of the organelles.

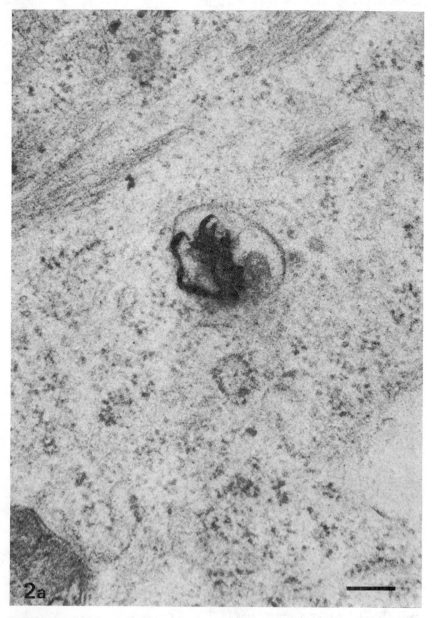

FIGURE 2. (a) Grain of radioactive VIP in a tubular multivesicular endosome. Bar, 200 nm.

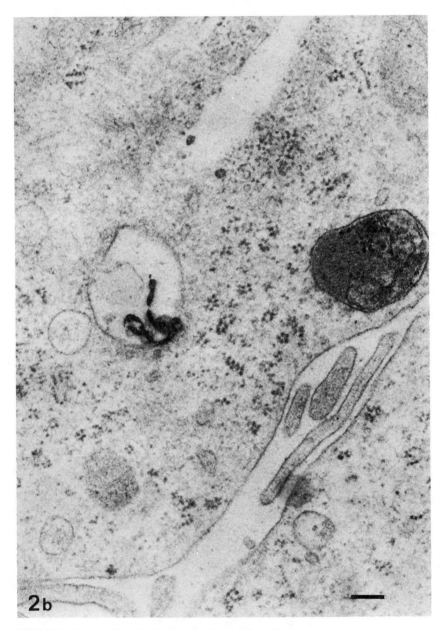

FIGURE 2. (b) Labeling of a C-shaped endosome. Bar, 200 nm.

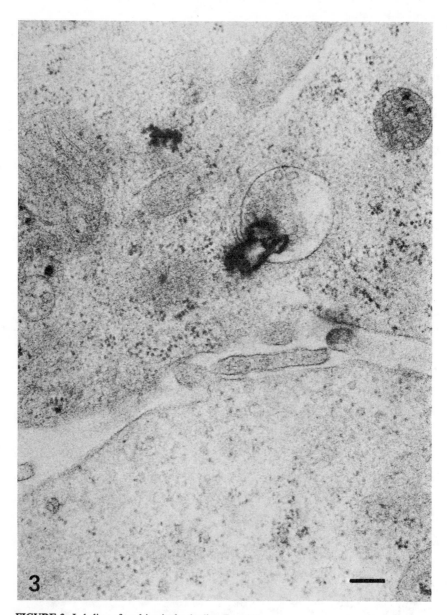

FIGURE 3. Labeling of multivesicular bodies. Bar, 200 nm.

might also be due to the association of the endosomal vesicles with small vesicles that come from the Golgi and contain lysosomal enzymes. Morphologically, however, the multivesicular bodies are clearly distinct from the multivesicular endosome because they are surrounded by a continuous membrane (FIG. 3). The multivesicular bodies might be clear or dense and are presumed to form a prelysosomal structure that contains degrading enzymes.[70] It is likely to correspond to the place where the VIP receptor degradation starts. The localization of internalized [^{125}I]VIP was investigated by Muller *et al.*[42] by subcellular fractionation techniques. It is likely that the multivesicular bodies observed in our preparation are a part of the low-density fraction that was obtained on discontinuous metrizamide gradients[42] and also contains large lysosomes with a major peak of acid phosphatase activity. The density of grains that we observed in these structures is low because our data (FIG. 2) were taken 10 minutes after exposure of the cell to VIP at 37°C. The appearance of radioactivity in the lysosomal fraction of Muller occurs later, 20 minutes after incubation at 37°C. In our data, the multivesicular endosome might be considered to be an intermediatory structure from which the VIP receptor might be either recycled to the cell surface or directed to the multivesicular lysosomal compartment.

TABLE 4. Recovery of the VIP Binding Site at the Cell Surface and of the VIP-Induced cAMP Stimulation at 37°C

| | Time (minutes) | | | | | | | |
	0	5	10	20	60	120	180	Controls[a]
Binding[b]	0.04	0.07	0.08	0.15	0.23	0.25	0.24	0.36
cAMP[c]	1.4	2.3	10	18	24	33	36	65

[a] Controls are incubated under the same conditions as the tested cells, but in the absence of a preexposure desensitizing dose (10^{-8} M) of VIP.
[b] Binding was performed after the removal of VIP at the recovery period of time indicated, by addition of 4×10^{-11} M VIP. Quantity bound is in fm/10^6 cells.
[c] Maximally stimulated levels of cAMP was obtained by the addition of 10^{-8} M VIP at the recovery period of time indicated. Results are in picomoles of cAMP produced/10^6 cells (stimulated-basal).

The recovery of the VIP receptor was tested by removing VIP from the medium; the cell layers are thereafter incubated at different temperatures in a VIP-free medium (TABLE 4). At 37°C, the reappearance of the [^{125}I]VIP binding site during the recovery is rapid with a half-time of 10 minutes. However, the reversal of the receptor disappearance is partial, even after a 180-minute incubation, since [^{125}I]VIP binding represents 70% of that observed in control cells. Lowering the temperature of the recovery step resulted in decelerating the recovery and no reversal of the VIP-bound receptor internalization was observed at a temperature of 10°C.[45] Parallel study on the magnitude of the recovery of the VIP-inducing cyclic AMP stimulation indicates that VIP binding sites retain their ability to be coupled and reactivate the subunits of the cyclase. This recovery is not dependent on protein synthesis since the cycloheximide, added in all the buffers used throughout the experiments, did not suppress recovery of the binding site.[45]

From our study, a general pattern of the regulation of the VIP receptor in this cell might be proposed (FIG. 4). After the activation, the VIP-bound receptor is internalized in clear endosomal vesicles with a half-time of about three minutes at

37°C. The internalized receptor is functionally and likely structurally detached from the adenylyl cyclase. Most the internalized binding sites are not altered. VIP remains bound to the receptor, then is progressively detached. The undegraded receptors are recycled to the cell surface within a half-time of 10 minutes from the endosomal vesicles and probably in part from the multivesicular endosomes. The ligand appears degraded in the medium whereas the recycled receptor is coupled again to the adenylyl cyclase components. Some of the VIP receptor molecules are directed from the multivesicular endosome to the multivesicular bodies and the lysosomes where they are degraded. This degradation does not exceed 30% of the receptor after three hours of VIP (10^{-8} M) exposure at 37°C.

From these data as well as from the literature, it appears that the desensitization to VIP is related to several different processes. The chemical desensitization that was demonstrated to be associated to a phosphorylation of the catecholamine receptor

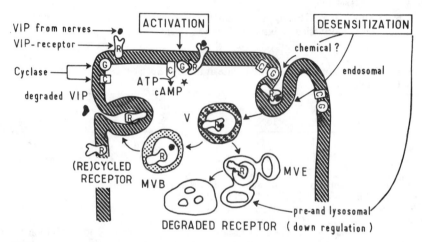

FIGURE 4. VIP (●) and VIP receptor (R) cycle in the cell. G, guanyl regulatory protein; C, catalytic subunit of the cyclase; V, vesicles; MVE, multivesicular endosome; MVB, multivesicular bodies.

might operate for VIP as suggested by the phorbol ester experiment quoted above.[34] Desensitization to VIP is also related to the removal of the cell surface receptor into the endosomes. This process accounts for a short-time desensitization and is fully operative for maximally effective doses of VIP leading to total occupancy of the receptor. Indeed, the complete cycle of internalization and recovery of the receptor do not exceed a half-time of 13 minutes. The desensitization related to this cycle may be also shorter if an endogenous pool of VIP receptor is present in the cells. Such a pool has been described in the case of the insulin receptors.[71] Desensitization is also due to the destruction of part of the receptor into the prelysosomal and lysosomal compartments. This mechanism accounts for the long-term desensitization also called "downregulation" and lasts for as long a time as is required for the biosynthesis and the process of new VIP receptor to the cell surface.

The regulation of the VIP receptor biosynthesis is not known. However, several models exist where the density and/or the activity of the VIP receptor was found to be dramatically modified according to the evolution of the cells. In the gut axis, the development of VIP receptor was shown to be associated with the differentiation of pancreatic[72] or colonic[73] cancerous cells in culture. On the other hand, a decrease in the VIP effect was observed following the differentiation of the human cancerous colonic cell in culture (HT-29) or during the maturation of intestinal cells in fetal and neonates.[74] A receptor-dependent decrease in the VIP effect has been also noticed during the proliferation of intestinal epithelium following intestinal resection[75] after ligation of pancreatic and bile ducts.[76] The affinity of VIP receptor is decreased in the membranes from the regenerating liver cells following hepatectomy.[77] Dissimilar results were also obtained with neural tissues or cells. The VIP effect has been shown to increase with maturation of forebrain[78] or the development of cortical neurons (Staun-Olsen, unpublished data). In other types of cells, such as the striatal neuron,[79] a decrease in the VIP effect was observed with the differentiation.

REFERENCES

1. SAID, S. I. 1986. Vasoactive intestinal peptide. J. Endocrinol. Invest. **9:** 191-200.
2. ROSSELIN, G. 1986. The receptors of the VIP family peptides (VIP, secretin, GRF, PHI, PHM, GIP, glucagon and oxyntomodulin). Specificities and identity. Peptides 7(Suppl. 1): 89-100.
3. CHRISTOPHE, J., M. SVOBODA, M. LAMBERT, M. WAELBROECK, J. WINND, J. P. DEHAYE, M. C. VANDERMEERS-PIRET, A. VANDERMEERS & P. ROBBERECHT. 1986. Effector mechanisms of peptides of the VIP family. Peptides 7(Suppl. 1): 101-107.
4. SIBLEY, D. R. & R. J. LEFKOWITZ. 1985. Molecular mechanisms of receptor desensitization using the beta-adrenergic receptor-coupled adenylate cyclase system as a model. Nature **317:** 124-129.
5. PASTAN, I. & M. C. WILLINGHAM, EDS. 1985. Endocytosis. Plenum Press. New York.
6. YANAIHARA, C., Y. HASHIMOTO, H. MANAKA & N. YANAIHARA. 1985. Opposite effects of N- and C-terminal PHI fragments upon glucose-induced insulin release. Regul. Peptides Suppl. **3:** S69.
7. VELICELEBI, G., S. PATTHI & E. T. KAISER. 1986. Design and biological activity of analogs of growth hormone releasing factor with potential amphiphilic helical carboxyl termini. Proc. Natl Acad. Sci. USA **83:** 5397-5399.
8. WAELBROECK, M., P. ROBBERECHT, D. H. COY, J. C. CAMUS, P. DENEEF & J. CHRISTOPHE. 1985. Interaction of growth hormone-releasing factor (GRF) and 14 GRF analogs with vasoactive intestinal peptide (VIP) receptors of rat pancreas. Discovery of (N-Ac-Tyr^1,D-Phe^2)-GRF(1-29)-NH$_2$ as a VIP antagonist. Endocrinology **116:** 2643-2649.
9. PANDOL, S. J., K. DHARMSATHAPHORN, M. S. SCHOEFFIELD, W. VALE & J. RIVIER. 1986. Vasoactive intestinal peptide receptor antagonist (4Cl-DPhe^6, Leu^{17}) VIP. Am. J. Physiol. **250:** G553-G557.
10. TURNER, J. T., S. B. JONES & D. B. BYLUND. 1986. A fragment of vasoactive intestinal peptide, VIP (10-28), is an antagonist of VIP in the colon carcinoma cell line, HT29. Peptides **7:** 849-854.
11. ROSSELIN, G., M. LABURTHE, D. BATAILLE, J. C. PRIETO, C. DUPONT, B. AMIRANOFF, J. P. BROYART & J. BESSON. 1980. Receptors and effectors of vasoactive intestinal peptide in cell function and differentiation. In Hormones and Cell Regulation. J. Dumont & J. Nunez, Eds. Vol. **4:** 311-330. Elsevier/North Holland. Amsterdam, the Netherlands.
12. BATAILLE, D., C. GESPACH, M. LABURTHE, B. AMIRANOFF, K. TATEMOTO, N. VAUCLIN, V. MUTT & G. ROSSELIN. 1980. Porcine peptide having N-terminal histidine and C-terminal isoleucine amide (PHI). Vasoactive intestinal peptide (VIP) and secretin-like effects in different tissues from the rat. FEBS Lett. **114:** 240-242.
13. LABURTHE, M., A. COUVINEAU & C. ROUYER-FESSARD. 1986. Study of species specificity in growth hormone-releasing factor (GRF) interaction with vasoactive intestinal peptide

(VIP) receptors using GRF and intestinal VIP receptors from rat and human: Evidence that AC-Tyr¹hGRF is a competitive VIP antagonist in the rat. Mol. Pharmacol. **29:** 23-27.

14. ARILLA, E., J. C. PRIETO, J. M. LOPEZ-MARTINEZ & R. GOBERNA. 1981. Somatostatin action on insulin secretion induced by chicken and porcine vasoactive intestinal peptide in the perfused rat pancreas. Horm. Metab. Res. **13:** 314-317.

15. GOURDJI, D., D. BATAILLE, N. BUISSON & A. TIXIER-VIDAL. 1985. GH rat pituitary cell strains as target models for regulatory peptides: Interaction of peripheral hormones with TRH and VIP. *In* Regulatory Peptides in Digestive, Nervous and Endocrine Systems. J. M. J. Lewin & S. Bonfils, Eds.: 125-133. Elsevier/North Holland. Amsterdam, the Netherlands.

16. O'DORISIO, M. S., N. Q. HERMINA, T. M. O'DORISIO & S. P. BALCERZAK. 1981. Vasoactive intestinal polypeptide modulation of lymphocyte adenylate cyclase. J. Immunol. **127:** 2551-2554.

17. ROSTÈNE, W. H. 1984. Neurobiological and neuroendocrine functions of the vasoactive intestinal peptide (VIP). Progr. Neurobiol. **22:** 103-129.

18. VAN CALKER, D., M. MULLER & B. HAMPRECHT. 1980. Regulation by secretin, vasoactive intestinal peptide and somatostatin of cyclic AMP accumulation in cultured brain cells. Proc. Natl Acad. Sci. USA **77:** 6907-6911.

19. ROSTÈNE, W. H., M. DUSSAILLANT & G. ROSSELIN. 1982. Rapid inhibition by somatostatin of vasoactive intestinal peptide-induced prolactin secretion by rat pituitary cells. FEBS Lett. **146:** 213-216.

20. CARTER, R. F., K. N. BITAR, A. M. ZFASS & G. MAKHLOUF. 1978. Inhibition of VIP-stimulated intestinal secretion and cyclic AMP production by somatostatin in the rat. Gastroenterology **74:** 726-730.

21. DORFLINGER, L. J. & A. SCHONBRUNN. 1983. Somatostatin inhibits basal and vasoactive intestinal peptide-stimulated hormone release by different mechanisms in GH pituitary cells. Endocrinology **113:** 1551-1558.

22. CHNEIWEISS, H., J. GLOWINSKI & J. PRÉMONT. 1984. Vasoactive intestinal polypeptide receptors linked to an adenylate cyclase, and their relationship with biogenic amine- and somatostatin-sensitive adenylate cyclase on central neuronal and glial cells in primary cultures. J. Neurochem. **44:** 779-786.

23. KOCH, B. D., L. J. DORFLINGER & A. SCHONBRUNN. 1985. Pertussis toxin blocks both cyclic AMP-mediated and cyclic AMP-independent actions of somatostatin. J. Biol. Chem. **260:** 13138-13145.

24. YAJIMA, Y., Y. AKITA & T. SAITO. 1986. Pertussis toxin blocks the inhibitory effects of somatostatin on cAMP-dependent vasoactive intestinal peptide and cAMP-independent thyrotropin releasing hormone-stimulated prolactin secretion of GH₃ cells. J. Biol. Chem. **261:** 2684-2687.

25. LUINI, A., D. LEWIS, S. GUILD, D. CORDA & J. AXELROD. 1985. Hormone secretagogues increase cytosolic calcium by increasing cAMP in corticotropin-secreting cells. Proc. Natl Acad. Sci. USA **82:** 8034-8038.

26. TATTER, D., G. CHARPENTIER, J. BESSON, G. ROSSELIN & J. P. BERCOVICI. 1983. Le VIP lève l'inhibition de la sécrétion de prolactine induite par la dopamine chez les sujets présentant un prolactinome. C.R. Acad. Sci. Paris **297:** 331-334.

27. OLIVA, D., L. VALLAR, G. GIANNATTASIO, A. SPADA & S. NICOSIA. 1984. Combined effects of vasoactive intestinal peptide and dopamine on adenylate cyclase in prolactin-secreting cells. Peptides **5:** 1067-1070.

28. WEISS, S., M. SEBBEN, J. A. GARCIA-SAINZ & J. BOCKAERT. 1985. D₂-dopamine receptor-mediated inhibition of cyclic AMP formation in striatal neurons in primary culture. Mol. Pharmacol. **27:** 595-599.

29. PACHTER, J. A. & D. MAN-KIT LAM. 1986. Interactions between vasoactive intestinal peptide and dopamine in the rabbit retina stimulation of a common adenylate cyclase. J. Neurochem. **46:** 257-264.

30. MAGISTRETTI, P. J. & M. SCHORDERET. 1984. VIP and noradrenaline act synergistically to increase cyclic AMP in cerebral cortex. Nature **308:** 280-282.

31. BOIGE, N., A. MUNCK & M. LABURTHE. 1984. Adrenergic versus VIPergic control of cyclic AMP in human colonic crypts. Peptides **5:** 379-383.

32. TURNER, J. T., C. RAY-PRENGER & D. B. BYLUND. 1985. Alpha$_2$-adrenergic receptors in the human cell line, HT29. Characterization with the full agonist radioligand [^{3}H]UK-13,304 and inhibition of adenylate cyclase. Mol. Pharmacol. **28:** 422-430.
33. NAKAKI, T., T. NAKADATE, S. YAMAMOTO & R. KATO. 1983. Alpha$_2$-adrenergic receptor in intestinal epithelial cells. Identification by ^{3}H-yohimbine and failure to inhibit cyclic AMP accumulation. Mol. Pharmacol. **23:** 228-234.
34. QUILLIAM, L. A., P. R. M. DOBSON & B. L. BROWN. 1985. Modulation of cyclic AMP accumulation of GH$_3$ cells by a phorbol ester and thyroliberin. Biochem. Biophys. Res. Commun. **129:** 898-903.
35. FISCHER, S. K., P. D. KLINGER & T. K. HARDEN. 1983. Muscarinic agonist binding and phospholipid turnover in brain. J. Biol. Chem. **258:** 7358-7363.
36. ONALI, P., C. EVA, M. C. OLIANAS, J. P. SCHWARTZ & E. COSTA. 1983. In GH$_3$ cells, acetylcholine and vasoactive intestinal peptide antagonistically modulate adenylate cyclase, cyclic AMP content and prolactin secretion. Mol. Pharmacol. **24:** 189-194.
37. AUDIGIER, S., C, BARBERIS & S. JARD. 1986. Vasoactive intestinal polypeptide increases inositol phospholipid breakdown in the rat superior cervical ganglion. Brain Res. **376:** 363-367.
38. MALLAT, A., C. PAVOINE, M. DUFOUR, S. LOTERSZTEJN, D. BATAILLE & F. PECKER. 1987. A glucagon fragment is responsible for the inhibition of the liver Ca^{2+} plump by glucagon. Nature **325:** 620-622.
39. ROTSZTEJN, W. H., M. DUSSAILLANT, F. NOBOU & G. ROSSELIN. 1981. Rapid glucocorticoid inhibition of vasoactive intestinal peptide-induced cyclic AMP accumulation and prolactin release in rat pituitary cells in culture. Proc. Natl. Acad. Sci. USA **78:** 7584-7588.
40. SCHUSDZIARRA, V., R. SCHMID & M. CLASSEN. 1986. Effect of insulin on secretion of bombesin-like immunoreactivity and gastrin from the isolated rat stomach in response to acetylcholine, VIP and leucine-enkephalin. Neuropeptides **7:** 51-62.
41. BOISSARD, C., G. HEJBLUM, J. C. MARIE, C. GESPACH & G. ROSSELIN. 1984. Désensibilisation au VIP par rétro-régulation des récepteurs de ce peptide dans les cellules transformées HT-29 de l'épithélium colique humain en culture. C.R. Acad. Sci. Paris **299:** 795-798.
42. MULLER, J. M., A. EL-BATTARI, E. AH-KYE, J. LUIS, F. DUCRET, J. PICON & J. MARVALDI. 1985. Internalization of the vasoactive intestinal peptide (VIP) in a human adenocarcinoma cell line (HT29). Eur. J. Biochem. **152:** 107-114.
43. MARIE, J. C., D. HUI BON HOA, G. HEJBLUM & G. ROSSELIN. 1986. Cycle of VIP in the human transformed colonic epithelial cells (HT-29) in culture. Peptides **7:** 129-135.
44. LUIS, J., J. M. MULLER, B. ABADIE, J. M. MARTIN, J. MARVALDI & J. PICHON. 1986. Cycle of the vasoactive intestinal peptide and its binding site in a human adenocarcinoma cell line (HT 29). Eur. J. Biochem. **156:** 631-636.
45. BOISSARD, C., J. C. MARIE, G. HEJBLUM, C. GESPACH & G. ROSSELIN. 1986. Vasoactive intestinal peptide receptor regulation and reversible desensitization in human colonic carcinoma cells in culture. Cancer Res. **46:** 4406-4413.
46. HOHMANN, E. L., L. LEVINE & A. H. TASHJIAN. 1983. Vasoactive intestinal peptide stimulates bone resorption via a cyclic 3',5'-monophosphate-dependent mechanism. Endocrinology **112:** 1233-1239.
47. GESPACH, C., S. EMANI & G. ROSSELIN. 1984. Gastric inhibitory peptide (GIP), pancreatic glucagon and vasoactive intestinal peptide (VIP) are cAMP-inducing hormones in the human gastric cancer cell line HGT-1. Homologous desensitization of VIP receptor activity. Biochem. Biophys. Res. Commun. **120:** 641-649.
48. HOHMANN, E. & A. H. TASHJIAN. 1984. Functional receptors for vasoactive intestinal peptide on human osteosarcoma cells. Endocrinology **114:** 1321-1327.
49. ROUSSET, M., M. LABURTHE, G. CHEVALIER, C. BOISSARD, G. ROSSELIN & A. ZWEIBAUM. 1981. Vasoactive intestinal peptide (VIP) control of glycogenolysis in the human colon carcinoma cell line HT-29 in culture. FEBS Lett. **126:** 38-40.
50. GANZ, P., A. W. SANDROCK, S. C. LANDIS, J. LEOPOLD, M. A. GIMBRONE & R. W. ALEXANDER. 1986. Vasoactive intestinal peptide: Vasodilation and cyclic AMP generation. Am. J. Physiol. **250:** H755-H760.

51. OTTAWAY, C. A. 1984. *In vitro* alteration of receptor for vasoactive intestinal peptide changes the *in vivo* localization of mouse T cells. J. Exp. Med. **160:** 1054-1069.

52. PHILLIS, J. W., J. R. KIRKPATRICK & S. I. SAID. 1978. Vasoactive intestinal polypeptide excitation of central neurons. Can. J. Physiol. Pharmacol. **56:** 337-340.

53. STAUN-OLSEN, P., B. OTTESEN, P. D. BARTELS, M. H. NIELSEN, S. GAMMELTOFT & J. FAHRENKRUG. 1982. Receptors for vasoactive intestinal polypeptide on isolated synaptosomes from rat cerebral cortex. Heterogeneity of binding and desensitization of receptors. J. Neurochem. **39:** 1242-1251.

54. KAKU, K., M. TSUCHIYA, M. MATSUDA, Y. INOUE, T. KANEKO & N. YANAIHARA. 1985. Light and agonist after vasoactive intestinal peptide binding and intracellular accumulation of adenosine 3',5'-monophosphate in the rat pineal gland. Endocrinology **117:** 2371-2375.

55. KREJS, G. J. Personal communication.

56. MANDEL, K. G., K. DHARMSATHAPHORN & J. A. MCROBERTS. 1986. Characterization of a cyclic AMP-activated Cl⁻ transport pathway in the apical membrane of a human colonic epithelial cell line. J. Biol. Chem. **261:** 704-712.

57. FORGUE-LAFITTE, E., G. ROSSELIN, M. LABURTHE, J. C. CÉZARD, A. ZWEIBAUM & A. J. MOODY. 1981. Peptidic regulation of gut epithelium; relationship with specific receptors in normal and cancerous cells. *In* Colonic Carcinogenesis. R. A. Malt & R. C. N. Williamson, Eds.: 339-353. MTP Press. Lancaster/Boston/the Hague.

58. KITABGI, P., C. POUSTIS, A. ZWEIBAUM & P. FREYCHET. 1979. Peptide receptors in colonic tumor cells; specific binding of epidermal growth factor to the HT 29 cell line. *In* Hormone Receptors in Digestion and Nutrition. G. Rosselin, P. Fromageot & S. Bonfils Eds.: 255-260. Elsevier/North Holland. Amsterdam, the Netherlands.

59. SCEMAMA, J. L., C. RUELLAN, P. CLERC, F. CLEMENTE & A. RIBET. 1984. Dopamine receptors in a human colonic cancer cell line (HT29). Some receptor-related biological effects of dopamine. Int. J. Cancer **34:** 675-679.

60. COUVINEAU, A., M. ROUSSET & M. LABURTHE. 1985. Molecular identification and structural requirement of vasoactive intestinal peptide (VIP) receptors in the human colon adenocarcinoma cell line HT-29. Biochem. J. **231:** 139-143.

61. COUVINEAU, A. & M. LABURTHE. 1985. The human vasoactive intestinal peptide receptor: Molecular identification by covalent cross-linking in colonic epithelium. J. Clin. Endocr. Metab. **61:** 50-55.

62. DICKINSON, K. E., M. SCHACHTER, C. M. M. MILES, D. H. COY & P. S. SEVER. 1986. Characterization of vasoactive intestinal peptide (VIP) receptors in mammalian lung. Peptides **7:** 791-800.

63. WOOD, C. L. & M. S. O'DORISIO. 1985. Covalent cross-linking of vasoactive intestinal polypeptide to its receptors on intact lymphoblasts. J. Biol. Chem. **260:** 1243-1247.

64. EL BATTARI, A., J. LUIS, J. M. MARTIN, F. FANTINI, J. M. MULLER, J. MARVALDI & J. PICHON. 1987. The vasoactive intestinal peptide receptor on intact human colonic adenocarcinoma cells (HT29-D4). Biochem. J. **242:** 185-191.

65. NGUYEN, T. D., J. A. WILLIAMS & G. M. GRAY. 1986. Vasoactive intestinal peptide receptor on liver plasma membranes: Characterization as a glycoprotein. Biochemistry **25:** 361-368.

66. DALY, J. W. 1984. Forskolin, adenylate cyclase and cell physiology: An overview. Adv. Cyclic Nucl. Protein Phosphor. Res. **17:** 81-89.

67. BOUHELAL, R., G. GUILLON, V. HOMBURGER & J. BOCKAERT. 1985. Forskolin-induced change of the size of adenylate cyclase. J. Biol. Chem. **260:** 10901-10904.

68. HEJBLUM, G., A. M. DOWNS & J. P. RIGAUT. 1986. ARGIA: A user-friendly image analyser-based package for autoradiograph evaluation by the crossfire method. Acta Stereol. **5:** 245-249.

69. HEJBLUM, G., P. GALI, C. BOISSARD, A. ASTÉSANO, J. C. MARIE, A. ANTEUNIS, D. HUI BON HOA & G. ROSSELIN. 1988. Cellular processing of VIP and VIP receptors in cultured cells: A combined ultrastructural and biochemical study. To be published.

70. ANTEUNIS, A. 1974. Origin and fate of the multivesicular bodies in PHA stimulated lymphocytes. Cell Tissue Res. **149:** 497-511.

71. CHVATCHKO, Y., E. VAN OBBERGHEM & M. FEHLMANN. 1984. Internalization and recycling of insulin receptors in hepatoma cells. Absence of regulation by receptor occupancy. Biochem. J. **222:** 111-117.

72. ESTIVAL, A., P. MOUNIELOU, V. TROCHERIS, J. L. SCEMAMA, F. CLEMENTE, E. HOLLANDE & A. RIBET. 1983. Presence of VIP receptors in a human pancreatic adenocarcinoma cell line, modulation of the cAMP response during cell proliferation. Biochem. Biophys. Res. Commun. **111:** 958-963.

73. RUELLAN, C., J. L. SCEMAMA, P. CLERC, P. FAGOT-REVURAT, F. CLEMENTE & A. RIBET. 1986. VIP regulation of a human pancreatic cancer cell line: Capan-1. Peptides 7(Suppl. 1): 267-271.

74. CHASTRE, E., C. GESPACH, G. ROSSELIN & Y. BROER. 1985. Récepteurs fonctionnels et spécifiques du peptide intestinal vasoactif dans les entérocytes isolés chez le rat à l'âge foetal ou adulte. C.R. Acad. Sci. Paris **300:** 399-404.

75. FERNANDEZ-MORENO, M. D., J. L. DIAZ-JUAREZ, E. ARILLA & J. C. PRIETO. 1985. Effect of resection of small intestine on the interaction of vasoactive intestinal peptide with rat colonic epithelial cells. Horm. Metab. Res. **17:** 289-292.

76. DIAZ-JUAREZ, J. L., E. ARILLA & J. C. PRIETO. 1985. Influence of ligation of pancreatic and bile ducts on the interaction of vasoactive intestinal peptide with rat duodenum epithelial cells. Comp. Biochem. Physiol. **82:** 479-482.

77. PRIETO, J. C., J. L. DIAZ-JUAREZ & E. ARILLA. 1986. VIP interaction with intestinal epithelial cells in liver plasma membranes from hepatectomized rats. Peptides 7(Suppl. 1): 273-278.

78. ROTH, L. B. & M. B. BEINFELD. 1985. The postnatal development of VIP binding sites in rat forebrain and hindbrain. Peptides **6:** 27-30.

79. WEISS, S., M. SEBBEN, D. E. KEMP & J. BOCKAERT. 1986. Vasoactive intestinal peptide actions on cyclic AMP levels in cultured striatal neurons. Peptides 7(Suppl. 1): 187-192.

Vasoactive Intestinal Peptide Receptors in Pancreas and Liver

Structure-Function Relationship[a]

JEAN CHRISTOPHE,[b] MICHAL SVOBODA, MAGALI
WAELBROECK, JACQUES WINAND, AND PATRICK
ROBBERECHT

Department of Biochemistry and Nutrition
Medical School, Université Libre de Bruxelles
Brussels, B-1000 Belgium

INTRODUCTION

Activation of Adenylate Cyclase by VIP Proceeds through the Coupling of VIP
Receptors to N_s

Vasoactive intestinal peptide (VIP) control starts with the binding of VIP to its receptor (R). A bimolecular collision then allows the floating VIP-R complex to interact with N_s loaded with GDP. N_s (G_s) is a guanyl nucleotide binding heterotrimer made of three subunits: alpha$_s$, beta, and a small 8-kDa gamma subunit. The alpha$_s$ subunit may exist in two forms (e.g., of 50 and 42 kDa, in pancreatic acinar cells[1]); it carries the GTP-GDP binding site and is capable of hydrolyzing GTP into GDP and P_i. The formation of the high-affinity ternary complex VIP-R-NsGDP is followed by a first-order "slow" conformational change that accelerates the exchange of GDP with GTP in the alpha$_s$ subunit of N_s. There results: (1) a dissociation of alpha$_s$ from the beta-gamma subunits of N_s, (2) the hydrolysis of GTP to GDP + P_1 in alpha$_s$, and (3) a low-affinity state of R for VIP. This is why direct binding studies of VIP are more difficult in the presence than in the absence of GTP: The rapid dissociation of [^{125}I]VIP is due to GTP provoking low binding of the radioligand at equilibrium.

[a] Aided by Grant 5 ROI-AM 17010-9 from the National Institutes of Health (USA) and Grant 3.4504.81 from the Fonds de la Recherche Scientifique Médicale (Belgium).

[b] Address for correspondence: Dr. Jean Christophe, Department of Biochemistry and Nutrition, Medical School, Université Libre de Bruxelles, 115 Boulevard de Waterloo, Brussels, B-1000 Belgium.

Heterogeneity of Pancreatic VIP-Secretin Receptors and Subheterogeneity of Hepatic VIP-Preferring Receptors

When comparing the ability of VIP, secretin, and related peptides to interact with receptors and the accompanying adenylate cyclase system, a distinction between "VIP-preferring" and "secretin-preferring" receptors may be required when these two types of functional receptors coexist as observed in the pancreas from rat and guinea pig.[2-5] Besides, when "VIP-preferring receptors" only are present, they must often be sub-divided into two subtypes: for example, in rat liver membranes, displacement curves of [125I]VIP binding by VIP and VIP analogues develop on more than three logarithms and are clearly multiphasic (see below).

The direct demonstration of such a receptor heterogeneity obviously requires (a) the availability of highly selective agonists and antagonists for each (sub)class and (b) the chemical characterization of distinct receptor species.

Basis of the Molecular Pharmacology Applied to VIP Receptors in Pancreatic and Hepatic Plasma Membranes

Analysis of the Dose-Effect Curve of Adenylate Cyclase Activation by a Stimulatory VIP Agonist

Intrinsic activity (I.A.) can be calculated; it is defined as the relative efficacy of the analogue as compared to that of a maximal concentration of VIP used as reference. The intrinsic activity of a VIP agonist to activate adenylate cyclase, in the presence of GTP, reflects how easily the preliminary ternary complex agonist-R-N_s(GDP) is formed and allows a rapid GDP-GTP exchange reaction, so that N_s(GTP) is then available for adenylate cyclase activation (see above). A 20% change in I.A. with reference to VIP is highly significant already when considering the precision of the I.A. representation on an arithmetic scale.

Potency, $K_{act} = EC_{50}$, can be obtained, that is, the peptide concentration required for half-maximal adenylate cyclase stimulation. A difference between two K_{act} values is significant only when higher than threefold: this is due to the relative imprecision of the logarithmic scale used for representing the data.

When a VIP analogue is inactive or very poorly active and provided that it binds to receptors, it is of interest to examine the specificity and potency ($K_i = IC_{50} =$ concentration required to inhibit half-maximally) of its possible inhibitory action on adenylate cyclase activation by VIP. An efficient VIP antagonist is clearly unable to form an operative ternary complex with N_s(GDP) but has a low K_i, that is, keeps a high affinity (potency) for VIP receptors.

K_D Value

The K_D value, or the ligand concentration required to occupy 50% of the receptors when competing for binding with [^{125}I]VIP on plasma membranes, can be easily quantified, provided that enough binding sites are present for [^{125}I]VIP. If the competition curve with the radioligand is multiphasic, the ligand is assumed to recognize two (or even three) subclasses of receptors and the program developed by Richardson and Humrich is utilized.[6]

A useful comparison can be made when binding and enzymatic data are collected under the same conditions, that is, when using exactly the same medium composition. There is usually a good correlation between receptor occupancy and the ability of an *antagonist* to inhibit agonist effects. By contrast, the correlation between the potency of *agonist* binding (K_D) and the potency of the biological response (EC_{50}) may point out some intricacies due to postreceptor amplification, even in a system as simple as adenylate cyclase where the probe explores what immediately follows the binding step. Indeed, an agonist may: (a) recognize several classes of receptors with different affinities in which each class is not necessarily coupled to adenylate cyclase (see below), or (b) bind to different functional states of the same receptor. Its I.A. then usually correlates with its ability to induce a high-affinity receptor complex. Besides, agonist binding studies are more difficult under conditions allowing adenylate cyclase activation, that is, when GTP, a mandatory agent for hormone stimulation of adenylate cyclase, is present in the medium and induces a rapid dissociation of the radioligand from its receptor.

Pitfalls and Solutions

The study of binding sites in both dispersed acini and semi-purified plasma membranes from the rat pancreas is complicated by the fact that all ligands at hand (except one, see below) are relatively unspecific, each of them interacting with all binding sites, and moderate changes in experimental conditions affecting ligand selectivity (e.g., the presence of guanine nucleotides in the incubation medium of pancreatic plasma membranes). This is why the advance of our knowledge in this field will depend on:

1. A good strategy for the tailoring of peptide analogues, highly specific for each receptor, that might act as: (a) superagonists, that is, be more potent, efficient, and stable than VIP; (b) full antagonists retaining high affinity for the receptor. We will see that, among the several synthetic VIP and GRF analogues we tested recently, some are efficient VIP antagonists *in vitro*, but none is 100% selective; (c) radioligands serving as tracer to identify, quantify, and examine separately the regulation of VIP as opposed to secretin receptors. Again the challenge is to synthesize analogues conserving (or increasing) their specificity for the corresponding receptors.

2. The study of the molecular architecture of pancreatic VIP and secretin receptors associated or not with regulatory proteins. An analogue, characterized as defined above, could be used to full advantage if its affinity is high enough for cross-linking experiments (see section on molecular characterization of VIP receptors).

The long-term goal of this type of research is to obtain analogues that might be longer-acting and more potent *in vivo*.

FUNCTIONAL CHARACTERISTICS OF COEXISTENT VIP AND SECRETIN RECEPTORS IN THE EXOCRINE PANCREAS

In Dispersed Rat Pancreatic Acini

VIP and secretin receptors in dispersed rat pancreatic acini represent a complex model due to the coexistence of at least four binding sites and of biological responses when each (sub)class of receptor is occupied.[7-10] Our data indicate the binding of VIP and secretin to four functionally distinct classes of binding sites: (1) A high-affinity class binds secretin and allows a small increase in cyclic AMP (in centro-acinar cells?). (2 and 3) Two intermediate affinity classes of receptors, preferring VIP and secretin, respectively, are responsible for the large increase in cyclic AMP, most of the phosphorylation of 33-kDa, 25-kDa, and 21-kDa particulate proteins, modest stimulus-secretion coupling (tested by amylase secretion) when used alone but also for an efficient potentiation of the secretory effect of CCK-8 (COOH-terminal octapeptide of cholecystokinin) acting through its own receptors. (4) A fourth population of receptors with low affinity for secretin is unable to bind VIP and to raise cyclic AMP but is responsible for most of the secretory effect of secretin when used alone.

In Rat Pancreatic Plasma Membranes

VIP-preferring receptors and secretin-preferring receptors coexist also in purified rat pancreatic plasma membranes.[2,4] With coexistent receptors endowed with somewhat overlapping affinities and dose-effect curves of adenylate cyclase activation extending over more than two logarithms, it is not clear whether functional high- and low-affinity receptors for VIP and secretin represent two states for each receptor species or whether high-affinity VIP-preferring receptors are low-affinity secretin receptors and low-affinity VIP-receptors are in fact secretin-preferring receptors.

Specificity of VIP Analogues as Agonists for VIP-Preferring Receptors

The only VIP agonist available that appears to be totally selective for VIP receptors in rat pancreatic plasma membranes is (D-Phe^4)PHI.[11] While VIP, PHI, and secretin inhibit the binding of both [^{125}I]VIP and [^{125}I]secretin in a wide concentration range, (D-Phe^4)PHI inhibits [^{125}I]VIP binding only (with an IC$_{50}$ of 7 nM). With all the other VIP agonists we tested, except that one, the slope of dose-effect curves on adenylate cyclase develops on more than three logarithms, suggesting interaction with two classes of receptors. These peptides are thus able to occupy functional VIP-preferring as well as secretin-preferring receptors. To the contrary, the dose-effect curve of (D-Phe^4)PHI activation of adenylate cyclase is monophasic, and competitively modified by (D-Phe^2)VIP (a VIP antagonist[12]) but not by secretin$_{7-27}$ (a secretin antagonist[2,4]).

When compared to the previous compounds, helodermin and helospectin, two agonists extracted from the venom of two helodermae lizards,[13-17] interact with near equal potency with VIP and secretin receptors in rat pancreatic acini.[7,15] In rat pancreatic membranes, they also inhibit [^{125}I]VIP and [^{125}I]secretin binding with the same EC_{50} (10 nM) and increase adenylate cyclase activity through both VIP and secretin receptors, as demonstrated by the ability of the VIP analogue (D-Phe^2)VIP (a VIP antagonist) and secretin$_{4-27}$ (a secretin antagonist) to inhibit helodermin- and helospectin-stimulated adenylate cyclase[16] (see also Vandermeers et al., this volume). Thus, these peptides secreted by the venomous glands of lizards cannot distinguish between VIP and secretin receptors and act as aspecific agonists on the rat pancreas, in sharp contrast with (D-Phe^4)PHI. It is tempting (see TABLE 1 and Vandermeers[16]) to attribute the unspecificity of the lizard peptides to the simultaneous presence of alanine in position 4 (that recalls the presence of Ala^4 in VIP) and of glutamic acid in position 9 (that recalls Glu^9 in secretin).

Identity of VIP and GRF Receptors

In rat pancreatic plasma membranes, GRF$_{1-29}$-NH$_2$ and GRF$_{1-40}$-OH are partial VIP agonists, with relatively low intrinsic activity on adenylate cyclase[18] perhaps because Ala^4 in GRF, like Ala^4 in VIP, favors VIP receptor recognition. The proof that the stimulatory effect of GRF is due to the occupancy of VIP-preferring receptors, not that of GRF-preferring or secretin-preferring receptors, relies on the fact that (N-Ac-Tyr^1, D-Phe^2)-, (His^1, D-Ala^2, D-Ser^3, NLeu^{27})-, and (His^1, D-Ala^2, D-Thr^7, NLeu^{27})GRF$_{1-29}$-NH$_2$ inhibit dose-dependently the VIP- as well as the GRF-stimulated adenylate cyclase with the same potency (K_i of 1-3 μM) but not the secretin-stimulated adenylate cyclase.[18,19] Thus, VIP and GRF receptors are indistinguishable in the rat pancreas. The same holds true in the guinea pig pancreas.[20]

Structural Requirements for VIP Receptor Occupancy and Subsequent Adenylate Cyclase Activation

VIP, PHI (peptide histidine-isoleucinamide), secretin, GRF (human growth hormone-releasing factor) and glucagon are structurally related peptides (TABLE 1). Adenylate cyclase activation by this family of peptides and the final biological response depend critically on the NH$_2$-terminal part, a region where Phe^6 and Thr^7 are common to all amino acid sequences. D. H. Coy et al.[21] have established Chou-Fasman structural predictions for ligands of this type that are likely to represent the most common ligand species in the presence of a specific receptor domain (FIG. 1). Accordingly, VIP and PHI may have a first beta-bend in the 1-4 region and, in addition, a second beta-bend in the 6-10 region. In position 4 (at the beginning of a beta sheet), L-alanine (in VIP) may maintain chirality whereas glycine (in PHI or secretin: TABLE 1) may bind to receptors in either a pseudo-D or pseudo-L conformation so that introducing a D-isomer may affect the biological activity. The discovery[11] of (D-Phe^4)PHI as a specific VIP agonist (see above) shows that replacing Gly^4 in PHI by a highly hydrophobic phenylalanine residue of the D series makes a VIP analogue more specific than VIP itself for VIP-preferring receptors. The hydrophobicity of Val

TABLE 1. The VIP-PHI-Secretin-GRF-Glucagon Family of Peptides

Species[a]	Peptide	Sequence (1 · · · 5 · · · 10 · · · 15 · · · 20 · · · 25 · · · 30 · · · 35 · · · 40 · · · 45)
p	VIP	H-S-D-A-V-F-T-D-N-Y-T-R-L-R-K-Q-M-A-V-K-K-Y-L-N-S-I-L-N-*
p	PHI	H-A-D-G-V-F-T-S-D-F-S-R-L-L-G-Q-L-S-A-K-K-Y-L-E-S-L-I-*[b]
r	PHI	H-A-D-G-V-F-T-S-D-Y-S-R-L-L-G-Q-I-S-A-K-K-Y-L-E-S-L-I-*
p	Secretin	H-S-D-G-T-F-T-S-E-L-S-R-L-R-D-S-A-R-L-Q-R-L-L-Q-G-L-V-*
p	Glucagon	H-S-Q-G-T-F-T-S-D-Y-S-K-Y-L-D-S-R-R-A-Q-D-F-V-Q-W-L-M-N-T
h	GRF$_{1-44}$	Y-A-D-A-I-F-T-N-S-Y-R-K-V-L-G-Q-L-S-A-R-K-L-L-Q-D-I-M-S-R-Q-Q-G-E-S-N-Q-E-R-G-A-R-A-R-L-*
g	Helodermin	H-S-D-A-I-F-T-E-E-Y-S-K-L-L-A-K-L-A-L-Q-K-Y-L-A-S-I-L-G-S-R-T-S-P-P-*

[a] g: Gila monster; h: human; p: porcine; r: rat.
[b] Underlining indicates fragments that are identical to VIP.

in position 5 in VIP and PHI may also be important for VIP-PHI receptor recognition.[2,4,5] There is no preferred conformation for residues 1 to 3 in native GRF, while residues 4 to 6 allow a beta sheet leading to a reverse turn between residues 6 and 10. Finally, in secretin, there appears to be a single beta-bend in the 1-4 area.[21]

The rationale for testing amino acid substitutions among the first amino acids is that such substitutions may alter the ability of the resulting analogue to couple the VIP receptor with the adenylate cyclase system more than it affects binding affinity.

We observed that the intrinsic activity and K_{act} of VIP analogues modified in the first position decrease in the following order[11,12,22]: VIP > (Ac-His[1])VIP > (3-Me-His[1])VIP = (Phe[1])VIP > (D-His[1])VIP. Beforehand, N-acetylation was considered

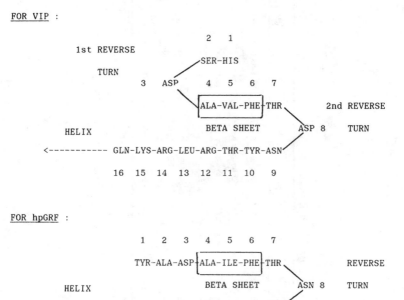

FIGURE 1. Chou-Fasman structural predictions for VIP and human pancreatic (hp)GRF.[21]

useful for protecting VIP against N-aminopeptidase activities, but the position and ionization of the His residue is obviously important for binding and activation. In VIP the pK_a values for the free alpha-amino group and the imidazole function of His[1] are, respectively, 7.88 and 7.59, so that both groups are ionizable over the physiological pH range.[23] It is possible that, upon VIP binding to its receptor, the pK_a value of the alpha-amino group is lowered by the receptor that induces an increased hydrogen bonding capacity for the deprotonated imidazole group.[23]

The six D-amino substituted VIP analogues we tested are less potent than VIP itself, their *potency* decreasing gradually when D-substitutions are closer to the NH₂-terminus: VIP > (D-Ala[4])VIP > (D-Asp[3])VIP > (D-Ser[2])VIP > (D-His[1])VIP.[11,12]

(D-Arg^2)-VIP and (D-Phe^2)-VIP are partial agonists with an I.A. of respectively, 0.35 and 0.09, as compared to that of VIP, which is equal to 1.0. These results demonstrate the highly unfavorable role of increasing hydrophobicity or basicity in position 2 (FIG. 1). (D-Phe^2)VIP is of such a low I.A. as a VIP agonist that it is in fact capable of competitively inhibiting the VIP-stimulated enzyme with a K_i of 0.1 μM but not the secretin-stimulated enzyme.[11,12]

Examining closely the inhibition of the VIP-stimulated enzyme by (D-Phe^2)-VIP, it appears that this inhibition is limited to the first major high-affinity component of the curve. In mirror, the secretin antagonist secretin$_{7-27}$ inhibits the second, low-affinity component of the VIP stimulation curve. Thus, the extra 25% activity of VIP when compared to (D-Phe^4)PHI represents the capacity of VIP to occupy secretin-preferring receptors at high concentrations.[11]

In dispersed acini from guinea pig pancreas (D-(Cl^4)Phe^6, Leu^{17})VIP inhibits VIP-stimulated increases in cellular cyclic AMP but has no effect on secretin-induced increases in cyclic AMP, indicating specificity for the VIP receptor.[24]

Using GRF$_{1-29}$-NH$_2$ and VIP as peptides of reference, we compared[18,19] the ability of 30 GRF analogues substituted in positions 1 to 10 to stimulate or inhibit adenylate cyclase activity and to inhibit [^{125}I]VIP binding in purified rat pancreatic plasma membranes.

In GRF, a free alpha-NH$_2$ group (as opposed to the N-Ac-Tyr^1 derivative) and the L-conformation of position 1 (L-Tyr^1 as opposed to D-Tyr^1), but not the phenolic function of Tyr^1, is important for optimal intrinsic activity. By contrast, the replacement of Ala^2 by D-Ala^2 (in GRF as well as in the N-acetylated Tyr^1 derivative) increases the intrinsic activity. However, substitutions of Ala^2 in (N-Ac-Tyr^1)GRF$_{1-29}$-NH$_2$ by the bulkier D-amino acid D-Phe^2 leads to (N-Ac-Tyr^1, D-Phe^2)GRF$_{1-29}$-NH$_2$, one of the first described VIP antagonists active *in vitro* in the micromolar concentration range (see above).

The L-conformation of Asp^3 is also critical, (D-Asp^3)GRF$_{1-29}$-NH$_2$ presenting only 22% of the intrinsic activity of GRF. Substitution in GRF (or its N-acetylated derivative) of Ala^4 by D-Ala^4 reduces the intrinsic activity whereas substitution of the natural L-amino acid residue by more hydrophobic D-Phe^4 gives a superagonist: (D-Phe^4)GRF$_{1-29}$-NH$_2$, when interacting with VIP receptors in both rat pancreatic and liver (see below) membranes is more potent than GRF itself.

Changes of Phe^6 for D-Phe^6 or pCl-Phe^6, and of Thr^7 for D-Thr^7 in the native peptide, and substitution of Phe^6 by Trp^6 in the N-Ac-Tyr^1 derivative give analogues with markedly reduced affinity and intrinsic activity.

Importance of Disulfide Bonds in VIP Receptors

Functional VIP receptors coupled to adenylate cyclase are very susceptible toward 2-mercaptoethanol.[25] Among VIP receptors, those with high affinity for VIP are already altered by simple exposure to 5 mM 2-mercaptoethanol, during pancreas homogenization at 5°C. The importance of disulfide bonds for functional integrity is also evident when testing VIP receptors with [^{125}I]VIP, after a preincubation of rat pancreatic plasma membranes with dithiothreitol: a low 1-2 mM dithiothreitol concentration suffices already to reduce the number of VIP receptors: at higher dithiothreitol concentration, the affinity of the remaining VIP receptors is also reduced.[25]

RAT LIVER VIP RECEPTORS

Several investigators have shown that VIP stimulates adenylate cyclase activity in rat hepatic membrane preparations through high-affinity VIP receptors.[26–29] This coupling with adenylate cyclase presents, however, several peculiarities: (a) it depends less on the presence of GTP than glucagon-stimulated coupling[28]; (b) despite the presence of a high number of VIP receptors and the high sensitivity of adenylate cyclase toward VIP stimulation, the efficacy of enzyme stimulation (i.e., the amount of cyclic AMP produced) is low[28]; (c) in intact cells the occupancy of receptors is followed, at high VIP concentration, by a modest increase of intracellular cyclic AMP,[30,31] this effect on hepatocytes and nonparenchymal cells being equally mediocre,[32] whereas glucagon efficiently increases cyclic AMP levels in both cell populations. The metabolic effects of VIP observed at high peptide concentrations are, however, qualitatively identical to those triggered by other hormonal agents acting through adenylate cyclase activation, for example, glycogenolysis and gluconeogenesis.[30,31,33] Considering the low efficacy of VIP as a stimulant of cyclic AMP accumulation, it has been hypothesized that the main role of liver VIP receptors is to initiate the degradation of the peptide extracted from portal blood[34] and/or to exert (unknown) cyclic AMP-independent effects on nonparenchymal hepatic cells.[32]

High- and Low-Affinity VIP Receptors with Distinct Coupling Characteristics

Rat liver membranes possess VIP-preferring receptors but no secretin-preferring receptors. These VIP-preferring receptors cross-react (poorly) with secretin: Secretin inhibits [^{125}I]VIP binding but is only about 1 % as potent as unlabeled VIP. Competition curves using [^{125}I]VIP and unlabeled VIP develop over more than two logarithms of concentrations so that the K_D estimated for two subclasses of VIP receptors are, respectively, 0.3 nM and 12nM.[35–37]

[^{125}I]Helodermin, the radioiodinated form of a parent peptide of VIP purified from the venom of the Helodermae lizard Gila monster (see above), binds specifically to one subclass of VIP binding sites and the competition curve with unlabeled VIP indicates a K_D of 0.3 nM.[35,36] Thus, [^{125}I]helodermin recognizes specifically high-affinity VIP receptors in these membranes. By contrast, unlabeled helodermin occupies all (including low affinity) VIP receptors, indicating that the properties of helodermin are modified by iodine atom(s), in line with previous data on iodinated glucagon[38] and iodinated VIP.[39,40] Besides, we have already seen that helodermin binds to both VIP-preferring and secretin-preferring receptors in the rat pancreas being aspecific in that respect on the latter organ.

([^{125}I]His^1, D-Ala^2, NLeu^{27})GRF$_{1–29}$-NH$_2$ binding on rat liver membranes is qualitatively similar to that of [^{125}I]helodermin; this tracer binds also to the single high-affinity class of VIP receptors (K_D for VIP of 0.1 nM).[41]

Dithiothreitol reduces the number of high-affinity VIP receptors as it decreases [^{125}I]helodermin binding without altering the K_D of VIP. Besides, guanyl nucleotides accelerate the dissociation rate of both [^{125}I]helodermin, ([^{125}I]His^1, D-Ala^2, NLeu^{27})GRF$_{1–29}$-NH$_2$, and [^{125}I]VIP bound to their receptors, but IC$_{50}$ values for guanyl nucleotides indicate that the high-affinity VIP receptors specifically labeled by the first two radioligands are more efficiently coupled to the guanyl nucleotide regulatory binding protein N_s than those occupied collectively by [^{125}I]VIP.[36]

Concerning stimulus-effector coupling, despite the presence of a high number of VIP receptors in fresh rat hepatic membranes, the VIP-stimulated adenylate cyclase activity remains low as compared to the glucagon response. The potency of VIP is, however, remarkably high, making rat hepatic adenylate cyclase one of the most sensitive models for VIP. Recent data from Couvineau *et al.*[42] on solubilized liver VIP receptors suggest that several VIP receptors interact with N_s. Our data on fresh membranes reflect the presence of a sizeable proportion of well-coupled VIP receptors and not a general lack of N_s and/or catalytic units.

In line with this topic, VIP and several VIP analogues display almost the same intrinsic activity in fresh rat liver membranes, the VIP analogues distinguishing themselves by their reduced potency.[12] Since the major difference observed in the rat pancreas between VIP and these VIP analogues pertains to their intrinsic activity (see above), we may conclude that high-affinity VIP receptors are highly coupled to adenylate cyclase in liver while VIP receptors are poorly coupled in the pancreas. In liver membranes the occupancy of a small percentage of VIP receptors suffices to induce maximal (but limited) adenylate cyclase activation. By contrast, in the pancreas, a maximal response is obtained only by full occupancy of all VIP receptors by VIP, so that a VIP analogue—inducing feeble coupling with adenylate cyclase—will never activate the enzyme maximally. In other terms, the same VIP analogue with reduced potency may act as full agonist in a tightly coupled system (the liver) and as a partial VIP agonist in a poorly coupled system (the pancreas).

This unique profile of coupling of VIP receptors to adenylate cyclase in freshly prepared rat liver membranes depends, at least partly, on the physical state of membranes (Robberecht *et al.*, unpublished data). Indeed, after freezing and thawing, the capacity of VIP to stimulate adenylate cyclase greatly increases and dose-effect curves are then compatible with the coexistence of two (sub)classes of receptors coupled to the enzyme: a high-affinity-low-capacity one, identical to that found in fresh membranes, and a new low-affinity-higher capacity component revealed only after freezing and thawing. The total binding capacity of [^{125}I]VIP bound, and the K_D and relative proportions of the two [^{125}I]VIP binding sites are not affected by freezing so that there is now an excellent correlation between the two K_{act} of VIP stimulation of adenylate cyclase and the K_D values of the two VIP binding sites in the thawed membranes. The data obtained with [^{125}I]helodermin (that labels specifically the high-affinity VIP binding sites) confirm the stability of the two classes of VIP receptors after freezing and thawing. This observation, made on rat liver membranes only, and for VIP receptors only, suggests that freezing facilitates mobility, making possible a better association between VIP receptors, N_s, and the catalytical unit. Of course, the absence of coupling between the low-affinity VIP receptors and adenylate cyclase observed before freezing leaves these receptors without a known effector system in the "fresh" state.

Structure-Activity Relationship of VIP and VIP Analogues on Rat Liver Membranes

Six VIP analogues inhibit [^{125}I]VIP and [^{125}I]helodermin binding to high-affinity VIP receptors in rat hepatic membranes. They also stimulate adenylate cyclase activity through these receptors, their decreasing order of potency being: VIP > (D-Ala^4)VIP

=(D-Asp³)VIP > (D-Ser²)VIP > (D-His¹)VIP > (D-Phe²)VIP > (D-Arg²)VIP.
Thus (D-Phe²)VIP shows a slightly better affinity than (D-Arg²)VIP for high- and
low-affinity hepatic VIP receptors[12] but has a lower intrinsic activity. When used as
an inhibitor, its inhibition is selective for the VIP-stimulated enzyme (K_i 0.1 μM)
and secretin stimulation is unaffected. Atypically, COOH-terminal helodermin fragments lacking several first amino acid residues are still capable of activating the
enzyme.[37]

As well as in rat pancreatic membranes, GRF activates hepatic adenylate cyclase
through interaction with VIP receptors in rat liver membranes.[19] For GRF analogues,
the nature of the first amino acid is of reduced importance: analogues with Tyr¹,
Phe¹, and His¹ are equipotent. However, iodination of Tyr¹ gives a very poor GRF
analogue (making it unsuitable for receptor identification in binding studies) and the
acetylation of the free NH_2 group drastically decreases the peptide efficacy.

Concerning position two (D-Ala²)GRF$_{1-29}$-NH₂ is a superagonist while (D-Arg²)-
or (D-Phe²)-derivatives are very poor activators or inhibitors. Replacement of the
acidic aspartate residue in position three by the D-isomer of serine suppresses adenylate
cyclase activation through VIP receptors. By contrast, substitution of alanine in
position four by phenylalanine increases both the efficacy and potency of the GRF
derivative on VIP receptors. Finally, substitution of phenylalanine 6 and threonine 7
by their D-isomer leads to analogues that are inactive on VIP receptors.

DISTINCT STRUCTURAL REQUIREMENTS IN VIP AND GRF FOR VIP RECEPTOR OCCUPANCY IN PANCREATIC AND LIVER MEMBRANES [12-19]

The nature of the amino acid and the chemical function present in position one
in VIP is critical for VIP receptor occupancy on pancreatic membranes, not on liver
membranes.[22] Pancreatic VIP receptors do not distinguish (D-His¹)VIP from (D-
Ser²)VIP and (D-Asp³)VIP, but they clearly discriminate (D-Asp³)VIP from D-
Ala⁴)VIP; in general, they display a lower affinity than liver VIP receptors. Liver
VIP receptors discriminate (D-His¹)VIP from (D-Ser²)VIP, and (D-Ser²)VIP from
(D-Asp³)VIP and (D-Ala⁴)VIP, but they do not discriminate (D-Asp³)VIP from (D-
Ala⁴)VIP. Their occupancy by COOH-terminal fragments of helodermin is already
sufficient for stimulation of adenylate cyclase.[37]

The data obtained with GRF analogues substituted in positions one and three also
suggest different requirements for optimal activation of hepatic versus pancreatic VIP
receptors: (a) Acetylation of the NH_2 function of the NH_2-terminal amino acid
(tyrosine as in human GRF or histidine in rat GRF) reduces less drastically the I.A.
of the peptide derivatives on rat liver membranes: (b) a change in the stereospecificity
of aspartate-3 by using the D-isomer is much less unfavorable for the activation of
hepatic as compared to pancreatic adenylate cyclase. In conclusion, the well-coupled
VIP receptors of fresh rat liver membranes stimulate (modestly) adenylate cyclase at
low ligand concentration, and their specificity requirements are lower than those of
pancreatic VIP receptors.

MOLECULAR CHARACTERIZATION OF VIP RECEPTORS

At present, there is no evidence that the functionally distinct classes of VIP-secretin receptors in the exocrine pancreas and in subclasses of VIP receptors in liver differ in their primary structure. They might as well be structurally related but functionally different, depending on their localization, conformation and/or receptor-effector coupling.

As a first partial approach, the molecular architecture of VIP receptors in the pancreas can be probed by the covalent cross-linking of [^{125}I]VIP, followed by SDS-PAGE and autoradiography, thereby giving the molecular mass of covalent radiolabeled ligand-receptor complex(es). This chemical VIP cross-linking to receptors was described for the first time by Laburthe *et al.*[42] in rat intestinal epithelial membranes, using 3,3'-dithiobis(succinimidylpropionate) (DSP) as cross-linker. Since then, the cross-linking of VIP to receptors has been documented in several other preparations including rat liver membranes.[43,44] (See also other reports in this volume.)

In our experiments on dispersed rat pancreatic acini (M. Svoboda *et al.*, unpublished data), BSOCOES (bis(2-(succinimidooxycarbonyloxy)ethyl)sulfone) tends to preferentially cross-link [^{125}I]VIP to a 66-kDa band while DSP provokes a comparable labeling of 66- and 80-kDa bands. This may be the reason why DSP is a better cross-linker than BSOCOES (FIG. 2, lanes 7 and 11) in intact rat acini where the 80-kDa peptide is the only labeled band. In FIGURE 3, inhibitions of [^{125}I]VIP cross-linking by increasing concentrations of VIP are compared at 0°C in intact acini from rat (FIG. 3A) and guinea pig (FIG. 3B). In rat acini a high-M_r smearing material (in the 130-150 kDa range) coexists with a major 80-kDa radioactive band and variable proportions of a 66-kDa band, while in guinea pig acini there exists a main 160-kDa band. These differences, at the molecular level, between VIP receptors in intact acini of rat and guinea pig, are reminiscent of functional differences.[2,45,46]

The densitometric scannings of the autoradiographs indicate that the specific labeling of all bands is inhibited by VIP, and IC$_{50}$ values being comparable to those of VIP on [^{125}I]VIP binding in simple competitive binding assays conducted in parallel on the same preparations. This suggests that the chemically cross-linked bands correspond to VIP receptors. The specificity of labeling is obvious in the presence of VIP, secretin, (D-Phe^4)PHI (a specific VIP agonist), helodermin, and GRF, all offered at a 1 μM concentration: All peptides reduce the labeling, but GRF is less efficient.

Even under nonreducing conditions, the 80-kDa band is accompanied by 66- and 35-kDa bands of variable intensity in purified rat pancreatic plasma membranes. The migration rate of the 66-kDa band is curtailed by 4% after reduction, taking into account the fact that the migration rate of the bovine serum albumin standard decreases even more (by 16%) after reduction. This decrease in the apparent molecular mass of the 66-kDa band to 63 kDa suggests that intrachain disulfide bonds maintain some folded conformation in native pancreatic VIP receptors but not to the same extent as the abundant disulfide bonds do for albumin.

Taken together, our observations suggest a molecular mass of 80-kDa for the main VIP binding site in intact rat acini. This native 80-kDa receptor species is conceivably converted into the 66-kDa band during membrane preparation and/or membrane incubation, even under nonreducing conditions, by analogy with the easy conversion of the native VIP cross-linked 80-kDa band into a 56-kDa band in rat liver membranes.[44] The 85-kDa species in intact rat acini resembles a 77-86-kDa species in rat liver membranes.[42-44] By contrast, the 66-kDa peptide is heavier than the 51-56-kDa VIP binding site of rat liver membranes.[43]

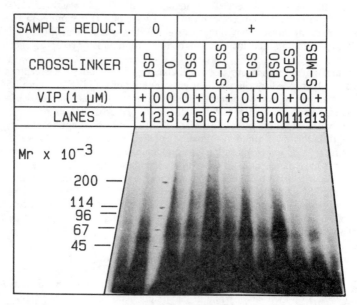

FIGURE 2. Covalent labeling of crude rat pancreatic membranes by [^{125}I]VIP induced with six cross-linkers. Dispersed pancreatic acini were washed in phosphate buffered saline (10 mM phosphate buffer (pH 7.4), 145 mM NaCl, 5 mM KCl), then disrupted by sonication (3 × 5 sec, 120 W) in buffer A made of 20 mM Tris-Cl (pH 7.5) enriched with 0.25 M sucrose and a protease inhibitor mix (1 mM EDTA, 1 mg/ml bacitracin, 0.1 mg/ml soybean trypsin inhibitor, and 1 mM phenylmethylsulfonyl fluoride). The lysate was centrifuged for five minutes at 500 g and the supernatant centrifuged for 30 minutes at 50,000 g. The pellet was homogenized in buffer A to a 5 mg protein/ml concentration.

These membranes (0.7 mg protein) were incubated for 15 minutes at 37°C with 0.1 nM [^{125}I]VIP (0.5-1 μCi/ml) in 50 mM Tris-maleate buffer (pH 7.5), 2 mM MgCl$_2$, 0.5% bovine serum albumin, 500 units/ml Trasylol (Bayer), and 0.2 mg/ml bacitracin, and in the absence or presence of 1 μM VIP. Membrane pellets obtained after centrifugation for 10 minutes at 50,000 g were washed twice by homogenization-centrifugation in phosphate-buffered saline then rehomogenized in 1.2 ml of 50 mM phosphate buffer (pH 7.5) and distributed in six aliquots. Cross-linking was induced by adding 2 μl of 0.1 M double agent in dimethylsulfoxide. After 10 minutes at 0°C, 5 μl of 1.0 M ethanolamine was added. Membranes were precipitated by acetone then solubilized by sonication in an electrophoresis sample buffer made of 0.125 M Tris-Cl (pH 6.8) containing 5% (wt/vol) SDS, 10% (wt/vol) sucrose and 0.02% (wt/vol) bromophenol blue, and enriched—when reducing conditions were sought (lanes 4 to 13)—with 1% (wt/vol) dithiothreitol and 4% (wt/vol) 2-mercaptoethanol. SDS-PAGE analysis was performed on 5-20% gradient polyacrylamide gels (80 × 80 × 1.5 mm). Autoradiography was conducted for one week at −70°C. Abbreviations: BSOCOES, bis(2-(succinimidooxycarbonyloxy)ethyl)sulfone; DSP, dithiobis(succini-midylpropionate); DSS, disuccinimidyl suberate; EGS, ethylene glycolbis-(succinimidylsuccinate); S-DDS, bis(sulfosuccinimidyl)suberate; S-MBS, m-maleimidobenzoylsulfosuccinimide ester.

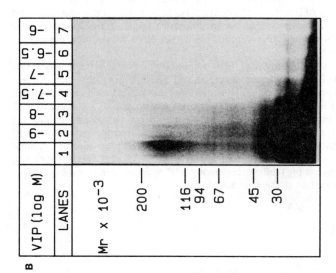

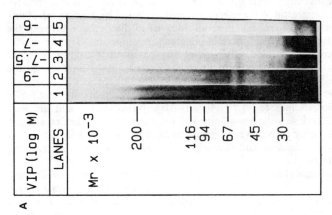

FIGURE 3. Covalent labeling of rat (panel **A**) and guinea pig (panel **B**) pancreatic acini by [^{125}I]VIP cross-linking with DSP. Inhibition by VIP. Acini were incubated for 45 minutes at 37°C in the presence of 0.1 nM [^{125}I]VIP (0.25 µCi/ml) and various concentrations of unlabeled VIP. They were washed three times by centrifugation-resuspension in phosphate-buffered saline and resuspended in Hepes-buffered Hank's balanced salt medium at a 50 mg wet weight/ml concentration. The cross-linker DSP was added to a final 1 mM concentration for 10 minutes at 0°C. After quenching excess cross-linker with 10 mM ethanolamine and centrifugation, the pelleted acini were disrupted by sonication in a lysis buffer made of 10 mM Tris-Cl (pH 7.4), 5 mM MgCl$_2$ and 20 µg/ml DNAse I (Grade I, Boehringer, Mannheim, F.R.G.). After 15 minutes at 0°C, solubilized acini were analyzed by SDS-PAGE performed under nonreducing conditions on 5–20% gradient polyacrylamide gels (180 × 200 × 3 mm). Autoradiography was conducted for four weeks at −70°C.

The broad, higher mass band could represent the cross-linking of the [^{125}I]VIP-labeled receptor to other nearby membrane component(s) such as N_s, that resists the conditions of SDS-PAGE. Couvineau et al.[46] have indeed demonstrated that solubilized liver VIP receptors remain partly associated to N_s and can be cross-linked to N_s, forming a labeled 150-kDa peptide. Our cross-linking experiments in FIGURES 2 and 3 were performed at 0°C so that any noncovalent association of VIP receptors with N_s and/or other components must obviously preexist in pancreatic membranes and intact acinar cells before cross-linking. As an alternative proposal, the 160-kDa smear could correspond to native VIP receptors highly sensitive to cleavage during the manipulations.

Species differences concerning pancreatic acini are well documented in physiological terms: while VIP is a poor secretagogue and secretin a much more efficient secretagogue on rat pancreatic acini, VIP is more potent than secretin and as efficient a secretagogue on guinea pig acini (for review, see Christophe & Robberecht[2] and Gardner[47]). The present covalent cross-linking experiments on rat and guinea pig pancreatic preparations offer some evidence for a chemical heterogeneity among VIP receptors that suggests that species dissimilarities in VIP receptor-effector coupling may be concerned with the receptor itself. Thus, tissue (pancreas versus liver) and species (rat versus guinea pig) differences among VIP receptors are becoming evident at the molecular as well as at the pharmacological level.

SUMMARY

In purified rat pancreatic plasma membranes, (D-Phe⁴)PHI interacts as a selective VIP agonist for rat pancreatic VIP-preferring receptors, based on binding selectivity and adenylate cyclase activation, therefore allowing us to discriminate between the participation of VIP-preferring and secretin-preferring receptors in VIP stimulation. VIP-preferring receptors also bind GRF. They rely on disulfide bridges for their functional integrity. Their coupling with adenylate cyclase, based on the intrinsic activity of VIP analogues, is poor when compared to that of hepatic VIP receptors.

In fresh rat liver plasma membranes, high-affinity VIP receptors are specifically labeled with [^{125}I]helodermin and [^{125}I]His¹, D-Ala², NLeu²⁷)GRF and are well coupled to adenylate cyclase while low-affinity VIP receptors are not. The first subtype of VIP receptors is highly responsive to guanyl nucleotides and is easily altered by dithiothreitol. Only after freezing and thawing are low-affinity hepatic VIP receptors coupled to adenylate cyclase.

Concerning the chemical characterization of VIP receptors, 66- and 35-kDa peptides are detected after specific [^{125}I]VIP cross-linking with double agents in rat pancreatic membranes. In contrast, in intact pancreatic acini, the main source of radioactivity has a molecular mass of 130–180 kDa (with no contribution of intramolecular disulfide bridges), and an 80-kDa peptide is also detectable. The 66-kDa species in membranes can conceivably derive from the 80-kDa species observed in intact cells. Its molecular mass is higher than that of the 56-kDa [^{125}I]VIP cross-linked protein previously observed in rat liver membranes. Besides, species differences between rat and guinea pig pancreas are also evident.

ACKNOWLEDGMENTS

We are deeply indebted to Dr. D. H. Coy (Peptide Research Laboratories, Department of Medicine, Tulane University, School of Medicine, New Orleans, LA) for his generous gift of VIP and GRF analogues that allows our collaborative efforts with his laboratory.

REFERENCES

1. SVOBODA, M., J. FURNELLE & J. CHRISTOPHE. 1981. The differential detergent solubilization of adenylate cyclase and polypeptide ADP-ribosylated with cholera toxin suggests an excess of G/F protein relative to adenylate cyclase in rat pancreatic plasma membranes. FEBS Lett. **135:** 207-211.
2. CHRISTOPHE, J. & P. ROBBERECHT. 1982. Effect of VIP on the exocrine pancreas. *In* Vasoactive Intestinal Peptide. S. I. Said, Ed.: 235-252. (In the series, Advances in Peptide Hormone Research.) Raven Press. New York.
3. CHRISTOPHE, J., M. SVOBODA, M. LAMBERT, M. WAELBROECK, J. WINAND, J.-P. DEHAYE, M. C. VANDERMEERS-PIRET, A. VANDERMEERS & P. ROBBERECHT. 1986. Effector mechanisms of peptides of the VIP family. Peptides 7(Suppl. 1): 101-107.
4. ROBBERECHT, P., P. CHATELAIN, M. WAELBROECK & J. CHRISTOPHE. 1982. Heterogeneity of VIP-recognizing binding sites in rat tissues. *In* Vasoactive Intestinal Peptide. S. I. Said, Ed.: 323-332. (In the series, Advances in Peptide Hormone Research.) Raven Press. New York.
5. ROBBERECHT, P., M. WAELBROECK, M. NOYER, P. CHATELAIN, P. DE NEEF, W. KÖNIG & J. CHRISTOPHE. 1982. Characterization of secretin and vasoactive intestinal peptide receptors in rat pancreatic plasma membranes using the native peptides, secretin-(7-27) and five secretin analogues. Digestion **23:** 201-210.
6. RICHARDSON, A. & A. HUMRICH. 1984. A microcomputer program for the analysis of radioligand binding curves and other dose-response data. Trends Pharmacol. Sci **5:** 47-49.
7. DEHAYE, J. P., J. WINAND, C. DAMIEN, F. GOMEZ, P. POLOCZEK, P. ROBBERECHT, A. VANDERMEERS, M. C. VANDERMEERS-PIRET, M. STIÉVENART, & J. CHRISTOPHE. 1986. Receptors involved in helodermin action on rat pancreatic acini. Am. J. Physiol. **251:** G602-G610.
8. BISSONNETTE, B. M., M. J. COLLEN, H. ADACHI, R. T. JENSEN & J. D. GARDNER. 1984. Receptors of vasoactive intestinal peptide and secretin on rat pancreatic acini. Am. J. Physiol. **246:** G710-G717.
9. CHRISTOPHE, J., M. C. VANDERMEERS-PIRET, J. RATHÉ, J. P. DEHAYE, N. D. BUI-NGUYEN, J. WINAND & A. VANDERMEERS. 1984. A comparison of the phosphorylation of M_r = 33K, 21K, and 25K membrane-bound proteins in the rat pancreas, submitted to various secretagogues. *In* Proceedings of the IUPHAR 9th International Congress of Pharmacology. W. Paton, J. Mitchell & P. Turner, Eds. Vol. **2:** 147-156. Macmillan Press Ltd. London, England.
10. VANDERMEERS, A., M. C. VANDERMEERS-PIRET, J. RATHÉ, J. P. DEHAYE, J. WINAND & J. CHRISTOPHE. 1984. Phosphorylation of three particulate proteins in rat pancreatic acini in response to vasoactive intestinal peptide (VIP), secretin and cholecystokinin (CCK-8). Peptides **5:** 359-365.
11. ROBBERECHT, P., D. COY, P. DE NEEF, J.-C. CAMUS, A. CAUVIN, M. WAELBROECK & J. CHRISTOPHE. 1987. (D-Phe⁴)-Peptide histidine isoleucinamide ((D-Phe⁴)-PHI), a highly selective vasoactive intestinal peptide (VIP) agonist, discriminates VIP-preferring

from secretin-preferring receptors in rat pancreatic membranes. Eur. J. Biochem. **165:** 243-249.

12. ROBBERECHT, P., D. H. COY, P. DE NEEF, J. C. CAMUS, A. CAUVIN, M. WAELBROECK & J. CHRISTOPHE. 1986. Interaction of vasoactive intestinal peptide (VIP) and N-terminally modified VIP analogs with rat pancreatic hepatic and pituitary membranes. Eur. J. Biochem. **159:** 45-49.

13. VANDERMEERS, A., M. C. VANDERMEERS-PIRET, P. ROBBERECHT, M. WAELBROECK, J. P. DEHAYE, J. WINAND & J. CHRISTOPHE. 1984. Purification of a novel pancreatic secretary factor (PSF) and a novel peptide with VIP- and secretin-like properties (helodermin) from Gila monster venom. FEBS Lett. **166:** 273-276.

14. HOSHINO, M., C. YANAIHARA, J. M. HONG, S. KISHIDA, Y. KATSUMARU, A. VANDER-MEERS, M. C. VANDERMEERS-PIRET, P. ROBBERECHT, J. CHRISTOPHE & N. YANAI-HARA. 1984. Primary structure of helodermin, a VIP-secretin-like peptide isolated from Gila monster venom. FEBS Lett. **178:** 233-239.

15. ROBBERECHT, P., M. WAELBROECK, J. P. DEHAYE, J. WINAND, A. VANDERMEERS, M. C. VANDERMEERS-PIRET & J. CHRISTOPHE. 1984. Evidence that helodermin, a newly extracted peptide from Gila monster venom, is a member of the secretin/VIP/PHI family of peptides with an original pattern of biological properties. FEB Lett. **166:** 277-282.

16. VANDERMEERS, A., P. GOURLET, M.-C. VANDERMEERS-PIRET, A. CAUVIN, P. DE NEEF, J. RATHE, P. ROBBERECHT & J. CHRISTOPHE. 1987. Chemical, immunological and biological properties of vasoactive intestinal peptide-peptide histidine isoleucinamide (VIP-PHI)-like peptides extracted from the venom of two lizards (*Heloderma horridum* and *Heloderma suspectum*). Eur. J. Biochem. **164:** 321-327.

17. PARKER, D. S., J. P. RAUFMAN, L. O'DONOHUE, M. BLEDSOE, M. YOSHIDA & J. J. PISANO. 1984. Amino acid sequences of helospectins, new members of the glucagon superfamily, found in Gila monster venom. J. Biol. Chem. **259:** 11751-11755.

18. WAELBROECK, M., P. ROBBERECHT, D. H. COY, J. C. CAMUS, P. DE NEEF & J. CHRIS-TOPHE. 1985. Interaction of growth hormone-releasing factor (GRF) and 14 GRF analogs with rat pancreatic VIP receptors. Discovery of (N-AC-TYR[1], D-PHE[2])-GRF(1-29)-NH$_2$ as a vasoactive intestinal peptide (VIP) antagonist. Endocrinology **116:** 2643-2649.

19. ROBBERECHT, P., M. WAELBROECK, D. H. COY, P. DE NEEF, J.-C. CAMUS & J. CHRIS-TOPHE. 1986. Comparative structural requirements of thirty GRF analogs for occupancy of GRF- and VIP receptors and coupling to adenylate cyclase in rat adenopituitary, liver and pancreas. Peptides 7(Suppl. 1): 53-59.

20. PANDOL, S. J., H. SEIFERT, M. W. THOMAS, J. RIVIER & W. VALE. 1984. Growth hormone-releasing factor stimulates pancreatic enzyme secretion. Science **225:** 326-328.

21. COY, D. H., W. A. MURPHY, J. SUEIRAS-DIAZ, E. J. COY & V. A. LANCE. 1985. Structure-activity studies on the N-terminal region of growth hormone releasing factor. J. Med. Chem. **28:** 181-185.

22. ROBBERECHT, P., M. WAELBROECK, J. C. CAMUS, P. DE NEEF, D. COY & J. CHRISTOPHE. 1984. Effects of His[1] modifications on the ability of vasoactive intestinal peptide to stimulate adenylate cyclase from rat and human tissues. Peptides **5:** 877-881.

23. HEFFORD, M. A., R. M. EVANS, G. ODA & H. KAPLAN. 1985. Unusual chemical properties of N-terminal histidine residues of glucagon and vasoactive intestinal peptide. Biochemistry **24:** 867-874.

24. PANDOL, S. J., K. DHARMSATHAPHORN, M. S. SCHOEFFIELD, W. VALE J. RIVIER. 1986. Vasoactive intestinal peptide receptor antagonist (4Cl-D-Phe[6]), Leu[17]VIP, Am. J. Physiol. **250:** G553-G557.

25. ROBBERECHT, P., M. WAELBROECK, J. CAMUS, P. DE NEEF, & J. CHRISTOPHE. 1984. Importance of disulfide bonds in receptors for vasoactive intestinal peptide (VIP) and secretin in rat pancreatic plasma membranes. Biochem. Biophys. Acta **773:** 271-278.

26. BATAILLE, D., P. FREYCHET & G. ROSSELIN. 1974. Interactions of glucagon, gut glucagon, vasoactive intestinal peptide, and secretion with liver and fat cell plasma membranes: Binding to specific sites and stimulation of adenylate cyclase. Endocrinology **95:** 713-721.

27. DESBUQUOIS, B. 1974. The interaction of vasoactive intestinal polypeptide and secretin with liver-cell membranes. Eur. J. Biochem. **46:** 439-450.

28. AMIRANOFF, B., M. LABURTHE & G. ROSSELIN. 1980. Differential effects of guanine nucleotides on the first step of VIP and glucagon action in membranes from liver cells. Biochem. Biophys. Res. Commun. 96: 463-468.

29. WAELBROECK, M., P. ROBBERECHT, P. DE NEEF, P. CHATELAIN & J. CHRISTOPHE. 1985. Binding of vasoactive intestinal peptide and its stimulation of adenylate cyclase through two classes of receptors in rat liver membranes. Effects of 12 secretin analogues and 2 secretin fragments. Biochem. Biophys. Acta 678: 83-90.

30. SOUQUET, J. C., J. P. RIOU, M. BEYLOT, J. A. CHAYVIALLE & R. MORNEX. 1982. Effects of VIP on glucose and lactate metabolism in isolated rat liver cells. FEBS Lett. 145: 115-120.

31. FELIU, J. E., M. MOJENA, R. A. SILVESTRE, L. MONGE & J. MARCO. 1983. Stimulatory effect of VIP on glycogenolysis and gluconeogenesis in isolated rat hepatocytes: Antagonism by insulin. Endocrinology 112: 2120-2125.

32. GARDNER, D. F., M. S. KILBERG, M. M. WOLFE, J. E. McGUIGAN & R. I. MISBIN. 1985. Preferential binding of vasoactive intestinal peptide to hepatic nonparenchymal cells. Am. J. Physiol. 248: G663-G669.

33. LEISER, J. & J. J. BLUM. 1984. Effects of VIP and forskolin on alanine metabolism in isolated hepatocytes. FEBS Lett. 173: 407-413.

34. GAMMELTOFT, S., P. STANN-OLSEN, B. OTTESEN & J. FAHRENKRUG. 1984. VIP receptors in pig liver cells: Binding characteristics and role in degradation. Peptides 5: 367-370.

35. ROBBERECHT, P., M. WAELBROECK, P. DE NEEF, J. C. CAMUS, A. VANDERMEERS, M.-C. VANDERMEERS-PIRET & J. CHRISTOPHE. 1984. Specific labelling by [^{125}I]helodermin of high-affinity VIP receptors in rat liver membranes. FEBS Lett. 172: 55-58.

36. ROBBERECHT, P., A. VANDERMEERS, M.-C. VANDERMEERS-PIRET, P. DE NEEF, J. C. CAMUS, M. WAELBROECK, D. H. COY & J. CHRISTOPHE. 1985. Specific labelling of high-affinity VIP receptors in rat liver and lung membranes by [^{125}I]helodermin. *In* Regulatory Peptides in Digestive, Nervous and Endocrine Systems. M. J. M. Lewin & S. Bonfils, Eds. INSERM Symposium n° 25: 149-152. Elsevier Science Publishers. Amsterdam, the Netherlands.

37. ROBBERECHT, P., N. YANAIHARA, C. YANAIHARA, P. DE NEEF, J.-C. CAMUS, A. VANDERMEERS, M.-C. VANDERMEERS-PIRET & J. CHRISTOPHE. 1986. Interaction of synthetic N- and C-terminal fragments of helodermin with rat liver VIP receptors. Peptides 7(Suppl. 1): 79-82.

38. DESBUQUOIS, B. 1975. Iodoglucagon. Preparation and characterization. Eur. J. Biochem. 53: 569-580.

39. MARIE, J-C., D. H. B. HOA, R. JACKSON, G. HEJBLUM & G. ROSSELIN. 1985. The biological relevance of HPLC-purified vasoactive intestinal polypeptide monoiodinated at tyrosine 10 or tyrosine 22. Reg. Peptides 12: 113-123.

40. MARTIN, J-L., K. ROSE, G. J. HUGHES & P. J. MAGISTRETTI. 1986. [mono[^{125}I]iodo-Tyr^{10},MetO^{17}-]-Vasoactive intestinal polypeptide. Preparation, characterization, and use for radioimmunoassay and receptor binding. J. Biol. Chem. 261: 5320-5327.

41. ROBBERECHT, P., D. H. COY, P. DE NEEF, J.-C. CAMUS, M. WAELBROECK & J. CHRISTOPHE. 1986. Specific labelling of high-affinity vasoactive intestinal peptide receptors in rat liver membranes by a growth hormone-releasing factor analog. Neuroendocrinology 44: 108-111.

42. LABURTHE, M., B. BREANT & C. ROUYER-FESSARD. 1984. Molecular identification of receptors for vasoactive intestinal peptide in rat intestinal epithelium by covalent cross-linking. Evidence for two classes of binding sites with different structural and functional properties. Eur. J. Biochem. 139: 181-187.

43. COUVINEAU, A. & M. LABURTHE. 1985. The rat liver vasoactive intestinal peptide binding site. Molecular characterization by covalent cross linking and evidence for difference from the intestinal receptor. Biochem. J. 225: 473-479.

44. NGUYEN, T. D., J. A. WILLIAMS & G. M. GRAY. 1986. Vasoactive intestinal peptide receptor on liver plasma membranes: Characterization as a glycoprotein. Biochemistry 25: 361-368.

45. CHRISTOPHE, J., J. P. CONLON & J. GARDNER. 1976. Interaction of porcine vasoactive-intestinal peptide with dispersed pancreatic acinar cells from the guinea pig: Binding of radioiodinated peptide. J. Biol. Chem. 251: 4629-4634.

46. COUVINEAU, A., B. AMIRANOFF & M. LABURTHE. 1986. Solubilization of the liver vasoactive intestinal peptide receptor. Hydrodynamic characterization and evidence for an association with a functional GTP regulatory protein. J. Biol. Chem. **261:** 14482-14489.
47. GARDNER, J. D. 1979. Regulation of pancreatic exocrine function *in vitro:* Initial steps in the actions of secretagogues. Ann. Rev. Physiol. **41:** 55-66.

Characterization of Vasoactive Intestinal Peptide Receptors in Nervous and Immune Systems[a]

M. S. O'DORISIO,[b,c] T. M. O'DORISIO,[d] C. L. WOOD,[d]
J. C. BRESNAHAN,[e] M. S. BEATTIE,[e] AND
L. B. CAMPOLITO[c]

[c]Department of Pediatrics
[d]Department of Medicine and
[e]Department of Anatomy
Ohio State University
Columbus, Ohio 43205

Initial observations of VIP immunoreactivity in mast cells and neutrophils[1,2] led to the hypothesis that lymphocytes might possess receptors for VIP and suggested that this neuropeptide-leukocyte interaction might serve as a model for delineation of a more extensive neuroimmune axis.[3] Neuropeptide modulation of the immune response, first postulated nearly 30 years ago on the basis of phenomenological studies,[4] has now been confirmed by demonstrations of receptors for enkephalins, somatostatin, substance P, and VIP on immune effector cells.[5–8] An afferent arm of this putative neuroimmune axis is also being delineated with the demonstration of receptors for thymosin, interleukins, and antigen recognition in central nervous system.[9–11]

Vasoactive intestinal peptide may play a central role in communication between the nervous and immune systems. Neutrophils, eosinophils, and mast cells synthesize or concentrate a VIP-immunoreactive peptide, while lymphocytes possess specific high-affinity receptors for VIP that are linked to the adenylate cyclase-cAMP dependent protein kinase network.[1,2,8,12–14] Functional studies suggest that VIP may modulate natural killer cell activity,[15] lymphocyte proliferation,[16] or lymphocyte trafficking in gut-associated lymphoid tissue.[17,18]

Whether the mechanism by which VIP modulates the immune response is similar to the mechanism involved in neurotransmission remains to be elucidated. Accordingly, these experiments were designed to compare the kinetics, molecular structure, and second messenger system of VIP receptors in nervous and immune tissues.

[a]This research was supported by grants from the National Cancer Institute (RO1CA 41997), Ohio Cancer Research Associates, and the Childrens' Hospital Research Foundation.

[b]Address for correspondence: Dr. M. S. O'Dorisio, Department of Pediatrics, Children's Hospital, 700 Children's Drive, Columbus, OH 43205.

257

METHODS

Cell Culture

Molt 4b lymphoblasts were originally obtained from Roswell Park.[19] They were grown in RPMI 1640 with 15% calf serum 1% L-glutamine, 10 U/ml penicillin and 10 mg/ml streptomycin. All culture supplies were purchased from GIBCO. The cells were placed in tissue culture flasks (Corning), incubated at 37°C, and cultures divided every three days. They were used three days after the final split. Before usage, the cells were washed twice with RPMI 1640 with L-glutamine, 25 mM Hepes buffer (GIBCO), and 2% human serum albumin (Travenol). The cells were enumerated by Coulter count. Viability was 95% as tested by trypan blue exclusion.

Frontal Cortex Dissection

The frontal cortex (anterior to bregma) was dissected from brains obtained from female Lewis rats weighing 250-325 g, lightly anesthetized with ketamine and xylazine. After decapitation, brains were quickly removed (within 1 min) and placed onto crushed dry ice. After freezing, the brains were separated into left and right halves with a saggital cut, and the anterior cortex was removed from the underlying white matter. Tissue was then stored at −70°C until membrane preparations were made.

Preparation of Plasma Membrane

Membranes were prepared by a modification of the technique of Kaslow and coworkers.[20] Cells or tissue were suspended in buffer A (20 mM Hepes, 2 mM MgCl$_2$, 5 mM EDTA, 1 mM 2-mercaptoethanol, 150 mM NaCl, 50 μg/ml phenylmethyl-sufonylflouride, pH 7.4) at a concentration of 50 × 10^6 cells or 10 mg tissue/ml buffer. Tissue was disrupted in a Brinkman polytron followed by centrifugation at 750 g for 5 minutes. The pellet was resuspended in one-half the original volume of buffer A and polytroned for 30 seconds. After a second 750 g spin, the two supernatant fractions were combined and centrifuged 20 minutes at 48,000 g. The resulting particulate fraction was washed in the original volume of buffer A and centrifuged 48,000 g for 20 minutes. The particulate membrane fraction was resuspended in buffer A and stored at −80°C until use.

Membrane Binding

Binding studies were performed using 100-500 μg membrane protein in buffer A. Competition experiments for estimation of receptor affinity (K_D) and number (B$_{max}$)

were performed with radiolabeled VIP ± increasing concentrations of unlabeled VIP or homologous peptide in a total volume of 0.5 ml. Reactions were started by the addition of membrane and the vials then kept in a shaking, controlled-temperature water bath. The reaction was stopped by layering triplicate 0.15-ml aliquots of binding mixture over 1 ml buffer A containing 0.2% bovine serum albumin (BSA) followed by filtration over GF/C filters presoaked in 0.3% polyethyleneimine. Radioactivity bound to filters was determined in a Beckman Gamma 5500. For every data point, triplicates for both total and nonspecific binding were run in parallel. Specific binding was calculated as the difference between the means of determinations of total binding and of binding in the presence of excess unlabeled VIP ($1\mu M$). B_{max} and K_D were determined by SAS nonlinear computer analysis using the equation of Akera and Cheng.[21]

Adenylate Cyclase Assay

This was done as previously described.[12] Briefly, cells were disrupted by sonication in 5 mM Tris/0.25 M sucrose, pH 7.4. The enzyme reaction was initiated by addition of 25-50 µg cell protein to assay media containing 1 mM ATP, 2 mM MgCl$_2$, 10mM phosphocreatine, 3 U creatine kinase, and 100 mM Tris-HCl, pH 7.7 in a total volume of 0.1 ml. Adenylate cyclase activity was measured at 37°C in a 30-minute assay. The reaction was terminated by addition of 0.1 ml of 0.1 M sodium acetate, pH 4.0, followed by heating at 90°C for three minutes; cAMP generated in the reaction was quantified by radioimmunoassay using specific antisera generated in our laboratories.

Cross-Linking

Membranes were incubated with [^{125}I]VIP under the optimal binding conditions for each tissue. Disuccinimidyl suberate (in dimethyl sulfoxide) was added at a final concentration of 5 mM. Control samples received solvent only. Samples were allowed to react at room temperature for 20 minutes; glycine (final concentration 40 mM) was added to consume any unreacted cross-linker, and samples centrifuged to recover the cell pellet. Pellets (300 µg) were solubilized in 0.5 ml lysis buffer (9 M urea, 2% Nonidet P-40, 100 mM dithiothreitol) and mixed vigorously. Then 0.5 ml of treatment buffer (120 mM Tris-HCl, pH 6.8, 20% glycerol, 80 mM dithiothreitol, 4% SDS, and a trace of bromophenol blue) was added followed by mixing. The samples were stored at −80°C.

After thawing, the samples were centrifuged for two minutes at 7,000 × g to remove debris; 75-µl samples were electrophoresed according to Laemmli.[22] The stacking gel was 10% acrylamide, 0.125 M Tris-HCl, pH 6.8, and 0.1% SDS. The separating gel was 10% acrylamide, 0.375 M Tris-HCl, pH 8.8, and 0.1% SDS. The acrylamide to bisacrylamide ratio was 36.5 : 1, and the gel thickness 1.5 mm. The tank buffer was 0.025 M Tris, pH 8.3, 0.0192 M glycine, 0.1% SDS. Electrophoresis was carried out at 20 mA constant current for 30 minutes and then at 60 mA until the tracking dye approached the bottom of the gel. Gels were fixed two hours in 9% acetic acid, 50% methanol, stained one hour in 0.2% Coomassie brilliant blue, 7% acetic acid,

30% methanol, and dried onto Whatman No. 1 filter paper. Autoradiography was conducted at −80°C with Kodak XAR-5 film and a Dupont Lighting Plus intensifying screen, for three to five days. Molecular weights were estimated by comparison of mobilities with those of the standard proteins electrophoresed in different lanes on the same gel.

Antibody Production

Molt 4b lymphoblasts (5×10^7 cells) were solubilized in lysis buffer and cellular proteins separated by SDS polyacrylamide gel electrophoresis. The gel was incubated two hours in 200 ml of renaturing solution (2 mM EDTA, 4 M urea, 0.13 M NaCl, 10 mM Tris, pH 8.0). The 45,000 to 50,000 M_r fraction was cut from the gel and emulsified 1 : 1 with Freund's complete adjuvant; 2 ml of the emulsion was injected subcutaneously into New Zealand white rabbits; animals were boosted every 10 days with 1 ml emulsion. The immunoglobulin fraction of serum was isolated by NH_4SO_4 precipitation.

RESULTS AND DISCUSSION

High-affinity binding sites for VIP have been demonstrated in both lymphocytes and brain,[8,16,17,23,24] but whether these binding sites constitute a single class or a family of homologous receptors has not been studied. In this study the binding kinetics for VIP receptors were compared in lymphoblasts and frontal cortex using competitive binding techniques. A single high-affinity binding site was found in membrane prepared by both lymphoblasts and frontal cortex with binding affinities in the nanomolar range (TABLE 1) in good agreement with earlier studies on intact lymphoblasts[25] and rat brain membranes.[23] The maximum number of binding sites per mg membrane protein appears to be greater in lymphoblasts than in frontal cortex (TABLE 1); this difference may reflect the fact that the lymphoblastic cell line is clonal in origin whereas the frontal cortex is a heterogeneous cell population, only a subpopulation of which possess

TABLE 1. Comparison of VIP Binding Kinetics in Molt 4b Lymphoblasts and Rat Frontal Cortex[a]

| Membrane | Binding Kinetics | |
	K_D (nM)	B_{max} (nmoles/mg)
Molt 4b (13)	8.0 ± 1.2	3.9 ± 0.79
Frontal cortex (10)	7.0 ± 1.5	.68 ± 0.12[b]

[a] Membranes were prepared from each tissue and competitive binding experiments performed as described in methods. Affinity (K_D) and number of binding sites (B_{max}) were calculated by computer-assisted fit nonlinear using the equation of Akera and Cheng.[21] Values are mean ± SEM with number of experiments in parentheses.
[b] $p < 0.01$ compared to Molt 4b.

TABLE 2. Specificity of VIP Binding in Immune and Nervous Tissues[a]

Membrane	K_D (nM)		
	VIP	PHI	GHRF
Molt 4b lymphoblast	11.9 ± 2.5	131 ± 41[b]	97 ± 20[b]
Rat frontal cortex	6.30 ± 0.8	105 ± 21[b]	62 ± 6.3[b]

[a] Membranes were prepared as described in Methods. Competitive binding experiments were performed using 200 μg membrane protein and 100 pM [125I]VIP ± increasing concentrations of competing unlabeled peptide from 1 pM to μM. Affinity constants were calculated using computer assisted one-site modeling. Values are mean ± SEM for three independent experiments.

[b] $p < 0.01$ compared to VIP.

the VIP receptor. This interpretation is supported by observations of several investigators that the apparent number of binding sites for VIP is greater on the Molt 4b lymphoblastic cell line than on peripheral blood T lymphocytes[8,25] and greater on murine T cells than on unseparated mononuclear cells.[17]

In both lymphoblasts and brain, the binding is highly specific with a greater affinity for VIP than for peptide histidine isoleucine (PHI), which shares 13 amino acid sequence homology with VIP[26] or growth hormone releasing factor (GHRF), which has an 11 amino acid homology.[27]

TABLE 2 demonstrates that lymphoblasts and brain have 11- and 17-fold greater affinity, respectively, for VIP than for PHI. Similarly, both lymphoblasts and brain demonstrate an 8-10-fold greater affinity for VIP than for GHRF.

Constitutive adenylate cyclase activity is 37-fold higher in brain than in Molt cells (36.7 versus 0.99 pmol cAMP generated/mg protein/min), but in both tissues, VIP induces a two- to threefold stimulation over the basal activity (TABLE 3). PHI activates adenylate cyclase in membranes prepared from Molt cells, a finding that is in agreement with our earlier observations demonstrating PHI-mediated increases in cAMP in viable lymphoblasts.[14] PHI does not, however, activate adenylate cyclase in brain. GHRF does not activate adenylate cyclase in either lymphoblasts or brain. Maximum stimulation of adenylate cyclase activity in both tissues is seen in the presence of GppNHp, a nonhydrolyzable GTP analogue that catalyzes stimulatory guanine nucleotide binding protein activation of the catalytic unit of adenylate cyclase.[28]

Both the kinetic studies and the enzymatic studies described above suggest great similarities between the VIP receptors in immune and nervous tissues. In order to compare the molecular structure of the receptors, rabbits were immunized with the putative receptor protein isolated from Molt 4b lymphoblasts by polyacrylamide gel electrophoresis. The immunoglobulin fraction of immune serum was then tested for its ability to inhibit binding of [125I]VIP to Molt membranes (FIG. 1). VIP binding was inhibited by 95% at a 1 : 20 dilution of the antiserum. In three experiments, binding to membranes of Molt lymphoblasts was inhibited 95 ± 3% while binding to rat frontal cortex membranes was inhibited 89 ± 6%.

The antiserum was then tested for its ability to inhibit covalent cross-linking of [125I]VIP to membranes from both lymphoblasts and frontal cortex. In agreement with our earlier studies with viable Molt 4b lymphoblasts, the major cross-linked species in membranes prepared from these cells is a 50,000 M_r species (FIG. 2, lanes 1 and 2). The major cross-linked species in frontal cortex is also a 50,000 M_r species (FIG. 2, lanes 6 and 7). In both brain and lymphocytes, the putative receptor protein appears to be a 47,000 M_r species (50,000 = MW of VIP). Cross-linking of [125I]VIP

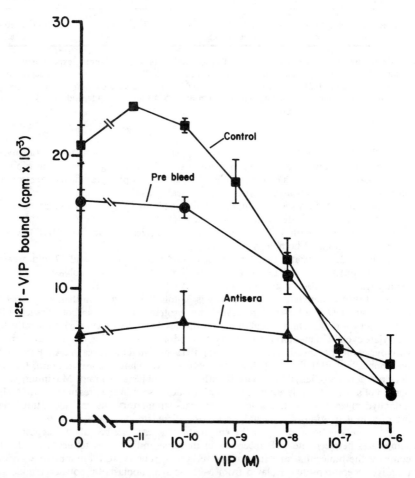

FIGURE 1. Effect of immune rabbit serum on binding of [^{125}I]VIP to membranes of Molt 4b lymphoblast. Membrane was preincubated one hour at 4°C in medium alone, preimmune serum or immune serum (1 : 20 dilution) followed by washing in RPMI-1640 and centrifugation at 48,000 × *g*. Competitive binding experiments were then performed using 200 µg of membrane protein, 100 p*M* [^{125}I]VIP and indicated concentrations of unlabeled VIP. Values are mean ± SD for triplicates from one of three experiments.

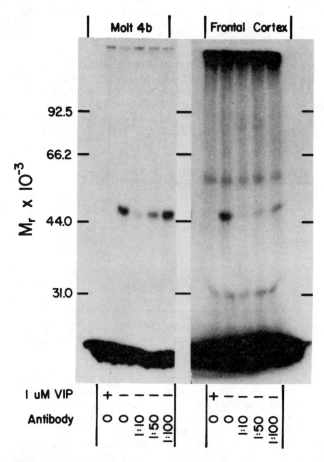

FIGURE 2. Effect of immune rabbit serum on putative VIP receptor identified by covalent cross-linking. Membranes were incubated one hour at 4°C in medium alone or indicated concentration of immune rabbit serum followed by washing of membrane protein and centrifugation at 48,000 × *g*. Cross-linking of [^{125}I]VIP to each membrane was performed as described in Methods.

to both lymphoblasts and brain is blocked in a dose-dependent manner by the putative anti-receptor antisera (FIG. 2, lanes 3-5 and 8-10). These cross-linking experiments, like the kinetic and adenylate cyclase data, suggest homologous, if not identical, VIP receptors in nervous and immune tissue.

Cross-linking experiments in other tissues suggest heterogeneity of VIP receptors including cross-linked species of 150,000,[29] 86,000,[30] and 67,000[31] in addition to the 47,000 M_r component.[32-34] In all of these studies, the 47,000 M_r species appears to comprise the entire ligand binding component of the receptor with the higher molecular weight species representing the receptor protein in association with carbohydrate moities[30,31] or the stimulatory guanine nucleotide binding protein.[29,35]

In summary, lymphoblasts and frontal cortex appear to contain homologous VIP receptors based on kinetic studies of their affinity and specificity for VIP. In both immune and nervous tissues, this receptor appears to be linked to adenylate cyclase via guanine nucleotide binding proteins. The molecular structure of the VIP receptor also appears to be homologous, with both tissues demonstrating a 47,000 M_r protein comprising or being associated with the ligand binding site. Minor differences in the

TABLE 3. VIP Activation of Adenylate Cyclase in Lymphoblasts and Brain[a]

| | Adenylate Cyclase Activity (pmol cAMP/mg protein/min) | |
	Lymphoblast	Brain
Basal	0.99 ± 0.10	36.7 ± 29
VIP	3.12 ± 0.32	76.1 ± 8.8
PHI	3.60 ± 0.34	35.8 ± 3.1
GHRF	1.03 ± 0.15	40.4 ± 6.7
GppNHp	8.69 ± 0.47	298 ± 25

[a] Adenylate cyclase activity was measured using 25 μg membrane protein as described in Methods. Concentration of each neuropeptide was 1 μM; GppNHp was 10 μM. Values are mean ± SD, $n = 3$.

amount or composition of the associated carbohydrate may account for the apparent heterogeneity among different tissues. Such differences may allow development of tissue-specific VIP agonists or antagonists.

Taken together, these studies support the existence of a neuroimmune axis in which VIP released from nerve endings in such tissues as thymus, spleen, or Peyer's patches may modulate the function of immune effector cells via specific, high-affinity receptors. Whether VIP-immunoreactive peptides present in neutrophils, eosinophils, or mast cells can be released to modulate function in immune or nervous tissue remains an exciting area for future investigation.

ACKNOWLEDGMENTS

The authors are grateful to Daniel Fleshman and Todd Brown for excellent technical assistance and to Marjorie Miller for editorial assistance.

REFERENCES

1. CUTZ, E., W. CHAN, N. TRACK, A. GOTH, & S. SAID. 1978. Nature **275:** 661.
2. O'DORISIO, M. S., T. M. O'DORISIO, S. CATALAND, & S. P. BALCERZAK. 1980. J. Lab. Clin. Med. **96:** 666.
3. O'DORISIO, M. S., C. L. WOOD & T. M. O'DORISIO. 1985. J. Immunol. **135:** 792s.
4. FILIPP, G. & A. SZENTIVANYI. 1958. Ann. Allergy **16:** 306.
5. WYBRAN, J., T. APPLEBOOM, J. FAMAEY & A. GOVAERTS. 1979. J. Immunol. **123:** 1068.
6. BHATHENA, S., J. LOUIS, G. SCHECTER, R. REDMAN, L. WAHL & L. RECANT. 1981. Diabetes **30:** 127.
7. PAYAN, D. B., DR. BREWSTER, A. MISSIRIAN-BASTIAN & E. J. GOETZL. 1984. J. Clin. Invest. **74:** 1532.
8. DANEK, A., M. S. O'DORISIO, T. M. O'DORISIO, & J. M. GEORGE. 1983. Immunol. **131:** 1173.
9. PALASZYNSKI, E. W., T. W. MOODY, T. L. O'DONAHUE, & A. L. GOLDSTEIN. 1983. Peptides **4:** 463.
10. BESEDOVSKY, H., A. DELREY, E. SORKIN & C. DINARELLO. 1986. Science **233:** 652.
11. MADDON, P. J., A. G. DALGLEISH, J. S. MCDOUGAL, P. R. CLAPHAM, R. A. WEISS & R. AXEL. 1986. Cell **47:** 333.
12. O'DORISIO, M. S., N. HERMINA, S. P. BALCERZAK & T. M. O'DORISIO. 1981. J. Immunol. **127:** 2551.
13. WOOD, C. L. & M. S. O'DORISIO. 1985. J. Biol. Chem. **260:** 1243.
14. O'DORISIO, M. S., C. L. WOOD, G. D. WENGER & L. M. VASSALO. 1985. J. Immunol. **134:** 4078.
15. ROLA-PLESZCZYNKI, M., D. BOLDUC & S. ST. PIERRE. 1986. J. Immunol. **135:** 2569.
16. KRCO, C. J., A. GORES & V. L. W. GO. 1986. Clin. Immunol. Immunopathol. **39:** 309.
17. OTTAWAY, C. A. & G. R. GREENBERG. 1984. J. Immunol. **132:** 417.
18. OTTAWAY, C. A. 1984. J. Exp. Med. **160:** 1054.
19. MINOWADA, J., T. OHNUMA & G. E. MOORE. 1972. J. Natl. Cancer Inst. **49:** 891.
20. KASLOW, H. R., Z. FARFEL, G. L. JOHNSON & H. R. BOURNE. 1979. Mol. Pharmacol. **15:** 472.
21. AKERA, T. & V. CHENG. 1979. Biochem. Biophys. Acta **4790:** 412.
22. LAEMMLI, U. K. 1970. Nature **227:** 680.
23. TAYLOR, D. P. & C. B. PERT. 1979. Proc. Natl. Acad. Sci. USA **76:** 660.
24. GUERRERO, J. M., J. C. PRIETO, F. L. ELORZA, R. RAMIREZ & R. GOBERNA. 1983. Endocrinology **21:** 151.
25. BEED, E. A., M. S. O'DORISIO, T. S. GAGINELLA & T. M. O'DORISIO. 1983. Regul. Peptides **6:** 1.
26. ITOH, N., K. OBATA, N. YAMAHARA & H. OKAMOTO. 1983. Nature **304:** 547.
27. GUILLEMIN, R. 1982. Science **218:** 585.
28. GILMAN, A. G. 1984. Cell **36:** 577.
29. COUVINEAU, A., B. AMIRANOFF & M. LABURTHE. 1986. J. Biol. Chem. **261:** 14482.
30. NGUYEN, T. D., J. A. WILLIAMS & G. M. GRAY. 1986. Biochemistry **25:** 361.
31. BATTARI, E., J. LUIS, J. M. MARTIN, J. FANTANI, J. M. MULLER, J. MARVALDI & J. PICHON. 1987. Biochem. J. **242:** 185.
32. COUVINEAU, A. & M. LABURTHE. 1985. Biochem. J. **225:** 473.
33. MCARTHUR, K. E., C. L. WOOD, M. S. O'DORISIO, J. D. GARDNER & R. T. JENSEN. Am. J. Physiol. In press.
34. WOOD, C. L., M. S. O'DORISIO, L. M. VASSALO, W. B. MALARKEY & T. M. O'DORISIO. 1985. Regul. Peptides **12:** 237.
35. PAUL, S. & S. I. SAID. 1987. J. Biol. Chem. **262:** 158.

Structural Characterization of Vasoactive Intestinal Peptide Receptors from Rat Lung Membranes

GÖNÜL VELIÇELEBI,[a] SARASWATHI PATTHI,
SALLY PROVOW, MICHAEL AKONG, AND
SUSAN SIMERSON

Salk Institute Biotechnology/Industrial Associates, Inc.
La Jolla, California 92037

The presence of specific receptors for vasoactive intestinal peptide (VIP) in numerous cell and membrane preparations has been well documented.[1] The binding of VIP to cell-surface receptors correlates with the stimulation of adenylate cyclase activity and elevation of intracellular concentration of cAMP, leading to the biological effects of the peptide.[2] Hence, structural and functional characterization of VIP receptors will be integral to understanding the molecular mechanism of action of VIP.

Our studies have focused on the characterization of VIP receptors from rat lung. There is evidence that the lung may be an important target organ for the actions of VIP based on the demonstration of VIP innervation associated with airways and pulmonary vessels,[3] bronchodilatory effects of VIP in humans,[4] and its relaxant effects on pulmonary vascular smooth muscle.[5]

In this study, we describe characterization of VIP receptors from rat lung membranes both in the membrane-bound and detergent-solubilized states. In the former case, rat lung membrane proteins were covalently labeled with [125I]VIP using a bifunctional cross-linker and a 55-kDa species was identified as a ligand-binding unit of rat lung VIP receptors. Cross-linking studies have been reported in greater detail elsewhere.[6] In the latter case, [125I]VIP-labeled, membrane-bound receptors were solubilized in Triton X-100 and studied by gel filtration and sucrose density gradient sedimentation, yielding an apparent molecular weight of 270,000 for the [125I]VIP-receptor complex in Triton X-100 solution.

[a]Address for correspondence: Dr. Gönül Veliçelebi, Salk Institute Biotechnology/Industrial Associates, Inc., 505 Coast Blvd., S., La Jolla, California 92037.

MATERIALS AND METHODS

Materials

The materials used in the experiments were obtained from the following sources: VIP and atrial natriuretic factor (ANF) from Peninsula Laboratories; rat and human growth hormone-releasing factors (rGHRF and hGHRF) from Clayton Laboratories for Peptide Biology; [^{125}I]VIP and Triton X-100 from New England Nuclear; ethylene glycolbis (succinimidylsuccinate) (EGS) from Pierce Chemical Co.; bovine serum albumin (BSA) from Miles Laboratories; guanine nucleotides from Boehringer Mannheim Biochemicals; wheat germ agglutinin (WGA)-Sepharose, N-acetyl-D-glucosamine (NAG), and marker proteins used in gel filtration and sucrose density gradients from Sigma Chemical Co.; and sodium dodecyl sulfate-polyacrylamide gel electrophoresis (SDS-PAGE) protein standards from BioRad.

Binding and Cross-Linking of [^{125}I]VIP to Rat Lung Membrane Receptors

Rat lung membranes were prepared according to the procedure described by Leroux *et al.*[7] [^{125}I]VIP was bound and cross-linked to rat lung membrane receptors as detailed before.[6] Briefly, 480 μg of rat lung membrane protein was incubated [^{125}I]VIP (20 pM for binding studies, 200 pM for cross-linking studies) in the presence of varying concentrations of unlabeled VIP in 1.2 ml of assay buffer (25 mM Tris-HCl, 5 mM MgCl$_2$, 0.1% bacitracin, and 0.1% BSA, pH 7.4) for 20 minutes at 37°C by gentle rocking. At the end of the binding incubation, the assay mixture was spun down for three minutes in a Beckman 12 microfuge and each pellet was washed twice with 1 ml each of cold buffer without BSA. The final pellet was resuspended in 450 μl of this buffer and EGS was added to a final concentration of 5 mM (50 mM stock in dimethyl sulfoxide). The cross-linking reaction was carried out for 20 minutes at room temperature and was subsequently quenched by addition of glycine (50 mM final). The membrane suspension was spun down in the microfuge and washed once with one milliliter of cold assay buffer, and the final pellet was resuspended in 100 μl of assay buffer.

Solubilization of Rat Lung Membranes Labeled with [^{125}I]VIP

Membranes were labeled with [^{125}I]VIP before incubation with 1.5% (wt/vol) Triton X-100 for 30 minutes at room temperature by gentle rocking. Subsequently, the membrane-detergent suspension was centrifuged at 100,000 × g for one hour at 4°C and the supernatant was analyzed by gel filtration and sucrose density gradient sedimentation.

Gel Filtration of Solubilized VIP Receptors

400 μl of detergent-solubilized preparation of [^{125}I]VIP-labeled rat lung receptors was applied on a Sepharose 4-B column (1.5 $\times$ 50 cm). The column was preequilibrated with 25 mM Tris, 5 mM MgCl$_2$, pH 7.4 containing 0.1% Triton X-100. The flow rate of the column was maintained at 5 ml/h and 1-ml fractions were collected. The fractions were counted for [^{125}I]VIP as well as analyzed by SDS-PAGE. The column was calibrated by applying the following marker proteins with known Stokes radii: β-galactosidase (*E. coli*), 6.9 nm[9]; apoferritin, 6.1 nm[10]; catalase (bovine liver), 5.2 nm[9]; and BSA, 3.55 nm.[10] Blue dextran and K$_2$Cr$_2$O$_7$ were used to determine void volume (V$_0$) and total volume (V$_t$), respectively.

Sucrose Density Gradient Sedimentation

Five to twenty percent linear sucrose density gradients were prepared in 25 mM Tris-HCl, 5 mM MgCl$_2$, pH 7.4 containing 0.1% Triton X-100. Two hundred microliters of solubilized receptors prelabeled with [^{125}I]VIP was applied to a 5-ml gradient. The following marker proteins with known sedimentation coefficient (s$_{20,w}$) values[9] were included to calibrate each gradient run: β-galactosidase, 15.9 s; catalase, 11.3 s; fumarase, 9.0 s; lactate dehydrogenase, 7.3 s, and BSA, 4.7 s. The gradients were sedimented using a Beckman SW 50.1 rotor by centrifuging for 16 hours at 34,000 rpm for H$_2$O gradients and at 44,000 rpm for D$_2$O gradients. Each gradient was fractionated using a peristaltic pump, and the fractions were counted for [^{125}I]VIP and analyzed by SDS-PAGE to determine the positions of the marker proteins as well as the covalently labeled receptor species.

SDS-PAGE Analysis and Autoradiography

Samples were analyzed by SDS-PAGE using the Laemmli system[11] after denaturation by the addition of sample buffer (final concentration of 10% glycerol, 5% SDS, 65 mM Tris, 0.05% bromophenol blue, pH 6.8). The following proteins were used as molecular weight standards: myosin, 200,000; β-galactosidase, 116,000; phosphorylase b, 92,500; BSA, 66,200; ovalbumin, 45,000; carbonic anhydrase, 31,000. The gels were stained, destained, and dried onto Whatman 3M filter paper. Autoradiographs were obtained by exposing the dried gels with Kodak XAR-5 film using a Kronex intensifying screen.

Affinity Chromatography on WGA-Sepharose

Five hundred microliters of [^{125}I]VIP-labeled rat lung membrane extract were incubated by gentle rocking for 16 hours at 4°C with one ml of WGA-Sepharose that had been extensively washed with 25 mM Tris-HCl, 5 mM MgCl$_2$, 0.1% bacitracin,

0.1% Triton X-100, pH 7.4. At the end of the incubation, the beads were spun down in a table-top centrifuge and washed with 50 ml of the buffer above before transferring into a small column for elution. The elution was carried out using 0.5 ml aliquots of 0.3 M NAG in 25 mM Tris-HCl, 5 mM MgCl$_2$, 0.1% Triton X-100, pH 7.4. The fractions were collected, rapidly counted for [^{125}I]VIP, and analyzed by SDS-PAGE.

RESULTS

Characterization of Membrane-Bound Receptors

The binding of [^{125}I]VIP to rat lung membranes was quite rapid as indicated by the results of time course studies shown in FIGURE 1. Maximal binding was reached within 20 minutes, one hour, and six hours at 37, 20, and 4°C, respectively. The rate of binding increased with increasing temperature, as shown for early time points in the figure inset. Maximal level of specific binding remained steady at $\sim$ 40% of total [^{125}I]VIP up to 24 hours at 20°C and 4°C (data not shown). Furthermore, the extent of degradation during the course of binding at all three temperatures was assayed by testing for precipitability in 10% trichloroacetic acid. No significant degradation of [^{125}I]VIP was observed during the binding incubation in the presence of 0.1% bacitracin that was included in the assay buffer.

Competitive Binding Studies and Scatchard Analyses

The binding of [^{125}I]VIP to rat lung membrane receptors was carried out in the presence of increasing concentration of unlabeled VIP to determine the K_D, the dissociation constant for the binding reaction, as well as the binding capacity (B.C.) of the membrane preparation. The results of a typical competition curve are shown in FIGURE 2A. VIP inhibited the binding of [^{125}I]VIP with an overall IC$_{50}$ $\sim$ 750 pM. rGHRF and hGHRF, two peptides structurally related to VIP, and ANF, an unrelated peptide, were also tested for their ability to displace bound [^{125}I]VIP to determine the peptide specificity of rat lung VIP receptors. rGHRF, which has been demonstrated to interact with VIP receptors in rat pancreas,[12] bound to rat lung VIP receptors with $\sim$20 times lower affinity than VIP (IC$_{50}$ $\simeq$ 20 nM) whereas hGHRF was significantly less potent (IC$_{50}$ $\simeq$ 1μM). ANF did not exhibit any detectable cross-reactivity with rat lung VIP receptors, as indicated by the lack of displacement of bound [^{125}I]VIP. Scatchard analysis of VIP binding data (FIG. 2B) indicated the presence of two classes of binding sites: 0.28 $\pm$ 0.11 pmoles/mg protein of Class I binding sites with K_D = 79.2 $\pm$ 26.4 pM and 3.3 $\pm$ 0.9 pmoles/mg protein of Class II binding sites with lower binding affinity (K_D = 4.8 $\pm$ 2.1 nM).

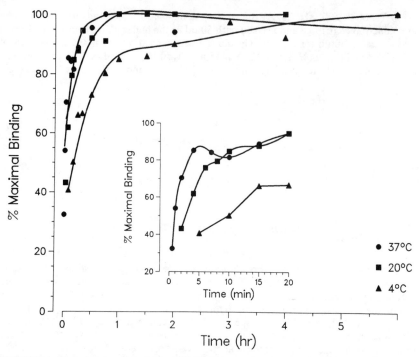

FIGURE 1. Time course of binding of [^{125}I]VIP to rat lung membranes at three temperatures. Rat lung membranes (400 μg protein/ml) were incubated with [^{125}I]VIP (20 pM final) in the absence (total binding) and presence (nonspecific binding) of 0.5 μM unlabeled VIP at 4, 20, and 37°C. At the indicated time points, duplicate aliquots were removed from each binding mixture and centrifuged. The pellets were washed twice and counted. Specific binding was determined by subtracting nonspecifically bound counts from total bound counts and expressed as percent of maximal specific binding. Under maximal conditions, 60-70% of total counts were bound in the absence of unlabeled VIP, of which approximately 6% was not displaced in the presence of 0.5 μM unlabeled VIP, that is, was nonspecifically bound.

Effects of Guanine Nucleotides on the Binding of [^{125}I]VIP

The stimulation of adenylate cyclase activity in lung membranes by VIP has been reported,[14,15] suggesting that lung VIP receptors may be coupled to the stimulatory guanine nucleotide-binding regulatory protein (N_s) of hormone-sensitive adenylate cyclase system. To demonstrate this coupling directly, we investigated the effect of nonhydrolyzable GTP analogues on the binding of [^{125}I]VIP to rat lung receptors. The results, shown in FIGURE 3, indicated that guanosine-5′-O-(3-thiotriphosphate) (GTPγS), guanosine-5′-O-(2-thiodiphosphate) (GDPβS), and guanylylimidophosphate (GppNHp) inhibited the binding of [^{125}I]VIP in a dose-dependent fashion, with potency order of GTPγS > GDPβS > GppNHp. Competitive binding in the presence of GTPγS (FIG. 4A) indicated that the overall IC$_{50}$ for VIP was shifted to a higher

VIP concentration (2 and 3 nM in the presence of 1 and 100 μM GTPγS, respectively). Scatchard analysis of the competitive binding data (FIG. 4B) revealed that the shift in overall affinity was primarily due to the decreased number of higher affinity (Class I) binding sites.

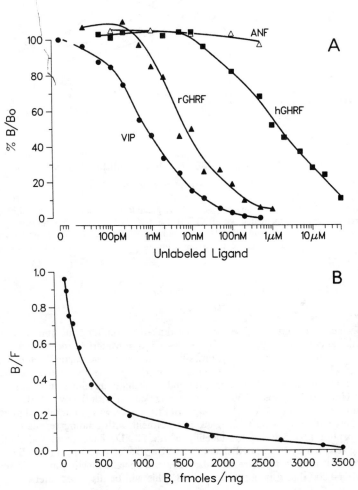

FIGURE 2. Competitive binding of [^{125}I]VIP to rat lung membranes (peptide specificity, Scatchard analysis). (A) 400 μg/ml of rat lung membrane protein was incubated with 20 pM [^{125}I]VIP and increasing concentration of unlabeled VIP, rGHRF, hGHRF, and ANF for 20 minutes at 37°C. Nonspecific binding, that is, binding in the presence of 0.5 μM VIP, was subtracted from binding observed at each other concentration of VIP and other peptides. Specific binding thus calculated was expressed as percent of that obtained in the absence of unlabeled VIP.

(B) Specific binding data were analyzed by the method of Scatchard.[13]

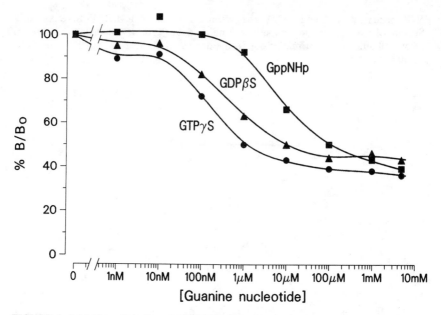

FIGURE 3. Inhibition of binding of [^{125}I]VIP by guanine nucleotides. 400 μg/ml of rat lung membrane protein was incubated with [^{125}I]VIP (20 pM) in the presence of increasing concentrations of GTPγS, GDPβS, and GppNHp with and without 0.5 μM VIP for 20 minutes at 37°C. Specific binding was calculated and plotted as a function of guanine nucleotide concentration.

Cross-Linking of [^{125}I]VIP to Rat Lung Receptors

Specifically bound [^{125}I]VIP was cross-linked to rat lung membranes using the bifunctional cross-linking agent, EGS, as described in Materials and Methods. Optimization and characterization of the cross-linking reaction was carried out as described in detail elsewhere.[6] Specific labeling of a 58-kDa species was observed that was inhibited by unlabeled VIP in a dose-dependent fashion, as shown in FIGURE 5. IC_{50} for inhibition by VIP was ~750 pM, in close agreement with the overall IC_{50} observed in binding studies (FIG. 2A). The labeling of this species was also inhibited by rGHRF (FIG. 5A) with IC_{50} ~30 nM, again in agreement with binding results (FIG. 2A). Thus, peptide specificity of the labeling of the 58-kDa band paralleled that of the binding reaction and indicated that the 58-kDa species was a ligand-binding unit of rat lung VIP receptors. There was also covalent, specific labeling in a diffuse region around 160,000 that was not well resolved. This will be discussed later.

Characterization of Solubilized Receptors

[^{125}I]VIP-labeled rat lung receptors were solubilized in Triton X-100 as described in Materials and Methods. Under these conditions, typically 35% of total protein and

45% of [^{125}I]VIP-receptor complexes were solubilized. Triton X-100 solubilized [^{125}I]VIP-receptor complexes were characterized by gel filtration on Sepharose 4B and sucrose density gradient sedimentation through 5-20% linear sucrose density gradients in H_2O and D_2O.

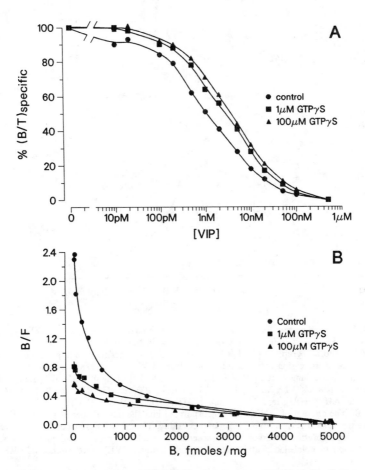

FIGURE 4. Competitive binding of [^{125}I]VIP in the presence of GTPγS. Rat lung membrane protein (400 μg) was incubated with 20 pM [^{125}I]VIP and the indicated concentration of unlabeled VIP in the presence of 1 μM (filled squares) and 100 μM GTPγS (filled triangles) and in the absence of GTPγS (filled circles). Binding was carried out for 20 minutes at 37°C.

(A) Plot of specific binding (expressed as percent of maximal specific binding) versus the concentration of VIP.

(B) Scatchard analysis of the binding data displayed in part A.

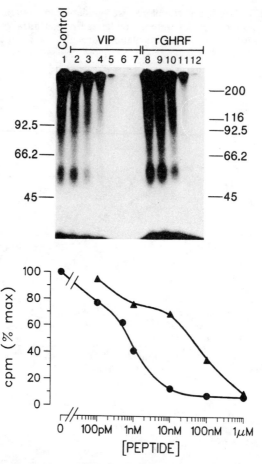

FIGURE 5. Specific cross-linking of [^{125}I]VIP to rat lung VIP receptors. [^{125}I]VIP was bound and cross-linked to rat lung membranes as described in Materials and Methods.

(A) Autoradiograph of [^{125}I]VIP-labeled rat lung membranes. Binding was carried out in the presence of increasing concentrations of unlabeled VIP and rGHRF as follows: lane 1, no unlabeled peptide; lane 2, 100 pM VIP; lane 3, 500 pM VIP; lane 4, 1 nM VIP; lane 5, 10 nM VIP; lane 6, 100 nM VIP; lane 7, 1 $\mu$$M$ VIP; lane 8, 100 pM rGHRF; lane 9, 1 nM rGHRF; lane 10, 10 nM rGHRF; lane 11, 100 nM rGHRF; lane 12, 1 $\mu$$M$ rGHRF.

(B) The amount of radioactivity incorporated into the labeled species was quantitated by excising the labeled region from the gel and counting. The results were calculated as percent of maximal incorporation observed in the absence of unlabeled peptide and plotted versus the concentration of unlabeled peptide present during binding. (VIP, filled circles; rGHRF, filled triangles)

Gel Filtration Chromatography

When chromatographed on a Sepharose 4B gel filtration column, Triton X-100 solubilized [^{125}I]VIP-receptor complexes eluted as a single peak of radioactivity, well separated from the free [¹²⁵I]VIP peak that eluted at ~V_t (FIG. 6). Values (1-K_{ave}) for the marker proteins were plotted versus their known Stokes radii and the Stokes radius of the labeled species was determined to be 6.1 ± 0.4 nm ($n = 6$) by interpolation, as shown in the figure inset. SDS-PAGE analysis of the peak at 6.1 nm displayed the presence of the labeled 58-kDa species (data not shown).

Sucrose Density Gradient Sedimentation

When Triton X-100 extract of [¹²⁵I]VIP-labeled rat lung membranes was analyzed by sedimentation through 5-20% linear sucrose density gradients, the [¹²⁵I]VIP-labeled receptor sedimented as a single peak of radioactivity with an apparent sedimentation coefficient of ~7.0 s (FIG. 7A). This peak was also well resolved from the peak corresponding to free [¹²⁵I]VIP which sedimented toward the top of the gradient. Gradient fractions were analyzed by SDS-PAGE to determine the sedimentation profile of the labeled 58-kDa species. The results, shown in FIG. 7B, indicated the 58-kDa labeled species was a component of the peak sedimenting at ~7 s but not the peak corresponding to free [¹²⁵I]VIP, confirming that the 7 s peak represented [¹²⁵I]VIP-receptor complexes. Also contained in the 7 s peak was a covalently-labeled 159-kDa species that sedimented identically to the 58-kDa species. Results of similar

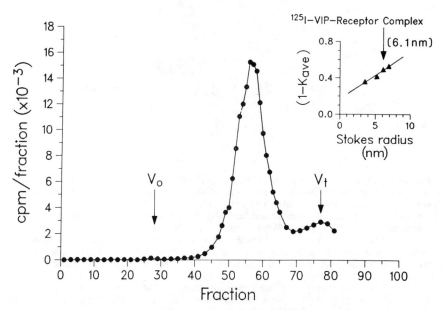

FIGURE 6. Gel filtration of Triton X-100 extract of [¹²⁵I]VIP-labeled rat lung membranes. Rat lung membranes were covalently labeled with [¹²⁵I]VIP, solubilized in Triton X-100, and chromatographed on a Sepharose 4B column as described in detail in Materials and Methods. β-Galactosidase, catalase, and BSA were used as marker proteins. Void volume (V_o) and total volume (V_t) were determined using blue dextran and $K_2Cr_2O_7$, respectively.

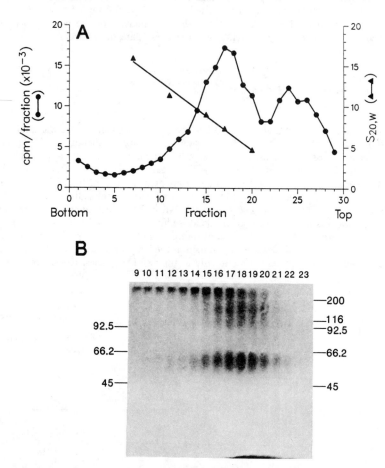

FIGURE 7. Sucrose density gradient sedimentation of Triton X-100 extract of [^{125}I]VIP-labeled rat lung membranes. [^{125}I]VIP-labeled rat lung membranes were extracted in Triton X-100 and analyzed by sucrose density gradient sedimentation on 5-20% linear sucrose density gradients prepared in H$_2$O (details in Materials and Methods). β-Galactosidase, catalase, fumarase, lactate dehydrogenase, and BSA were included as markers in each gradient.

(A) Sedimentation profile of [^{125}I]VIP counts. Each gradient was fractioned in identical fashion using a peristaltic pump and the fractions were counted for [^{125}I]VIP. The positions of the marker proteins were determined by SDS-PAGE analysis of the protein content of each fraction.

(B) Autoradiograph of the gradient fractions analyzed by SDS-PAGE: Gradient fractions were analyzed by SDS-PAGE using a 10% separating gel in the Laemmli system.[11] The gels were dried down and exposed with Kodak XAR film to obtain the autoradiograph shown. The lane numbers correspond to numbers of gradient fractions.

analyses carried out using sucrose solutions prepared in D_2O (data not shown) yielded an apparent sedimentation coefficient of 6.0 s for the [^{125}I]VIP-receptor complex.

Hydrodynamic Properties of [^{125}I]VIP-Receptor Complexes Solubilized in Triton X-100

The data from sucrose density gradients were analyzed as described by Clarke[16] to yield the values for densities in H_2O and D_2O (ρ_H and ρ_D, respectively), viscosities in H_2O and D_2O (η_H and η_D, respectively) and sedimentation coefficients in H_2O and D_2O (s_H and s_D, respectively). These values were used to determine partial specific volume (ν) and sedimentation coefficient ($s_{20,w}$), which were subsequently used to determine the molecular weight of the [^{125}I]VIP-receptor complex. Hydrodynamic parameters calculated according to Clarke[16] are tabulated in TABLE 1. These calculations yielded 270,000 ± 35,000 for the size of [^{125}I]VIP-receptor complexes solubilized in Triton X-100.

Partial Purification by WGA-Sepharose Affinity Chromatography

[^{125}I]VIP-labeled, Triton X-100 extract was incubated with WGA-Sepharose and specifically eluted by 0.3 M NAG. The results of SDS-PAGE analysis (FIG. 8) indicated that the material that was specifically eluted contained most of the labeled 58-kDa [^{125}I]VIP-receptor unit complex. The flow-through consisted mainly of [^{125}I]VIP. The material eluted from WGA-Sepharose column was further analyzed by sucrose density gradient sedimentation, during which it displayed the same sedimentation characteristics as the cruder extract (data not shown).

DISCUSSION

We have demonstrated that rat lung membranes contain specific receptors for VIP with a significantly high total binding capacity of 3.3 pmoles/mg membrane protein. Binding of [^{125}I]VIP to rat lung membrane receptors was rapid and saturable. Peptide specificity for binding of peptides related to VIP was as follows: VIP > rGHRF > > hGHRF. Unrelated peptides such as ANF did not exhibit any specific binding to these receptors. Nonhydrolyzable GTP analogues, GTPγS, GDPβS, and GppNHp, inhibited the binding of [^{125}I]VIP to rat lung membrane receptors at submicromolar doses, indicating the coupling of these receptors to N_s, consistent with reports of stimulatory effect of VIP on adenylate cyclase in the lung reported by others.[14,15] The order of effectiveness for the three guanine nucleotides that were studied paralleled that reported for their effects on other N_s-coupled peptide receptors, for example, the parathyroid hormone receptor.[17]

VIP receptors in rat lung membranes appeared to belong to two classes with different specific binding characteristics: Class I binding sites displayed higher binding

TABLE 1. Hydrodynamic Properties of [^{125}I]VIP-Receptor Complexes Solubilized from Rat Lung Membranes in Triton X-100

Stokes radius (a)	6.1 ± 0.4 nm ($n = 6$)
Apparent sedimentation coefficients	
in H$_2$O	6.9 ± 0.6 s ($n = 8$)
in D$_2$O	5.8 ± 0.3 s ($n = 6$)
Partial specific volume (ν)	0.81 ml/g^a
Sedimentation coefficient ($s_{20,w}$)	7.35 ± 0.45 s^b
Molecular weight of receptor-detergent	
complex, M_c	$270,000 \pm 35,000^c$
Molecular weight of receptor, M_p	$159,000^d$

^{a} Calculated from the following equation[16]:

$$\nu = \{(s_H\eta_H/s_D\eta_D) - 1\} / \{\rho_D(s_H\eta_H/s_D\eta_D) - \rho_H\}$$

where the values for ρ_H, ρ_D, s_H, s_D, η_H, and η_D were determined experimentally.

^{b} Calculated from all possible pairings of the H$_2$O and D$_2$O gradient runs according to the following equation[16]:

$$s_{20,w} = \{s_H(\eta_H/\eta_{20,w}) (1 - \nu\rho_{20,w})\} / (1 - \nu\rho_H)$$

^{c} Calculated from the following equation:

$$M_r = 6\pi N\eta_{20,w} \, a \, s_{20,w} / (1 - \nu\rho_{20,w})$$

where, N = Avogadro's number; $\eta_{20,w}$ = viscosity of H$_2$O at 20°C (0.01002 g/cm s) $\rho_{20,w}$ = density of H$_2$O at 20°C (0.99823 g/ml).

^{d} Calculated from: $M_p = M_c/(1 + \delta)$ where $\delta = (\nu_p - \nu_c)/(\nu_c - \nu_d)$ See text for discussion.

affinity ($K_D = 79.2 \pm 26.4$ pM) and lower binding capacity (B.C. = 0.28 pmole/mg protein) while Class II sites bound [^{125}I]VIP with a $K_D = 4.8 \pm 2.1$ nM and B.C. = 3.3 ± 0.9 pmoles/mg protein. The presence of two classes of binding sites had been reported by Leroux et al.[7] but their values for K_D and B.C. were significantly lower than the ones determined in our study due to the significantly higher concentration of [^{125}I]VIP used in their study. When the competitive binding studies were carried out in the presence of GTPγS, the overall IC$_{50}$ for the inhibition of [^{125}I]VIP binding by VIP was shifted to higher VIP concentration. Scatchard analyses of the data revealed that the number of Class I binding sites was significantly reduced in the presence of GTPγS, suggesting differential coupling of higher affinity (Class I) receptors to N$_s$.

Structural information about rat lung VIP receptors was obtained through covalent labeling of membrane-bound receptors with [^{125}I]VIP using the bifunctional cross-linker, EGS. A 58-kDa species was specifically labeled, with a peptide specificity and dose-dependence that was identical to that observed for binding to the membranes. We had shown in an earlier report[6] that the labeling of the 58-kDa species was also inhibited by GTPγS in a similar fashion to that observed for the inhibition of binding. These results collectively indicated that the 58-kDa species was a unit of the functional VIP receptor. Thus, if we assume a 1 : 1 stoichiometry for the binding of VIP, subtraction of the molecular weight of the peptide yields an apparent size of 55-kDa for the ligand-binding unit of the rat lung VIP receptor.

In order to determine the total size of rat lung VIP receptors, [^{125}I]VIP-labeled membrane-bound receptors were solubilized using the nondenaturing detergent Triton X-100 and analyzed by gel filtration chromatography and sucrose density gradient sedimentation. [^{125}I]VIP-receptor complexes behaved as one major species in both analyses with an estimated Stokes radius (a) of 6.1 ± 0.4 nm and sedimentation coefficient ($s_{20,w}$) of 7.35 ± 0.45 s. SDS-PAGE analyses of gel filtration and gradient fractions revealed that the [^{125}I]VIP-labeled 58-kDa unit was a component of this species. These values and the estimated partial specific volume (0.81 ml/g) were used to calculate an apparent molecular mass of 270 kDa ± 35 kDa for [^{125}I]VIP-receptor complex in Triton X-100 solution.

Estimation of the real size of the VIP receptor requires subtraction of the amount of detergent bound to the protein from this estimate of 270,000 representing the detergent-protein complex. δ, Grams of detergent bound per g of protein, can be calculated from the following equation[18]:

$$\delta = (\nu_p - \nu_c)/(\nu_c - \nu_d)$$

where ν_p, ν_c, and ν_d refer to partial specific volume of protein, protein-detergent complex, and detergent, respectively. ν_c was determined experimentally to be 0.81 ml/g as described above, ν_d is reported to be 0.91,[9] and we can assume a value of

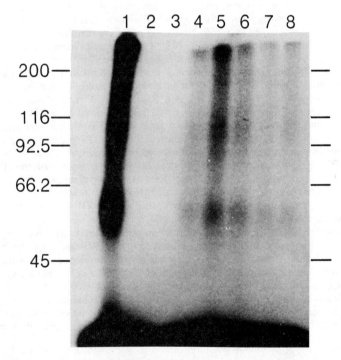

FIGURE 8. Autoradiograph of WGA-Sepharose affinity chromatography on Triton X-100 extract of [^{125}I]VIP-labeled rat lung membranes. Rat lung membranes were labeled with [^{125}I]VIP by cross-linking, extracted in 1% Triton X-100, and bound to and eluted from WGA-Sepharose as described in Materials and Methods. The lanes correspond to the following samples: lane 1, total extract; lanes 2-3, flow-through from WGA-Sepharose; lanes 4-8, fractions collected during specific elution with 0.3 M NAG.

0.74 for v_p, which is a typical value for many proteins and has been determined on the basis of amino acid composition for another adenylate cyclase-coupled receptor with similar subunit size, the β-adrenergic receptor.[18] Using these values, δ was calculated as 0.7. Next, the size of the receptor protein, M_p, can be determined using the estimates for δ and M_c, the size of the protein-detergent complex, by the following relationship:

$$M_p = M_c/(1 + \delta)$$

This calculation yields a molecular weight of $\sim 159,000$ for the VIP receptor. As mentioned above, we have occasionally observed covalent labeling of a 159-kDa species with [^{125}I]VIP, which displayed identical sedimentation properties to the more predominant 58-kDa unit on 5-20% linear sucrose density gradients (FIG. 7A). It is possible that this higher molecular weight species represents a cross-linked complex of the 58-kDa ligand-binding unit with a regulatory component of the VIP receptor that is not easily accessible for cross-linking. An alternative explanation would be the formation of a complex between the VIP receptor unit and N_s, as was also suggested by Couvineau et al.[10]

The results reported here are comparable to and subject to similar uncertainties as those contained in three recent reports[10,19,20] describing characterization of detergent-solubilized VIP receptors. Two of these studies[10,19] were carried out with liver VIP receptors solubilized in Triton X-100. Nguyen et al.[19] have observed a major 200-kDa and a minor 47-kDa unit upon analysis of [^{125}I]VIP-receptor complexes by gel permeation chromatography. Couvineau et al.[10] have analyzed [^{125}I]VIP-receptor complexes by gel filtration and sucrose density gradient sedimentation and observed a major heavy and a minor light component with apparent molecular weights of 150,000 and 52,000, respectively. In the third report, Paul and Said[20] have described solubilization of guinea pig lung VIP receptors in CHAPS followed by gel filtration chromatography and reported two fractions that bound [^{125}I]VIP with Stokes radii of 5.9 nm and 2.3 nm. The hydrodynamic properties of [^{125}I]VIP-receptor complexes we have determined correlate with those of the major component reported by several workers.[10,29,20] However, we have not observed the minor component under the conditions used in our studies. Nguyen et al.[19] have concluded that the smaller 47-kDa unit seen in their analyses was an artifact of the solubilization process. Precise determination of the size and oligomeric structure of the VIP receptor must await purification of the protein to homogeneity.

We have carried out preliminary purification attempts by using WGA-Sepharose affinity chromatography. Our results indicated that [^{125}I]VIP-labeled solubilized receptors bound quite effectively to WGA-Sepharose and were specifically eluted with a sharp profile, in agreement with the results of Nguyen et al.[19] Preliminary hydrodynamic characterization of WGA-eluted [^{125}I]VIP-receptor complexes yielded similar results to those obtained with the total extract. Thus, it seems that rat lung VIP receptors contain complex N-linked carbohydrate chains and WGA-Sepharose affinity chromatography may be utilized as an initial step in ultimate purification of the protein.

[Note added in proof: Since the presentation of these results describing characterization of VIP receptors solubilized in Triton X-100, we have also determined the hydrodynamic parameters of VIP receptors solubilized in another nondenaturing detergent, n-octyl-β-D-glucopyranoside (Patthi, S., M. Akong & G. Velicelebi. 1987. J. Biol.

Chem. **262**: 15740-15745). Using two sets of complete hydrodynamic data obtained in Triton X-100 and n-octyl-β-D-glucopyranoside, it was possible to estimate directly the amount of bound detergent, yielding a corrected molecular weight of 55,000 for the VIP receptor. Since this species included the 55K binding unit, as also shown here, we concluded that the VIP receptor is a glycoprotein consisting of a single 55K polypeptide chain.]

REFERENCES

1. SAID, S. I. 1984. Peptides **5**: 143-150.
2. SAID, S. I. 1982. *In* Advances in Peptide Hormone Research. S. I. Said, Ed. Vol. **1**: 1-512. Raven Press. New York.
3. DEY, D. A., W. A. SHANNON & S. I. SAID. 1981. Cell Tissue Res. **220**: 231-238.
4. MORICE, A., R. J. UNWIN & P. S. SEVER. 1984. Peptides **5**: 439-440.
5. SAID, S. I. 1982. Exp. Lung Res. **3**: 343-348.
6. PROVOW, S. & G. VELICELEBI. 1987. Endocrinology **120**: 2442-2452.
7. LEROUX, P., H. VAUDRY, A. FOURNIER, S. ST-PIERRE & G. PELLETIER. 1984. Endocrinology **114**: 1506-1512.
8. LOWRY, O. H., N. J. ROSEBROUGH, A. L. FARR & R. J. RANDALL. 1951. J. Biol. Chem. **193**: 265-275.
9. AIYER, R. A. 1983. J. Biol. Chem. **258**: 14992-14999.
10. COUVINEAU, A., B. AMIRANOFF & M. LABURTHE. 1986. J. Biol. Chem. **261**: 14482-14489.
11. LAEMMLI, U. K. 1970. Nature **227**: 680-685.
12. WAELBROECK, M., P. ROBBERECHT, D. H. COY, J.-C. CAMUS, P. DE NEEF & J. CHRISTOPHE. 1985. Endocrinology **116**: 2643-2649.
13. SCATCHARD, G. 1949. Ann. N. Y. Acad. Sci. USA **51**: 660-672.
14. ROBBERECHT, P., P. CHATELAIN, P. DE NEEF, J. C. CAMUS, M. WAELBROECK & J. CHRISTOPHE. 1981 Biochim. Biophys. Acta **678**: 76-82.
15. TATON, G., M. DELHAYE, J. C. CAMUS, P. DE NEEF, P. CHATELAIN, P. ROBBERECHT & J. CHRISTOPHE. 1981. Pflugers Arch. **391**: 178-182.
16. CLARKE, S. 1975. J. Biol. Chem. **250**: 5459-5469.
17. NISSENSON, R. A., E. MANN, J. WINER, A. P. TEITELBAUM & C. D. ARNAUD. 1986. Endocrinology **118**: 932-939.
18. SHORR, R. G. L., D. R. McCASLIN, M. W. STROHSACKER, G. ALIANELL, R. REBAR, J. M. STADEL & S. T. CROOKE. 1985. Biochemistry **24**: 6869-6875.
19. NGUYEN, T. D., J. A. WILLIAMS & G. M. GRAY. 1986. Biochemistry **25**: 361-368.
20. PAUL, S. & S. I. SAID. 1987. J. Biol. Chem. **262**: 158-162.

Regulatory Aspects of the Vasoactive Intestinal Peptide Receptor in Lung[a]

SUDHIR PAUL,[b] JOANNE CHOU,[c] AND
SAMI I. SAID[d]

Department of Medicine
Oklahoma University Health Sciences Center and
Veterans Administration Medical Center
Oklahoma City, Oklahoma 73190

Receptor molecules bind ligand and activate signal-transducing pathways. Previous reports have documented the presence of high-affinity receptors for vasoactive intestinal peptide (VIP) in membranes prepared from the lungs of man, rat, and guinea pig.[1,2] Binding of VIP to lung membranes is accompanied by cyclic AMP synthesis, suggesting that the VIP receptors are coupled to adenylate cyclase.[1,3] To obtain a better understanding of the molecular events leading to the physiologic actions of vasoactive intestinal peptide (VIP), we are studying the structural and regulatory characteristics of VIP receptors. An additional incentive for these studies is the potential role of the VIP-receptor in disease: (1) VIP is a likely factor in the autonomic regulation of airway smooth muscle tone,[4,5] and VIP-receptor dysfunction may result in airway hyperreactivity; and (2) the VIP receptor, like receptors for some other endogenous agents,[6,7] may serve as the binding site for certain viral coat proteins and permit entry of virus (including HIV) particles into host cells.

The membrane environment of the receptors is a complex milieu of structural and regulatory components. Experiments on receptor function in membrane or cell preparations do not permit, therefore, a clear distinction between receptor properties originating from environmental modulation and those intrinsic to the receptor. Similarly, structural characterization of receptors, required to obtain a molecular understanding of their function, is difficult to perform in intact membranes. Solubilization and purification of receptors, and investigation of their function in defined environments, constitute major aims in receptor research. In this paper, we describe: (1) the solubilization of active VIP receptors from guinea pig lung and chromatographic separation of two molecular species of the receptors; (2) a role for phospholipids and GTP-binding proteins (G-proteins) in conferring high affinity and VIP selectivity to

[a] Supported by National Institutes of Health Grants HL-35506 (S.P.) and HL-35656 (S.I.S.) and Veterans Association research funds (S.I.S.).

[b] Current address: Department of Pharmacology, University of Nebraska Medical Center, Omaha, NE 68105-1065.

[c] Current address: VA West Los Angeles Medical Center, Los Angeles, CA 90073.

[d] Current address: Department of Medicine, University of Illinois, P.O. Box 6988, Chicago, IL 60680.

the receptors; and (3) some of the characteristics of VIP-receptor coupling with adenylate cyclase.

METHODS

$[^{125}I]VIP$

Purified porcine VIP was labeled with $Na^{125}I$ by the chloramine-T method and purified to a specific activity of 2.26 Ci/μmole by reverse-phase HPLC.[8]

Lung Membranes

Crude membranes from guinea pig lung were prepared according to Paul and Said,[9] except that: (1) before homogenization, the lungs were perfused[10] *in situ* with Krebs buffer, pH 7.4, (8 ml/min; total volume 50-100 ml) through the pulmonary artery, using a Harvard pump (Model 1045) and rodent respirator (Model 680) supplying room air enriched with 95% O_2/5% CO_2; and (2) homogenization of lungs was in five volumes of 10 mM Trizma, pH 7.2, containing 0.25 M sucrose, 100 units aprotinin/ml, 5 μM pepstatin A (Sigma, St. Louis, MO), 100 μM phenylmethylsulfonyl fluoride (Sigma) and 1 mM EDTA (sodium salt), by two 30-second bursts of a Biohomogenizer (10,000 rpm, Model M133/1281-0; Biospec Products, Bartlesville, OK).

Solubilization and Chromatography of VIP Receptors

Lung membranes (10-15 mg protein/ml) were treated with the detergent 3-[(3-cholamidopropyl)dimethylammonio]-1-propanesulfonate](CHAPS; 9 mM) as described previously.[9] The detergent was diluted to 3 mM, the soluble extract was centrifuged (160,000 $\times$ g, 30 min at 4°C) and the supernatent passed through a 0.22 μM Millipore filter. Chromatography of this soluble extract was on a high-performance Protein-pak 300 sw column (Waters, Milford, MA) in buffers containing different concentrations of CHAPS.[11] The column was calibrated with marker proteins [ferritin, catalase, aldolase, bovine serum albumin (BSA), ovalbumin, and ribonuclease] using the chromatographic conditions employed for the soluble lung extract.

$[^{125}I]VIP$ Receptor Binding

$[^{125}I]$VIP binding to membrane and solubilized receptor fractions was assayed in triplicate as described previously.[9,11] The binding was corrected for nonspecifically associated radioactivity determined in the presence of 1 μM VIP for the membrane and solubilized 5.9 nm Stokes radius fraction, and 10 μM VIP or 3 μM rat GRF for the 2.3-nm Stokes radius fraction. Pretreatment of the membrane preparations (10 mg protein/ml of homogenization buffer) with an equal volume of phospholipase A_2 (*Crotalus durissus terrificus* venom; Sigma) or phospholipase C (*Bacillus cereus*, Grade 1; Boehringer Mannheim GmbH, W. Germany) dissolved in 50 mM Trizma, pH 7.2, containing 5 mM MgCl$_2$ and 1% BSA (RIA grade; Sigma) was for 10 minutes at 23°C. Phospholipase pretreatment of the solubilized receptors was done similarly, except that the receptor fractions (200-400 μg protein/ml) were in 50 mM Trizma, pH 7.2, containing 5 mM MgCl$_2$ and 3 mM or 9 mM CHAPS. The enzyme-treated receptor preparations were then assayed directly for specific VIP binding.

Cyclic AMP Synthesis

Lung membranes (~20 μg protein) or solubilized lung extracts (~50 μg protein) were incubated in quadruplicate for 10 minutes at 37°C in a shaking bath in a final volume of 100 μl of 50 mM Trizma, pH 7.4, containing 5 mM MgCl$_2$, 1 mM EDTA, 2 mM IBMX, 10 mM phospho(enol)pyruvate, 0.2 mM ATP, 40 units pyruvate kinase/ml and 100 nM GTP. In some experiments, forskolin (Sigma) was included in the incubation mixture. Blanks consisted of incubation without lung membranes or solubilized extracts. The reaction was terminated by addition of 250 μl each of 0.1 M zinc sulfate and 0.1 M sodium carbonate, and the tubes kept for 3-18 hours at -80°C. The samples were then thawed at 37°C and centrifuged at 2,000 $\times$ g. Aliquots (250 μl) of the supernatants were withdrawn and the cyclic AMP was acetylated with 15 μl of an acetic anhydride : triethylamine mixture (1 : 2). The cyclic AMP was measured by radioimmunoassay. For this purpose, a radioactive tracer was prepared by mixing 20 μl 0.5 M sodium phosphate, pH 7.4, 1 mCi Na^{125}I (NEN, Boston, MA), 0.8 μg 2′O-succinyl cyclic AMP tyrosine methyl ester (TME-ScAMP; Sigma) dissolved in 20 μl 5 mM sodium acetate, pH 4.75, and 5 μg chloramine T(5 μl) for 60 seconds. Fifty micrograms sodium metabisulfite (50 μl) was then added, and the iodination mixture passed through a Seppak-C18 cartridge (Waters) that had been preequilibrated with 5 ml 60% methanol in 5 mM sodium phosphate, pH 4.0 (solvent B) followed by 10 ml 5 mM sodium phosphate, pH 4.0 (solvent A). The cartridge was washed with 10 ml solvent A, and bound radioactivity eluted with 3 ml solvent B. The eluate was concentrated to 0.5 ml under dry air, and then chromatographed on a Novapak C18 column (Waters) using a gradient of 10% to 65% methanol over 40 minutes. Radioactivity in the effluent was measured by a flow-through Beckman detector (Model 170) attenuated with one piece of lead foil. The purified [^{125}I]cyclic-AMP analogue fractions were pooled and stored in aliquots at -80°C. Radioimmunoassay (RIA) of cyclic AMP[12] was in a final volume of 400 μl of 50 mM sodium acetate, pH 4.75, containing 10 mg/ml BSA, using doubling concentrations from 0.039 to 10 pmol/ml cyclic AMP (Sigma; acetylated under the conditions used for the samples) as standard, 10-15 $\times$ 10^3 CPM [^{125}I]TME-ScAMP tracer and 1 : 100K (final dilution) of a specific sheep antiserum to TME-ScAMP conjugated to BSA. The RIA tubes were incubated for 18-24 hours at 4°C. One milliliter of 0.02% dextran T-70 (Pharmacia, Piscataway, NJ), 8 mg/ml charcoal (Norit A; Pfanstiehl, Waukegan, IL), and 10 mg/ml BSA in 100 mM potassium phosphate, pH 6.3, was added, the tubes incubated for 20 minutes at 40°C, centrifuged (2,000 $\times$ g, 10 min). The supernatants, separated by careful decantation, were counted for radioactivity. Data reduction was with a DP-5500 computer (Model 5500). Unknown values were obtained from the standard curve constructed by plotting logit B/BO versus log dose.

RESULTS AND DISCUSSION

Solubilization of VIP Receptors

We used a zwitterionic detergent, CHAPS, to solubilize VIP receptors from guinea pig lung.[9] Maximal solubilization of specific VIP-binding activity occurred by brief treatment (15 min) of lung membranes with 12 mM CHAPS. The solubilized binding activity was best preserved by diluting CHAPS to 3 mM before recovery of the solubilized fraction by ultracentrifugation. Detergent solubilization of receptors takes place by progressive displacement of receptor-bound phospholipids by detergent molecules. Phospholipid moieties are probably crucial in maintaining receptor activity (see below), and it is not surprising that prolonged treatment of the solubilized material at high CHAPS concentration produced a loss in VIP-receptor activity.

Receptor Size and Affinity

The solubilized lung extracts contained two discrete forms of specific VIP-binding activity that were separated by high-performance gel filtration chromatography.[11] The Stokes radii of the two receptor species, deduced from a comparison with the elution position of marker proteins, were 5.9 nm and 2.3 nm. When decreased CHAPS (9 mM instead of 12 mM) and membranes (10 mg/protein/ml) from perfused instead of unperfused lung were employed in the solubilization step, the binding activity appeared almost entirely as the 5.9 nm Stokes radius fraction after gel filtration in 3 mM CHAPS (TABLE 1). A decreased detergent to membrane protein ratio during solubilization appears to favor recovery of the intact 5.9-nm receptor species, therefore. Pretreatment of the solubilized extract at 9 mM CHAPS (10 min at 23°C) followed by gel filtration in eluent containing 9 mM CHAPS, caused most of the VIP binding (93%) to appear in the 2.3-nm Stokes radius fraction. The use of 6 mM CHAPS during pretreatment and chromatography resulted in nearly evenly distributed binding activity in the two fractions. The 5.9-nm receptor species was stable enough to rechromatograph in 3 mM CHAPS, but when rechromatographed in 9 mM CHAPS, it was partially dissociated to produce the 2.3-nm species.[11]

[^{125}I]VIP binding by the two receptor fractions was saturable, as shown by competition with progressively increasing concentrations of unlabeled VIP.[11] Scatchard analysis of the competition data suggested a high VIP-binding affinity for the 5.9-nm species (K_D: 300 pM), and a very low affinity for the 2.3-nm species (K_D: 957 nM). The Scatchard plots were linear, suggesting a single class of binding sites in each of the receptor fractions. These observations suggest: (1) the low-affinity 2.3-nm complex is produced by dissociation of the high-affinity 5.9-nm complex; (2) the high-affinity complex, a stable species if detergent treatment is held low, may represent the VIP-

TABLE 1. Characteristics of Solubilized VIP Receptors[a]

Stokes Radius[b]	IC$_{50}$, nM[1]		Inhibition by GTP, Percent[b]	Percent Preponderance[c] in:		
	VIP	GRF		3 mM CHAPS	6 mM CHAPS	9 mM CHAPS
5.9 nm	0.2	5.5	61	93	39	8
2.3 nm	1203.0	53.0	0	4	61	90

[a] The solubilized lung extract, originally in 3 mM CHAPS, was kept at different detergent concentrations for 10 minutes (23°C) in a shaking bath and then chromatographed on a Protein-pak 300SW gel filtration column. The concentration of CHAPS in the eluent was the one employed for pretreatment. Stokes radii of the specific VIP-binding fractions were deduced from a comparison of elution positions with marker proteins. IC$_{50}$ values were from competition experiments using unlabeled peptides to displace [^{125}I]VIP binding. Percent inhibition of specific binding by GTP was obtained by inclusion of a 10^{-4} M concentration of the nucleotide in the receptor assay.
[b] From Paul & Said.[11]
[c] Represents specific binding as percent of total binding activity recovered in the Protein-pak 300SW column fractions.

responsive receptor complex present on cell membranes *in situ;* and (3) dynamic receptor transitions *in situ,* analogous to the observed conversion of the solubilized high-affinity receptor complex to a disaggregated receptor, may account for the two affinity states of the VIP receptor detected[13,15] in cell and membrane preparations.

Receptor Affinity and Selectivity: Modulation by G-Proteins and Phospholipids

VIP was more potent than rat GRF in displacing high-affinity [^{125}I]VIP binding to the solubilized 5.9-nm complex, whereas GRF was more potent than VIP in displacing the low-affinity binding to the disaggregated 2.3-nm species (TABLE 1). Thus, the 2.3-nm receptor is GRF-preferring, although it is the apparent binding subunit in the VIP-preferring 5.9-nm complex. Several investigators[16–19] have observed that GTP and phospholipase treatment decrease the binding of VIP and other ligands to membrane preparations. Solubilization and disaggregation can be expected to reduce or disturb interactions of the VIP-binding subunit with G-proteins and phospholipids. To compare receptor interactions with these regulatory agents in the two solubilized fractions, we measured VIP binding with and without treatment of the receptors with GTP, phospholipase A$_2$ (PLA$_2$), or phospholipase C (PLC). Increasing GTP concentrations progressively reduced the VIP binding by the 5.9-nm fraction, apparently due to a decrease in binding affinity.[11] On the other hand, the nucleotide was without effect on VIP binding by the 2.3-nm fraction. Pretreatment with PLA$_2$ or PLC decreased the binding by the 5.9-nm complex, and the effect of PLA$_2$ was enhanced in the presence of 5 mM CaCl$_2$ (FIG. 1). In contrast, pretreatment with either enzyme increased the binding by the 2.3-nm receptor (FIG. 2), and the increases became progressively greater with increasing concentration of CaCl$_2$. The CaCl$_2$ itself was inhibitory for receptor binding. The magnitude of changes in VIP binding by the 5.9-

nm and the 2.3-nm receptors increased with increasing concentration of PLA_2 (5-160 μg/ml) and PLC (1-30 units/ml) used during pretreatment (not shown). Scatchard analyses of data obtained from competitive inhibition experiments suggested that the PLA_2 pretreatment decreased the binding affinity of the 5.9-nm complex, and increased the receptor number in the 2.3-nm fraction. The above observations indicate distinct receptor : G-protein : phospholipid interactions in the 5.9-nm and 2.3-nm binding fractions. This may account for the different affinity and selectivity characteristics of the two receptor fractions.

The presence of CHAPS in the above experiments was a potential confounding factor, since differential detergent binding may be a factor in the observed VIP-binding properties of the solubilized receptors. To assess the impact of G-proteins on phospholipids under more native conditions, we switched to intact lung membranes as the source of receptors. Specific [^{125}I]VIP binding to lung membranes was inhibited by 52% upon inclusion of 0.1 mM GTP in the assay mixture, and by 66% upon pretreatment of the membranes with 20 μg/ml PLA_2. The potency of VIP and rat GRF in displacing [^{125}I]VIP binding to membranes was measured without and with GTP or PLA_2 pretreatment. The ligand selectivity index (SI) of the receptor-binding was obtained as: (IC_{50} GRF/IC_{50} VIP). The IC_{50} of VIP using untreated membranes was lower than that of GRF (SI: 26.3), reflecting the VIP-preferring nature of native receptors (TABLE 2). Exposure of the membranes to GTP or PLA_2 increased the

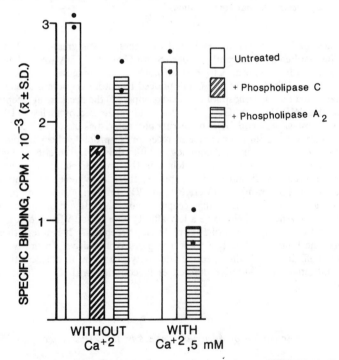

FIGURE 1. Effect of pretreatment with phospholipase C and A_2 on [^{125}I]VIP binding by the 5.9-nm Stokes radius receptor complex. Pretreatment with phospholipase A_2 was done in the absence and presence of 5 mM $CaCl_2$ (see Methods). The values are means of four replicates.

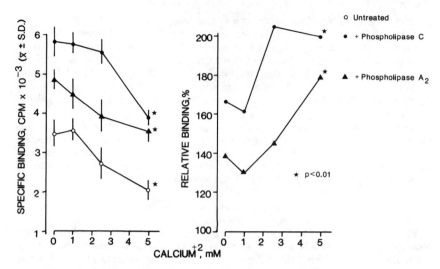

FIGURE 2. Increased [^{125}I]VIP binding by phospholipase C or phospholipase A_2 pretreated 2.3-nm Stokes radius receptors: effect of calcium chloride. The values in the right panel are expressed as percent of the binding obtained without phospholipase A_2 pretreatment at the corresponding calcium chloride concentration.

IC_{50} values for VIP as well as GRF, but the increase was greater for VIP than for GRF. This resulted in significantly reduced SI for GTP- and PLA_2-treated membranes, compared to native membranes ($p < 0.005$). These data suggest: (1) receptor affinity for VIP and GRF is decreased by GTP-induced receptor/G-protein uncoupling, and PLA_2-catalyzed removal phospholipid head groups; (2) the decrease in receptor affinity is greater for VIP than for GRF; (3) this renders the receptors less VIP selective; and (4) the low-affinity and GRF-preferring characteristics of solubilized 2.3-nm VIP receptors may arise from interference in receptor/G-protein/phospholipid coupling.

VIP shows strong amino acid homologies with GRF, PHI, secretin, and glucagon.[20] Although more needs to be done to delineate the precise relationships between the receptors that bind VIP and related peptides, there is evidence for isotypy among these receptors. For example, (1) GRF binds VIP-preferring receptors in the lung[15] and pancreas,[23] but GRF-preferring receptors have been described in the pituitary;[24] and (2) PHI is generally held to be a low-affinity agonist for VIP receptors,[22] but the rat liver contains a population of PHI-preferring receptors.[21] It is interesting to speculate that the binding subunit of these receptors is a relatively primitive molecule, whose high affinity and distinct peptide selectivity properties in different tissues result from quantitative or qualitative differences in coupling with G-proteins and phospholipids.

Activation of Adenylate Cyclase by the VIP Receptor

Previous reports have shown that the binding of VIP to its receptors in cell and membrane preparations is usually accompanied by synthesis of cyclic AMP.[3,22] We measured VIP-responsive cyclic AMP production by guinea pig lung membranes in the absence and presence of GTP, and a recently described[25] VIP antagonist. For this purpose, the membranes were incubated with the test agents in an ATP-regenerating system and a phosphodiesterase inhibitor (IBMX). Cyclic AMP was measured by radioimmunoassay, using an HPLC-purified [^{125}I]cyclic-AMP derivative (Inset, FIG. 3) and a specific antiserum raised against this cyclic AMP derivative. The IC_{50} of this assay was 1.18 ± 0.19 pmol cyclic AMP/ml and sensitivity was 57 ± 26 fmol cyclic AMP/ml ($n = 28$ assays).

Increasing GTP concentration (10^{-8} to 10^{-4} M) progressively stimulated cyclic AMP production by the lung membranes in the absence and presence of VIP (FIG. 4). The stimulation of cyclic AMP production by VIP was greater in the presence of GTP than in its absence. This potentiation of VIP-stimulated cyclic AMP production by GTP indicates that the G-protein coupled to the VIP receptor is Gs (an adenylate cyclase stimulatory G-protein). The stimulation of cyclic AMP production increased progressively with increasing VIP concentrations (IC_{50} 3.3 nM) (FIG. 5). In the presence of an analogue of VIP, [4Cl-D-Phe^6-Leu^{17}]VIP (10 μM), the potency of VIP in stimulating cyclic AMP production was decreased by 9.8-fold (TABLE 3). The VIP analogue displaced [^{125}I]VIP binding to lung membranes with a potency 394-fold lower than that of VIP itself (TABLE 3). These observations suggest: (1) [4Cl-D-Phe^6-Leu^{17}]VIP is a low-affinity antagonist for the VIP receptor expressed in the lung, and (2) cyclic AMP synthesis is at least one of the signals generated by the receptor. The VIP-antagonist was nearly equipotent in displacing [^{125}I]VIP binding by the lung membranes and the solubilized 5.9-nm and 2.3-nm receptor species (IC^{50}: 205 nM). On the other hand, VIP was considerably more potent in displacing [^{125}I]VIP binding to the lung membranes (IC_{50}: 520 pM) and the solubilized 5.9-nm complex (IC_{50}: 240 pM) compared to the 2.3-nm receptor (IC_{50}: 1.2 μM) (TABLE 3). The high VIP-binding affinity of lung membranes and the solubilized 5.9-nm complex is attributable, at least in part, to receptor coupling with G-proteins.[11] In contrast, low-affinity VIP binding by the 2.3-nm receptor appears to be uncoupled from G-protein influence. The observed equipotency of the VIP-analogue in displacing [^{125}I]VIP binding by membranes and the solubilized 5.9-nm complex on the one hand, and the 2.3-nm receptor on the other, suggests that G-proteins do not modulate receptor affinity for the analogue. This conclusion is supported by preliminary observations that the VIP-analogue displaces [^{125}I]VIP binding to lung membranes with nearly equivalent po-

TABLE 2. Ligand Selectivity of VIP Receptors in the Lung: Modulation by G-Proteins and Phospholipids[a]

Membrane Preparation	IC_{50}, nM[b] VIP	GRF	Selectivity Index[c]
Untreated	0.6	15.8	26.3 ± 2.5
GTP-treated[d]	4.0	24.0	5.9 ± 2.0
Phopholipase[e] A$_2$-pretreated	3.4	35.6	10.4 ± 2.6

[a] Values are means of three or more experiments.
[b] Concentration giving 50% inhibition of specific [^{125}I]VIP binding.
[c] (IC_{50} GRF)/(IC_{50} VIP).
[d] 10^{-4} M GTP was included in the receptor assay.
[e] 20 μg/ml; pretreatment was for 10 minutes at 23°C.

tency in the absence and presence of 10^{-4} M GTP. Since activation of G-proteins is generally associated with GTP-mediated reduction in receptor binding, the observed insensitivity of binding of the VIP analogue suggests a lack of G-protein activation. This is the likely molecular mechanism for the antagonist action of the VIP analogue. Conversely, these considerations reinforce the importance of receptor-G-protein interactions in expression of the biologic effects of VIP.

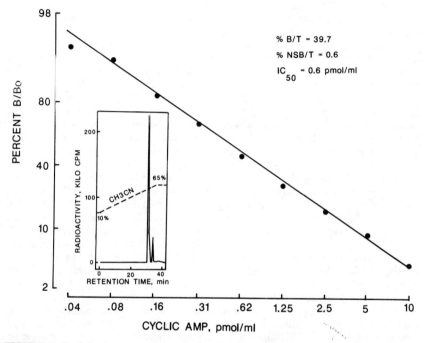

FIGURE 3. Radioimmunoassay for cyclic AMP: a plot showing displacement of [^{125}I]-2'O-succinyl cyclic AMP tyrosine methyl ester ([^{125}I]TME-ScAMP) by increasing concentrations of unlabeled cyclic AMP. Inset shows the purification of [^{125}I]TME-ScAMP by reverse-phase HPLC. The larger, earlier eluting peak of radioactivity (retention time 32.3 min) was used as tracer in the RIA.

Stability of Receptor-G-Protein Coupling

The GTP-sensitive VIP-receptor complex appears to be a stable species if the detergent is maintained at low concentrations. This suggests a stable association of the VIP receptor with a G-protein, probably the G_s (see above). Activation of G_s by the receptor *in situ* may, therefore, be independent of the restricted diffusional opportunities available in the plasma membrane. This would promote fast and efficient signal transduction by the receptor, since random collision between Gs and the receptor would not be a prerequisite for activation of cyclic AMP synthesis. In preliminary

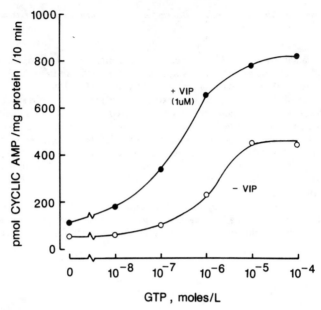

FIGURE 4. Effect of increasing concentrations of GTP on basal and VIP-stimulated cyclic AMP production by lung membranes. Values are means of four replicates from a representative experiment.

experiments, we observed that pretreatment with phospholipase A_2 or C attenuates the inhibitory effect of GTP on specific VIP binding by lung membranes. This suggests that the receptor-G-protein coupling is phospholipid-dependent. Detergents delipidate the receptors, and high detergent concentrations render the solubilized VIP receptors refractory to inhibition by GTP. These considerations are consistent with a critical role for phospholipids in maintaining stable VIP receptor-G-protein coupling.

TABLE 3. Receptor Binding and Antagonist Properties of the VIP Analogue, [4Cl-D-Phe[6]-Leu[17]] VIP[a]

| Receptor Fraction | IC$_{50}$, nM | | SD$_{50}$, nM VIP | |
	VIP	VIP Analogue[b]	Without VIP Analogue	With VIP Analogue[a]
Membranes	0.5	336	3.3	32.3
5.9 nm[b]	0.2	202		
2.3 nm[b]	1203.0	216		

[a] Values are means of two or more experiments each. IC$_{50}$ and ED$_{50}$ values are, respectively, the concentrations giving 50% inhibition of specific [^{125}I]VIP binding and 50% stimulation of cyclic AMP production (SD$_{50}$).

[b] Stokes radius of solubilized receptors.

[c] 10 μM.

Receptor-Adenylate Cyclase Interaction in Solubilized Lung Extracts

Because an apparently stable VIP receptor-G-protein (R : G) complex was present in the solubilized lung extract, it was of interest to investigate functional coupling of R : G to the catalytic activity of adenylate cyclase (AC). For this purpose, cyclic AMP produced by the solubilized lung extract in the absence and presence of sodium fluoride, forskolin, GTP, and/or VIP was measured. Successful solubilization of AC was indicated by a progressive increase in cyclic AMP levels with increasing incubation period (FIG. 6), and by an increase in cyclic AMP levels in the presence of forskolin or sodium fluoride (16 mM). These agents stimulate AC directly, bypassing G-proteins and receptors. Neither VIP (FIG. 6) nor GTP (10^{-8} to 10^{-3} M) stimulated cyclic AMP production by the solubilized extract. VIP was also without effect on cyclic AMP production in the presence of forskolin, an agent that is reported to potentiate adenylate cyclase stimulation by other hormones.[26] These data suggest that the solubilized R : G complex (or G alone) was unable to stimulate AC. This may reflect inactivation or nonsolubilization of essential factors required for coupling of AC with R : G or G.

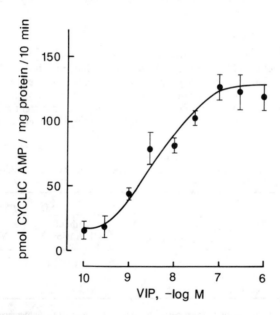

FIGURE 5. Effect of increasing concentrations of VIP on cyclic AMP production by lung membranes. Values, means ± SD from a representative experiment, are corrected for the basal cyclic AMP level measured in the absence of VIP (43 pmol/mg protein/10 min).

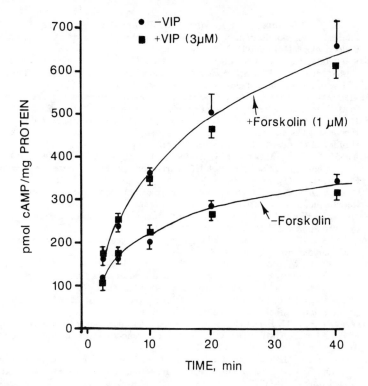

FIGURE 6. Cyclic AMP production by the solubilized lung extract: lack of effect of VIP. Values are means of six replicates ± SD.

ACKNOWLEDGMENTS

Antibody to cyclic AMP was generously provided by Dr. J. Linden, and the VIP antagonist by Dr. J. Rivier. Dr. L. Olansky helped in standardization of the cyclic AMP RIA. Drs. L. Liu and T. Iwanaga provided the perfused lungs. Skilled technical assistance by Jerry Currie, Nicolas Dominguez, and Georgia Koren, manuscript preparation by Janet Cottrell and Jan Gamble, and preparation of illustrations by Suzie Carter and George O'Shea is acknowledged.

REFERENCES

1. ROBBERECHT, P., K. TATEMOTO, P. CHATELAIN, M. WAELBROECK, M. DELHAYE, G. TATON, P. DE NEEF, J -C. CAMUS, D. HEUSE & J. CHRISTOPHE. 1982. Effects of PHI on vasoactive intestinal peptide receptors and adenylate cyclase activity in lung membranes. A comparison in man, rat, mouse and guinea pig. Regul. Pept. **4:** 241-250.

2. LEROUX, P., H. VAUDRY, A. FOURNIER, S. ST.-PIERRE & G. PELLETIER. 1984. Characterization and localization of vasoactive intestinal peptide receptors in the rat lung. Endocrinology **114:** 1506-1512.

3. ROBBERECHT, P., P. CHATELAIN, P. DE NEEF, J.-C. CAMUS, M. WAELBROECK & J. CHRISTOPHE. 1982. Presence of vasoactive intestinal peptide receptors coupled to adenyl cyclase in rat lung membranes. Biophys. Biochem. Acta **678:** 76-82.

4. MATSUZAKI, Y., Y. HAMASAKI & S. I. SAID. 1980. Vasoactive intestinal peptide: A possible transmitter of non-adrenergic relaxation of guinea pig airways. Science **210:** 1252-1253.

5. SAID, S. I. & DEY, R. D. 1988. VIP in the airways. *In* The Airways: Neural Control in Health and Disease. M. A. Kaliner & P. Barnes, Eds.: 395-416. *In* Lung Biology in Health and Disease. C. Lenfant, Exec. Editor. Marcel Dekker, Inc. New York.

6. RUFF, M. R., B. M. MARTIN, E. I. GINNS, W. L. FARRAR & C. B. PERT. 1987. CD4 receptor binding peptides that block HIV infectivity cause human monocyte chemotaxis. FEBS Lett. **211(1):** 17-22.

7. GAULTON, G. N. & M. I. GREENE. 1986. Idiotypic mimicry of biological receptors. Ann. Rev. Immunol. **4:** 253-280.

8. PAUL, S., K. WOOD & S. I. SAID. 1984. Purification of [^{125}I]-vasoactive intestinal peptide by reverse-phase HPLC. Peptides **5:** 1085-1087.

9. PAUL, S. & S. I. SAID. 1986. Solubilization of active receptors for VIP from guinea pig lung. Peptides **7**(Suppl. 1): 147-149.

10. HAMASAKI, Y., M. MOJARAD, T. SAGA, H. TAI & S. I. SAID. 1984. Platelet activating factor raises airway and vascular pressures and induces edema in lungs perfused with platelet free solution. Am. Rev. Respir. Dis. **129:** 742-746.

11. PAUL, S. & S. I. SAID. 1987. Characterization of receptors for vasoactive intestinal peptide from the lung. J. Biol. Chem. **262:** 158-162.

12. HARPER, J. F. & G. BROOKER. 1975. Femtomole sensitive radioimmunoassay of cyclic AMP and cyclic GMP after 2'O acetylation by acetic anhydride in aqueous solution. Adv. Cyclic Nucleotide Res. **1:** 207-218.

13. BISSONNETTE, B. M., M. J. COLLEN, H. ADACHI, R. T. JENSEN & J. D. GARDNER. 1984. Receptors for vasoactive intestinal peptide and secretin on rat pancreatic acini. Am. J. Physiol. **246:** G710-G717.

14. INOUE, Y., K. KAKU, T. KANEKO, N. YANAIHARA & T. KANNO. 1985. Vasoactive intestinal peptide binding to specific receptors on rat parotid acinar cells induces amylase secretion accompanied by intracellular accumulation of cyclic adenosine 3'-5'-monophosphate. Endocrinology **116:** 686-692.

15. DICKINSON, K. E. J., M. SCHACHTER, C. M. M. MILES, D. H. COY & P. S. SEVER. 1986. Characterization of vasoactive intestinal peptide (VIP) receptors in mammalian lung. Peptides **7:** 791-800.

16. RAMIREZ-CARDENAS, R., J. C. PRIETO, J. M. GUERRERO & R. GOBERNA. 1981. Guanyl nucleotide regulation of vasoactive intestinal peptide interaction with rat liver membranes. Revista Espanola de Fisiologia **37:** 9-16.

17. LEVITZKI, A. 1984. Receptor to effector coupling in the receptor-dependent adenylate cyclase system. J. Recept. Res. **4:** 399-409.

18. SARRIEAU, A., N. BOIGE & M. LABURTHE. 1985. Role of phospholipids in the binding activity of vasoactive intestinal peptide receptors. Experientia **41:** 631-633.

19. MCCALEB, M. L. & D. B. DONNER. 1981. Affinity of the hepatic insulin receptor is influenced by membrane phospholipids. J. Biol. Chem. **256:** 11051-11057.

20. MILLER, R. J. 1984. PHI and GRF: Two new members of the glucagon/secretin family. Med. Biol. **61:** 159-162.

21. PAUL, S., J. CHOU, E. KUBOTA & S. I. SAID. 1987. High-affinity peptide-histidine-isoleucine preferring receptors in rat liver membranes. Life Sci. **41:** 2373-2380.

22. DESBUQUOIS, B. 1985. Receptors for gastrointestinal peptides. *In* Receptors and Ligands in Intercellular Communication. B. Cinader & B. I. Posner, Eds. **4:** 419-479. Marcel Dekker, Inc. New York.

23. PANDOL, S. J., H. SEIFERT, M. W. THOMAS, J. RIVIER & W. VALE. 1984. Growth hormone-releasing factor stimulates pancreatic enzyme secretion. Science **225:** 326-328.

24. SEIFERT, H., M. PERRIN, J. RIVIER & W. VALE. 1985. Binding sites for growth hormone releasing factor on rat pituitary cells. Nature **313:** 487-489.
25. PANDOL, S. J., K. DHARMSATHAPHORN, M. SCHOEFFIELD, W. VALE & J. RIVIER. 1986. Vasoactive intestinal peptide receptor antagonist [4Cl-D-Phe^6,Leu^{17}]VIP. Am. J. Physiol. **250:** G553-G557.
26. DALY, W. 1984. Forskolin, adenylate cyclase and cell physiology: An overview. Adv. Cyclic Nucleotide Protein Phosphor. Res. **17:** 81-89.

Molecular Analysis of Vasoactive Intestinal Peptide Receptors

A Comparison with Receptors for VIP-Related Peptides

MARC LABURTHE AND ALAIN COUVINEAU

Equipe de Neuroendocrinologie du Système Digestif
Institut National de la Santé et de la Recherche Médicale
INSERM U1 78
94807 Villejuif Cedex, France

The vasoactive intestinal peptide (VIP) is a neuropeptide with widespread distribution and action in the organism.[1] In consonance with the ubiquitous role of VIP as an information-bearing peptide, VIP receptors have been identified in many tissues where they are positively coupled to adenylate cyclase.[1] By using membrane fusion techniques, VIP receptors from one cell line have been transferred to adenylate cyclase of another cell line devoid of VIP receptors demonstrating that receptors and adenylate cyclase are two physically distinct proteins.[2] For activating the enzyme, VIP receptors communicate with G proteins.[3] Indeed, GTP enhances the dissociation of VIP from its receptors[4] and is a mandatory cofactor for VIP stimulation of adenylate cyclase.[5] VIP receptors have undergone extensive physiological and pharmacological characterization,[1] but their molecular properties have been investigated only recently.

MOLECULAR IDENTIFICATION OF VIP RECEPTORS BY COVALENT CROSS-LINKING

Preliminary work involving attack of plasma membranes by proteases[6] and phospholipases[7] or modification of membrane fluidity[8] indicated that VIP receptors are proteins whose activity is modulated by membrane phospholipids.

At the same time, cross-linking procedures have been developed to analyze the molecular characteristics of VIP receptors in rat intestinal epithelium[9] and thereafter in several other target tissues (TABLE 1). Various cross-linking patterns have been reported with regard to the molecular weight of the major VIP binding protein and

---

[a] Address for correspondence: Dr. Marc Laburthe, Equipe de Neuroendocrinologie du Système Digestif, Institut National de la Santé et de la Recherche Médicale, INSERM U178, 16 avenue Paul Vaillant Couturier, 94807 Villejuif Cedex, France.

TABLE 1. Molecular Characteristics of VIP Receptors from Different Tissues and Species: Analysis by Covalent Cross-Linking

Tissue	Species	Cross-linker[a]	Molecular Weight[b]		Reference
			Major	Minor	
Intestinal epithelium (Membranes)	Rat	DTSP	73 (high affinity)	33 (low affinity)	9
Colonic epithelium (Membranes)	Human	DTSP	63 (high affinity)	30 (low affinity)	10
Liver (Membranes)	Rat	DTSP	48	86	11
	Rat	DTSP, DSS, HSAB	53	77	12
Brain (Membranes)	Rat	DTSP	46	57	13
	Rat	DSS	47	72	14
Lymphoblast (Molt 4bT) (Cells)	Human	DSS, EGS SANAH	47		15
Colon cancer (HT-29) (Membranes)	Human	DTSP	63		16
(Cells)		DTSP	64	117; 31	17
Pituitary tumor (GH₃) (Cells)	Rat	DSS, EGS	47		18
Lung (Membranes)	Human	DSS	62		19
	Rat		53		
	Rabbit		61		
	Guinea pig		63; 57		

[a] Abbreviations used: DTSP, dithiobis(succinimidyl propionate); DSS, dissuccinimidyl suberate; HSAB, N-hydroxysuccinimidyl 4-azidobenzoate; EGS, ethylene glycol bis(succinimidyl succinate); SANAH, N-succinimidyl 6-(4'-azido-2'-nitrophenylamino)hexanoate.

[b] After covalent cross-linking of [^{125}I]VIP to membrane proteins, SDS-PAGE analysis of solubilized proteins often reveals the presence of several bands corresponding to specific [^{125}I]VIP-protein complexes. We have indicated here the molecular weights (expressed in kDa) of the major and minor VIP binding proteins after substraction of the VIP molecular weight (3 kDa) assuming that one molecule of VIP is cross-linked per binding protein.

the presence of minor binding components. Major binding proteins have molecular weights ranging from 46,000 to 73,000 depending on tissues and species (TABLE 1) and display the high affinity and peptide specificity of the VIP receptor. The significance of minor components may be different depending on the models studied. In intestinal epithelium, minor binding proteins display the properties of a low-affinity binding site (TABLE 1). In rat liver, Nguyen et al.[12] suggested that a M_r 77,000 component is the true VIP receptor that would generate a M_r 53,000 product through proteolysis. Alternatively, we have suggested that the minor M_r 86,000 component identified in rat liver (see TABLE 1) could be the M_r 48,000 receptor cross-linked to a subunit of a G protein or to a still unknown polypeptide closely associated with the receptor.[11]

It is not yet clear whether the different cross-linking patterns observed are related to the various experimental conditions used or indicate actual heterogeneity of receptor proteins. As far as experimental conditions are concerned, it may be stressed that: (1) Proteolysis or deglycosylation of receptors may occur during preparation and/or incubation of biological samples.[12] (2) The use of various cross-linkers with different spans, reactive moeities, or abilities to permeate membranes may result or not in the cross-linking of receptors to neighboring proteins. However, this may not explain why different results are obtained using the same cross-linkers (TABLE 1). (3) The use of different biological preparations, for example membranes versus intact cells, may also play a role.[20] Recent experiments performed on membrane-bound and solubilized receptors emphasize the importance of receptor environment and accessibility for cross-linking reactions.[21] Alternatively, cross-linking experiments may have revealed authentic molecular heterogeneity of VIP receptors according to tissues and/or species. This may be due to a number of possible conditions. (1) Several different proteins may bear the VIP recognition site. A definitive answer for this possibility has to wait for the complete purification of receptors or the determination of gene structure encoding for receptors from various sources. (2) Differentially glycosylated forms of the same receptor may be present in situ. This is suggested by the fact that treatment with neuraminidase of different forms of lung receptors results in a single homogeneous form.[19] Different glycosylation of the insulin receptor in different tissues has been previously demonstrated.[22] (3) There may be covalent alteration of receptors, such as in phosphorylation. A recent observation indicating that VIP receptors are regulated by phorbol ester, an activator of protein kinase C, suggests that they may be phosphorylated under physiological conditions.[23] Other receptor-coupled adenylate cyclase systems such as the beta-adrenergic receptor have been shown to undergo phosphorylation, thereby altering their mobility in SDS-polyacrylamide gels.[24]

Although further experiments are needed to assess whether or not VIP receptors are structurally heterogeneous, various observations point out their functional heterogeneity. Thus, they display different pharmacological properties according to tissues[25] and species.[26,27] Furthermore, their coupling with the adenylate cyclase system is different from one tissue to another. For example, VIP is moderately efficient, though very potent, in activating adenylate cyclase in rat liver, whereas it is an efficient activator of the enzyme in rat intestine (reviewed in Couvineau & Laburthe[11]).

The cross-linking technique has been a fruitful approach in the molecular analysis of VIP receptors but displays several limitations for ultimate purification of functional receptors. Cross-linking of peptides to their receptors usually has a low yield, that is, $< 10\%$,[9,28] which is poorly compatible with further purification of the covalent peptide-receptor complex. Moreover, such irreversible complexes are not physiologically relevant and are usually analyzed in denaturing detergent solutions by SDS-PAGE (TABLE 1). Therefore, in order to document the nature and molecular form(s) of VIP receptors in a functional state and with the ultimate goal of purifying the receptor, we have recently developed the solubilization of functional receptors in nondenaturing detergent solutions.[21]

SOLUBILIZATION OF FUNCTIONAL VIP RECEPTORS

Liver is a convenient organ for studies aimed at the solubilization and purification of VIP receptors since this tissue contains a high concentration of receptors above 1 pmol/mg of membrane protein.[12,29] We have therefore tried to solubilize VIP-receptor complexes from rat liver plasma membranes.[21] Membranes are incubated with 3 nM [^{125}I]VIP at equilibrium and membrane proteins are then solubilized with 1% Triton X-100. Chromatography of solubilized material on Sephacryl S-300 (FIG. 1) reveals two peaks of radioactivity: a major one (80%) and a minor one (20%) with Stokes radii of 5.8 nm and 3.0 nm, respectively. Both components are specifically labeled since they almost completely disappear when 0.3 μM unlabeled VIP is added with [^{125}I]VIP (FIG 1). The sedimentation coefficient ($s_{20,w}$) of each component is determined by ultracentrifugation on sucrose gradients (FIG. 2). The major component migrates with a $s_{20,w}$ of 6.0 s while the minor one migrates with a $s_{20,w}$ of 4.0 s. Identical results are obtained from gradients made up in D_2O suggesting that the two components have bound a small amount of detergent.[21] From these results it is possible to calculate the molecular weight of the two components, that is, 150,000 (heavy) and 52,000 (light) for the major and minor one, respectively (FIG. 3). Their biological significance has been investigated using GTP, which regulates VIP binding to liver membranes.[29,30] GTP induces a rapid dissociation of [^{125}I]VIP from the heavy component, whereas it does not affect the stability of the light one (FIG. 4). Similarly, when GTP is added with each component in sucrose gradients, the heavy one ($s_{20,w}$ = 6.0 s) is no longer observed after ultracentrifugation, whereas the light one ($s_{20,w}$ = 4.0 s) is unaffected (FIG. 2). These results and other observations[21] suggest that the heavy species of M_r 150,000 consists of the VIP receptor of M_r 52,000 associated with a G protein, probably G_s. This is further supported by the ability of the M_r 150,000 species to generate the M_r 52,000 one after mild urea treatment.[21] Furthermore, the G_s protein specifically labeled by cholera toxin-catalyzed [^{32}P]ADP ribosylation is coeluted with the M_r 150,000 species on Sephacryl S-300.[21]

The solubilization of [^{125}I]VIP-labeled liver membranes has revealed the existence of a major ternary complex (M_r 150,000) consisting of VIP, the receptor and a G protein.[21] The GTP-induced dissociation of VIP from this ternary complex (FIG. 2) demonstrates the functional properties of both receptor and G protein and their physical interaction in solution. A minor VIP-receptor complex of M_r 52,000 that is not sensitive to GTP is also observed (FIG. 3). It is very similar to the putative VIP binding protein of M_r 51,000 (including VIP) identified by SDS-PAGE analysis after cross-linking of [^{125}I]VIP to liver membranes.[11] When the cross-linking reaction is carried out on the Triton-solubilized material from membranes preloaded with [^{125}I]VIP, this M_r 51,000 component becomes minor while a major M_r 150,000 band is observed (FIG. 5), likely corresponding to the VIP-receptor-G protein complex described above. The difference observed in the two conditions can be tentatively ascribed to the fact that the site of interaction between the receptor and the G protein is not freely accessible to the cross-linker in intact membranes.[21] Whatever the conditions of cross-linking, a minor M_r 89,000 band is observed (FIG. 5), but its nature remains conjectural (see above).

Two groups have recently reported the solubilization of unoccupied VIP receptors.[31,32] [^{125}I]VIP was shown to bind solubilized material obtained from Lubrol-treated rat liver membranes.[31] The M_r of the binding protein has been estimated at 80,000 by chromatography on Sepharose 6B.[31] Unfortunately, these results cannot be compared to our results since molecular sieving alone often yields a very imprecise estimate of molecular mass for hydrophobic membrane proteins.[33] Furthermore the sensitivity to GTP of the solubilized protein has not been investigated.[31] At any rate, these experiments support the possibility of solubilizing active, unoccupied VIP receptors. In a recent work, VIP receptors from guinea pig lung have been solubilized using the detergent CHAPS.[32] By molecular sieving two binding components are identified with Stokes radii of 5.9 nm and 2.3 nm. The major 5.9-nm component has a high affinity for VIP and, in the presence of high detergent concentration, generates the 2.3-nm

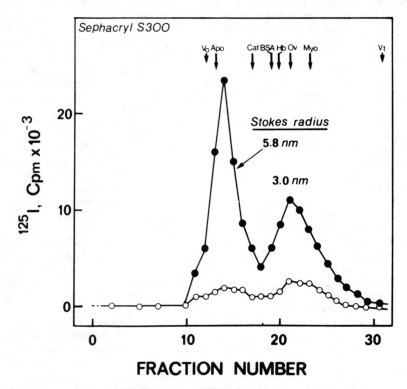

FIGURE 1. Chromatography of solubilized [^{125}I]VIP-receptor complexes on Sephacryl S-300. Rat liver membranes are incubated with [^{125}I]VIP in the absence (●) or presence (○) of 0.3 μM unlabeled VIP. Membranes proteins solubilized with 1% Triton X-100 are then applied to a Sephacryl S-300 column (60 × 0.9 cm) and fractions of 1 ml are collected. The column is calibrated with proteins of known Stokes radius, apoferritin (Apo), 6.1 nm; catalase (Cat), 5.2 nm; bovine serum albumin (BSA), 3.55 nm; hemoglobin (Hb), 3.2 nm; ovalbumin (Ov), 3.05 nm; and myoglobin (Myo), 1.9 nm. For details see Couvineau et al.[21]

component, which has a low affinity for the peptide. GTP inhibits the binding of [^{125}I]VIP to the 5.9-nm component but not the 2.3-nm one.[32] Although sedimentation coefficients and the amount of receptor-bound detergent are not determined,[32] the major component solubilized from guinea pig lung by CHAPS compares well, with respect to Stokes radius and sensitivity to GTP, to the ternary complex of M_r 150,000 (Stokes radius = 5.8 nm) solubilized from rat liver by Triton[21] (also this paper). Therefore, direct solubilization of unoccupied VIP receptors may also result in a

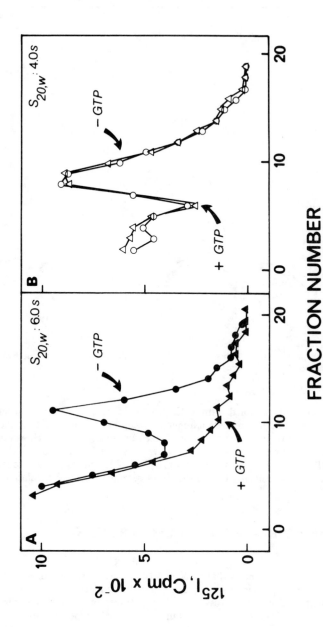

FIGURE 2. Sucrose density gradient ultracentrifugation of [^{125}I]VIP-receptor complexes. The two peaks obtained after gel filtration on Sephacryl are, centrifuged separately in the absence ($\bullet$, $\bigcirc$) or presence ($\blacktriangle$, $\triangle$) of 0.1 mM GTP through a 5–20% sucrose gradient for 16 hours at 43,000 rpm. Fractions of 180 μl are collected from the top of the gradients and their radioactivity determined. Panel A: profile obtained after ultracentrifugation of the [^{125}I]VIP-receptor complex of Stokes radius 5.8 nm. Panel B: profile obtained after ultracentrifugation of the [^{125}I]VIP-receptor complex of Stokes radius 3.0 nm (see Fig. 1). The sedimentation coefficients ($s_{20,w}$) are estimated from a standard curve obtained with proteins of known $s_{20,w}$, that is, cytochrome C (1.71 s); bovine serum albumin (4.6 s); bovine gamma-globin (7.2 s); and catalase (11.4 s). For details, see Couvineau et al.[21]

Parameters	Major Form 80 %	Minor Form 20 %
Stokes Radius , nm	5.8	3.0
Sedimentation Coefficient , S	6.0	4.0
MOLECULAR WEIGHT	150 000	52 000
GTP Regulation	+	−
MODELS		

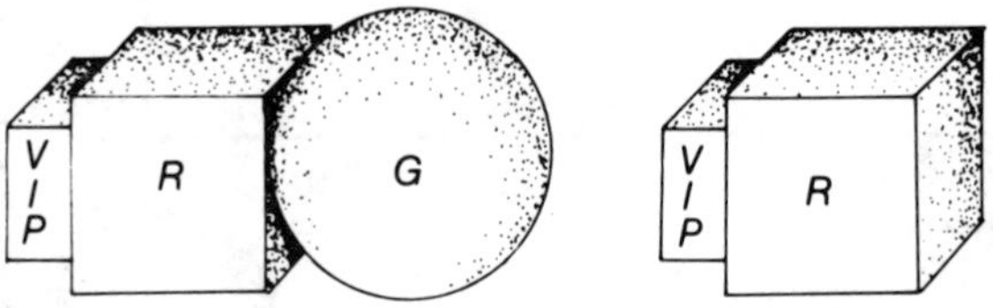

FIGURE 3. Molecular parameters and models of VIP receptors solubilized from rat liver membranes. For details see Couvineau *et al.*[21]

binding protein functionally coupled with a G protein. This could be somewhat surprising since previous studies of beta-adrenergic receptors[34] indicated that the presence of an agonist is a requisite for coupling of receptors to G_s proteins. However this may indicate that VIP receptors are already physically coupled with G proteins in the absence of VIP and the occupancy of receptors by VIP only confers the functional coupling with G protein and thereby the sensitivity of receptors to GTP regulation.

THE VIP RECEPTOR: A GLYCOPROTEIN

Following initial studies indicating that rat liver VIP receptors are glycoproteins,[12] we have analyzed their glycoproteic moiety by using immobilized lectins with different carbohydrate specificities. Solubilized cross-linked [^{125}I]VIP-receptor complexes from rat liver are bound by Pea, WGA, and ConA but not retained by peanut, soybean, and winged Pea (FIG. 6). The interaction with the three former lectins is specific since (1) there is no binding to Sepharose 6B alone; (2) the radioactivity retained on lectins is dramatically decreased in the presence of 0.3 M appropriate sugar (FIG. 6).

The material eluted from active lectins by incubation with specific sugars has been analyzed on SDS-PAGE (FIG. 7). Two components of M_r 51,000 and 89,000 are observed. Similar results are obtained when the cross-linked VIP-receptor complexes from liver membranes are directly submitted to SDS-PAGE (FIG. 7), suggesting that the existence of these two components is not related to qualitative differences in their carbohydrate moiety. The various lectins do not inhibit [125I]VIP binding to liver membranes (not shown) supporting the supposition that the lectin binding sites and the VIP recognition site on VIP receptors are different. Several conclusions may be drawn from our results: (1) The carbohydrate moiety of VIP receptors contains N-acetylglucosamine, mannose, and/or glucose. (2) Galactose, N-acetylgalactosamine, and fucose are absent or not accessible to lectins. Although WGA is generally accepted as rather specific for N-acetylglucosamine or its 1-4 oligomers, it may also interact with sialoglycoproteins,[35] suggesting that sialic acid may be present on VIP receptors. Treatment of cross-linked VIP-receptor complexes from mammalian lung[19] and human colon adenocarcinoma cells[36] with neuraminidase supports this view more directly. An N-glycosidic linkage between N-acetylglucosamine and receptor proteins may exist, the possible presence of mannose favoring this hypothesis. This has been demonstrated by the ability of N-glycosidases to alter the electrophoretic mobility of receptors from rat liver[12] or HT-29 cells.[36] Moreover, the absence of N-acetylgalactosamine residues suggests that no O-linked carbohydrate chain occurs in rat liver VIP receptors in consonance with the absence of effect of endo-H on their electrophoretic mobility.[12]

We have further investigated the use of immobilized lectins in a one-step method for preliminary purification of the liver VIP receptor. FIGURE 8 shows that WGA-Sepharose retains up to 50% of [125I]VIP-receptor complexes solubilized with Triton X-100 as described[21] (also, see above). Thereafter, they can be eluted from WGA by

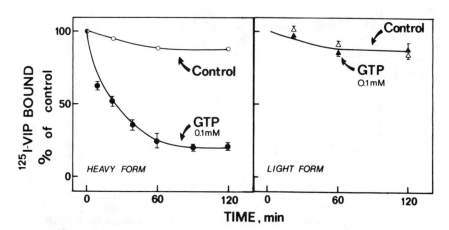

FIGURE 4. Effect of GTP on the dissociation of solubilized [125I]VIP-receptor complexes. Rat liver membranes are incubated with [125I]VIP, solubilized with Triton and separated on Sephacryl S-300 to obtain the solubilized heavy and light components (see FIGS. 1 & 3). Dissociation is initiated by adding to the heavy component (left) or light component (right) 0.3 μM native VIP without ($\triangle$ $\bigcirc$) or with ($\blacktriangle$, $\bullet$) 0.1 mM GTP. Samples are incubated at 30°C for the indicated times and the radioactivity remaining bound to the macromolecular components determined by chromatography on Sephadex G-50 as described by Couvineau et al.[21] Each point is the mean $\pm$ SE of three determinations.

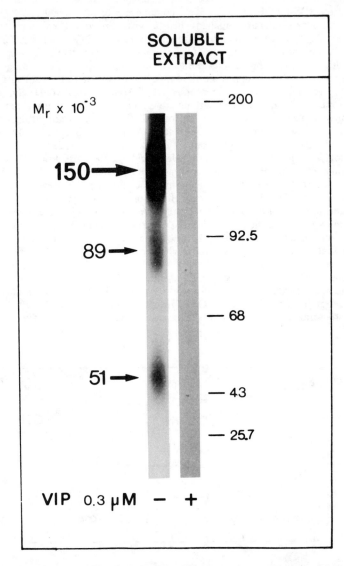

FIGURE 5. Affinity cross-linking of solubilized [^{125}I]VIP-receptor complexes. Rat liver membranes are incubated with [^{125}I]VIP and the material solubilized with 1% Triton is then treated with the cross-linker DTSP (1 mM) for 15 minutes at 4°C. The samples are then prepared as described by Couvineau et al.[21] for SDS-PAGE analysis on a 5-15% polyacrylamide slab gel with a 3% stacking gel. The gel is calibrated with proteins of known molecular weight.

incubation with N-acetylglucosamine (FIG. 8, left). Chromatography of the eluted material on Sephacryl S-300 (FIG. 8, right) shows the presence of two components, that is, a major one (Stokes radius = 5.8 nm) and a minor one (Stokes radius = 3.0 nm) corresponding to the ternary VIP-receptor-G protein complex and the VIP-receptor complex, respectively (see above). The material eluted from WGA-Sepharose displays a 5-10-fold enrichment in [^{125}I]VIP-labeled receptors per milligram of protein. Such a technique can therefore be used in a preliminary purification of VIP receptors and, together with other procedures, may lead to complete purification of the receptor. Such studies are currently in progress.

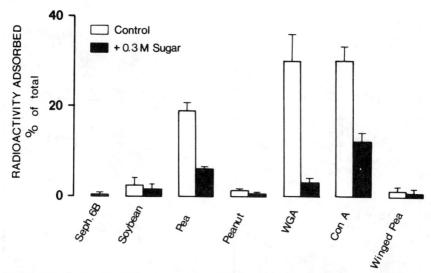

FIGURE 6. Binding of solubilized cross-linked [^{125}I]VIP-receptor complexes to various lectins-coupled to Sepharose. Covalent [^{125}I]VIP-receptor complexes obtained from rat liver membranes, as previously described,[11] are solubilized with 1% Triton. One hundred microliters of solubilized complexes are then incubated with 300 μl of lectin coupled to Sepharose beads (about 2 mg of protein/ml of settled gel) in the presence or absence of 0.3 M specific sugar for 30 minutes at 25°C. After washing, the radioactivity bound to lectin agarose beads is counted. The following specific sugars are used: N-acetylgalactosamine (soybean); alpha-methyl-mannopyranoside (pea and ConA); galactose (peanut); N-acetylglucosamine (WGA); fucose (winged pea). Results represent the mean ± SE of four determinations.

RECEPTORS FOR VIP AND RELATED PEPTIDES: A FAMILY OF RECEPTORS?

VIP belongs to a superfamily of regulatory peptides including secretin, glucagon, gastric inhibitory polypeptide (GIP), growth hormone-releasing factor (GRF), peptide histidine isoleucine amide (PHI), and helodermin (reviewed in Laburthe[37]). It is generally accepted that such a structural family of peptides has appeared during evolution through successive events of gene duplication giving redundant copies of a gene coding for an original peptide.[38] While the original peptide continues to carry out its functional role, the duplicate gene is free to mutate, and thereby its product may acquire the structural properties necessary to interact with a different set of receptors. However this diversification of information-bearing peptides has been only possible because membrane proteins responsible for the recognition of peptides, that is, receptors, have also become different, permitting the unequivocal recognition of each peptide. Thus we have proposed that a family of receptors for VIP-related peptides has evolved parallel to the family of peptides during evolution through successive

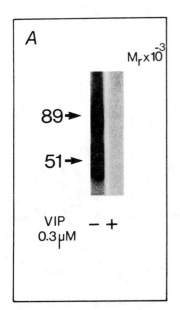
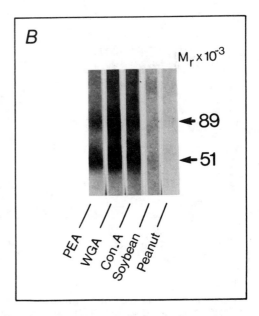

FIGURE 7. SDS-PAGE analysis of cross-linked [¹²⁵I]VIP-receptor complexes solubilized from liver membranes and eluted from various lectins. Panel A: Membranes are incubated with [¹²⁵I]VIP in the presence or absence of 0.3 μM native VIP, washed, treated with 1 mM cross-linker (DTSP), solubilized with SDS and submitted to SDS-PAGE as previously described.[11]

Panel B: Membranes are incubated with [¹²⁵I]VIP, washed, treated with 1 mM DTSP and solubilized with 1% Triton. The solubilized [¹²⁵I]VIP-receptor complexes are bound to the indicated lectins coupled to Sepharose and eluted from the beads by specific sugars (see FIG. 6), adjusted to 3% SDS and submitted to SDS-PAGE as previously described.[11]

events of gene duplication followed by mutation.[37] This hypothesis is based on the comparison of pharmacological, functional, and even molecular properties of receptor for VIP-related peptides showing striking similarities.

Specific receptors have been identified for VIP (TABLE 1), glucagon,[39] secretin,[40–42] GIP,[43–45] and GRF.[46,47] To date, no specific receptors for PHI and helodermin have been demonstrated but these peptides bind with a low affinity to VIP and secretin receptors.[26,40,42,48–52]

Two functional domains can be characterized in a peptide receptor: (1) the recognition site responsible for the specific binding of the peptide; and (2) the coupling

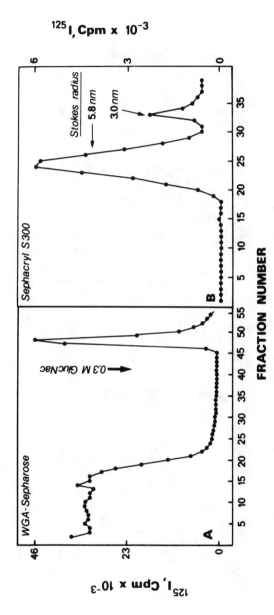

FIGURE 8. Binding of Triton-solubilized [^{125}I]VIP-receptor complexes to WGA Sepharose and elution by N-acetylglucosamine. Panel A: Liver membranes preloaded with [^{125}I]VIP are treated by 1% Triton X-100. The solubilized material is incubated with WGA-Sepharose (see FIG. 6) and then eluted from the beads by 0.3 M N-acetylglucosamine.

Panel B: The material eluted from WGA-Sepharose by N-acetylglucosamine is chromatographed by Sephacryl S-300 as described in the legend to FIGURE 1.

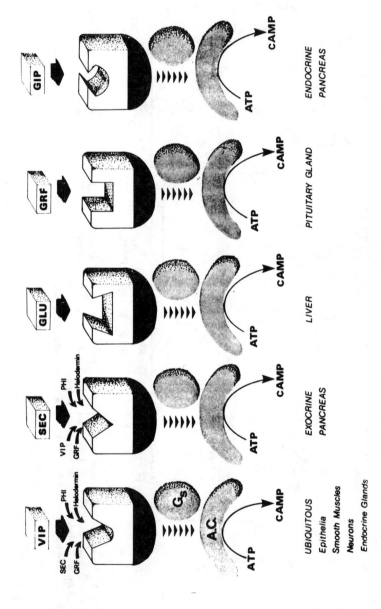

FIGURE 9. Schematic representation of receptors for VIP, secretin (SEC), glucagon (GLU), GIP, and GRF in their respective target cells.

TABLE 2. Molecular Identification of Receptors for VIP-Related Peptides (Glucagon, GIP, Secretin, GRF) by Covalent Cross-Linking

Peptide	Tissue	Cross-Linking Technique[a]	Molecular Weight of Receptor[b]	References
Glucagon	Rat liver membranes	Chemical (HSAB)	50	54
	" " "	Photoaffinity	49–67	55
	" " "	Ultraviolet irradiation	59	56
	" " "	Chemical (HSAB)	60	57
GIP	Hamster pancreatic beta cell membranes	Chemical (DTSP)	59	58
		Ultraviolet irradiation	59	59
Secretin	Rat gastric membranes	Chemical (DTSP)	60	60
GRF	Bovine pituitary membranes	Chemical (DSS)	70	61
	Rat pituitary cells	Chemical (DSS)	21	62

[a] Abbreviations of cross-linkers are the same as in TABLE 1.
[b] We have indicated the molecular weights (expressed in kDa) of peptide binding units after substraction of the ligand molecular weight assuming that one molecule of ligand is bound per binding protein.

site responsible for the coupling of the receptor with an effector system in the plasma membrane.

As far as the recognition site is concerned, some receptors for VIP-related peptides display common pharmacological characteristics. Thus, VIP and secretin receptors recognize the same panel of peptides (FIG. 9), that is, VIP, secretin, PHI, GRF, and helodermin.[26,40,42,48-53] On a pharmacological basis, they are distinguishable from each other only by their ability to bind VIP with a higher affinity than other peptides, that is, VIP receptors or secretin with a higher affinity than other peptides, that is, secretin receptors. These similar pharmacological properties strongly suggest that the recognition sites of the two receptors are not structurally very different. In contrast, other receptors are more specialized and do not recognize other peptides of the structural family (FIG. 9).

As far as the coupling site is concerned, it is most interesting to observe that all these receptors are positively coupled with the production of cAMP (FIG. 9) which appears to be a common second messenger of VIP-related peptides in their respective target cells.[1,3,39,40,42,44,46]

These observations suggest that the functional diversification of receptors for VIP-related peptides has been achieved through the specialization of recognition sites. This contrasts with the remarkable preservation of the coupling site. Therefore, the repeated events of duplication-mutation of a gene encoding for an ancestral receptor would have only concerned the receptor domain responsible for recognition of peptides. This view is compatible with the molecular identification of receptor binding units for glucagon, GIP, secretin, and GRF (TABLE 2). Indeed, the M_r of these receptors (range: 49,000-70,000) compares well, in most studies, with that of VIP receptors (TABLE 1), supporting the idea that receptors for VIP-related peptides have similar overall structures. It is therefore tempting to speculate that when the structure of genes encoding for these receptors will be described, striking homologies will appear in their amino-acid sequences.

REFERENCES

1. SAID, S. I., Ed. 1982. Advances in Peptide Hormone Research, Vol. 1: Vasoactive Intestinal Peptide. Raven Press. New York.
2. LABURTHE, M., G. ROSSELIN, M. ROUSSET, A. ZWEIBAUM, M. KORNER, Z. SELINGER & M. SCHRAMM. 1979. Transfer of the hormone receptor for vasointestinal peptide to an adenylate cyclase system in another cell. FEBS Lett. 98: 41-43.
3. LABURTHE, M. & B. AMIRANOFF. 1988. Peptide receptors in the intestinal epithelium. In Handbook of Physiology. (Vol. on Neuroendocrinology of the Gut.) G. M. Makhlouf, Ed. American Physiological Society. Bethesda, MD. In press.
4. AMIRANOFF, B., M. LABURTHE & G. ROSSELIN. 1980. Characterization of specific binding sites for vasoactive intestinal peptide (VIP) in rat intestinal epithelial cell membranes. Biochim. Biophys. Acta 267: 215-224.
5. AMIRANOFF, B., M. LABURTHE & G. ROSSELIN. 1980. Potentiation by guanine nucleotides of the VIP-induced adenylate cyclase stimulation in intestinal epithelial cell membranes. Life Sci. 26: 1905-1911.
6. SARRIEAU, A., M. LABURTHE & G. ROSSELIN. 1983. Intestinal VIP receptors: Differential effect of trypsin on the high-and low-affinity binding sites. Mol. Cell. Endocrinol. 31: 301-313.
7. SARRIEAU, A., N. BOIGE & M. LABURTHE. 1985. Role of phospholipids in the binding activity of VIP receptors. Experientia 41: 631-633.

8. EL BATTARI, A., E. AH-KYE, J. M. MULLER, H. SARI & J. MARVALDI. 1985. Modification of HT-29 cell response to the vasoactive intestinal peptide (VIP) by membrane fluidization. Biochimie **67:** 1217-1224.

9. LABURTHE, M., B. BREANT & C. ROUYER-FESSARD. 1984. Molecular identification of receptors for vasoactive intestinal peptide in rat intestinal epithelium by covalent cross-linking. Eur. J. Biochem. **139:** 181-187.

10. COUVINEAU, A. & M. LABURTHE. 1985. The human vasoactive intestinal peptide receptor: Molecular identification by covalent cross-linking in colonic epithelium. J. Clin. Endocrinol. Metab. **61:** 50-55.

11. COUVINEAU, A. & M. LABURTHE. 1985. The rat liver vasoactive intestinal peptide (VIP) binding site: Molecular characterization by covalent cross-linking and evidence for differences from the intestinal receptor. Biochem. J. **225:** 473-479.

12. NGUYEN, T. D., J. A. WILLIAMS & G. M. GRAY. 1986. Vasoactive intestinal peptide receptor on liver plasma membranes: Characterization as a glycoprotein. Biochemistry **25:** 361-368.

13. COUVINEAU, A., S. GAMMELTOFT & M. LABURTHE. 1986. Molecular characteristics and peptide specificity of vasoactive intestinal peptide receptors from rat cerebral cortex. J. Neurochem. **47:** 1469-1475.

14. VASILOFF, J., M. S. O'DORISIO, L. B. CAMPOLITO, J. C. BRESNAHAN, M. S. BEATTIE & T. M. O'DORISIO. 1986. Vasoactive intestinal polypeptide receptors in rat brain: Characterization by binding and covalent cross-linking. Can. J. Physiol. Pharmacol. (Symposium on Gastrointestinal Hormones) Abstr. **461:** 172.

15. WOOD, C. L. & M. S. O'DORISIO. 1985. Covalent cross-linking of vasoactive intestinal polypeptide to its receptors on intact human lymphoblasts. J. Biol. Chem. **260:** 1243-1247.

16. COUVINEAU, A., M. ROUSSET & M. LABURTHE. 1985. Molecular identification and structural requirement of vasoactive intestinal peptide (VIP) receptors in the human colon adenocarcinoma cell line HT-29. Biochem. J. **231:** 139-143.

17. MULLER, J. M., J. LUIS, J. FANTINI, B. ABADIE, F. GIANNELLINI, J. MARVALDI & J. PICHON. 1985. Covalent cross-linking of vasoactive intestinal peptide (VIP) to its receptor in intact colonic adenocarcinoma cell in culture (HT-29). Eur. J. Biochem. **151:** 411-417.

18. WOOD, C. L., M. S. O'DORISIO, L. M. VASSALO, W. B. MALARKEY & T. M. O'DORISIO. 1985. Vasoactive intestinal peptide effects on GH_3 pituitary tumor cells: High affinity binding, affinity labeling, and adenylate cyclase stimulation. Comparison with peptide histidine isoleucine and growth hormone releasing factor. Regul. Peptides. **12:** 237-248.

19. DICKINSON, K. E. J., M. SCHACHTER, C. M. M. MILES, D. H. COY & P. S. SEVER. 1986. Characterization of vasoactive intestinal peptide (VIP) receptors in mammalian lung. Peptides **7:** 791-800.

20. MARVALDI, J., J. LUIS, J. M. MULLER, A. EL BATTARI, J. FANTINI, J. M. MARTIN, B. ABADIE, A. TIRARD & J. PICHON. 1986. Characterization of the vasoactive intestinal peptide (VIP) binding sites: A biochemical and an immunological approach. Peptides 7(Suppl. 1): 137-145.

21. COUVINEAU, A., B. AMIRANOFF & M. LABURTHE. 1986. Solubilization of the liver VIP receptor: Hydrodynamic characterization and evidence for an association with a functional GTP regulatory protein. J. Biol. Chem. **261:** 14482-14489.

22. HEIDENRICH, K. A., N. R. ZAHNISER, P. BERHANU, D. BRANDENBURG & J. M. OLEFSKY. 1983. Structural differences between insulin receptors in the brain and peripheral target tissues. J. Biol. Chem. **258:** 8527-8530.

23. BOZOU, J. C., A. COUVINEAU, C. ROUYER-FESSARD, M. LABURTHE, J. P. VINCENT & P. KITABGI. 1987. Phorbol ester induces loss of VIP stimulation of adenylate cyclase and VIP-binding sites in HT-29 cells. FEBS Lett. **211:** 151-154.

24. STADEL, J. M., P. NAMBI, R. G. L. SHORR, D. F. SAWYER, M. G. CARON & R. J. LEFKOWITZ. 1983. Catecholamine-induced desensitization of turkey erythrocyte adenylate cyclase is associated with phosphorylation of the beta-adrenergic receptor. Proc. Natl. Acad. Sci. USA **80:** 3173-3177.

25. ROBBERECHT, P., D. H. COY, P. DE NEEF, J. C. CAMUS, A. CAUVIN, M. WAELBROECK & J. CHRISTOPHE. 1986. Interaction of vasoactive intestinal peptide (VIP) and N-terminally modified VIP analogs with rat pancreatic, hepatic and pituitary membranes. Eur. J. Biochem. **159:** 45-49.

26. LABURTHE, M., B. AMIRANOFF, N. BOIGE, C. ROUYER-FESSARD, K. TATEMOTO & L. MORODER. 1983. Interaction of GRF with VIP receptors and stimulation of adenylate cyclase in rat and human intestinal epithelial membranes. Comparison with PHI and secretin. FEBS Lett. **159:** 89-92.

27. LABURTHE, M., A. COUVINEAU & C. ROUYER-FESSARD. 1986. Study of species specificity in growth hormone-releasing factor (GRF) interaction with vasoactive intestinal peptide (VIP) receptors using GRF and intestinal VIP receptors from rat and human: Evidence that Ac-Tyr¹h GRF is a competitive VIP antagonist in the rat. Mol. Pharmacol. **29:** 23-27.

28. PILCH, P. F. & M. P. CZECH. 1979. Interaction of cross-linking agents with the insulin effector system of isolated fat cells. J. Biol. Chem. **254:** 3375-3381.

29. DESBUQUOIS, B. 1974. The interaction of vasoactive intestinal polypeptide and secretin with liver cell membranes. Eur. J. Biochem. **46:** 439-450.

30. AMIRANOFF, B., M. LABURTHE & G. ROSSELIN. 1980. Differential effects of guanine nucleotides on the first step of VIP and glucagon action in membranes from liver cells. Biochem. Biophys. Res. Commun. **96:** 463-468.

31. GUERRERO, J. M., J. R. CALVO, M. R. GARRIDO, P. MOLINERO, C. OSUNA, J. JIMENEZ & R. GOBERNA. 1986. Vasoactive intestinal peptide (VIP) binding to solubilized material from rat liver plasma membranes. Biosci. Rep. **6:** 39-44.

32. PAUL, S. & S. I. SAID. 1987. Characterization of receptors for vasoactive intestinal peptide solubilized from the lung. J. Biol. Chem. **262:** 158-162.

33. DAVIS, A. 1984. Determination of the hydrodynamic properties of detergent-solubilized proteins. *In* Molecular and Chemical Characterization of Membrane Receptors. J. C. Venter & L. C. Harrison, Eds.: 161-178. Alan R. Liss, Inc. New York.

34. LIMBIRD, L. E., D. M. GILL & R. J. LEFKOWITZ. 1980. Agonist-promoted coupling of the beta-adrenergic receptor with the guanine nucleotide regulatory protein of the adenylate cyclase system. Proc. Natl. Acad. Sci. USA **77:** 775-779.

35. BHAVANANDAN, V. P. & A. W. KATLIC. 1979. The interaction of wheat germ agglutinin with sialoglycoproteins. The role of sialic acid. J. Biol. Chem. **254:** 4000-4008.

36. EL BATTARI, A., J. M. MARTIN, J. FANTINI, J. M. MULLER, J. MARVALDI & J. PICHON. The vasoactive intestinal peptide (VIP) receptor on intact human colonic adenocarcinoma cells (HT-29-D4). Evidence for its glycoprotein nature. Biochemistry. In press.

37. LABURTHE, M. 1985. The vasoactive intestinal peptide (VIP): An ubiquitous neuropeptide member of a structural family of regulatory peptides. Biochimie **67:** XI-XVIII.

38. NIALL, H. D. 1982. The evolution of peptide hormones. Ann. Rev. Physiol. **44:** 615-624.

39. RODBELL, M., H. M. J. KRANS, S. L. POHL & L. BIRNBAUMER. 1971. The glucagon sensitive adenyl cyclase in plasma membrane of rat liver. J. Biol. Chem. **246:** 1861-1869.

40. JENSEN, R. T., C. G. CHARLTON, H. ADACHI, S. W. JONES, T. L. O'DONOHUE & J. D. GARDNER. 1983. Use of ¹²⁵I-secretin to identify and characterize high-affinity secretin receptors on pancreatic acini. Am. J. Physiol. **245**(Gastrointest. Liver Physiol. 8): G186-G195.

41. FREMEAU, R. T., T. R. JENSEN, C. G. CHARLTON, R. L. MILLER, T. T. O'DONOHUE & T. W. MOODY. 1983. Secretin: Specific binding to rat brain membranes. J. Neurosci. **3:** 1620-1625.

42. GESPACH, C., D. BATAILLE, N. VAUCLIN, L. MORODER, E. WUNSCH & G. ROSSELIN. 1986. Secretin receptor activity in rat gastric glands. Binding studies, cAMP generation and pharmacology. Peptides 7(Suppl. 1): 155-163.

43. MALETTI, M., B. AMIRANOFF, M. LABURTHE & G. ROSSELIN. 1983. Mise en évidence de récepteurs spécifiques du peptide inhibiteur gastrique (GIP). C.R. Acad. Sci. (Paris) **297:** 563-566.

44. AMIRANOFF, B., N. VAUCLIN-JACQUES & M. LABURTHE. 1984. Functional GIP receptors in a hamster pancreatic beta cell line, In111: Specific binding and biological effects. Biochem. Biophys. Res. Commun. **123:** 671-676.

45. AMIRANOFF, B., N. VAUCLIN-JACQUES & M. LABURTHE. 1985. Interaction of gastric inhibitory polypeptide (GIP) with the insulin-secreting pancreatic beta cell line, In111: Characteristics of GIP binding sites. Life Sci. **36:** 807-813.

46. SEIFERT, H., M. PERRIN, J. RIVIER & W. VALE. 1985. Binding sites for growth hormone releasing factor on rat anterior pituitary cells. Nature **313:** 487-489.

47. VELICELEBI, G., T. M. SANTA CROCE & M. M. HARPOLD. 1985. Specific binding of synthetic human pancreatic growth hormone releasing factor (1-40-OH) to bovine anterior pituitaries. Biochem. Biophys. Res. Commun. **126:** 33-39.
48. BATAILLE, D., C. GESPACH, M. LABURTHE, B. AMIRANOFF, K. TATEMOTO, N. VAUCLIN & G. ROSSELIN. 1980. Porcine peptide having N-terminal histidine and C-terminal isoleucine amide: VIP-like and secretin-like effect in different tissues from rat. FEBS Lett. **114:** 240-242.
49. LABURTHE, M., A. COUVINEAU, C. ROUYER-FESSARD & L. MORODER. 1985. Interaction of PHM, PHI, and 24-glutamine PHI with human VIP receptors from colonic epithelium. Life Sci. **36:** 991-995.
50. AMIRANOFF, B., N. VAUCLIN-JACQUES, N. BOIGE, C. ROUYER-FESSARD & M. LABURTHE. 1983. Interaction of Gila Monster venom with VIP receptors in intestinal epithelium of human: A comparison with rat. FEBS Lett. **164:** 299-302.
51. RAUFMAN, J. P., R. T. JENSEN, V. E. SUTLIFF, J. J. PISANO & J. D. GARDNER. 1982. Actions of Gila monster venom on dispersed acini from guinea pig pancreas. Am. J. Physiol. **242:** G470-G474.
52. ROBBERECHT, P., M. WAELBROECK, P. DE NEEF, J. C. CAMUS, A. VANDERMEERS, M. C. VANDERMEERS-PIRET & J. CHRISTOPHE. 1984. Specific labeling by ^{125}I-helodermin of high affinity VIP receptors in rat liver membranes. FEBS Lett. **172:** 55-58.
53. WAELBROECK, M., P. ROBBERECHT, P. DE NEEF, P. CHATELAIN & J. CHRISTOPHE. 1985. Interaction of growth hormone-releasing factor (GRF) and 14 GRF analogs with vasoactive intestinal peptide (VIP) receptors of rat pancreas. Endocrinology **116:** 2643-2649.
54. JOHNSON, G. L., V. I. MAC ANDREW & P. F. PILCH. 1981. Identification of the glucagon receptor in rat liver membranes by photoaffinity cross-linking. Proc. Natl. Acad. Sci. USA **78:** 875-878.
55. DEMOLIOU-MASON, C. & R. M. EPAND. 1982. Identification of the glucagon receptor by covalent labeling with a radiolabeled photoreactive glucagon analogue. Biochemistry **21:** 1996-2004.
56. IWANIJ, V. & K. C. HUR. 1985. Direct cross-linking of ^{125}I-labeled glucagon to its membrane receptor by UV irradiation. Proc. Natl. Acad. Sci. USA **82:** 325-329.
57. IYENGAR, R. & J. T. HERZBERG. 1984. Structural analysis of the hepatic glucagon receptor. Identification of a guanine nucleotide sensitive hormone-binding region. J. Biol. Chem. **259:** 5222-5229.
58. COUVINEAU, A., B. AMIRANOFF, N. VAUCLIN-JACQUES & M. LABURTHE. 1984. The GIP receptor on pancreatic beta cell tumor: covalent cross-linking and molecular characterization. Biochem. Biophys. Res. Commun. **122:** 283-288.
59. AMIRANOFF, B., A. COUVINEAU, N. VAUCLIN-JACQUES & M. LABURTHE. 1986. Gastric inhibitory polypeptide receptor in hamster pancreatic beta cells. Direct cross-linking, solubilization and characterization as a glycoprotein. Eur. J. Biochem. **159:** 353-358.
60. GESPACH, C., W. BAWAB, J. C. MARIE, E. CHASTRE, G. ROSSELIN & N. YANAIHARA. 1986. VIP and secretin (SEC) receptors in human and rat gastric glands, pharmacology and molecular identification by covalent cross-linking. In Purification, Biosynthesis and Regulation of Membrane-Bound Receptors. Cap d'Agde, France. September 8-12, Abstract, p. 125.
61. VELICELEBI, G., S. PATTHI, S. PROVOW & M. AKONG. 1986. Covalent cross-linking of growth hormone-releasing factor to pituitary receptors. Endocrinology **118:** 1278-1283.
62. ZYSK, J. R., M. J. CRONIN, J. M. ANDERSON & M. O. THORNER. 1986. Cross-linking of a growth hormone releasing factor-binding protein in anterior pituitary cells. J. Biol. Chem. **261:** 16781-16784.

Anatomical Distribution of Vasoactive Intestinal Peptide Binding Sites in Peripheral Tissues Investigated by *in Vitro* Autoradiography[a]

R. F. POWER,[b] A. E. BISHOP,[b] J. WHARTON,[b]
C. O. INYAMA,[b] R. H. JACKSON,[c] S. R. BLOOM,[d] AND
J. M. POLAK [b,e]

[b]Department of Histochemistry and
[d]Department of Medicine
Royal Postgraduate Medical School
London W12 OHS, United Kingdom and
[c]Department of Labelled Compounds
Amersham International PLC
Amersham, Bucks JP7 9LL, United Kingdom

INTRODUCTION

Vasoactive intestinal polypeptide (VIP) has a widespread distribution in the central and peripheral nervous systems, as demonstrated by radioimmunoassay and immunohistochemistry, and considerable information is available on the physiological and pharmacological actions of VIP within the body (for a review, see Said[1]). While there is increasing evidence to support a role for VIP as a neurotransmitter or neuromodulator within these systems,[2-4] precise proof is lacking. VIP is thought to be released locally to act on target cells,[5] and, as with other regulatory molecules, its effects are produced by interaction with specific receptors (for example, Laburthe *et al.*[5]). Binding studies using isolated membrane preparations have demonstrated specific receptors in a variety of tissues,[5-8] in different species including man, but their precise anatomical localization in many tissues has not been reported. We investigated the anatomical localization of VIP binding sites in some adult guinea pig and rat peripheral tissues, where VIP is known to have an effect, using [^{125}I]VIP, by means of *in vitro* autora-

[a]This work was supported in part by the Wellcome Trust.

[e]Address for correspondence: Professor Julia M. Polak, Department of Histochemistry, Royal Postgraduate Medical School, Du Cane Road, London W12 OHS, United Kingdom.

diography. In order to compare the distribution of binding sites with that of VIP-containing nerves, parallel immunocytochemical studies were made.

MATERIALS AND METHODS

Autoradiography

Tissues under study were rapidly dissected from adult Wistar rats and Dunkin Hartley guinea pigs that had been killed by an overdose of ether. Tissues were macroscopically normal, and unfixed cryostat blocks were prepared. Sections were cut at 15 μm and thaw-mounted onto poly-L-lysine-coated slides.[9] After drying, sections were preincubated for 15 minutes at room temperature in 50 μM Tris-HC1 buffer (pH 7.4) in an attempt to remove impurities and uncouple endogenously bound VIP. Preliminary results were recorded to determine the optimal conditions of binding. By varying the length of incubation, concentration of ligand, and the temperature at which the procedure was carried out, it was possible to maximize the differences between specific and nonspecific binding and saturation of binding sites. Thus, sections were incubated with 1 nM [125I]VIP in the same buffer containing 1% bovine serum albumin, 4 mg/ml leupeptin and 40 mg/ml bacitracin. Radiolabeled VIP was obtained from Amersham International (England). The ligand was prepared by iodination of VIP using sodium iodide-125 and chloramine T and purified by high-performance liquid chromatography. To determine nonspecific binding, sections were incubated in the presence or absence of 1 μM unlabeled VIP. Incubation was terminated by two washes of five minutes each in 50 μM Tris-HCl at 4°C followed by a rinse in distilled water at 0°C. Washing was followed by rapidly drying the sections under a stream of cold air. Dried sections were either apposed to LKB [3H]Ultrofilm at 4°C for four days[10] or attached for two weeks at 4°C to coverslips[11] previously coated with Ilford K5 emulsion. After exposure, the image on both film and coverslips was developed using Kodak D19 at 20°C (five minutes for the film and three minutes for the coverslips). Sections attached to coverslips were stained with hematoxylin and eosin. Both Ultrofilm and coverslips were viewed using dark-field and light-field microscopy.

Immunocytochemistry

The tissues for immunocytochemistry were taken from areas adjacent to those used for autoradiography and were fixed by immersion in a 0.4% solution of *p*-benzoquinone in 0.1 M phosphate-buffered saline (PBS, pH 7.2-7.4), for two hours.[12] After thorough washing in PBS containing 0.1% sodium azide and 15% sucrose, cryostat blocks were prepared. Sections were cut at 10 μm and thaw-mounted onto poly-L-lysine-coated slides and allowed to dry at room temperature for one hour. The primary antiserum to synthetic porcine VIP was applied at a dilution of 1/10,000 and the indirect immunofluoresence technique performed.[13] Photographs were taken using FP4 black and white film (Ilford Ltd., ASA 125).

RESULTS

Localization of Binding Sites

Autoradiograms demonstrated specific labeling over discrete structures in rat and guinea pig respiratory, gastrointestinal, and genital tracts. In both species, in the respiratory tract, labeling was present over respiratory epithelium and smooth muscle of bronchi and dense labeling over alveolar walls (FIG. 1). It was not possible to determine the precise anatomical localization of the binding in the latter owing to the present lack of resolution with the technique. In addition, labeling was also seen over the smooth muscle of pulmonary blood vessels.

In the gastrointestinal tract, specific labeling was evident over the gastric, and colonic mucosa of the guinea pig, ileal, and a low density of binding was apparent over the muscularis propria (FIG. 2).There was also an apparent lack of binding in all areas of the rat gastrointestinal tract examined.

Moderate to dense labeling of the epithelial linings of fallopian tube, uterus (FIG. 3), cervix, and vagina was seen in both guinea pig and rat. In the males of both species, high levels of binding were seen in the glandular epithelium of the prostate (FIG. 4). Moderate binding was seen in the epithelial lining of the seminal vesicle and low levels in the testes. There was a lack of binding in the ovary, epididymus, vas deferens, and penis. In both sexes, in both species, there was also an apparent lack of binding in smooth muscle, including that of blood vessels.

Specific binding was abolished in the presence of a 1 μM concentration of unlabeled VIP (FIG. 3b).

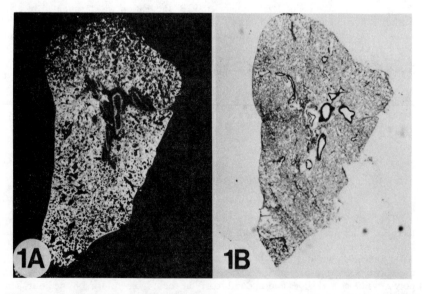

FIGURE 1. Distribution of [^{125}I]VIP binding in rat lung. (**a**) Cryostat section of rat lung incubated with [^{125}I]VIP showing dense labeling over the lung parenchyma. (**b**) Adjacent (non-serial) section stained with hematoxylin and eosin.

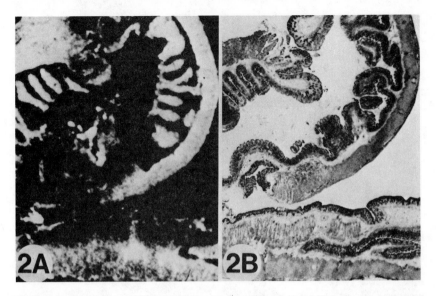

FIGURE 2. Distribution of [^{125}I]VIP binding in guinea pig colon. (a) Ultrofilm autoradiograph of a section of guinea pig colon incubated with [^{125}I]VIP showing labeling in the mucosa and low binding in the muscularis propria. (b) Hematoxylin and eosin stain of a section of guinea pig colon.

Distribution of Nerve Fibers

In the lung of both species, VIP nerve fibers were seen around submucous glands and smooth muscle fibers of major airways and blood vessels. Very few fibers were seen in smaller airways or in alveolar walls.

A similar distribution of VIP-immunoreactive nerve fibers and ganglion cells was observed in all areas of gastrointestinal tract examined. The two major locations of fibers were the circular muscle coat and the mucosa, where the fibers surrounded blood vessels and lay just beneath the epithelium. Fibers were seen in both the myenteric and submucous plexuses, but immunoreactive ganglion cells were seen only in the latter.

In both the male and female genital tracts, a wide distribution of VIP-immunoreactive fibers was seen. In the male, VIP-immunoreactive fibers were present in the erectile tissue, around blood vessels, and beneath the urethral epithelium of the penis. The prostate, seminal vesicle, epididymus, and vas deferens also demonstrated VIP fibers in the smooth muscle and subepithelial connective tissue close to the epithelium. Only a few VIP-containing fibers were seen in the testis, usually just within the testicular capsule.

In the female, a dense supply of fibers was seen in the vagina, in the smooth muscle, around blood vessels, and in the subepithelial connective tissue close to the surface squamous epithelium. A similar distribution was seen in the cervix and corpus uteri; VIP-immunoreactive fibers were seen in close association with muscle cells, around parametrial, endometrial, and endocervical blood vessels and in the endometrial

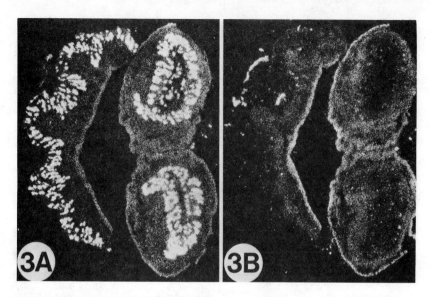

FIGURE 3. Distribution of [^{125}I]VIP binding in guinea pig uterus. (a) Cryostat section of guinea pig uterus incubated with [^{125}I]VIP showing dense labeling in the endometrium that is abolished by the presence of 1 μM unlabeled VIP (b).

stroma running close to the basal segment of the uterine glands. In the oviduct, VIP nerve fibers were scattered throughout all layers of the wall including the adventitia. Only a few fibers were seen in the ovary, mainly associated with blood vessels.

DISCUSSION

The purpose of this study was to identify specific binding sites for VIP by *in vitro* autoradiography and to correlate their distribution with that of VIP-containing nerves and with the known effects of the peptide.

In vitro autoradiography was originally developed by Young and Kuhar[11] in 1979, and since then has been used extensively in the detailed analysis of the distribution of peptide receptors in many tissues, but particularly in the brain.[14-18] While the use of high-affinity radioligand binding techniques allows the characterization of binding sites and study of the structure-activity relationship of peptide action,[19,20] it does not permit anatomical resolution and thus does not reveal the localization of receptor sites at the microscopic level. To overcome this problem, *in vivo* labeling was used initially, but this proved to be of limited value in the study of peptide receptors. Ligands of very high affinity, low nonspecific binding, and metabolic stability are required; this excludes many peptides that are easily degraded. In addition, peptides are unable to cross organ and tissue barriers encountered in *in vivo* labeling. *In vitro* autoradiography permits the labeling of tissue sections mounted onto microscope slides. Conditions of binding can be controlled or modified, anatomical barriers are circumvented, and the metabolism of the ligand can be controlled, thus permitting the use of ligands such as peptides.

Using this technique, we have shown, in both rat and guinea pig lung, dense labeling over the alveolar walls in both species and moderate labeling over the smooth muscle of major airways and pulmonary vessels. VIP-immunoreactive nerve fibers were seen around submucous glands and blood vessels of major airways and smooth muscle bundles. Very few VIP-containing nerve fibers were seen innervating alveoli. The results of our studies on the distribution of VIP-immunoreactive nerve fibers agree with that of other workers.[21,22]

VIP receptors in the lung have previously been demonstrated both by membrane binding studies[23,24] and autoradiography.[25,26] Robberecht *et al.*[23,24] used lung homogenates, from several species including humans, to demonstrate receptors by direct binding techniques; this, however, gave no information on their anatomical localization. Binding sites have been demonstrated by autoradiography in human, guinea pig, and rat lung.[25-27] In these studies binding sites were localized to alveolar walls and smaller airways; larger airways, arteries, and veins were labeled in the human and guinea pig, but these structures remained unlabeled in the rat lung.

In the larger airways, VIP binding sites were demonstrated on submucous glands, over the epithelium and over the smooth muscle. This corresponds with the known effects of VIP in the lung. It has been known that VIP stimulates mucus secretion in the dog[28] and ferret,[29] and although its effect in the species presently under study is not known, the presence of binding sites on mucous glands and surface epithelium would support a previous suggestion that VIP may play a part in regulating mucociliary transport.[26] VIP has a relaxing effect on airway smooth muscle[30-32] and has a potent vasodilator effect on pulmonary vessels,[33-35] the demonstration of binding sites on both

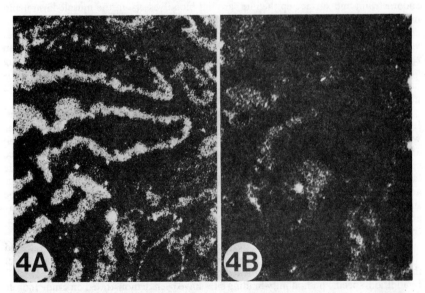

FIGURE 4. Localization of VIP binding sites in the rat prostate. (a) Ultrofilm autoradiograph of a section of rat prostate incubated with [^{125}I]VIP, (b). Section incubated in the presence of 1 μM of unlabeled VIP.

these structures supports a direct role for VIP at these sites. No effect of VIP on alveolar function has yet been described.

VIP was originally isolated from porcine duodenum,[36] and VIP immunoreactivity is present in nerves throughout the gastrointestinal tract of man and many other animals.[37-42] Receptors for VIP have previously been characterized biochemically in detail[43,44] and have been shown for example on human colonic epithelium[45] and guinea pig small intestinal epithelial cells[46] by membrane binding studies. The localization of binding sites by *in vitro* autoradiography has not been reported previously. In our studies, there was a good correlation between the distribution of VIP-immunoreactive nerves and the localization of binding sites in the guinea pig. Binding sites were identified on guinea pig gastric, ileal, and colonic mucosa and to a lesser extent on the muscularis propria. The distribution in the epithelium fits with the known action of VIP as a stimulator of water and electrolyte secretion from intestinal mucosa[47,48] and suggests that this is a direct action. In addition, the direct relaxing effect of VIP on smooth muscle[49,50] is confirmed by our anatomical localization of binding sites to the muscularis propria. There was an apparent lack of labeling throughout all areas of rat gastrointestinal tract examined.

The reasons for this lack of binding are not clear. The peptide specificity of VIP receptors varies considerably between species, this has been shown by the different ability of receptors to identify partial VIP sequences and natural VIP agonists such as secretin.[51,52] There are differences, especially for the high-affinity binding sites, between human and rat epithelium,[45] and this may explain the apparent lack of binding in the rat gastrointestinal tract in the present study. Alternatively, there may be a subset of receptors that does not recognize the label used.

In the female genital tract, the highest density of binding sites was identified in the endometrial lining of the uterus and in the epithelial linings in the oviduct, cervix, and vagina. In general, immunocytochemistry revealed VIP nerve fibers beneath the endometrium and surface epithelium, around blood vessels, in the muscle layers, and in the adventitia. In the male genital tract, dense labeling was seen in the glandular epithelium of the prostate and moderate binding in the epithelium of the seminal vesicle. With the exception of the testes, which showed low labeling, there was an apparent lack of binding in other tissues examined. A rich network of VIP-containing nerves was seen in the prostate, seminal vesicle, vas deferens, epididymus, and penis both in the smooth muscle and close to the surface epithelium. In addition, VIP nerve fibers were also seen in the erectile tissue of the penis.

VIP-immunoreactive material has been described extensively in both the male and female genital tracts,[3,53-58] and the results of our studies agree with those of other workers. In the female, the highest concentrations occur at the utero-cervical junction and in the vagina. In general, immunoreactive fibers are located beneath the surface epithelium, close to or around blood vessels and seromucous glands, in the muscle layer and in the adventitia. In the male, VIP-immunoreactive fibers are most numerous around blood vessels in the corpus cavernosum of the penis, in the prostate (in the smooth muscle between prostatic glands), and in the seminal vesicle.[55,58] Precise anatomical localization of binding sites in these tissues, and at other sites in the genital tract, has been reported previously by us.[59]

The apparent lack of binding in uterine smooth muscle is surprising. VIP is released during electrical stimulation of isolated uterine muscle strips. This has a relaxing effect that is dose related and that is mimicked by the exogenous administration of VIP.[3,60,61] In addition, specific high-affinity binding sites have been demonstrated on crude muscle preparations of porcine uterus.[62] However, lack of binding here may reflect species differences in the character of the VIP receptor, or, alternatively, binding sites may have been present in low numbers. The lack of labeling on vascular smooth muscle in view of the known vasodilatory effect[63,64] of VIP is unexplained.

Exogenous administration of VIP is associated with endometrial secretion in isolated, everted guinea pig uterine horns.[65] The demonstration of specific binding sites on the endometrium, together with previous membrane binding studies on human endometrial cells,[66] supports the hypothesis that VIP has a direct effect at this site and elsewhere in the female genital tract. A similar situation probably exists for secretory epithelium in the male genital tract. Previous experiments have shown that prostatic contraction and secretion is induced in dogs by exogenous VIP[67]; high-affinity binding sites have been shown in isolated rat prostatic epithelial cells,[68] and this combined with the results of this study suggests a role for VIP in initiating or modulating secretory actions in the male genital tract.

There was a lack of correlation between the distribution of VIP nerve fibers and the anatomical localization of binding sites in some of the tissues examined. This apparent spatial mismatch is a problem that has been encountered in many studies particularly in the central nervous system (for reviews see Refs. 69, 70, and 71), and is the subject of much speculation. Explanations include differences in the finesse of the techniques used and the presence of low-affinity, occupied, or nonfunctional spare receptors. Furthermore, a neuropeptide may act in a neuroendocrine manner, and thus its target cell may be at a distance from the site of its release. Finally, it has been suggested that receptors may be expressed in a "coupled" form;[71] this is based on the discovery of the coexistence of neurotransmitters and neuropeptides in the same synapse.[72]

In conclusion, specific binding sites for VIP have been demonstrated in a variety of peripheral tissues in guinea pig and rat. The localization correlates to some extent with the distribution of VIP-containing nerves and their presence supports a direct role for the peptide in these tissues.

SUMMARY

Vasoactive intestinal polypeptide has a widespread distribution in the body, occurring in both the central and peripheral nervous systems and considerable information is available on its distribution, physiology, and pharmacological actions. Receptors for VIP have been demonstrated previously in peripheral tissues by conventional binding techniques using isolated membrane preparations. However, information on their precise localization is limited. We therefore localized binding sites in a variety of guinea pig and rat tissues by *in vitro* autoradiography and made a parallel study of the distribution of VIP nerves in these tissues using immunocytochemistry. [^{125}I]VIP was prepared by the chloramine T method and shown to be pharmacologically active. After a preincubation procedure to remove endogenously bound VIP, unfixed cryostat sections were incubated with 1 nM [^{125}I]VIP. To determine specific binding, sections were incubated in the presence or absence of 1 μM unlabeled VIP. Autoradiograms were generated by exposing the sections to LKB-Ultrofilm or emulsion-coated coverslips. Dense binding occurred in discrete locations within the gastrointestinal, respiratory, and genital tracts, correlating with known actions of VIP and, to various extents, with the distribution of VIP nerves. For example, there was precise localization to respiratory epithelium, smooth muscle of airways and blood vessels, and alveolar walls, in keeping with the effects of VIP on vascular and airway smooth muscle and mucus secretion.

REFERENCES

1. SAID, S. I. 1986. Vasoactive intestinal peptide. J. Endocrinol. Invest. **9:** 191-200.
2. FAHRENKRUG, J., U. HAGLUND, M. JODAL, O. LUNDGREN, L. OLBE & O. B. SCHAFFALITZKY DE MUCKADELL. 1978. Nervous release of vasoactive intestinal polypeptide in the gastrointestinal tract of cats: Possible physiological implication. J. Physiol. (London) **284:** 291-305.
3. OTTESEN, B. 1983. Vasoactive intestinal polypeptide as a neurotransmitter in the female genital tract. Am. J. Obstet. Gynecol. **147:** 208-224.
4. FAHRENKRUG, J. 1982. VIP as a neurotransmitter in the peripheral nervous system. *In* Vasoactive Intestinal Peptide. S. I. Said, Ed.: 361. Raven Press. New York.
5. LABURTHE, M., D. BATAILLE, M. ROUSSET, J. BESSON, Y. BROER, A. ZWEIBAUM & G. ROSSELIN. 1978. The expression of cell surface receptors for VIP, secretin, and glucagon in normal and transformed cells of the digestive tract. *In* Proceedings of the 11th Meeting of the Federation of European Biochemical Societies. **45:** 271. P. Nicholls, J. V. Moller, P. L. Jorgensen, A. J. Moody, Eds. Pergamon Press. New York.
6. LABURTHE, M., B. BREANT & C. ROUYER-FESSARD. 1984. Molecular identification of receptors for vasoactive intestinal peptide in rat intestinal epithelium by covalent cross-linking. Evidence for two classes of binding sites with different structural and functional properties. Eur. J. Biochem. **139:** 181-196.
7. SUZUKI, Y., D. MCMASTER, M. HUANG, K. LEDERIS & O. P. RORSTAD. 1985. Characterization of functional receptors for vasoactive intestinal peptide in bovine cerebral arteries. J. Neurochem. **45:** 890-899.
8. TAYLOR, D. P. & C. B. PERT. 1979. Vasoactive intestinal polypeptide: Specific binding to rat brain membranes. Proc. Natl. Acad. Sci. USA **76:** 660-664.
9. HUANG, W. M., S. J. GIBSON, P. FACER, J. GU & J. M. POLAK. 1983. Improved section adhesion for immunocytochemistry using high molecular weight polymers of L-lysine as a slide coating. Histochemistry **77:** 275-279.
10. UNNERSTALL, J. R., D. L. NIEHOFF, M. J. KUHAR, & J. M. PALACIOS. 1982. Quantitative receptor autoradiography using [³H]Ultrofilm: Application to multiple benzodiazepine receptors. J. Neurosci. Methods **6:** 59-63.
11. YOUNG III, W. S. & M. J. KUHAR. 1979. A new method for receptor autoradiography: [³H]opioid receptors in mounted tissue sections. Brain Res. **179:** 255-270.
12. BISHOP, A. E., J. M. POLAK, S. R. BLOOM, & A. G. E. PEARSE. 1978. A new universal technique for the immunocytochemical localization of peptidergic innervation. J. Endocrinol. **77:** 25-26.
13. COONS, A. H., H. H. LEDUC & J. M. CONNOLLY. 1955. Studies on antibody production. J. Exp. Med. **102:** 49-60.
14. POULIN, P., Y. SUZUKI, K. LEDERIS & O. P. RORSTAD. 1986. Autoradiographic localization of binding sites for vasoactive intestinal peptide (VIP) in bovine cerebral arteries. Brain Res. **381:** 382-384.
15. BESSON, J., M. DUSSAILLANT, J. C. MARIE, W. ROSTENE & G. ROSSELIN. 1984. *In vitro* autoradiographic localization of vasoactive intestinal peptide (VIP) bindings sites in the rat central nervous system. Peptide **5:** 339-340.
16. WYNN, P. C., R. L. HAUGER, M. C. HOLMES, M. A. MILLAN, K. J. CATT & G. AGUILERA. 1984. Brain and pituitary receptors for corticotropin releasing factor: Localization and differential regulation after adrenalectomy. Peptide **5:** 1077-1084.
17. SHAFFER, M. M. & T. W. MOODY. 1986. Autoradiographic visualization of CNS receptors for vasoactive intestinal peptide. Peptides **7:** 283-288.
18. DE SOUZA, E. B., H. SEIFERT & M. J. KUHAR. 1985. Vasoactive intestinal peptide receptor localization in rat forebrain by autoradiography. Neurosci. Lett. **56:** 113-120.

19. SYNDER, S. H. & J. P. BENNETT, JR. 1976. Neurotransmitter receptors in the brain: Biochemical identification. Ann. Rev. Physiol. **38:** 153-175.
20. UNDEN, A., L. L. PETERSON & T. BARTFAI. 1985. Somatostatin, substance P, vasoactive intestinal polypeptide and neuropeptide Y receptors: Clinical assessment of biochemical methodology and results. *In* International Review of Neurobiology. Vol. 27. J. R. Smythes & R. J. Bradley, Eds. Academic Press, Inc. New York.
21. BARNES, P. J., A. CADIEUX, J. R. CARSTAIRS, B. GREENBERG, J. M. POLAK, & K. RHODEN. 1986. VIP in bovine artery. Localization, function and receptor autoradiography. Br. J. Pharmacol. **89:** 157-162.
22. GHATEI, M. A., M. N. SHEPPARD, D. J. O'SHAUGHNESSY, T. E. ADRIAN, G. P. MC-GREGOR, J. M. POLAK & S. R. BLOOM. 1982. Regulatory peptides in the mammalian respiratory tract. Endocrinology **111:** 1248-1254.
23. ROBBERECHT, P., P. CHATELAIN, P. DE NEEF, J. C. CAMUS, M. WAELBROECK & J. CHRISTOPHE. 1981. Presence of vasoactive intestinal polypeptide receptors coupled to adenylate cyclase in rat lung membranes. Biochem. Biophys. Acta **678:** 76-82.
24. ROBBERECHT, P., K. TATEMOTO, P. CHATELAIN, M. WAELBROECK, J. C. CAMUS, D. HEUSE & J. CHRISTOPHE. 1982. Effects of PHI on vasoactive intestinal peptide receptors and adenylate cyclase activity in lung membranes. A comparison in man, rat, mouse and guinea pig. Reg. Peptides **4:** 241-250.
25. CARSTAIRS, J. R. & P. J. BARNES. 1986. Visualization of vasoactive intestinal peptide receptors in human and guinea pig lung. J. Pharmacol. Exp. Ther. **239:** 249-255.
26. LEROUX, P., H. VAUDRY, A. FOURNIER, S. ST. PIERRE & G. PELLETIER. 1984. Characterization and localization of vasoactive intestinal peptide receptors in the rat lung. Endocrinology **114:** 1506-1512.
27. LEYS, K., A. H. MORICE, O. MADONNA & P. S. SEVER. 1986. Autoradiographic localization of VIP receptors in human lung. FEBS Lett. **199:** 198-202.
28. COLES, S. J., K. R. BASRAR, D. D. O'SULLIVAN, D. DEFUDIF, K. H. NEILL, & L. M. REID. 1984. Neuropeptides and airway mucus. *In* Ciba Foundation Symposium. **109:** 40-54. Pitman. London, England.
29. PEATFIELD, A. C., P. J. BARNES, C. BRATCHER, J. A. NADEL & B. DAVIS. 1983. Vasoactive intestinal peptide stimulates tracheal submucosal gland secretion in ferret. Am. Rev. Respir. Dis. **128:** 89-93.
30. DIAMOND, L., J. L. SZARCK, M. N. GILLESPIE & R. J. ALTIERE. 1983. *In vivo* bronchodilator activity of vasoactive intestinal peptide in the cat. Am. Rev. Respir. Dis. **128:** 827-832.
31. COX, C. P., M. R. LERNER, J. H. WELLS & S. I. SAID. 1981. Inhaled vasoactive intestinal peptide (VIP) prevents bronchoconstriction induced by inhaled histamine (Abstract). Am. Rev. Respir. Dis. **127:** A249.
32. ALTIERE, J. P. & L. DIAMOND. 1983. Relaxant effects of vasoactive intestinal peptide and bethanecol in cat intrapulmonary artery. Eur. J. Pharmacol. **93:** 121-124.
33. HAMASAKI, Y. M., M. MOJARAD & S. I. SAID. 1983. Relaxant action of VIP on cat pulmonary artery. Comparison with acetylcholine, isoproterenal and PGE. J. Appl. Physiol. **54:** 1607-1611.
34. LUNDBERG, J. M., J. FAHRENKRUG, T. HÖKFELT, C. R. MARTLING, O. LARSSON, K. TATEMOTO & A. ÅNGGÅRD. 1984. Co-existence of peptide HI (PHI) and VIP in nerves regulating blood flow and bronchial smooth muscle tone in various mammals including man. Peptides **5:** 593-606.
35. NANDIWADA, D. A., D. J. KADOWITZ, S. I. SAID, M. MOJARAD & A. L. HYMAN. 1985. Pulmonary vasodilator responses to vasoactive intestinal peptide in the cat. J. Appl. Physiol. **28:** 1723-1728.
36. SAID, S. I. & V. MUTT. 1972. Isolation from porcine intestinal wall of a vasoactive octacosapeptide related to secretin and to glucagon. Eur. J. Biochem. **28:** 199-204.
37. POLAK, J. M. & S. R. BLOOM. 1977. Peptidergic innervation of the gastrointestinal tract. *In* Gastrointestinal Hormones and Pathology of the Digestive System. M. Grossman, V. Speranza, N. Basso & E. Lezoche, Eds.: 27-49. Plenum Press. New York; London, England.
38. POLAK, J. M. & S. R. BLOOM. 1979. The neuroendocrine design of the gut. Clin. Endocrinol. Metab. **8(2):** 313-329.

39. FAHRENKRUG, J. 1979. Vasoactive intestinal polypeptide: Measurement distribution and putative neurotransmitter function. Digestion 19: 149-169.
40. FAHRENKRUG, J. 1980. Vasoactive intestinal peptide. Clin. Gastroenterol. 9: 633-644.
41. POLAK, J. M. & S. R. BLOOM. 1981. Distribution and tissue localization of VIP in the central nervous system and in several peripheral organs. In Vasoactive Intestinal Peptide. Advance in Peptide Hormone Research Series. S. I. Said, Ed.: 107. Raven Press. New York.
42. MUTT, V. 1982. Isolation and structure of vasoactive intestinal polypeptide from various species. In Advances in Peptide Research. S. I. Said, Ed: New York. Raven Press. Vol. 1: 1.
43. BROYART, J. P. C. DUPONT, M. LABURTHE & G. ROSSELIN. 1981. Characterization of vasoactive intestinal peptide receptors in human colonic epithelial cells. J. Clin. Endocrinol. Metab. 52: 715-721.
44. AMIRANOFF, B., M. LABURTHE & G. ROSSELIN. 1980. Characterization of specific binding sites for vasoactive intestinal peptide in rat intestinal epithelial cell membranes. Biochim. Biophys. Acta 627: 215-224.
45. LABURTHE, M. & A. COUVINEAU. 1985. The human vasoactive intestinal peptide receptor: Molecular identification by covalent cross-linking in colonic epithelium. J. Clin. Endocrinol. Metab. 61: 50-55.
46. BINDER, H. J., G. F. LEMP & G. D. GARDNER. 1980. Receptors for vasoactive intestinal peptide and secretin on small intestinal epithelial cells. Am. J. Physiol. 238: G190-G196.
47. KREJS, G. R., R. M. BARKLEY, N. W. READ & J. S. FORDTRAN. 1978. Intestinal secretion induced by vasoactive intestinal polypeptide; a comparison with cholera toxin in the canine jejunum in vivo. J. Clin. Invest. 61: 1337-1345.
48. SCHWARTZ, C. J., D. V. KIMBERG, H. E. SHEERIN, M. FIELD & S. I. SAID. 1974. Vasoactive intestinal peptide stimulation of adenylate cyclase and active electrolyte secretion in intestinal mucosa. J. Clin. Invest. 54: 536-544.
49. SAID, S. I. & V. MUTT. 1970. Potent peripheral and splanchnic vasodilator peptide from normal gut. Nature 255: 863-864.
50. PIPER, P. J., S. I. SAID & J. R. VANE. 1970. Effects on smooth muscle preparations of unidentified vasoactive peptides from intestine and lung. Nature 225: 1144-1146.
51. LABURTHE, M., B. AMIRANOFF, N. BOIGE, C. ROUYER-FESSARD, K. TATEMOTO & L. MORODER. 1983. Interaction of GRF and VIP receptors and stimulation of adenylate cyclase in rat and human intestinal epithelial membranes. Comparisons with PHI and secretin. FEBS Lett. 159: 89-92.
52. COUVINEAU, A., C. ROUYER-FESSARD, A. FOURNIER, S. ST. PIERRE, R. PIPKORN & M. LABURTHE. 1984. Structural requirements for VIP interaction with specific receptors in human and rat intestinal membranes: Effect of nine partial sequences. Biochem. Biophys. Res. Commun. 121: 493-498.
53. HEINRICH, D., M. REINECKE & W. G. FORSSMANN. 1986. Peptidergic innervation of the human and guinea pig uterus. Arch. Gynecol. 237: 213-219.
54. HUANG, W. M., J. GU, M. A. BLANK, J. M. ALLEN, S. R. BLOOM & J. M. POLAK. 1984. Peptide-immunoreactive nerves in the mammalian female genital tract. Histochemistry 16: 1297-1310.
55. LARSEN, J.-J., B. OTTESON, J. FAHRENKRUG & L. FAHRENKRUG. 1981. Vasoactive intestinal polypeptide (VIP) in the male genito-urinary tract, concentration and motor effect. Invest. Urol. 19: 211-213.
56. LARSSON, L.-I. 1977. Occurrence of nerves containing vasoactive intestinal polypeptide immunoreactivity in the male genital tract. Life Sci. 21: 503-508.
57. POLAK, J. M., J. GU, S. MINA & S. R. BLOOM. 1981. VIPergic nerves in the penis. Lancet 2: 217-219.
58. ALM, P., J. ALUMETS, R. HAKANSON, CH. OWMAN, F. SUNDLER & B. WALLES. 1980. Origin and distribution of VIP (vasoactive intestinal polypeptide) nerves in the genito-urinary tract. Cell Tissue Res. 205: 337-341.
59. INYAMA, C. O., J. WHARTON, K. McFARTHING, R. H. JACKSON, S. R. BLOOM & J. M. POLAK. 1986. In vitro autoradiographic localization of VIP-binding sites to the epithelial linings of the guinea pig genital tract (Abstract.) J. Pathol. 149: 204A.

60. OTTESON, B., J. J. LARSEN, J. FAHRENKRUG, M. STJERNQUIST & F. SUNDLER. 1981. Distribution and motor effect of VIP in female genital tract. Am. J. Physiol. **240**: E32-E36.
61. BOLTON, T. B., R. J. LANG & B. OTTESEN. 1981. Mechanism of action of vasoactive intestinal polypeptide on myometrial smooth muscle of rabbit and guinea pig. J. Physiol. **318**: 41-55.
62. OTTESEN, B., P. STAUN-OLSEN, S. GAMMELTOFT & J. FAHRENKRUG. 1982. Receptors for vasoactive intestinal polypeptide on crude muscle membranes from porcine uterus. Endocrinology **110**: 2037-2043.
63. OTTESEN, B. & J. FAHRENKRUG. 1981. Effect of vasoactive intestinal polypeptide (VIP) upon myometrial blood flow in non pregnant rabbit. Acta Physiol. Scand. **112**: 195-201.
64. CARTER, A. M., N. EINER JENSEN, J. FAHRENKRUG & B. OTTESEN. 1981. Increased myometrial blood flow evoked by vasoactive intestinal polypeptide in the non-pregnant goat. J. Physiol. **310**: 471-480.
65. HAMMARSTRÖM, M. 1985. Autonomic nervous control of endometrial secretion in the guinea pig. Acta Physiol. Scand. **125**: 461-469.
66. PRIETO, J. C., J. M. GUERRORO, C. DE MIGUEL & R. GOBERNA. 1981. Interaction of vasoactive intestinal peptide with a cell line (HeLa) deprived from human carcinoma of the cervix: Binding to specific sites and stimulation of adenylate cyclase. Mol. Cell. Biochem. **37**: 167-176.
67. SMITH, E. R., T. B. MILLER, M. W. WILSON & M. C. APPEL. 1984. Effects of vasoactive intestinal peptide on canine prostatic contraction and secretion. Am. J. Physiol. **247**: R701-R708.
68. PRIETO, J. C. & J. M. CARMENA. 1983. Receptors for vasoactive intestinal peptide on isolated epithelial cells of rat prostate. Biochim. Biophys. Acta **163**: 408-413.
69. KUHAR, M. J. 1985. The mismatch problem in receptor mapping studies. Trends Neurosci. **8**: 190-191.
70. SHULTS, C. W., R. QUIRION, B. CHRONWALL, T. N. CHASE & T. L. O'DONOHUE. 1984. A comparison of the anatomical distribution of substance P and substance P receptors in the rat central nervous system. Peptides **5**: 1097-1128.
71. SCHULTZBERG, M. & T. HÖKFELT. 1986. The mismatch problem in receptor autoradiography and coexistence of multiple messengers. Trends Neurosci. **9**: 109-110.
72. LUNDBERG, J. M., J. FAHRENKRUG, O. LARSSON & A. ÅNGGARD. 1984. Co-release of vasoactive intestinal polypeptide and peptide histidine isoleucine in relation to atropine resistant vasodilation in cat submandibular salivary gland. Neurosci. Lett. **52**: 37-42.

Mechanism of VIP-Stimulated Chloride Secretion by Intestinal Epithelial Cells

RICHARD D. MCCABE AND
KIERTISIN DHARMSATHAPHORN [a]

University of California Medical School
University of California, San Diego
San Diego, California 92103

INTRODUCTION

Vasoactive intestinal peptide (VIP) causes water and electrolyte secretion from both large and small intestine.[1-4] This secretory effect, observed in animals and man, occurs as the result of Cl^- secretion. Our laboratory utilizes a human colonic cell line, T_{84}, as a model system to study the regulation of Cl^- secretion by VIP.[5-11] This cell line resembles colonic crypt cells morphologically[12,13] and secretes Cl^- in response to a variety of peptides or other regulatory substances.[5] Culture cells are homogenous and free of the influence of unknown regulatory peptides and other neurotransmitters normally present in the intestine. Therefore, the T_{84} cell line is a useful model system to investigate the mechanisms involved in this electrolyte transport process and its regulation. This paper summarizes the results obtained with T_{84} cells on the mechanism of Cl^- secretion induced by VIP.

METHODS

The approaches introduced by Dr. Hans Ussing[14] and others[15-20] have been applied with further modification by our group to T_{84} cells. These methods have been summarized in a recent review[21] and detailed methods have also been presented in other publications.[5-7, 9-11] Readers are referred to these sources for detailed methodology. In brief, T_{84} cell monolayers were grown on permeable supports suitable for transepithelial electrolyte flux measurements. Transepithelial electrolyte fluxes were measured in the modified Ussing chamber. This technique confirmed that VIP stimulates Cl^- secretion

---

[a]Address correspondence to: K. Dharmsathaphorn, M.D., Associate Professor of Medicine, Gastroenterology Division (H-811-D), University Hospital, 225 Dickinson Street, San Diego, CA 92103.

across the T_{84} monolayer and that Cl^- secretion accounted for the changes in short-circuit current (I_{sc}). The use of specific blockers of various transport pathways, for example, bumetanide, Ba^{2+} and anthracene-COOH derivatives, provide indirect evidence for the participation that Na^+,K^+,Cl^- cotransport, K^+ channel, and Cl^- channel demonstrate in the Cl^- secretory process.

RESULTS

T_{84} cells when grown on the permeable, collagen-coated Nucleopore filters and suspended over the culture dish to permit "bottom feeding," formed a confluent monolayer with a high electrical resistance. After five to six days in culture, the cells formed a columnar epithelial monolayer with their basolateral membrane firmly attached to the collagen-coated surface and their microvillus membrane facing the medium.[12–13] These monolayers maintained a stable transepithelial resistance (R) of ~ 1.5 k$\Omega \cdot$cm^2. The collagen-coated Nucleopore membrane that served as the attachment support for the cells had a resistance of $< 4\Omega \cdot$cm^2; thus, it contributed insignificantly to the overall resistance.

VIP-Stimulated Increase in Short Circuit Current Correlated with VIP Receptor Binding and Cellular Cyclic AMP Levels and Represents an Increase in Net Cl⁻ Secretion across T_{84} Monolayers

Transepithelial electrolyte transport studies were carried out in a modified Ussing chamber. For these Ussing chamber studies, we have denoted the basolateral membrane as serosal and microvillus membrane as mucosal surface, respectively. As illustrated in FIGURE 1, addition of $10^{-8} M$ VIP to the serosal bathing solution caused an increase in the I_{sc}. Mucosal addition of VIP had no effect (data not shown). Maximal response was reached ~ 15 minutes after the addition of VIP, and the effect persisted for over one hour. The effect of VIP was dose dependent. A concentration of $10^{-10} M$ VIP induced a detectable alteration in the I_{sc} while a maximal effect was observed at $\sim 10^{-8}$ M (FIG. 2). The changes in I_{sc} correlated well with VIP receptor binding and activation of cellular cyclic AMP as shown in FIGURE 2.

Isotopic flux experiments demonstrated that VIP-stimulated I_{sc} results from an increase in net Cl^- secretion across T_{84} monolayers. FIGURE 3 illustrates a representative experiment for a single set of paired monolayers. The results from six paired monolayers are illustrated in FIGURE 4. After the addition of VIP (10^{-8} M), the increase in net Cl^- secretion (illustrated by the open bars) totally accounted for the change in I_{sc}. Changes in the I_{sc} and net Cl^- secretion had an excellent correlation, $r = 0.90$, $p < 0.001$). After addition of VIP, both $J_{s\text{-}M}Cl^-$ and $J_{M\text{-}s}Cl^-$ increase; however, the increase in the $J_{s\text{-}M}Cl^-$ was consistently greater, resulting in net Cl^- secretion. No significant effects were observed on net Na^+ flux (illustrated by the solid bars).

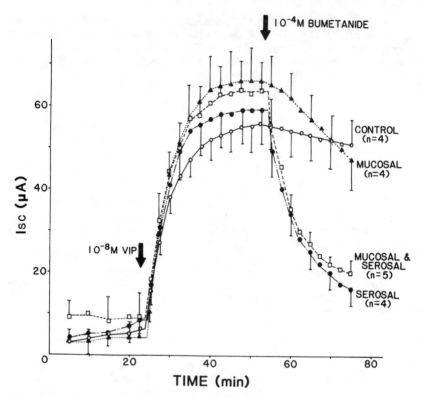

FIGURE 1. Reversal of VIP-stimulated I_{sc} by the serosal addition of bumetanide. T_{84} cell monolayers grown on permeable supports were mounted in the modified Ussing chambers. VIP ($10^{-8} M$) was added at 22.5 minutes to the serosal side. $10^{-4} M$ bumetanide was added at 57.5 minutes to the mucosal (▲), serosal (●) or to both sides (□) of the monolayers. Controls received an equivalent addition of dimethyl sulfoxide (○). Values are expressed as mean ± SE in μA/monolayer. The number of experiments (n) is indicated in parentheses. (From Dharmsathaphorn *et al.*[6] Used with permission from the *Journal of Clinical Investigation.*)

Participation of the Na^+,K^+,Cl^- Cotransport Pathway in VIP-Stimulated Cl^- Secretion

Transepithelial Studies Suggesting Stimulation of a Na^+,K^+,Cl^- Cotransport Mechanism during VIP-Stimulated Cl^- Secretion

Involvement of a basolaterally localized Cl^- cotransport pathway was suggested by: (1) the ability of bumetanide to inhibit VIP-stimulated Cl^- secretion when the compound was applied serosally. (Mucosal addition of bumetanide had little or no effect; Figs. 1 and 3.) (2) VIP's action was inhibited when the Ringer's solution was replaced by either a Na^+-, K^+-, or Cl^--free Ringer's solution. These studies suggest that the basolateral Cl⁻ entry step for VIP-induced Cl⁻ secretion is bumetanide-sensitive and requires the simultaneous presence of Na⁺, K⁺, and Cl⁻.

Radionuclide Uptake Studies Confirming the Existence of Na⁺,K⁺,Cl⁻ Cotransport on the Basolateral Membrane

The Ussing chamber studies described above suggest the Cl⁻ entry step at the basolateral membrane is either a Na⁺,K⁺,Cl⁻ cotransport system or Na⁺,Cl⁻ cotransport operating in close association with the Na⁺,K⁺-ATPase. To differentiate between these two possibilities, ion uptake into the cell were measured in the presence of ouabain. In the following section, uptake studies are described that were carried out on culture dish exposed to Ca²⁺-free media to allow access to the basolateral surface. Next we report on studies in which intact monolayers on permeable supports were used to determine the sidedness.

Verification of the Existence of a Bumetanide-Sensitive Na⁺,K⁺,Cl⁻ Cotransport System in T_{84} Cells. In the presence of ouabain, which inactivates the Na⁺,K⁺-ATPase pump, dependency of K⁺ or Rb⁺ on Cl⁻ uptake suggests a Na⁺,K⁺,Cl⁻ cotransport

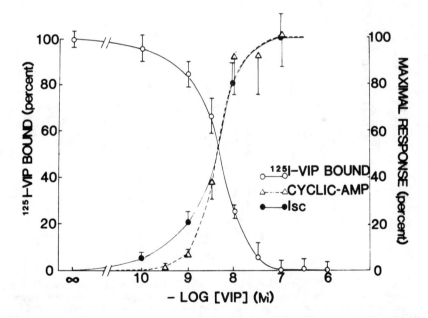

FIGURE 2. Comparison of competitive binding curve of [¹²⁵I]VIP, cellular cAMP production, and I_{sc} response at varying concentrations of VIP. Values represent mean ± SE of three to eight measurements. The scales were adjusted to 100% for comparison. Maximal binding of [¹²⁵I]VIP was 6.5 ± 0.2% with nonspecific binding being 3.9 ± 0.1%. Maximal cAMP level was 348 ± 51 pmol/mg of protein with basal cAMP level being 3 ± 1 pmol/mg of protein. Maximal I_{sc} response was 73 ± 8 μA/cm² with basal I_{sc} being zero. (From Mandel *et al*.[10] pp. 706–709. Used with permission of the *Journal of Biological Chemistry*.)

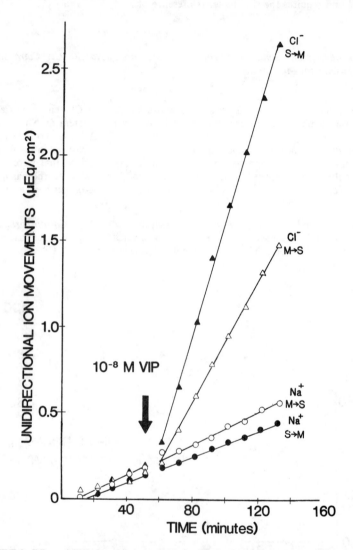

FIGURE 3. Effect of VIP on unidirectional Na$^+$ and Cl$^-$ flux across T$_{84}$ cell monolayers. This figure depicts the results for a representative pair of T$_{84}$ monolayers grown on the permeable support; the monolayers in this experiment had an initial conductance of 0.5 mS/cm^2 and ion flux was determined as described in Methods. VIP (10^{-8} M) was added 52 minutes after the addition of ^{22}Na$^+$ and ^{36}Cl$^-$ to the chambers. Samples were obtained at 10-minute intervals. $\triangle$, M → S Cl$^-$ movement; $\blacktriangle$, S → M Cl$^-$ movement $\bigcirc$, M → S Na$^+$ movement; and $\bigcirc$, S → M Na$^+$ movement. (From Mandel *et al.*[7] and Dharmsathaphorn *et al.*[6] Used with permission of the *American Journal of Physiology* and the *Journal of Clinical Investigation,* respectively.)

mechanism. [86]Rb^+ was used as a tracer for K^+ transport as it was found to be a reasonably good tracer for VIP or A23187-activated K^+ transport.[9] Results presented in FIGURE 5 indicate that Na^+,Rb^+, and Cl^- uptake into T_{84} cells are interdependent and highly sensitive to bumetanide. The interdependence of Na^+, Rb^+, and Cl^- uptake in the presence of ouabain suggests the presence of a bumetanide-sensitive Na^+,K^+,Cl^- cotransport in this cell line. [22]Na^+ uptake was only partially inhibited, because it is also taken up via the Na^+,H^+ antiporter.[21]

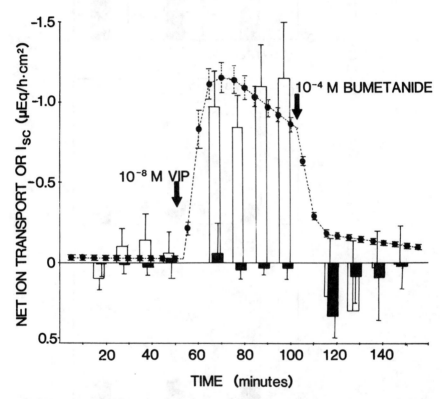

FIGURE 4. Time course of net Na^+ and Cl^- transport and correlation of net Cl^- secretion with the I_{sc}. The mean ± SE from six paired monolayers are illustrated. The circles and dotted line represent the I_{sc}; clear bars represent net Cl^- transport; and solid bars represent net Na^+ transport measured over 10-minute intervals. I_{sc} and flux rates are expressed as $\mu Eq \cdot h^{-1} \cdot cm^{-2}$. Values above the line indicate net secretion, and values below the line net absorption. (From Dharmsathaphorn et al.[6] Used with permission from the *Journal of Clinical Investigation*.)

To determine the stoichiometry of bumetanide-sensitive ion cotransport, the uptake of each of its three substrate ions, Na^+,Cl^-, and Rb^+ was determined in parallel studies using an identical assay buffer containing either [22]Na^+, [86]Rb^+, or [36]Cl^- (FIG. 6). The rates of bumetanide-sensitive uptake for each of the three ions were extrapolated to zero time by polynomial regression of the rates of uptake. Under these experimental conditions, the initial velocity of bumetanide-sensitive Na^+, Rb^+, and Cl^- uptakes

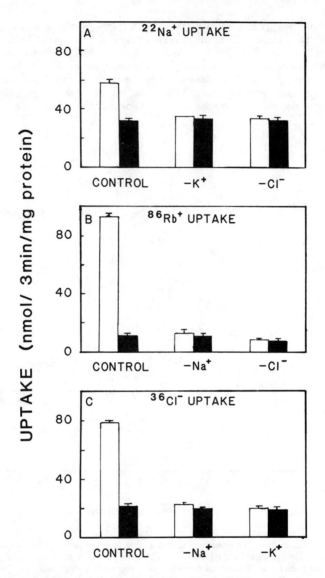

FIGURE 5. Interdependence of bumetanide-sensitive ^{22}Na$^+$, ^{86}Rb$^+$, and Cl$^-$ uptake. All experiments were carried out in the presence of 0.5 mM ouabain to inhibit the Na$^+$,K$^+$-ATPase pump. Clear bars represent uptake in the absence of bumetanide, and solid bars represent uptake in the presence of 0.2 mM bumetanide. T$_{84}$ monolayers attached to 35-mm culture dishes were preincubated as described in Dharmsathaphorn et al.[6] In the control experiments, uptake buffer contained 35 mM Na$^+$ gluconate, 35 mM K$^+$ gluconate, 70 mM N-methylglucamine Cl$^-$, 10 mM Tris-SO$_4$, pH 7.5, and 1.2 mM MgSO$_4$. In the ion substitution experiments, when Na$^+$,K$^+$, or Cl$^-$ were excluded from the uptake buffers, sucrose was added to maintain isotonicity. Experiments depicted in each panel were carried out on different days with different sets of confluent monolayers. (From Dharmsathaphorn et al.[6] Used with permission from the *Journal of Clinical Investigation.*)

were 9.8 ± 1.4, 11.5 ± 1.7, and 21.2 ± 2.5 nmol/min per mg protein, respectively. These uptake rates approached a ratio of 1 Na^+:1 Rb^+:2 Cl^-, similar to the Na^+,K^+,Cl^- cotransport systems reported in other cell types.

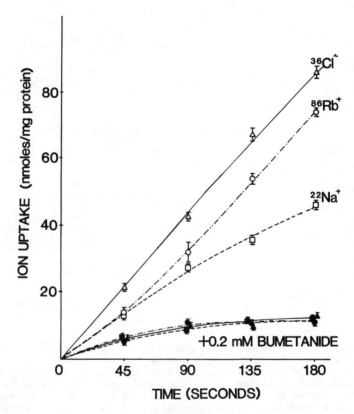

FIGURE 6. Stoichiometry of Na^+,K^+,Cl^- cotransport in T_{84} cells. The time course of bumetanide-sensitive $^{22}Na^+$, $^{86}Rb^+$, and $^{36}Cl^-$ uptake were studied to determine the initial ratios of uptake. A single set of confluent monolayers was preincubated as described in Dharmsathaphorn et al.[6] with the final preincubation buffer containing both 0.5 mM ouabain and 0.5 mM amiloride. Uptake buffer contained 70 mM choline chloride, 35 mM NaNO$_3$, 35 mM RbNO$_3$, 10 mM Tris-NO$_3$, pH 7.5, and 1.2 mM Mg(NO$_3$)$_2$, with trace amounts of either $^{86}Rb^+$ ($\bigcirc,\bullet$), $^{22}Na^+$ ($\square,\blacksquare$), or $^{36}Cl^-$ ($\triangle,\blacktriangle$). Uptakes were carried out in the presence ($\bullet,\blacksquare,\blacktriangle$) or absence ($\bigcirc,\square,\triangle$) of 0.1 m$M$ bumetanide for the given time intervals and terminated using the MgSO$_4$-sucrose wash, as described in Methods. Each point represents the mean $\pm$ SD of triplicate determinations. Zero time values (1-2 nmol/mg protein) have been subtracted from all data. (From Dharmsathaphorn et al.[6] Used with permission from the *Journal of Clinical Investigation*.)

Localization of the Na^+,K^+,Cl^- Cotransport to the Serosal Side of T_{84} Cells. Omission of Ca^{2+} from the incubation buffer in the experiments described above exposed the basolateral surface of the cells, as well as the brush-border surface, to the uptake medium. To determine the sidedness of the bumetanide-sensitive Na^+,K^+,Cl^- co-

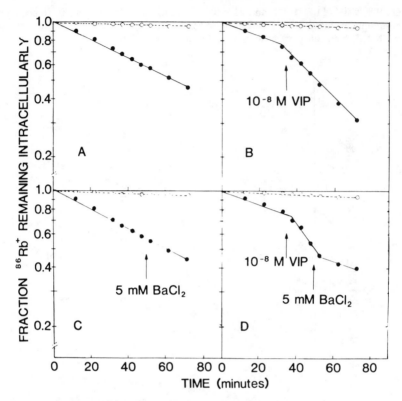

FIGURE 7. Evidence for a basolaterally localized K^+ efflux pathway stimulated by VIP and blocked by barium. $^{86}Rb^+$ efflux across the apical and basolateral membrane of T_{84} monolayers mounted in the Ussing chamber were measured simultaneously. For this set of experiments, monolayers were grown on collagen-coated Nucleopore filters, under conditions identical to those used in the isotopic flux studies described in FIGURE 3. Before use, the monolayers were equilibrated overnight with $^{86}Rb^+$ by adding 0.35 μCi/ml $^{86}Rb^+$ to the culture media ($\sim$4.3 mM K^+) and sterile filtering. The preincubated monolayers were washed rapidly in two changes of Ringer's solution, mounted in the Ussing chambers and voltage clamped. The washing and mounting procedure took approximately 15 seconds. Serial samples were taken simultaneously from the serosal and mucosal reservoirs (every 5 or 10 minutes for this study) with buffer replacement. Ten nM VIP or 5 mM BaCl$_2$ were added as indicated to both mucosal and serosal reservoirs. The data were corrected for sampling volume (0.5 ml of a 5 ml reservoir) and previous sampling loss due to buffer replacement. The results for serosal and mucosal $^{86}Rb^+$ efflux were analyzed independently using the closed three-compartment system with the assumption that $^{86}Rb^+$ acts as a perfect tracer for K^+. The rate of return flux back into the cell from either compartment was negligibly small as compared to the rate of $^{86}Rb^+$ efflux.[7] Therefore, the differential equations describing the three-compartment system (Solomon, Adv. Biol. Med. Phys. **3:** 65, 1953) can be reduced to those describing simple decay. The apparent rate constants for serosal (k_s) and mucosal (k_m) efflux were determined for each sampling time using the relationships:

$$K_s = \frac{\Delta Q}{t} \qquad \frac{1}{Po - R - Q} \qquad K_s = \frac{\Delta R}{t} \qquad \frac{1}{Po - R - Q}$$

transport system, uptake studies were carried out on cell monolayers grown on permeable supports identical to those used for the Ussing chamber studies. Either the brush-border or basolateral surface was exposed to the radionuclide in the uptake medium. As reported in Dharmsathaphorn et al.,[6] preferential bumetanide-sensitive uptakes of $^{22}Na^+$, $^{86}Rb^+$, and $^{36}Cl^-$ were observed only from the serosal side, thus localizing the bumetanide-sensitive Na^+,K^+,Cl^- cotransport pathway to the basolateral membrane. Similar basolateral localization was observed for ouabain-sensitive $^{86}Rb^+$ uptake, which was indicative of Na^+,K^+-ATPase.

Participation of a Basolateral K^+ Exit Pathway (K^+ Channels) in VIP-Stimulated Cl^- Secretion

Transepithelial K^+ and Cl^- transport studies in the Ussing chamber were summarized by Mandel et al.[7] VIP caused a small increase of serosal to mucosal movement of K^+. However, the net K^+ secretion observed was only 3.5% of net Cl^- secretion indicating that the bulk of K^+ that enters the cell along with Cl^- is not secreted and must be recycled. The studies in FIGURE 7 provide evidence for K^+ recycling at the basolateral membrane. Monolayers were loaded with $^{86}Rb^+$ by preincubating them in growth media overnight. $^{86}Rb^+$ efflux rates across both the apical and basolateral membranes of T_{84} monolayers were determined in the Ussing chamber while the change in I_{sc} was monitored. The results are shown in FIGURE 7. The rate of $^{86}Rb^+$ efflux into the mucosal bath was approximately one order of magnitude smaller than that into the serosal bath. The addition of VIP augmented the rate of $^{86}Rb^+$ efflux into the serosal bath two- to threefold. The increase in the rate of $^{86}Rb^+$ efflux into the mucosal bath was negligible in comparison with serosal efflux.

Involvement of K^+ channel in the K^+ efflux process was suggested by the ability of Ba^{2+} to inhibit serosal $^{86}Rb^+$ efflux as well as VIP-induced Cl^- secretion. As illustrated in FIGURE 8, addition of 1 mM Ba^{2+} at ~ 30 minutes following addition of VIP reversed the I_{sc} to near basal levels. Only Ba^{2+} added to the serosal side of

---

FIGURE 7. (Continued)
Where Po is the initial amount of $^{86}Rb^+$ in the cell, and R and Q are the amount of isotope in the mucosal and serosal compartments, respectively. Po was determined experimentally as the total amount of $^{86}Rb^+$ in replicate tissues and as the total amount in the experimental tissues at the end of the experiment plus the amount in the bathing media. The intracellular K^+ of the monolayers was estimated to be approximately 639 nmoles at the start of the experiment (derived from $^{86}Rb^+$ counts of the monolayers as compared to $^{86}Rb^+$ counts in the culture media with $[K^+]$ of 4.3 mM). Extracellular K^+ in the bathing reservoir was 26 μmoles (5 ml of solution with $[K^+]$ of 5.2 mM). The results of serosal efflux ($\bullet$——$\bullet$) and mucosal efflux ($\bigcirc$- - - -$\bigcirc$) are plotted as $1 - \dfrac{1}{Po-R-Q}$ for serosal efflux and $1 - \dfrac{1}{Po-R-Q}$ for mucosal efflux. The negative slope of the line over time represents the rate constant for $^{86}Rb^+$ efflux. 10^{-8} M VIP stimulated $^{86}Rb^+$ efflux across the basolateral membrane but has no effect on $^{86}Rb^+$ efflux across the apical membrane. $BaCl_2$, which by itself has no effect on $^{86}Rb^+$ efflux, effectively abolished VIP-stimulated efflux. (From Mandel et al.[10] pp. 710-712. Used with permission of the Journal of Biological Chemistry.)

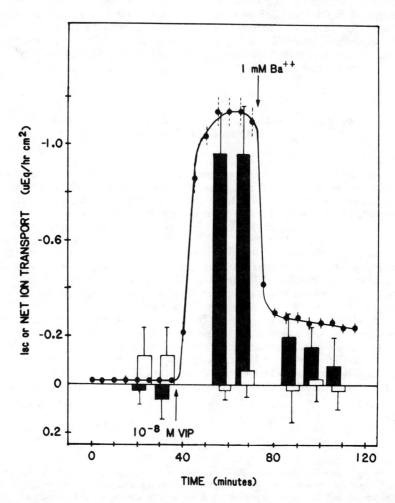

FIGURE 8. Inhibition of VIP-stimulated Cl^- secretion by barium. Time course for VIP-stimulated net Cl^- and Na^+ transport are shown together with the changes in short-circuit current (I_{sc}). T_{84} monolayers were grown on collagen-coated Nucleopore filters, and flux studies were carried out similar to those in FIGURE 4. Results are presented as means $\pm$ SE for eight pairs of monolayers. Net Na^+ flux rates (clear bars) and net Cl^- flux rates (solid bars) are indicated for sequential 10-minute periods. I_{sc} (filled circles) and flux rates are expressed as $\mu Eq \cdot h^{-1} \cdot cm^{-2}$. Values above the line indicate net secretion, and values below the line indicate net absorption. Barium applied serosally reversed VIP-stimulated Cl^- secretion.

the monolayers reversed VIP-induced I_{sc} suggesting that the Ba^{2+}-sensitive K^+ efflux mechanism is serosally localized.

Participation of an Apical Cl^- Exit Pathway (Cl^- Channel) in the Cl^- Secretory Mechanism Induced by VIP

Stimulation of apical Cl^- efflux by $10^{-7} M$ VIP was demonstrated [36]Cl^- preloaded T_{84} cells as shown in FIGURE 9. Dibutyryl cAMP (5 mM) similarly increased the rate of Cl^- efflux from T_{84} cells, and 1 mM N-phenylanthranilic acid inhibited VIP-accelerated Cl^- efflux.[10]

Since Cl^- movement via a Cl^- channel should be bidirectional, we tested for a stimulation of Cl^- uptake by VIP. Under steady-state conditions similar to those used in the Ussing chamber, addition of $10^{-7} M$ VIP to confluent T_{84} monolayers did accelerate the rate of [36]Cl^- uptake across the apical membrane.[10] Subsequently, Na^+-depleted, K^+-loaded cells were utilized in order to optimize the acceleration of Cl^- uptake by VIP, as well as to establish a standardized condition. FIGURE 10 shows that VIP dramatically increased the initial rate of [36]Cl^- uptake under this experimental condition. The uptake, similar to efflux, was inhibited by N-phenylanthranilic acid. Although our study does not directly prove that the Cl^- exit pathway is a Cl^- channel, results of our kinetic studies suggest that it is. Subsequently, Frizzell et al.[22] have demonstrated that the apical Cl^- exit pathway in this cell line is indeed a Cl^- channel.

Synergistic Effect between VIP-Stimulated Cl^- Secretion and Other Cl^- Secretory Mechanisms

VIP causes Cl^- secretion via a cyclic-AMP-dependent mechanism. Our study described above indicates that this process involves an uptake of Cl^- across the basolateral membrane via a Na^+,K^+,Cl^- cotransport pathway. The Na^+,K^+-ATPase pump, also on the basolateral membrane, provides energy for the Cl^- secretory process and recycles the Na^+ that enters the cell via the cotransporter. Cl^- exits across the apical membrane and K^+ exits across the basolateral membrane via their respective channels. Other cAMP-mediated Cl^- secretions, that induced by PGE_1 or adenosine, stimulate similar mechanisms.[23,24] cGMP-mediated Cl^- secretion induced by the heat-stable toxin of E. coli also acts by a similar mechanism involving the same transport pathways.[25] However, the Ca^{2+}-mediated Cl^- secretory response, which can be activated by carbachol, histamine, or A23187 acts via a different mechanism.[7,9,26,27] The latter involves a Ca^{2+}-activated K^+ channel less sensitive to Ba^{2+}[9] and does not appear to activate the cAMP-sensitive Cl^- channel.[10,26] Therefore, while cAMP- and cGMP-mediated responses are not additive to one another, both synergize with the Ca^{2+}-mediated response.[8,25,26] FIGURE 11 shows this synergistic phenomenon. When a threshold concentration of A23187 (0.3 μM) was tested in combination with a concentration of VIP that gave a maximal response (10 nM), the resulting net Cl^- secretion was significantly greater than predicted from the sum of their individual responses. The mechanism of this synergism has been addressed by Cartwright et al.[8], as well as in References 24-27.

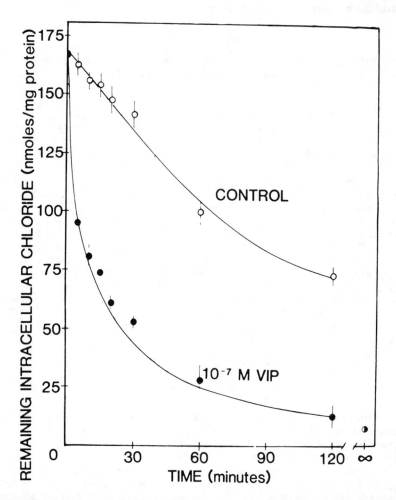

FIGURE 9. Acceleration of the rate of $^{36}Cl^-$ efflux from T_{84} cells by VIP. $^{36}Cl^-$ efflux studies carried out with monolayers on culture dishes as described in Mandel *et al.*[10] T_{84} monolayers were loaded with $^{36}Cl^-$ by a three-hour incubation at room temperature in KCl buffer (140 mM KCl, 10 mM Tris-SO$_4$, pH 7.5, 1 mM MgSO$_4$), washed twice with 2 ml of sucrose buffer (241 mM sucrose, 10 mM Tris-SO$_4$, pH 7.5, 1 mM MgSO$_4$), and incubated for one hour in 1 ml of sucrose buffer containing 0.5 mM ouabain and 0.1 mM bumetanide. Efflux was then initiated by aspiration of the sucrose-ouabain buffer and addition of 1 ml of a buffer containing 120 mM Na-gluconate, 10 mM K-gluconate, 10 mM NaCl, 20 mM Hepes-Tris, pH 7.5, 1 mM MgSO$_4$, 0.5 mM ouabain, and 0.1 mM bumetanide. The loss of intracellular isotope was measured in the presence (●) or absence (○) of 10^{-7} M VIP. At indicated times, efflux was terminated using the Mg-sucrose wash procedure. The results are presented as the mean remaining intracellular $^{36}Cl^-$ ± SD of triplicate monolayers versus time. $^{36}Cl^-$ efflux from T_{84} monolayers was accelerated by VIP. The results suggest that VIP opens a Cl^- efflux pathway in the T_{84} cells.

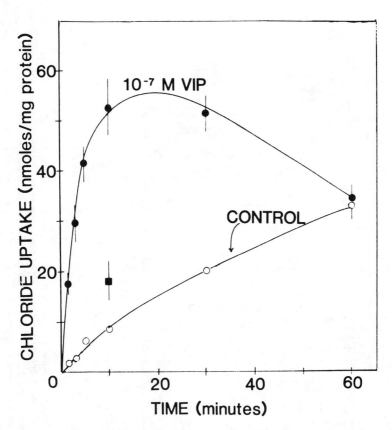

FIGURE 10. Stimulation of the initial rate of Cl$^-$ uptake by VIP. ^{36}Cl$^-$ uptake studies carried out with monolayers on culture dishes as described in Mandel *et al.*[10] Confluent monolayers grown on 35-mm dishes were washed twice and incubated in 1 ml of KCl buffer (140 mM KCl, 10 mM Tris-SO$_4$, pH 7.5, 1 mM MgSO$_4$) for two hours at room temperature. Cells were then washed with three changes of sucrose buffer (241 mM sucrose, 10 mM Tris-SO$_4$) and incubated in 1 ml of this buffer containing 0.5 mM ouabain and 0.1 mM bumetanide with or without 10^{-7} M VIP. After a five-minute preincubation, this buffer was aspirated and replaced with 0.7 ml Na-gluconate uptake buffer (140 mM Na-gluconate, 10 mM Tris-SO$_4$, pH 7.5, 1 ml MgSO$_4$, 0.5 mM ouabain, 0.1 mM bumetanide, and 1.0 μCi/ml ^{36}Cl$^-$). The final ^{36}Cl$^-$ concentration was approximately 2 mM with or without 10^{-7} M VIP. Uptakes were terminated and intracellular isotope counted as described in the text. The results shown represent the mean ± SD of triplicate measurements. ^{36}Cl$^-$ uptake was accelerated by VIP. The results suggest that the VIP-regulated pathway functions in both efflux and uptake directions.

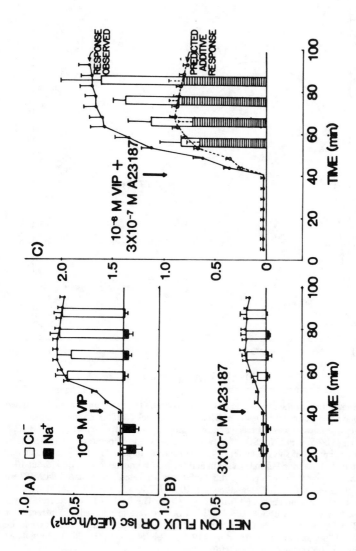

FIGURE 11. Synergism between cAMP- and calcium-mediated Cl⁻ secretory mechanisms. Time course of the effect of VIP (A), A23187 (B), and VIP plus (C) on net ion transport and I_{sc} across T_{84} cell monolayers are shown. Open bars represent net Cl⁻ transport and solid bars, net Na⁺ transport over a 10-minute flux period. Circles and lines represent I_{sc}. In C, the hatched bars, open circles, and dashed line represent the predicted additive response from results shown in A and B. Results are expressed as mean ± SE in $\mu Eq \cdot h^{-1} \cdot cm^{-2}$; values above the line represent net secretion and those below the line, net absorption. (Reprinted from Dharmsathaphorn & Madara,[21] p. 61. Used with permission of Academic Press.)

DISCUSSION

Cl^- Secretory Response of T_{84} Monolayers to VIP

Confluent T_{84} cell monolayers retain polarity, form tight junctions between cells, and grow to confluence with the basolateral surface attached to the growth substratum and their microvillus membrane facing the medium. Addition of VIP to T_{84} cell monolayers mounted in a modified Ussing chamber stimulates secretion of Cl^- similar to the phenomenon observed in isolated intestine from animal and man.[1-4] The similarity of the physiological response has encouraged us to use the T_{84} cell line as a model system to study the mechanism of VIP-stimulated Cl^- secretion.

Na^+,K^+,Cl^- Cotransport Pathway

Our results demonstrate the presence of a basolateral-localized Na^+,K^+,Cl^- cotransport system in the T_{84} cells strongly suggest that VIP-induced Cl^- secretion requires a functional Na^+,K^+,Cl^- cotransporter for the Cl^- uptake step. This conclusion is drawn from the following observations. (1) In the Ussing chamber system, we have observed that the VIP-stimulated I_{sc} and Cl^- secretion are reversed or prevented by the serosal application of bumetanide, an established and specific inhibitor of Na^+,Cl^- cotransport or Na^+,K^+,Cl^- cotransport. (2) In the presence of ouabain to inactivate the Na^+,K^+-ATPase, the bumetanide-sensitive uptake of $^{22}Na^+$, $^{36}Cl^-$, and $^{86}Rb^+$ (used as a tracer for K^+) required the simultaneous presence of all three substrate ions, Na^+,Cl^-, and K^+ (or Rb^+). Omission of any one ion reduced the level of uptake to that observed in the presence of bumetanide. (3) The stoichiometry for the interdependent uptake of the three substrate ions approached a ratio of 1 Na^+ : 1 K^+ : 2 Cl^-. This is identical to that previously reported for electroneutral Na^+,K^+,Cl^- cotransport systems in other cells. (4) Radionuclide uptake studies on monolayers grown on a permeable support verified the localization of the bumetanide-sensitive Na^+,K^+,Cl^- cotransport system to the basolateral membrane. These results, obtained from both the Ussing chamber and cellular ion uptake studies, strongly suggest that the Cl^- entry step involved in VIP-induced Cl^- secretion is a Na^+,K^+,Cl^- cotransport system localized on the basolateral membrane.

K^+ Channels

Subsequently, we explored the fate of K^+, which enters the cells in symport with Cl^-. We found that (1) little K^+ was secreted along with Cl^-; (2) the secretagogues (VIP and A23187) activated $^{86}Rb^+$ (K^+) efflux across the basolateral membrane;

and (3) secretagogue-activated basolateral K^+ efflux and Cl^- secretion were inhibited by Ba^{2+}. Taken together, these results suggest that K^+ is recycled across the basolateral membrane during the Cl^- secretory process. In the secretory process, Cl^- would accumulate to levels above its electrochemical equilibrium by action of the Na^+,K^+,Cl^- cotransporter and exit across the apical membrane. Na^+ can be recycled by the Na^+,K^+-ATPase, which can also transport additional K^+ into the intracellular compartment. The basolateral membrane-localized, Ba^{2+}-sensitive K^+ transport pathway would then function in K^+ recycling. This K^+ recycling process should allow a favorable electrochemical gradient both for Cl^- entry into the cell via the Na^+,K^+,Cl^- cotransport system on the basolateral membrane, and for Cl^- exit via a Cl^- transport pathway on the brush-border membrane.

Our results also point to a regulatory role for this basolaterally localized K^+ efflux pathway in the Cl^- secretory process. Stimulation of this K^+ efflux pathway by VIP was concurrent with the activation of electrogenic Cl^- secretion. Conversely, inhibition of K^+ efflux by Ba^{2+} inhibited the Cl^- secretory process. The correlation between activation of basolateral K^+ efflux and Cl^- secretion, suggests that the Ba^{2+}-sensitive K^+ transport mechanism plays a regulatory role in the Cl^- secretory process. Other investigators have also identified Ba^{2+}-sensitive K^+ channels in other epithelia and studied the relation between these channels and the Cl^- secretory mechanism. Ba^{2+} has been reported to inhibit electrogenic Cl^- secretion in frog and piglet gastric mucosa,[28,29] and a Ba^{2+}-sensitive increase in basolateral K^+ conductance during Cl^- secretion has been reported for canine trachea.[30,31] Brown and Simmons,[32] using a cultured kidney cell line, have found that agents that increase Cl^- secretion also stimulated $^{86}Rb^+$ efflux, primarily across the basolateral membrane. Basolaterally localized K^+ channels have also been strongly implicated in the hormonal regulation of exocrine cell secretion.[33,34]

Cl⁻ Channel

Utilizing the ion uptake and efflux techniques, we describe a VIP-activated Cl^- exit pathway on the apical membrane of the T_{84} human colonic epithelial cell line which is distinct from the Na^+,K^+,Cl^- cotransporter or the Cl^-/HCO_3^- antiporter. Cl^- transport by this system was noncompetitively inhibited by N-phenylanthranilic acid, a putative Cl^- channel blocker. Recently, Frizzell et al., utilizing the patch technique, verified the presence of a cyclic AMP-sensitive Cl^- channel on the apical membrane of this cell line.[22]

Studies in other epithelia that secrete Cl^-, for example, the trachea, cornea, ciliary body, or shark rectal gland, have produced findings that are also compatible with our proposed mechanism for Cl^- secretion, and suggest that similar Cl^- transport mechanisms may be shared by many Cl^- secreting epithelia. In these epithelial tissues, hormonal activation of an apically localized Cl^- conductance pathway has been associated with an increase in electrogenic Cl^- secretion. Petersen and Reuss[35] have shown that cAMP increased the Cl^- permeability across the luminal membrane of Necturus gallbladder epithelium. This effect was observed in parallel with a rapid decrease in intracellular Cl^- activities that is similar to our observations with T_{84} cells under steady-state conditions. Studies by Welsh[36] and by Shorofsky et al.[37] have demonstrated the presence of an Cl^- conductance pathway on the apical membrane of canine tracheal epithelial cells.

Synergism between VIP-Stimulated Cl⁻ Secretion and Ca²⁺-Mediated Cl⁻
Secretion

The mechanism by which VIP (cAMP) and A23187 (intracellular Ca^{2+}) regulate Cl^- transport and the basis for their synergistic actions have been investigated in our studies. Intracellular cAMP and cytosolic Ca^{2+} may interact with each other or interact with other intracellular mediators that mediate or modulate their actions. On the other hand, the cAMP-and Ca^{2+}-dependent processes may occur independently. They may stimulate different transport pathways that have cooperative interactions and are dependent on one another in the Cl^- secretory process. Measurement of cAMP showed that A23187 did not augment cAMP response to VIP, suggesting that A23187 potentiates the action of VIP at a step distal to the VIP binding and cAMP production. It is possible that cAMP may mobilize intracellular stores of Ca^{2+} but this does not appear to be the case; we have shown that VIP did not alter free cytosolic Ca^{2+}.[26] Having also shown that A23187 did not augment cAMP production by VIP, our study then sought to identify the different transport pathways activated by VIP and A23187, and to determine whether interaction at the level of the transport pathways could explain the synergistic action. The results suggest that this might be the case.

The mechanisms of Cl^- secretion stimulated by VIP and A23187 appear to be different. VIP directly activates an apical membrane Cl^- transport pathway,[10] and also increases basolateral membrane K^+ efflux. A23187, in contrast to VIP, activates another basolateral K^+ efflux pathway but not the apically localized Cl^- transport pathway. We postulated that A23187, by inducing K^+ efflux across the basolateral membrane, hyperpolarizes the cells and increases the driving force for Cl^- exit across the randomly opened Cl^- channel apical membrane. The opening of the apically localized Cl^- transport pathway by VIP allowed the K^+ efflux induced by A23187 to become a more effective driving force because the Cl^- exit pathway is rate limiting. According to this study, synergism is therefore a result of the cooperative interaction between the opening of the Cl^- exit pathway on the apical membrane and the potassium exit pathways on the basolateral membrane.

REFERENCES

1. SCHWARTZ, C. J., D. V. KIMBERG, H. E. SHEERIN, M. FIELD, & S. I. SAID. 1974. Vasoactive intestinal peptide stimulation of adenylate cyclase and active electrolyte secretion in intestinal mucosal. J. Clin. Invest. **54:** 536-544.
2. RACUSEN, L. C. & H. J. BINDER. 1977. Alteration of large intestinal electrolyte transport by vasoactive intestinal polypeptide in the rat. Gastroenterology **73:** 790-796.
3. WALDMAN, D. B., J. D. GARDNER, A. M. ZFASS & G. M. MAKHLOUF. 1977. Effects of vasoactive intestinal peptide, secretin, and related peptides on rat colonic transport and adenylate cyclase activity. Gastroenterology **73:** 518-523.
4. DAVIS, G. R., C. A. SANTA ANA, S. G. MORAWSKI & J. S. FORDTRAN. 1981. Effect of vasoactive intestinal polypeptide on active and passive transport in the human jejunum. J. Clin. Invest. **67:** 1687-1694.
5. DHARMSATHAPHORN, K., K. G. MANDEL, J. A. MCROBERTS, L. D. TISDALE & H. MASUI. 1984. A human colonic tumor cell line that maintains vectorial electrolyte transport. Am. J. Physiol. **246:** G204-G208.

6. DHARMSATHAPHORN, K., K. G. MANDEL, H. MASUI & J. A. MCROBERTS. 1985. VIP-induced chloride secretion by a colonic epithelial cell line: Direct participation of a basolaterally localized Na^+, K^+, Cl^- cotransport system. J. Clin. Invest. **75:** 462-471.

7. MANDEL, K. G., J. A. MCROBERTS, G. BEUERLEIN, E. S. FOSTER & K. DHARMSATHA-PHORN. 1986. Ba^{2+} inhibition of VIP and A23187-stimulated Cl^- secretion by T_{84} cell monolayers. Am. J. Physiol. **250:** C486-C494.

8. CARTWRIGHT, C. A., J. A. MCROBERTS, K. G. MANDEL & K. DHARMSATHAPHORN. 1985. Synergistic action of cyclic AMP and calcium mediated chloride secretion in a colonic epithelial cell line. J. Clin. Invest. **76:** 1837-1842.

9. MCROBERTS, J. A., G. BEUERLEIN & K. DHARMSATHAPHORN. 1985. Cyclic AMP and Ca^{2+} activated K^+ transport in a human colonic epithelial cell line. J. Biol. Chem. **260:** 14163-14172.

10. MANDEL, K. G., K. DHARMSATHAPHORN & J. A. MCROBERTS. 1986. Characterization of a cyclic AMP-activated Cl^- transport pathway in the apical membrane of a human colonic epithelial cell line. J. Biol. Chem. **261:** 704-712.

11. DHARMSATHAPHORN, K., P. HUOTT, C. A. CARTWRIGHT, J. A. MCROBERTS, K. G. MANDEL & G. BEUERLEIN. 1986. Inhibition of Cl^- secretion by quinidine in a human colonic epithelial cell line. Am. J. Physiol. **250:** G806-G813.

12. MADARA, J. & K. DHARMSATHAPHORN. 1985. Occluding junction structure-function relationships in a cultured human colonic cell monolayer. J. Cell Biol. **101:** 2124-2133.

13. MADARA, J. L., J. STATFORD, K. DHARMSATHAPHORN & S. CARLSON. 1987. Structure analysis of a model human intestinal epithelial cell line. Gastroenterology **92:** 1133-1145.

14. USSING, H. H. & K. ZERAHN. 1951. Active transport of sodium as the source of electric current in the short-circuited isolated frog skin. Acta. Physiol. Scand. **23:** 110-127.

15. MURAKAMI, H. & H. MASUI. 1980. Hormonal control of human colon carcinoma cell growth in serum-free medium. Proc. Natl. Acad. Sci. USA. **77:** 3464-3468.

16. HANDLER, J. S., R. E. STEELE, M. K. SAHIB, J. B. WADE, A. S. PRESTON, N. L. LAWSON & J. P. JOHNSON. 1979. Toad urinary bladder epithelial cells in culture: Maintenance of epithelial structure, sodium transport, and response to hormones. Proc. Natl. Acad. Sci. USA **76:** 4151-4155.

17. CEREIJIDO, M., E. S. ROBBINS, W. J. DOLAN, C. A. ROTUNNO & D. D. SABATINI. 1978. Polarized monolayers formed by epothelial cells on a permeable and translucent support. J. Cell Biol. **77:** 853-880.

18. BINDER, H. J. & C. L. RAWLINS. 1973. Electrolyte transport across isolated large intestinal mucosa. Am. J. Physiol. **225:** 1232-1239.

19. RINDLER, M. J., J. A. MCROBERTS & M. H. SAIER, JR. 1982. (Na^+, K^+)-cotransport in the Madin-Darby canine kidney cell line. J. Biol. Chem. **257:** 2254-2259.

20. RINDLER, M. J. & M. H. SAIER, JR. 1981. Evidence for Na^+/H^+ antiport in cultured dog kidney cells (MDCK). J. Biol. Chem. **256:** 10820-10825.

21. DHARMSATHAPHORN, K. & J. L. MADARA. 1988. Established intestinal cell lines as model systems for electrolyte transport studies. *In* Methods in Enzymology: Biomembranes Biological Transport, Volume 5. Cellular and Subcellular Transport: Epithelial Cells. Sidney Fleisher and Becca Fleisher, Eds.: In press. Academic Press. Orlando, FL.

22. HALM, D., G. RECHKEMMER & R. FRIZZEL. 1986. Single-channel recording from a secretory epithelial cell line. Fed. Proc. **741**(Abstr.).

23. WEYMER, A., P. HUOTT, W. LIU, J. A. MCROBERTS & K. DHARMSATHAPHORN. 1985. Chloride secretory mechanism induced by prostaglandin E_1 in a colonic epithelial cell line. J. Clin. Invest. **76:** 1828-1836.

24. HUOTT, P., K. BARRETT, S. WASSERMAN & K. DHARMSATHAPHORN. 1986. Immune-related intestinal secretion. Role of mast cell products in colonic secretion. Gastroenterology **90:** 1792.

25. DHARMSATHAPHORN, K., W. LIU, R. A. GIANNELLA & P. HUOTT. 1988. The mechanism of *E. Coli* heat-stable enterotoxin in a human colonic cell. J. Clin. Invest. In press.

26. DHARMSATHAPHORN, K. & S. PANDOL. 1986. Mechanism of chloride secretion induced by carbachol in a colonic epithelial cell line. J. Clin. Invest. **77:** 348-354.

27. WASSERMAN, S., P. HUOTT, K. BARRETT, G. BEUERLEIN, M. KAGNOFF & K. DHARM-SATHAPHORN. 1988. Immune-related intestinal secretion: I. Chloride secretion induced by histamine in a human colonic cell line. Am. J. Physiol. **254:** C53-C62.

28. McLennan, W. L., T. E. Machen & T. Zeuthen. 1980. Ba^{2+} inhibition of electrogenic Cl^- secretion *in vitro* frog and piglet gastric mucosa. Am. J. Physiol. **239:** G151-G160.
29. Rangachari, P. K. 1975. Ba^{2+} on the resting frog stomach: Effects on electrical and secretory parameters. Am. J. Physiol. **228:** 511-517.
30. Smith, P. L. & R. A. Frizzell. 1984. Chloride secretion by canine tracheal epithelium IV. Basolateral membrane K permeability parallels secretion rate. J. Membr. Biol. **77:** 187-199.
31. Welsh, M. J. 1983. Barium inhibition of basolateral membrane potassium conductance in tracheal epithelium. Am. J. Physiol. **244:** F639-F645.
32. Brown, C. D. A. & N. L. Simmons. 1982. K^+ transport in "tight" epithelial monolayers of MDCK cells: Evidence for a calcium-activated K^+ channel. Biochim. Biophys. Acta **690:** 95-105.
33. Maruyama, Y., D. V. Gallacher & O. H. Peterson. 1983. Voltage and Ca^{2+}-activated K^+ channel in baso-lateral acinar cell membranes of mammalian salivary glands. Nature **302:** 827-829.
34. Maruyama, Y., O. H. Peterson, P. Flanagan & G. T. Pearson. 1983. Quantification of Ca^{2+}-activated K^+ channels under hormonal control in pig pancreas acinar cells. Nature **305:** 228-232.
35. Petersen, K.-U. & L. Reuss. 1983. Cyclic AMP-induced chloride permeability in the apical membrane of Necturus gallbladder epithelium. J. Gen. Physiol. **81:** 705-729.
36. Welsh, M. J., P. L. Smith & R. A. Frizzell. 1982. Chloride secretion by canine tracheal epithelium. II. The cellular electrical potential profile. J. Membr. Biol. **70:** 227-238.
37. Shorofsky, S. R., M. Field & H. A. Fozzard. 1982. The cellular mechanism of active chloride secretion in vertebrate epithelia: Studies in intestine and trachea. Philos. Trans. R. Soc. Lond. **299:** 597-607.

Neurotransmitter Regulation of Ionic Channels in Freshly Dissociated Smooth Muscle Cells[a]

STEPHEN M. SIMS,[b] MICHEL B. VIVAUDOU,
LUCIE H. CLAPP, NANCY L. LASSIGNAL,
JOHN V. WALSH, JR., AND JOSHUA J. SINGER

Department of Physiology
University of Massachusetts Medical School
Worcester, Massachusetts 01655

An extraordinary array of neurotransmitters, including neuropeptides, act on smooth muscle, making it an attractive preparation for the investigation of the diverse mechanisms of transmitter action. Moreover, contraction serves as a simple assay for the actions of these agents, and as a consequence smooth muscle has long been used by pharmacologists studying transmitter-receptor interactions. But smooth muscle has been accorded much less attention by membrane biophysicists interested in ionic channels because of major technical difficulties associated with electrical syncytia into which the cells are almost invariably coupled. In order to take advantage of this richness of transmitter-receptor interactions without the problems associated with an electrical syncytium, we have employed a preparation of single smooth muscle cells, freshly dissociated from their tissue. We shall demonstrate here the use of such isolated cells to study the effects of a number of transmitters and neuropeptides on one species of K^+ channel and also on voltage-dependent Ca^{2+} channels. The methods have been described in detail in earlier work.[1-3]

It is a straightforward task to establish that the cells employed, which are obtained by enzymatic digestion from the stomach of the toad *Bufo marinus,*[4-6] still respond to a variety of transmitters after being isolated. This can be done by using contraction as a simple assay in much the same way that it has long been done in tissue. FIGURE 1 illustrates the ability of a single cell to respond to a number of neuropeptides and also to acetylcholine, the major classical excitatory neurotransmitter for visceral smooth muscle. The action of inhibitory or "relaxing" agents can be demonstrated in a similar fashion. As an example, the ability of VIP to inhibit acetylcholine-induced contractions is shown in FIGURE 2. In each of these demonstrations the use of single cells permits us to conclude that the receptors for various agents are located on one and the same cell. Thus the opportunity exists to study the relationship between the different receptor mechanisms and the end points of their action. For example, it can

[a] The work of the authors reported here was supported by National Institutes of Health Grant DK31620 and National Science Foundation Grant DCB8511674.

[b] Present address: Department of Physiology, University of Western Ontario, London, Ontario, Canada, N6A 5C1.

be determined whether different excitatory agents, acting on distinct receptors, affect the same set of ionic channels. We shall deal with one such question below.

Between the ligand-receptor interaction and the contraction of the cell stand the electrical events at the membrane level. These events have now been investigated in considerable detail for a number of excitatory agents. A typical response to physalaemin,[7] a peptide related to substance P, is shown in FIGURE 3, which displays video images of a cell impaled with a conventional micropipette (FIG. 3A), the time course

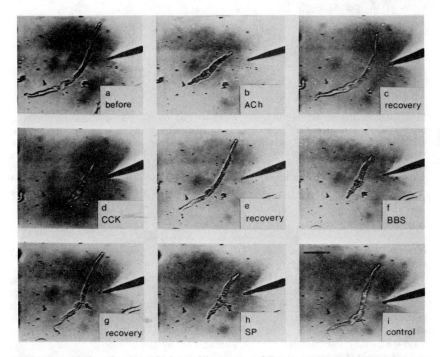

FIGURE 1. Single cell, relaxed in frame (**a**), contracts following 10-sec application of 10 μM acetylcholine (ACh) (**b**), 80 μM cholecystokinin-octapeptide (CCK) (**d**), 50 μM bombesin (BBS) (**f**), and 6 μM substance P (SP) (**h**). The concentrations given are those in the application pipette, which are necessarily higher than those at the cell surface. Application is made by applying a pulse of pneumatic pressure to the back of the pipette. Cell was allowed to relax four minutes between applications, as shown in frames (**c**), (**e**), and (**g**). Frame (**i**) shows that following application of control solution no change in length occurred. Bar, 50 μM. (From Lassignal *et al.*[1] Used with permission from the *American Journal of Physiology*.)

of the physalaemin-induced contraction (FIG. 3B), and the record of membrane potential (FIG. 3C). (Note that the time indicated by "0" on the abscissa in FIGURE 3B corresponds to the onset of physalaemin application in 3C). In response to physalaemin the membrane depolarizes and this depolarization, upon reaching a threshold level, results in the generation of action potentials. As we demonstrated some time ago,[8] these action potentials are pure Ca^{2+} "spikes", that is, the inward current that accounts for the rising phase of the action potential and the entry of positive charge

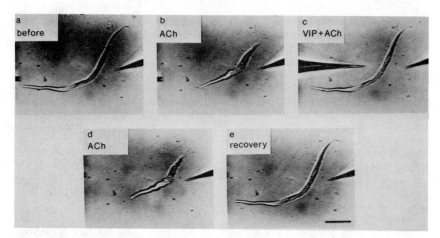

FIGURE 2. Inhibition of acetylcholine (ACh)-induced contraction by vasoactive intestinal peptide (VIP). (a) Relaxed cell before application of any agent; (b) peak contraction produced by a 10-sec pulse of ACh; (c) no response to same 10-sec pulse of ACh when preceded by 30-sec pulse of VIP; (d) recovery of cell responsiveness as shown by contraction caused by ACh application four minutes after time shown in c; (e) relaxed cell four minutes after time shown in d. Pipette on right contained 10 μM ACh, while pipette on left in frames a, b, and c contained 30 μM VIP. Bar, 50 μM. (From Lassignal et al.[1] Used with permission from the *American Journal of Physiology*.)

into the cell is carried by Ca ions. The existence of an action potential of this sort signals the presence of voltage-sensitive Ca^{2+} channels in the membrane.

The first change in membrane potential observed in the sequence displayed in FIGURE 3C is the depolarization that brings the membrane to the threshold level for action potential generation. We have investigated in detail the mechanism by which two excitatory agents, acetylcholine and the undecapeptide, substance P, cause this sort of depolarization.[2,7] In theory it can be caused in two fundamentally different ways—either by the opening of ionic channels or by their closing. As an example, ionic channels that permit the entry of Na^+ may be opened or those that permit the exit of K^+ may be closed by the action of the excitatory transmitter. In the case of both acetylcholine and substance P, the latter mechanism is at work in these cells.

The acetylcholine-induced closure of ionic channels that are selective for K ions was demonstrated by the type of experiment shown in FIGURE 4. As illustrated in FIGURE 4A, the membrane potential was maintained constant at the level indicated at the left of each of the four current traces displayed. Then muscarine was applied as a means of demonstrating that the cholinergic effects were mediated by muscarinic receptors, and the resulting change in current recorded. In this example the external solution contained 30 mM K^+ so that the equilibrium potential for K ions (E_K) was −40 mV. As can be seen, muscarine induced an *inward* current (seen as a downward deflection) above this potential and an *outward* current below it. Since the direction of the induced current is opposite to the direction expected for a K^+ current, muscarine must be causing the *closure* of K^+ channels. Furthermore, when the external $[K^+]$ was changed, the potential at which the induced current reversed direction conformed precisely to the K^+ equilibrium potential (FIG. 4B). Thus, the channels being closed are highly selective for K^+.

A second way to demonstrate this action on K^+ channels is shown in FIGURE 5. Here the membrane potential is rapidly shifted from one level to another while the resulting currents are recorded. (Note that the speed of the recording is changed to give better time resolution at the beginning and the end of the trace.) Upon examining the current trace at -36 mV, it can be seen that muscarine results in a downward deflection that may be caused either by more inward ionic current or less outward current. These alternatives, which are due to channel opening or channel closing, respectively, may be distinguished by examining the current in response to the rapid shifts in membrane potential. When the membrane potential is shifted from -36 to -65 mV, the initial rapid or ohmic jump in current provides a measure of the conductance of the membrane. Following application of muscarine, this jump is smaller in magnitude, indicating that the conductance of the cell has decreased as expected

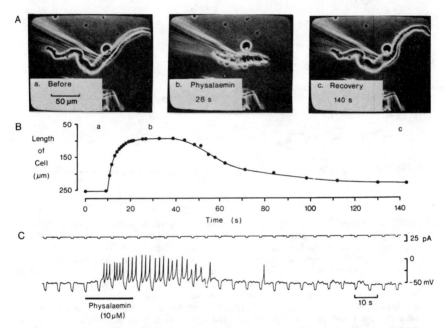

FIGURE 3. Simultaneous recording of contractile and electrical response to physalaemin, a peptide related to substance P. (**A**) video images show a smooth muscle cell before, during, and after a contraction elicited by physalaemin. Physalaemin was applied by pressure ejection from a pipette, seen in lower right of video images, slightly out of plane of focus. Recording microelectrode is in upper left of field, and circular object alongside muscle fiber is an erythrocyte. (**B**) measurements of cell length were made from video monitor at intervals throughout course of contraction, with time zero corresponding to onset of physalaemin application. Curve was fitted to points by eye. (**C**) membrane potential (lower trace) was recorded from cell shown in A, and constant current pulses (upper trace) were applied every six seconds through recording electrode. Physalaemin, applied for time indicated by bar below voltage trace (10 μM in application pipette), caused depolarization leading to action potentials. After a delay of one to two seconds, a burst of action potentials was accompanied by contraction of cell (see B), similar to that observed for other excitatory transmitter agents such as acetylcholine or substance P. Recovery is seen at right side of figure. (From Sims *et al.*[7] Used with permission from the *American Journal of Physiology.*)

upon closure of ionic channels. Thus one may conclude that muscarine has caused the closing of ionic channels carrying outward current as K^+ channels do over this range of potentials. This is precisely the same conclusion reached above using data of the sort illustrated in FIGURE 4.

The type of experimental paradigm shown in FIGURE 5 provides further insight into the nature of the K^+ channels acted on by acetylcholine or muscarine. Following the rapid jump in current when the membrane potential is stepped from -36 to -65 mV, there is a slow development or relaxation of the current to a new steady-state

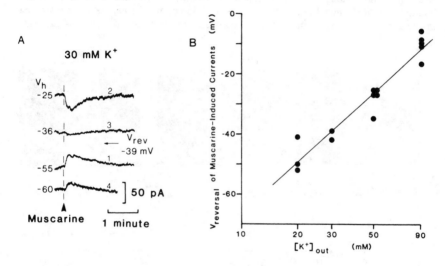

FIGURE 4. Reversal of muscarine-induced currents is dependent upon the external K^+ concentration ($[K^+]_{out}$). (**A**) Current records showing the responses to brief applications of muscarine were obtained at the holding membrane potentials indicated to the left of each trace. Muscarine application is indicated by the arrowhead and vertical lines. (The duration of muscarine application was two seconds, with 500 μM in the application pipette.) The order in which the measurements were made is given by the numbers at the right of the traces. Inward currents were observed positive to the reversal level, and outward currents at more negative potentials. The value of the reversal potential was determined by linear interpolation between the peak current changes found at each holding potential. (**B**) The reversal potentials ($v_{reversal}$) were dependent upon $[K^+]_{out}$, shifting positive with elevation of $[K^+]_{out}$. The relationship between $v_{reversal}$ and $[K^+]_{out}$ is plotted for 15 cells. The reversal potential shifted 58 mV positive per tenfold elevation of $[K^+]_{out}$ (determined by least squares regression), implicating a K^+ current in muscarinic responses. (From Sims *et al.*[9] Used with permission from *Trends in Pharmacological Science.*)

level. This relaxation is abolished when muscarine is applied, suggesting that it is due to the channels that are acted on by muscarine. The direction of this relaxation is consistent with the turning off of voltage-sensitive K^+ channels when the membrane potential is shifted to more negative levels. The relaxations are absent after muscarine application because the channels responsible for them have already been closed by muscarine. Thus these K^+ channels may be closed *either* by muscarine *or* by a sufficiently negative membrane potential.

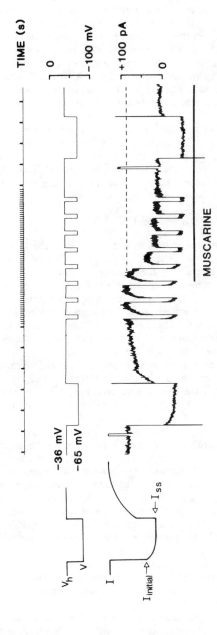

FIGURE 5. Cholinergic responses studied with voltage clamp. The membrane potential was periodically hyperpolarized for two seconds to the levels indicated to the left of the upper voltage trace. Membrane currents are shown in the lower trace, with inward currents downward. Upon hyperpolarization there was an initial rapid current jump ($I_{initial}$) followed by a slow inward current relaxation to a steady-state level (I_{ss}), which represents an outward K^+ current turning off. At the end of the two-second pulse, there was a smaller rapid current jump, followed by an outward current relaxation to baseline, which is the K^+ current turning back on again (see diagram at left). The speed of the chart recorder was reduced by a factor of ten at the onset of muscarine application (0.5 mM in the application pipette), as indicated by the timing trace. Muscarine caused a net inward current at both -36 and -65 mV. The expanded trace at the right shows that the current relaxations have been abolished and the initial rapid jump is smaller, the latter indicating a reduction of the conductance. One hundred pA, 100-msec calibration pulses (shown only for first and last current responses) preceded the current steps, but are off scale before the muscarine-induced baseline shift. (Modified from Sims *et al.*[2].)

If the interpretation of the relaxations offered above is correct, then the effects of acetylcholine or muscarine should be sensitive to membrane potential. This fact is demonstrated in experiments of the type shown in FIGURE 6, which also provide further information about the nature of the muscarine-sensitive K^+ channels. As shown in panel A, the membrane potential is stepped systematically through a series of levels resembling a staircase, and this paradigm is then repeated in the presence of muscarine. Each step in the staircase of potentials is maintained sufficiently long for the resulting current to reach a steady state. Then, as shown in panel B, the steady-state current is plotted against membrane potential for each step in the staircase. The difference in the plots obtained in the presence and absence of muscarine is shown by the dotted line, which indicates the magnitude of the current suppressed by muscarine at each potential.

Since we demonstrated above that the muscarine-sensitive current is carried by K^+ ions, the current displayed by the dotted line in panel B of FIGURE 6 can be corrected for the driving force on K^+, giving a measure of the K^+ conductance suppressed by muscarine at each potential as shown in FIGURE 6C. This plot provides a quantitative indication of the voltage sensitivity of the channels acted on by muscarine. Furthermore, the conductance, which may be designed g_M, is given by:

$$g_M = N \gamma P_o$$

where N is the total number of muscarine-sensitive channels in the membrane, γ is the unitary conductance of each channel and P_o is the probability of a channel being open. Since there appears to be relatively little change in γ at different potentials,[2] the plot of FIGURE 6C provides a measure of the effect of membrane potential on the probability of a muscarine-sensitive K^+ channel being open at each potential. The slope factor for this curve, which is a measure of its steepness, is consistently in the range of 7-11 mV. This means that the channel has a voltage sensitivity substantially less than the classical voltage-sensitive Na^+ channel but vastly greater than the nicotinic channels opened by acetylcholine in skeletal muscle.[10]

It should be noted that these muscarine-sensitive channels are *not* the same channels as the large-conductance Ca^{2+}-activated K^+ channels that are widely distributed throughout smooth muscle and have been characterized in detail in these cells.[11,12] Instead, the current carried by these K^+ channels resembles that originally discovered in bullfrog sympathetic ganglion by Adams, Brown, and Constanti, who designated it as M-current[13,14] for its sensitivity to muscarine, and seen since in a wide variety of preparations.[15,16] The "signature" of M-current is provided by the set of traces in FIGURE 5. In this characteristic pattern muscarine or acetylcholine, by closing K^+ channels, produce: (1) a net inward current at the less negative membrane potentials where the channels are open; (2) a decrease in the ohmic current jump; and (3) the elimination of the slow inward-going current relaxations seen upon hyperpolarization of the membrane. The functional significance of M-current is that it readily accounts for the initial depolarization of the membrane by acetylcholine, which leads in turn to generation of action potentials. Furthermore, no other effect of acetylcholine has been observed that can account for the this initial depolarization so that we can be fairly confident that it is caused by suppression of M-current.

The same sort of depolarization is also caused by the neuropeptides physalaemin (exemplified in FIG. 3), substance K, and substance P, which are excitatory for these cells.[7] Furthermore, one of the two major peptides found in immunohistochemical studies of the tissue from which these smooth muscle cells are dissociated is substance P, the other being VIP (M. Costa, personal communication). The question thus arises whether substance P acts on the same set of M-channels as acetylcholine. The type

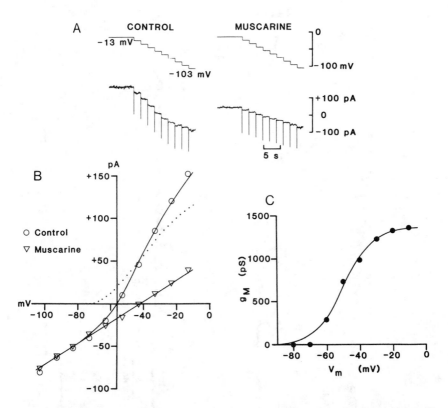

FIGURE 6. Steady-state current-voltage (I-V) relationships of a cell in the absence (control) and during (muscarine) application of muscarine reveal the muscarine-induced current. (**A**) Descending steps of command voltage are shown in the upper traces with membrane currents in the lower traces. Muscarine (0.5 mM in the application pipette) induced an inward current at the holding potential of -13 mV. (**B**) The current level at the end of each two-second voltage step is plotted against the command voltage, with the ordinate placed at the resting potential of the cell under control conditions. Muscarine caused a net inward current and reduced the slope conductance at potentials more positive than -70 mV. Values of I_m (dotted line) were obtained by taking the difference between the control I-V relationship and that measured in the presence of muscarine when I-V values were joined by straight lines. (**C**) The muscarine-sensitive conductance was determined as $g_m = I_m/(V_m - E_K)$. The continuous lines of the I-V curves in B were drawn according to a model where membrane conductance comprises a voltage-dependent G_M and a voltage-independent leak conductance. I_M for the control line was calculated at each voltage from the value of G_M predicted by the sigmoidal curve in C. G_M was set at 0 pS in the presence of muscarine. I_{leak} had an apparent reversal potential of -43 mV and a conductance of 1,240 pS when fitted by linear least-squares regression. (From Sims *et al.*[2] Used with permission from the *Journal of Physiology.*)

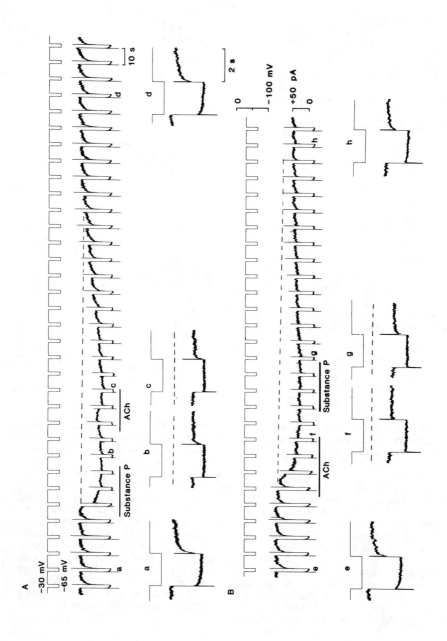

of experiment shown in FIGURE 7 indicates that this is in fact the case. As can be seen, substance P produces the same characteristic suppression of M-current as acetylcholine does. When, as shown, the dose of substance P is sufficient to produce complete suppression of M-current, then acetylcholine is without further effect. When the order is reversed and sufficient acetylcholine is applied to abolish the M-current, then substance P is without effect. Furthermore the action of acetylcholine is blocked by atropine whereas that of substance P is not, indicating, as expected, that the two agents act at distinct receptor sites. In summary, substance P and acetylcholine, acting at different receptor sites, suppress one and the same population of M-channels. Here again the smooth muscle cells resemble sympathetic ganglia where both acetylcholine, acting on muscarinic receptors, and a number of neuropeptides act to suppress M-current.[15,16] (We have not yet investigated whether in the smooth muscle cells other excitatory peptides such as bombesin and cholecystokinin affect M-current.)

An important functional consequence flows from the action of acetylcholine and substance P on M-current. Since the M-current channels are closed at negative potentials, these agents cannot cause the initial depolarization that leads to the chain of excitatory events when the membrane potential is sufficiently negative. This means that agents that have an inhibitory action by hyperpolarizing the membrane to levels of -80 mV or lower cannot have their effects offset by the action of excitatory agents that act exclusively on M-current.

It remains to be seen whether a mechanism resembling the suppression of M-current is a universal one in smooth muscle. In a different preparation of smooth muscle, a muscarinic excitatory mechanism involving a conductance increase has been described, but its ionic basis remains unknown and awaits detailed study.[17] In that preparation acetylcholine exerts a second effect, causing a decrease in outward K^+ current so that even when the M-current is apparently absent a different K^+ current is suppressed.[17,18]

The excitatory effect of acetylcholine or substance P on the smooth muscle cells would appear, at least in qualitative terms, to be satisfactorily explained by the suppression of M-current. Such M-current inhibition will drive the membrane toward the threshold for generation of Ca^{2+} action potentials and the resulting Ca^{2+} influx, if sufficient, will provide activator Ca^{2+} to trigger contraction. Nevertheless, it might also be that these agents have effects on other ionic channels that augment the excitatory effect of M-current suppression. Since augmentation of this sort might possibly be accomplished by an increase in the current through Ca^{2+} channels, we examined the effect of both acetylcholine and substance P on these channels.[3] To do so we used the tight seal, whole-cell recording method employing patch pipettes loaded with Cs^+ instead of K^+ to block all K^+ currents. The Ca^{2+} channels are activated

---

◄ **FIGURE 7.** Substance P and ACh effect same K^+ current. Ten minutes of continuous voltage-clamp recording from one cell are shown: There is no interruption between A and B. Voltage is shown in upper traces and membrane currents below. Some of the hyperpolarizing voltage jumps, indicated by letters, are shown on an expanded time scale (X10) below the continuous recording. Sequential application of substance P (6 μM in one application pipette) and ACh (10 μM in another pipette) revealed that when M-current was fully suppressed by either agonist, the other had no additional effect. As shown in A, substance P caused a net inward current, a membrane conductance decrease, and a suppression of current relaxations. After partial recovery from substance P, ACh also caused complete suppression of M-current. Recovery is shown in A and continued in B. As shown in B, ACh caused suppression of the M-current, and subsequent application of substance P caused no additional effect. (From Sims *et al.*[7] Used with permission from the *American Journal of Physiology*.)

when the membrane potential is stepped abruptly from a negative holding level to more positive levels. In contrast to the K^+ channels underlying M-current, the Ca^{2+} channels inactivate as the potential is maintained at the more positive level. This is illustrated in FIGURE 8B where the downward deflection of the current traces indicates the inward flow of current through the Ca^{2+} channels. Upon application of acetylcholine, the magnitude of the Ca^{2+} current increased and its inactivation or decay slowed. As can be seen in FIGURE 8A, the slowing is reflected by an increase in the

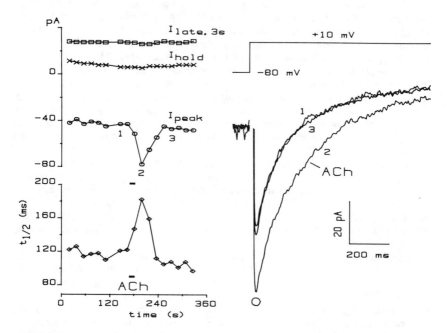

FIGURE 8. Effect of acetylcholine on voltage-activated inward current in the presence of normal external $[Ca^{2+}]$. This effect of acetylcholine was registered 11 minutes after rupture of the patch. A similar response was observed five minutes before this one. (**A**) Upper, increase in the peak inward current (o) following acetylcholine application and absence of effects on holding current (x) and late current ($\square$) are shown. Lower, effect on the $t_{1/2}$ ($\diamond$) of decay of the inward current is shown. Zero on the time axis is eight minutes after rupture of the patch. (**B**) Selected current traces showing control (1), maximum response (ACh) (2), and recovery (3) (50-Hz cut-off, 250-Hz effective sampling rate). Currents were elicited by three-second voltage pulses to 9 mV from a holding level of -78 mV repeated every 18 seconds. Acetylcholine concentration in application pipette was 50 μM. (From Clapp et al.[3] Used with permission from the *Proceedings of the National Academy of Sciences.*)

half time of decay. The effects outlasted the application of acetylcholine, and under the conditions of these experiments, where K^+ currents were blocked, no other currents were affected. Furthermore atropine blocked these effects and muscarine mimicked them.

The acetylcholine-induced slowing of the decay of the Ca^{2+} current might arise in several ways. For example, it might be caused by a selective increase in a subpopulation of voltage-activated Ca^{2+} channels with slower kinetics. Such an explanation is attractive since many kinds of cells possess two or three types of voltage-activated Ca^{2+} channels that differ in their kinetics and in other ways.[19-22] Not surprisingly, then, we found two types of voltage-activated Ca^{2+} current in the smooth muscle cells. One type of Ca^{2+} current displayed a low threshold of activation and inactivated rapidly, and the other had a high threshold of activation and inactivated slowly, a categorization common to a variety of cells. Acetylcholine appears to increase the current with a high threshold of activation and not the low-threshold current. That the slowing represents a selective effect on one type of channel is confirmed by multiexponential analysis of the decay of the current before and after acetylcholine application (not shown). The striking outcome of this analysis is that the time constants required to fit the decay did not change, but the weighting assigned to the time constants shifted in favor of the slower components.[23] This is the result to be expected if the kinetics of the several different types of Ca^{2+} channel are minimally affected but the total number of active channels with slower kinetics is increased.

Thus, acetylcholine selectively enhances one of two types of voltage-dependent Ca^{2+} current—an effect that appears to result, at least in part, from an increase in the number available to open of those channels with a higher threshold of activation and slower inactivation kinetics. As expected for smooth muscle, muscarinic receptors mediated these effects since they could be mimicked by muscarine and blocked by atropine. Moreover, substance P did the same,[23] augmenting and slowing the high threshold, slow Ca^{2+} current but not the low threshold, fast current. These actions of substance P were unaffected by atropine.

In summary, substance P and acetylcholine, the latter acting on muscarinic receptors, behaved in a similar fashion with respect to three different types of ionic current. Each suppressed M-current, which is carried by voltage-dependent K^+ channels; augmented the current subserved by the high threshold slow type of Ca^{2+} channel; and did not increase the current due to Ca^{2+} channels activated at lower threshold. Such precise correspondence between the effects of these two agents suggests that they act through a common intermediary, while the diversity of the shared effects suggests an intermediary that can act at a variety of sites. Neither Ca^{2+}, which does not appear to affect M-current, nor cAMP-dependent protein kinase, which is activated by β-adrenergic agents that *counter* the effects of acetylcholine, appear to satisfy the requirements for such an intermediary. Another possible intermediary is diacylglycerol, which might be generated by the muscarinic and substance P receptor systems in these cells and then exert its effects through C-kinase activation. Indeed this is our working hypothesis, which has now been supported by some preliminary findings.[24]

It will be of interest to see whether other excitatory peptides act in the same fashion as substance P and acetylcholine. An intriguing question is the significance of the existence in the same cell of receptor systems whose effects duplicate one another. Finally, although we have had little to say of the effects of inhibitory or "relaxing" agents on ionic currents in these cells, the results discussed above suggest a number of hypotheses. Most obvious is the possibility that agents such as isoproterenol and VIP that block the excitatory effects of acetylcholine in these cells do so by activating M-current, and preliminary findings suggest that this is the case at least for isoproterenol.[25,26] This is an exciting prospect because it should now be possible to study the interactions between the second messenger systems that mediate antagonistic effects on the same set of ionic channels.

[Note added in proof: Since this manuscript was submitted, a full account has appeared showing that isoproterenol is capable of inducing M-current and that this effect is mimicked by cAMP analogues (Sims, S. M., J. J. Singer & J. V. Walsh, Jr. 1988. Antagonistic adrenergic-muscarinic regulation of M-current in smooth muscle cells. *Science* **239:** 190-193). This report also showed that muscarinic suppression of the isoproterenol-induced M-current occurred at a point downstream in the β-adrenergic cascade from the control of cAMP levels. Furthermore, in another report we have provided evidence that acetylcholine increases the Ca^{2+} current by augmenting the slow-inactivating, high-threshold type of Ca^{2+} current but not the fast-inactivating, low-threshold type. We also demonstrated that this muscarinic effect is mimicked by a diacylglycerol analogue capable of activating protein kinase C but not by analogues that fail to activate this kinase (Vivaudou, M. B., L. C. Clapp, J. V. Walsh, Jr. & J. J. Singer. 1988. Diacylglycerol and acetylcholine regulate one type of Ca^{2+} current in smooth muscle cells. *FASEB Journal* **2(6):** In press). Thus, it may be that some muscarinic effects on ionic channels in smooth muscle cells are mediated by protein kinase C.]

REFERENCES

1. LASSIGNAL, N. L., J. J. SINGER & J. V. WALSH, JR. 1986. Multiple neuropeptides exert a direct effect on the same isolated single smooth muscle cell. Am. J. Physiol. **250:** C792-C798.

2. SIMS, S. M., J. J. SINGER & J. V. WALSH, JR. 1985. Cholinergic agonists suppress a potassium current in freshly dissociated smooth muscle cells of the toad. J. Physiol. **367:** 503-529.

3. CLAPP, L. H., M. B. VIVAUDOU, J. V. WALSH, JR. & J. J. SINGER. 1987. Acetylcholine increases voltage-activated Ca^{2+} current in freshly dissociated smooth muscle cells. Proc. Natl. Acad. Sci. USA **84:** 2092-2096.

4. BAGBY, R. M., A. M. YOUNG, R. S. DOTSON, B. A. FISHER & K. McKINNON. 1971. Contraction of single smooth muscle cells from *Bufo marinus* stomach. Nature **234:** 351-352.

5. FAY, F. S., R. HOFFMANN, S. LECLAIR & P. MERRIAM. 1982. Preparation of individual smooth muscle cells from the stomach of *Bufo marinus*. Methods Enzymol. **85:** 284-292.

6. SINGER, J. J. & J. V. WALSH, JR. 1980. Passive properties of the membrane of single freshly isolated smooth muscle cells. Am. J. Physiol. **239:** C153-C161.

7. SIMS, S. M., J. V. WALSH, JR. & J. J. SINGER. 1986. Substance P and acetylcholine both suppress the same K^+ current in dissociated smooth muscle cells. Am. J. Physiol. **251:** C580-C587.

8. WALSH, J. V., JR. & J. J. SINGER. 1980. Calcium action potentials in single freshly isolated smooth muscle cells. Am. J. Physiol. **239:** C162-C174.

9. SIMS, S. M., J. J. SINGER & J. V. WALSH, JR. 1986. A mechanism of muscarinic excitation in dissociated smooth muscle cells. Trends Pharmacol. Sci. **7(Suppl.):** 28-32.

10. HILLE, B. 1984. Ionic Channels of Excitable Membranes. Sinauer Associates. Sunderland, MA.

11. SINGER, J. J. & J. V. WALSH, JR. 1987. Characterization of calcium-activated potassium channels in single smooth muscle cells using the patch-clamp technique. Pflügers Arch. **408:** 98-111.

12. SINGER, J. J. & J. V. WALSH, JR. 1986. Large-conductance Ca^{2+}-activated K^+ channels in freshly dissociated smooth muscle cells. Membr. Biochem. **6:** 83-110.

13. ADAMS, P. R., D. A. BROWN & A. CONSTANTI. 1982. M-currents and other potassium currents in bullfrog sympathetic neurones. J. Physiol. **330:** 537-572.

14. ADAMS, P. R., D. A. BROWN & A. CONSTANTI. 1982. Pharmacological inhibition of the M-current. J. Physiol. **332:** 223-262.

15. ADAMS, P. R., S. W. JONES, P. PENNEFATHER, D. A. BROWN, C. KOCH & B. LANCASTER. 1986. Slow synaptic transmission in frog sympathetic ganglia. J. Exp. Biol. **124:** 259-286.

16. ADAMS, P. R. & M. GALVAN. 1986. Voltage-dependent currents of vertebrate neurones and their role in membrane excitability. *In* Advances in Neurology. A. V. Delgado-Escueta, A. A. Ward, Jr., D. M. Woodbury & R. J. Porter, Eds. **44:** 137-170. Raven Press. New York.

17. BENHAM, C. D., T. B. BOLTON & R. J. LANG. 1985. Acetylcholine activates an inward current in single mammalian smooth muscle cells. Nature **316:** 345-347.

18. SIMS, S. M., J. J. SINGER & J. V. WALSH, JR. 1987. Spontaneous transient K^+ currents in dissociated smooth muscle cells from cat esophagus are suppressed by acetylcholine. Biophys. J. **51:** 57a.

19. MCCLESKY, E. W., A. P. FOX, D. FELDMAN & R. W. TSIEN. 1986. Different types of calcium channels. J. Exp. Biol. **124:** 177-190.

20. MILLER, R. J. 1987. Multiple calcium channels and neuronal function. Science **235:** 46-52.

21. BEAN, B. P. 1985. Two kinds of calcium channels in canine atrial cells. Differences in kinetics, selectivity and pharmacology. J. Gen. Physiol. **86:** 1-30.

22. BEAN, B. P., M. STUREK, A. PUGA & K. HERMSMEYER. 1986. Calcium channels in muscle cells from rat mesenteric arteries: Modulation by dihydropyridine drugs. Circ. Res. **59:** 229-235.

23. VIVAUDOU, M. B., L. H. CLAPP, J. V. WALSH, JR. & J. J. SINGER. 1987. Multiple types of Ca^{2+} current in single smooth muscle cells and their regulation by substance P and acetylcholine. J. Gen. Physiol. **90:** 42a.

24. CLAPP, L. H., M. B. VIVAUDOU, J. J. SINGER & J. V. WALSH, JR. 1987. A diacylglycerol analogue mimics the action of acetylcholine and substance P on calcium currents in freshly dissociated smooth muscle cells. J. Gen. Physiol. **90:** 13a.

25. SIMS, S. M., J. V. WALSH, JR. & J. J. SINGER. 1987. Isoproterenol activates outward current that is suppressed by acetylcholine in freshly dissociated smooth muscle cells. Biophys. J. **51:** 58a.

26. SIMS, S. M., J. J. SINGER & J. V. WALSH, JR. 1987. Cyclic AMP analogues mimic isoproterenol by activating an acetylcholine sensitive K^+ current in gastric smooth muscle cells. J. Gen. Physiol. **90:** 38a.

Vasoactive Intestinal Peptide and Other Peptides as Neuromodulators of Colonic Motility in the Guinea Pig[a]

J. A. LOVE,[b] V. L. W. GO,[c] AND
J. H. SZURSZEWSKI [b]

[b]Department of Physiology and Biophysics
Mayo Medical School
Rochester, Minnesota 55905

[c]Gastroenterology Research Unit
Mayo Medical School
Rochester, Minnesota 55905

Kuntz and Saccomanno[1] suggested over 40 years ago that the abdominal, prevertebral ganglia participate in peripheral reflex activity. They found that distension of one segment of the intestine inhibited another segment even after the prevertebral ganglia were decentralized and all associated visceral afferent fibers issuing from the dorsal root were sectioned.[2,3] The basis for peripheral reflex activity between a prevertebral ganglion and a segment of the gastrointestinal tract was first obtained by Crowcroft, Holman, and Szurszewski.[4] In a preparation consisting of the inferior mesenteric ganglion and an attached segment of distal colon, they recorded asynchronous synaptic activity in neurons in the inferior mesenteric ganglion. The asynchronous activity, consisting of fast e.p.s.p.s. and action potentials, was blocked when a nicotinic receptor antagonist was superfused over only the ganglion and was abolished following transection of the lumbar colonic nerve trunk coursing between the colonic segment and ganglion. These observations suggested the existence of an afferent set of cholinergic fibers projecting from the colon onto sympathetic, noradrenergic neurons. Furthermore, spontaneous[5] and induced[4,6] increases in colonic intraluminal pressure led to an increase in the frequency and amplitude of the asynchronously occurring cholinergic e.p.s.p.s. As a result of these and other observations, it was suggested that the afferent, cholinergic neurons were mechanosensory neurons. The original observations by Crowcroft, Holman, and Szurszewski[4] were confirmed[5,6] and extended to include the entire chain of abdominal prevertebral ganglion in the guinea pig[7,8] as well as the inferior mesenteric ganglion of the rat,[9] mouse (Miller and Szurszewski, unpublished observations), and kitten (Szurszewski, unpublished observations). Thus, it is now well established that prevertebral ganglia participate in peripheral reflex activity connecting two regions of the same organ (i.e., the colo-colonic inhibitory reflex) and regions of different organs[8] (i.e., the gastroduodenal inhibitory reflex). The afferent limb of these

[a]This work was supported by National Institutes of Health Grant AM 17632.

peripheral reflexes consists of cholinergic, mechanosensory fibers and the efferent limb consists of noradrenergic, inhibitory neurons with synapses in the wall of the bowel.

The discovery of noncholinergic, excitatory postsynaptic potentials in bullfrog *para*vertebral sympathetic ganglia by Nishi and Koketsu[10] was the beginning of a new and now ever-expanding area of research in synaptic transmission mechanism in peripheral autonomic ganglia. The original observation by Nishi and Koketsu was confirmed by Jan and Jan[11] who also showed that the transmitter for the late slow e.p.s.p. was the peptide luteinizing hormone-releasing hormone. The observation that *pre*vertebral ganglia function as reflex centers and the observation that *para*vertebral ganglia contain peptidergic synapses led to the inevitable combination of both mechanisms in the same ganglion. Neild[12] was the first to provide convincing evidence for the existence of a noncholinergic slow e.p.s.p. in the inferior mesenteric ganglion of the guinea pig. His studies, combined with a vast literature on the immunohistochemistry of the prevertebral ganglia now make it evident that prevertebral ganglia serving the bowel have a rich peptidergic neuropil that participates in peripheral reflex activity alongside the cholinergic mechanosensory pathways. Although the picture is still incomplete, it is nevertheless clear that noncholinergic, peptidergic transmission in the inferior mesenteric ganglion participates in gastrointestinal reflexes and modulates cholinergic transmission.

Immunohistochemical studies have revealed a prominent collection of nerve terminals containing substance P (SP)-, enkephalin (ENK)-, cholecystokinin (CCK)-, vasoactive intestinal polypeptide (VIP)-, bombesin (BOM)-, neurotensin (NT)-, and dynorphin (DYN)-like immunoreactivity. SP terminals in prevertebral ganglia are *en passant* synapses belonging to primary afferent fibers. The cell bodies of these afferent fibers reside in the dorsal horn of the cord and the receptor element in the abdominal viscera.[13-16] In the inferior mesenteric ganglion of the guinea pig, electrical stimulation of the lumbar colonic nerves[17,18] and L_2 and L_3 dorsal roots[19] initiate the slow e.p.s.p. It appears likely that SP fibers mediate the late slow e.p.s.p. because exogenously applied SP mimics the slow e.p.s.p. caused by nerve stimulation, a SP antagonist blocks both the late slow e.p.s.p. and associated decrease in K conductance,[20,21] and both decentralization and treatment with capsaicin significantly reduce or abolish the late slow e.p.s.p. and immunoreactive-like SP.[19] Thus, the SP pathway provides a functional connection between sensory and autonomic neurons. The SP pathway appears to be a mechanosensory pathway because colonic distension causes, in a population of neurons, a depolarization and increase in membrane excitability that is capsaicin sensitive and is reduced by prior desensitization to exogenously administered SP.[22-24] Prolonged distension of the colon results in a decline of the distension-induced membrane depolarization in a similar time course as observed by tachyphylaxis of SP[24] In addition to mediating mechanosensory input, the SP pathway may also convey visceral nociception. It is not clear whether the same fibers convey both types of sensory information.[25]

ENK-like immunoreactive material is also present in terminals in the guinea pig inferior mesenteric ganglion. These terminals belong to axons whose cell bodies are located in the intermediolateral cell column of the spinal cord.[15,26,27] The ENK fibers leave the cord through the ventral roots and course to the prevertebral ganglia via the splanchnic nerves. The ENK-ergic system is a presynaptic inhibitory system that modulates the release of SP from primary afferent sensory fibers[28] and acetylcholine from preganglionic nerves.[18,19] In addition, exogenously applied enkephalins act presynaptically on the cholinergic mechanosensory pathway to depress ongoing mechanosensory afferent input.[30] Consequently, there is a decrease in the output from inhibitory noradrenergic neurons to the gut. The functional significance of the ENK-ergic pathway is to release the colon from the inhibitory effect of noradrenergic control.

Consequently, activation of the central ENK-ergic pathway would be expected to cause an increase in colonic motility, and this has been observed.[30]

Vasoactive intestinal polypeptide-like immunoreactivity is the third member of the septet of peptides so far known to be present in prevertebral ganglia. Unlike the situation for SP and ENK, the cell bodies of the VIP-containing fibers are located in the enteric ganglia.[31,32-35] The VIP fibers course to the prevertebral ganglia via the postganglionic nerve trunks.[33,34] A dense network of VIP fibers can be found in the inferior mesenteric ganglion and in the celiac ganglion.[31,32,34] Immunoelectron-microscopic studies have localized VIP to large dense core vesicles contained in axodendritic and axon-somatic synapses in the prevertebral ganglia.[34] The gut afferent VIP nerves projecting to the prevertebral ganglia apparently have specific target neurons because VIP nerves surround noradrenergic neurons containing somatostatin-(NA/SOM) but not noradrenergic neurons containing neuropeptide Y (NPY)-like immunoreactivity (NA/NPY).[36] VIP nerves also surround noradrenergic neurons containing a peptide which as yet has not been identified (see M. Costa, this volume). This selective innervation by VIP nerves may have functional significance. It is known that NA/NPY neurons selectively innervate vascular smooth muscle.[36] Since these neurons do not receive synaptic containing VIP-like material, they would not be expected to participate in peripheral gut reflexes utilizing the VIP pathway. Although the specific target for the NA/SOM neurons has not been settled, it may be the external smooth muscle layers of the gut. Thus, the peripheral VIP nerves have specific target neurons (NA/SOM) and the efferent target of the NA/SOM neurons may be the external smooth muscle layers of the gut.

It has been shown recently that the VIP pathway modulates cholinergic transmission by a postsynaptic action.[37] Exogenously applied VIP evoked a membrane depolarization in the majority of cells tested.[37] This VIP-induced depolarization was able to convert subthreshold, fast nicotinic e.p.s.p.s. due to colonic mechanoreceptors to action potentials. Thus, VIP increases the efficiency of cholinergic transmission thereby increasing noradrenergic inhibitory drive to the external muscularis of the intestines.

It has also been shown that the VIP pathway participates as a transmitter mediating mechanosensory information.[37] VIP-dependent slow e.p.s.p. can be evoked by lumbar colonic nerve stimulation and by radial distension of the colon. An example of each is shown in FIGURE 1 and FIGURE 2, respectively. In FIGURE 1, the lumbar colonic nerve trunk was selected for electrical stimulation because it contains most of the VIP-reactive nerve fibers that reach the inferior mesenteric ganglion.[32] Rabbit VIP anitserum was used to study the possible role of VIP in the noncholinergic slow e.p.s.p. In the experiment illustrated in FIGURE 1, hexamethonium ($2 \times 10^{-4} M$) and atropine ($2 \times 10^{-6} M$) were present to block cholinergic input. The amplitude of the slow e.p.s.p. in the untreated control (FIG. 1A) was 5 mV whereas in the same neuron the slow e.p.s.p. was reduced when VIP antiserum was present (FIG. 1C). In the presence of nonimmune rabbit anitserum, the amplitude of the slow e.p.s.p. was 4.5 mV. In three of seven other neurons tested with VIP antiserum, the amplitude of the slow e.p.s.p. was 3.6 ± 1.0 mV (mean $\pm$ SEM). In these same neurons, the amplitude without VIP antiserum was 5.8 ± 1.8 mV (mean $\pm$ SEM). The difference between the two means was significant ($p < 0.02$). It should be emphasized that the noncholinergic slow e.p.s.p. in some neurons was either insensitive to VIP antiserum or was only partially reduced by the antiserum indicating that other peptidergic transmitters are involved in mediating the noncholinergic slow e.p.s.p. SP[24] and cholecystokinin[38] are likely candidates for the non-VIP-mediated slow e.p.s.p.s induced by electrical stimulation of the lumbar colonic nerves.

Since colonic mechanosensory fibers travel in the lumbar colonic nerve trunk and in view of the results illustrated in FIGURE 1, we hypothesized that VIP fibers may mediate gastrointestinal reflexes. Thus, an *in vitro* preparation consisting of a segment of the distal colon attached to the inferior mesenteric ganglion was studied to determine

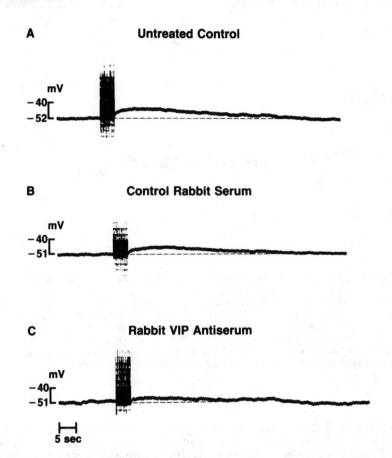

FIGURE 1. Effect of VIP antiserum on the slow noncholinergic e.p.s.p. evoked by lumbar colonic nerve stimulation. (**A**) Stimulation of the lumbar colonic nerves (20 Hz; 4 sec) evoked a slow, noncholinergic e.p.s.p. that was 5 mV in amplitude. (**B**) During application of nonimmune rabbit serum (pressure ejection, 900 msec, 20 psi, 0.15 Hz), the noncholinergic slow e.p.s.p. was 4.5 mV in amplitude. (**C**) During application of VIP antiserum, the slow e.p.s.p. was virtually abolished. All recordings made from the same neuron in the presence of hexamethonium (2 $\times$ 10^{-4} M) and atropine (2 $\times$ 10^{-6} M).

if radial distension of the segment of colon evoked a slow depolarization which was VIP-dependent. The effect of colonic distension on the membrane potential of a single neuron in the inferior mesenteric ganglion is shown in FIGURE 2. In panel A, distension evoked a 7-mV depolarization. In panel B, the distension-induced depolarization was

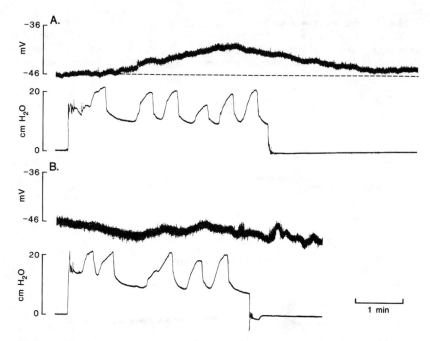

FIGURE 2. Effect of VIP antiserum on the slow e.p.s.p. evoked by distension of the distal colon. In each panel: top trace, intracellular recording from a neuron in the inferior mesenteric ganglion; bottom trace, intraluminal pressure in a segment of the distal colon. Throughout this experiment, hexamethonium ($2 \times 10^{-4} M$) and atropine ($2 \times 10^{-6} M$) were present in the Krebs solution bathing only the ganglion. In A, an increase in colonic intraluminal pressure caused a slow, noncholinergic depolarization which was 7 mV in amplitude. In B, pressure ejection (20 psi, 900 msec, 0.15 Hz) of VIP antiserum blocked, the distension induced slow depolarization. Recordings in A and B were made from the same neuron.

blocked when VIP antiserum was pressure ejected into the vicinity of the neuron from which the recording was made. It is apparent from these data that noncholinergic transmission in the inferior mesenteric ganglion participates in mediating gastrointestinal reflexes. A candidate transmitter for the noncholinergic mechanosensory pathway is VIP or a related peptide. It must be emphasized that distension-induced depolarizations in other neurons were either insensitive to or only partially reduced in amplitude by VIP antiserum. Thus, there are other transmitter candidates besides VIP for the peptidergic-mediated, distension-induced depolarization.

Based on electrophysiological and immunohistochemical data, the possible arrangement of gut VIP terminals and noradrenergic neurons in the inferior mesenteric ganglion can be schematically diagrammed as in FIGURE 3. The gut afferent VIP neurons projecting to the prevertebral ganglion synapse on noradrenergic neurons containing somatostatin (NA/SOM). Since the target tissue for the NA/SOM neurons is the external smooth muscle layers of the gut,[36] activation of the VIP mechanosensory pathway by radial distension of the gut leads to depolarization and an increase in the excitability of the NA/SOM neurons. During occurrence of fast, subthreshold e.p.s.p.s from cholinergic, colonic mechanoreceptors, the VIP-induced depolarization in NA/SOM neurons will convert these subthreshold events to action potentials. This in turn will lead to an increased inhibitory drive to the external muscle layers thereby reducing colonic motility. The apparent lack of VIP input to NA/NPY neurons[36] suggests that sympathetic tone to the intrinsic vascular supply to the gut is not affected by the VIP mechanosensory pathway.

In addition to the occurrence of SP, ENK and VIP, CCK,[15] NT,[39] DYN,[40] and BOM[15] are also known to be present in nerve terminals in the inferior mesenteric ganglion. Except for NT,[39] each of these peptides is contained in fibers in lumbar colonic nerves that synapse on neurons in the inferior mesenteric ganglion. With the exception of neurotensin,[40] the cell bodies of these neuronal types reside in the wall of the colon.[15,39] The cell bodies of the NT-ergic fibers are located in the central nervous system.[40] Thus, these peptidergic pathways may also be involved in colon-ganglion reflex activity. Preliminary evidence by Schumann and Kreulen[38] suggests that CCK afferents may be mechanosensory afferents. It is therefore likely that CCK plays an integral role in regulating colonic motility. The role of the other peptidergic systems remains to be determined.

The discovery of noncholinergic pathways running between the gastrointestinal tract and the prevertebral ganglia raises several important issues regarding visceral innervation of the abdominal ganglia. The functional significance of these numerous peptidergic pathways awaits further experimentation.

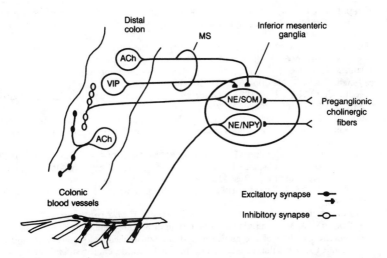

FIGURE 3. Schematic diagram of the relationship between the VIP afferent, mechanosensory fibers and two classes of noradrenergic neurons in the inferior mesenteric ganglion of the guinea pig. The projection of gut VIP fibers onto the class of noradrenergic neurons containing a peptide different from that of SOM and NPY is not shown. ACh, acetylcholine; VIP, vasoactive intestinal polypeptide; MS; colonic mechanosensory inputs; NE, norepinephrine; SOM, somatostatin; NPY, neuropeptide Y. *Closed symbol* synapses are excitatory, *opened symbol* synapses are inhibitory.

ACKNOWLEDGMENTS

The authors express their appreciation to Jan Applequist for her assistance in preparing this manuscript.

REFERENCES

1. KUNTZ, A. & C. J. SACCOMANNO. 1944. Reflex inhibition of intestinal motility mediated through decentralized prevertebral ganglia. J. Neurophysiol. 7: 163-170.
2. KUNTZ, A. L. 1938. The structural organization of the celiac ganglion. J. Comp. Neurol. 69: 1-12.
3. KUNTZ, A. 1940. The structural organization of the inferior mesenteric ganglion. J. Comp. Neurol. 72: 371-382.
4. CROWCROFT, P. J., M. E. HOLMAN & J. H. SZURSZEWSKI. 1971. Excitatory input from the distal colon to the inferior mesenteric ganglion in the guinea-pig. J. Physiol. (London) 219: 443-461.
5. WEEMS, W. A. & J. H. SZURSZEWSKI. 1978. An intracellular analysis of some intrinsic factors controlling neural output from inferior mesenteric ganglion of guinea pig. J. Neurophysiol. 41: 305-321.
6. KREULEN, D. L. & J. H. SZURSZEWSKI. 1979. Reflex pathways in the abdominal prevertebral ganglia: Evidence for a colo-colonic inhibitory reflex. J. Physiol. (London) 295: 21-32.
7. KREULEN, D. L. & J. H. SZURSZEWSKI. 1979. Nerve pathways in celiac plexus of the guinea pig. Am. J. Physiol. 237(Endocrinol. Metab. Gastrointest. Physiol. 6): E90-E97.
8. KREULEN, D. L., T. C. MUIR & J. H. SZURSZEWSKI. 1983. Peripheral sympathetic pathways to the gastroduodenal region of the guinea pig. Am. J. Physiol. 245(Gastrointest. Liver Physiol. 8): G369-375.
9. KREULEN, D. L. 1982. Intracellular recordings in the inferior mesenteric ganglion of the rat. Soc. Neurosci. Abstr. 8: 553.
10. NISHI, S. & K. KOKETSU. 1968. Early and late afterdischarges of amphibian sympathetic ganglion cells. J. Neurophysiol. 31: 109-118.
11. JAN, L. Y. & Y. N. JAN. 1982. Peptidergic transmission in sympathetic ganglion of the frog. J. Physiol. (London) 327: 219-246.
12. NEILD, T. O. 1978. Slowly developing depolarization of neurons in the guinea-pig inferior mesenteric ganglion following repetitive stimulation of the preganglionic nerves. Brain Res. 140: 231-239.
13. HÖKFELT, T., L.-G. ELFVIN, M. SCHULTZBERG, M. GOLDSTEIN & G. NILSSON. 1977. On the occurrence of substance P-containing fibers in sympathetic ganglia: Immunohistochemical evidence. Brain Res. 132: 29-41.
14. POLAK, J. M. & S. R. BLOOM. 1981. The peripheral substance P-ergic system. Peptides 2: 133-148.
15. DALSGAARD, C.-J., T. HÖKFELT, M. SCHULTZBERG, J. M. LUNDBERG, L. TERENIUS, G. J. DOCKRAY & M. GOLDSTEIN. 1983. Origin of peptide-containing fibers in the inferior mesenteric ganglion of the guinea pig: Immunohistochemical studies with antisera to substance P, enkephalin, vasoactive intestinal polypeptide, cholecystokinin and bombesin. Neuroscience 9(1): 191-211.
16. MATTHEWS, M. R. & A. C. CUELLO. 1984. The origin and possible significance of substance P immunoreactive networks in the prevertebral and related structures in the guinea-pig. Philos. Trans. R. Soc. London B306: 247-276.
17. DUN, N. J. & Z. G. JIANG. 1982. Non-cholinergic excitatory transmission in inferior mesenteric ganglia of the guinea-pig: Possible mediation by substance P. J. Physiol. (London) 325: 145-159.

18. KONISHI, S., A. TSUNOO & M. OTSUKA. 1979. Enkephalins presynaptically inhibit cholinergic transmission in sympathetic ganglia. Nature 282: 515-516.

19. TSUNOO, A., S. KONISHI & M. OTSUKA. Substance P as an excitatory transmitter of primary afferent neurons in guinea-pig sympathetic ganglia. Neuroscience 7: 2025-2037.

20. KONISHI, S., M. OTSUKA, K. FOLKERS & S. ROSELL. 1983. A substance P antagonist blocks non-cholinergic slow excitatory postsynaptic potential in guinea-pig sympathetic ganglia. Acta Physiol. Scand. 117: 157-160.

21. KRIER, J. & J. H. SZURSZEWSKI. 1982. Effect of substance P on colonic mechanoreceptors, motility and sympathetic neurons. Am. J. Physiol. 243(Gastrointest. Liver Physiol. 6): G259-G267.

22. PETERS, S. & D. L. KREULEN. 1984. A slow EPSP in mammalian inferior mesenteric ganglion persists after in vivo capsaicin. Brain Res. 303: 186-189.

23. PETERS, S. & D. L. KREULEN. 1986. Fast and slow synaptic potentials produced in a mammalian sympathetic ganglion by colon distension. Proc. Natl. Acad. Sci. USA 83: 1941-1944.

24. KREULEN, D. L. & S. PETERS. 1986. Non-cholinergic transmission in a sympathetic ganglion of the guinea-pig elicited by colon distension. J. Physiol. (London) 374: 315-334.

25. KING, B. F. & J. H. SZURSZEWSKI. Mechanoreceptor pathways from the distal colon to the autonomic nervous system in the guinea-pig. J. Physiol. (London) 350: 93-107.

26. DALSGAARD, C.-J., T. HÖKFELT, L.-G. ELFVIN & L. TERENIUS. 1982. Enkephalin-containing sympathetic preganglionic neurons projecting to the inferior mesenteric ganglion: Evidence from combined retrograde tracing and immunohistochemistry. Neuroscience 9: 2039-2050.

27. SCHULTZBERG, M., T. HÖKFELT, L. TERENIUS, L.-G. ELFVIN, J. M. LUNDBERG, J. BRANDT, R. P. ELDE & M. GOLDSTEIN. 1979. Enkephalin immunoreactive nerve fibers and cell bodies in sympathetic ganglia of the guinea-pig and rat. Neuroscience 4: 249-270.

28. BROWN, D. 1982. Peptidergic transmission in ganglia. Trends Neurosci. 5: 34-35.

29. KONISHI, S., A. TSUNOO & M. OTSUKA. 1981. Enkephalin as a transmitter for presynaptic inhibition in sympathetic ganglia. Nature 294: 80-82.

30. SHU, HUAI-DE, J. A. LOVE & J. H. SZURSZEWSKI. 1987. Effect of enkephalins on colonic mechanoreceptor synaptic input to inferior mesenteric ganglion. Am. J. Physiol. 252(Gastrointest. Liver Physiol. 15): G128-G135.

31. COSTA, M. & J. B. FURNESS. 1983. The origins, pathways and terminations of neurons with VIP-like immunoreactivity in the guinea-pig small intestine. Neuroscience 8: 665-676.

32. DALSGAARD, C.-J., T. HÖKFELT, M. SCHULTZBERG, J. M. LUNDBERG, L. TERENIUS, G. J. DOCKRAY & M. GOLDSTEIN. 1983. Origin of peptide-containing fibers in the inferior mesenteric ganglion of the guinea-pig: Immunohistochemical studies with antisera to substance P, enkephalin, vasoactive intestinal polypeptide, cholecystokinin and bombesin. Neuroscience 9: 191-211.

33. HÖKFELT, T., L.-G. ELFVIN, M. SCHULTZBERG, K. FUXE, S. I. SAID, V. MUTT & M. GOLDSTEIN. 1977. Immunohistochemical evidence of vasoactive intestinal polypeptide-containing neurons and nerve fibers in sympathetic ganglia. Neuroscience 2: 885-896.

34. KONDO, H. & R. YUI. 1982. An electron microscopic study on VIP-like immunoreactive nerve fibers in the celiac ganglion of guinea-pigs. Brain Res. 237: 227-231.

35. LERANTH, C. & E. FEHÉR. 1983. Synaptology and sources of vasoactive intestinal polypeptide and substance P containing axons of the cat celiac ganglion. An experimental electron microscopic immunohistochemical study. Neuroscience 3: 947-958.

36. LUNDBERG, J. M., T. HÖKFELT, A. ANGGARD, L. TERENIUS, R. ELDE, K. MACKEY, M. GOLDSTEIN & J. KIMMEL. 1982. Organization principles in the peripheral sympathetic nervous system: Subdivision by coexisting peptides (Somatostatin-, avian pancreatic polypeptide-, and vasoactive intestinal polypeptide-like immunoreactive materials). Proc. Natl. Acad. Sci. 79: 1303-1307.

37. LOVE, J. A. & J. H. SZURSZEWSKI. 1987. The electrophysiological effects of vasoactive intestinal polypeptide in the guinea-pig inferior mesenteric ganglion. J. Physiol. (London) 394: 67-84.

38. SCHUMANN, M. A. & D. A. KREULEN. 1986. Evidence that cholecystokinin is a neuro-

transmitter in the inferior mesenteric ganglion of guinea pig. Soc. Neurosci. Abstr. **12:** 1496.

39. REINECKE, M., W. G. FORSSMANN, G. THIEKÖTTER & J. TRIEPIL. 1983. Localization of neurotensin-immunoreactivity in the spinal cord and peripheral nervous system of the guinea pig. Neurosci. Lett. **37:** 37-42.

40. VINCENT, S. R., C.-J. DALSGAARD, M. SCHULTZBERG, T. HÖKFELT, I. CHRISTENSSON & L. TERENIUS. 1984. Dynorphin-immunoreactive neurons in the autonomic nervous system. Neuroscience **11:** 973-987.

Vasoactive Intestinal Peptide

Transmitter of Inhibitory Motor Neurons of the Gut[a]

J. R. GRIDER AND G. M. MAKHLOUF [b]

Departments of Medicine and Physiology
Medical College of Virginia
Richmond, Virginia 23298

The main, perhaps the only, neuropeptides with generalized relaxant activity are vasoactive intestinal peptide (VIP) and its cosynthesized homologue, PHI (or PHM in humans).[1,2] Other neuropeptides, for example, CGRP, cause relaxation of gastric[3] but not intestinal smooth muscle cells (J. R. Grider and G. M. Makhlouf, unpublished observations). Neurotensin, whose presence in intramural neurons of the gut remains uncertain, has a biphasic effect on colonic smooth muscle in some species[4] and a contractile effect on isolated intestinal smooth muscle cells. Other peptides with relaxant activity (e.g., secretin, glucagon, atriopeptins) are not present in intramural neurons of the gut. The unique properties of VIP entitle it to consideration as the mediator of inhibitory motor neurons of the gut. The evidence in favor of this view can be summarized as follows:

1. VIP is present in neurons of the myenteric plexus that project into circular muscle and specialized longitudinal muscle like tenia coli;[5,6]

2. VIP causes relaxation of muscle strips and isolated gastric and intestinal muscle cells;[7-11]

3. VIP is responsible for the dominant inhibitory neural background that normally masks myogenic phasic activity;[12]

4. Neurally induced VIP release is accompanied by a stoichiometric increase in relaxation that is inhibited by VIP antiserum and selective VIP antagonists;[8-11,13-15]

5. Selective release of VIP occurs during the descending relaxation phase of the peristaltic reflex; neutralization of VIP with VIP antiserum or blockade of its activity with VIP antagonists inhibits descending relaxation.[16,17]

[a] Supported by Grants DK-15564, DK-28300, and DK-34153 from the National Institute of Diabetes, Digestive and Kidney Disease.

[b] Address correspondence to: G. M. Makhlouf, M.D., Ph.D., Box 711, MCV Station, Medical College of Virginia, Richmond, Virginia 23298-0001.

INNERVATION OF CIRCULAR MUSCLE BY VIP/PHI NEURONS

The colocalization of VIP and PHI/PHM in neurons of the myenteric plexus has been described extensively and appears to be well conserved in mammals.[18,19] VIP neurons of the myenteric plexus project caudad into the plexus as well as directly into the underlying circular muscle layer.[5,6] PHI is cosynthesized within the same precursor but appears to be more extensively processed in all regions of the gut.[18,19] The molar ratio of VIP to PHI varies from three to five. This together with the lower potency of PHI as a relaxant agent (5-10 times less than VIP) suggests that its contribution to neurally induced relaxation is minor and may not exceed 5%.

VIP CAUSES DIRECT RELAXATION OF SMOOTH MUSCLE CELLS

VIP and its homologues (PHI, secretin, glucagon) cause relaxation of isolated gastric and intestinal smooth muscle cells.[7] Relaxation is mediated by high-affinity VIP receptors that have been characterized immunochemically in isolated gastric muscle cells using [^{125}I]VIP.[20] The relaxant effect of VIP is augmented by subthreshold concentrations of phosphodiesterase inhibitors and is accompanied by a significant increase in intracellular levels of cyclic AMP.

VIP and its homologues cause similar relaxation in intact muscle strips derived from the circular muscle layer in various regions of the gut (stomach,[8] small and large intestine,[9,12] muscularis mucosae,[11] and various sphincters such as lower esophageal and internal anal sphincters[10,14,15]). The contractile effect of VIP on longitudinal muscle strips with intact myenteric plexus is due to release of acetylcholine from cholinergic neurons supplying longitudinal muscle.[21]

VIP: MEDIATOR OF BACKGROUND INHIBITORY NEURAL TONE

Opioid peptides and the axonal blocker tetrodotoxin induce phasic contraction of intestinal circular smooth muscle, an effect that is attributable to blockade of the dominant inhibitory neural tone that normally masks myogenic phasic activity in the gut.[22,23] Evidence that VIP is the transmitter responsible for the background inhibitory neural tone is based on the following. In rat colonic strips, for example, the effect of tetrodotoxin can be mimicked by a variety of opioid agonists that suppress selectively the activity of inhibitory motor neurons.[12] Both tetrodotoxin and [Met]enkephalin cause a significant decrease in basal VIP release.[12] Neutralization of background VIP with VIP antiserum induces a concentration-dependent increase in phasic contraction that closely mimics that induced by tetrodotoxin or [Met]enkephalin.[12] A threshold concentration of VIP antiserum (1 : 960) potentiates the phasic response to TTX or [Met]enkephalin. Conversely, exogenous VIP inhibits phasic contraction in a concentration-dependent manner. The results suggest that elimination of background VIP initiates and enhances phasic contraction on which the contractile component of the peristaltic reflex is superimposed. Conversely, an increase in VIP release suppresses phasic contraction and induces the descending relaxation component of the peristaltic reflex (see below).

VIP: MEDIATOR OF NEURALLY INDUCED RELAXATION

Mediation of neurally induced relaxation by VIP has been studied extensively in guinea pig gastric (fundic) muscle and tenia coli.[8,9] In these preparations, neurally induced relaxation is accompanied by a stoichiometric increase in VIP release.[13] Apamin causes a decrease in neurally induced relaxation and a proportionate decrease in VIP release.[13] Neurally induced relaxation is inhibited by VIP antiserum and by selective VIP antagonists (e.g., VIP_{10-28}, [4-Cl-D-Phe^6,Leu^{17}]VIP and [Ac-Tyr^1, D-Phe^2]GRF$_{1-29}$), but is not affected by photoactivated 3'-0-(4-benzoyl)benzoyl ATP, a photoaffinity analogue of ATP that is capable of inhibiting the relaxant response to exogenous ATP (FIGS. 1 and 2 and TABLE 1).[8,9,24] The inhibitory effect of VIP antiserum has been demonstrated also in preparations from various regions of the gut (cat lower esophageal and rabbit internal anal sphincters and dog muscularis mucosae).[10,11,14,15]

VIP: MEDIATOR OF DESCENDING RELAXATION COMPONENT OF PERISTALTIC REFLEX

A preparation devised by Costa and Furness[17] consisting of an isolated small intestinal or colonic segment on which graded radial stretch can be applied has been used to characterize separately the ascending contraction and descending relaxation components of the peristaltic reflex.[16] Stretch of the caudad end produces ascending contraction only, whereas stretch of the orad end produces descending relaxation only. In rat and guinea pig colonic segments, VIP is released during descending relaxation only.[16] VIP antiserum inhibits descending relaxation and augments ascending contraction in a concentration-dependent manner (range of antiserum concentrations 1 : 480 to 1 : 60; FIG. 3, TABLE 1). The effects of VIP antiserum are mimicked by addition of VIP antagonists[24] (see above). Similar results have been recently obtained using the same VIP antagonists in flat sheet preparations of human and canine intestine to which graded radial stretch can be applied[25] (TABLE 1).

FACILITATORY INFLUENCE OF SOMATOSTATIN NEURONS ON VIP NEURONS

Somatostatin neurons of the myenteric plexus project caudad within the plexus but not into the underlying circular muscle. Somatostatin itself has no direct effect

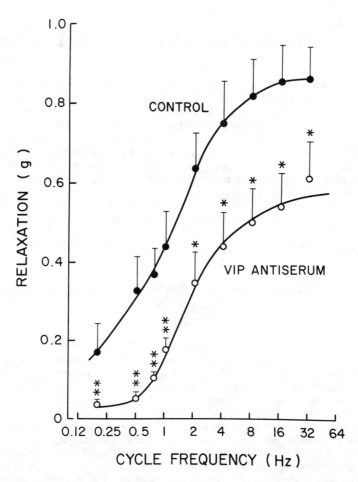

FIGURE 1. Relaxation induced by field stimulation (80 V, 1 msec, 0.2-32 Hz) in muscle strips from the gastric fundus of guinea pig. Data obtained in the presence of normal serum ● and VIP antiserum (final dilution 1 : 120) ○. Values are means ± SEM. Asterisks denote significance of difference from corresponding control values.**p < 0.01; p* < 0.05.

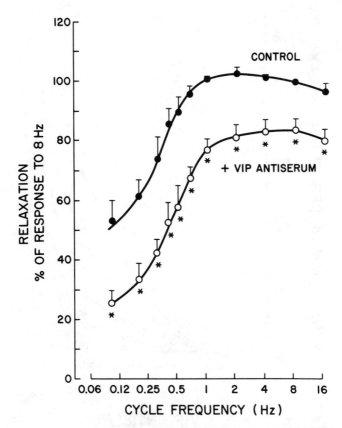

FIGURE 2. Relaxation induced by field stimulation (80 V, 0.5 msec, 0.1-16 Hz) in strips from tenia coli of guinea pig. Data obtained in the presence of normal serum ● and VIP antiserum (final dilution 1 : 60) ○. Values are means ± SEM. Asterisks denote significance of difference from corresponding control values. *p < 0.01. (From Grider *et al.*[9] Used with permission from *Gastroenterology.*)

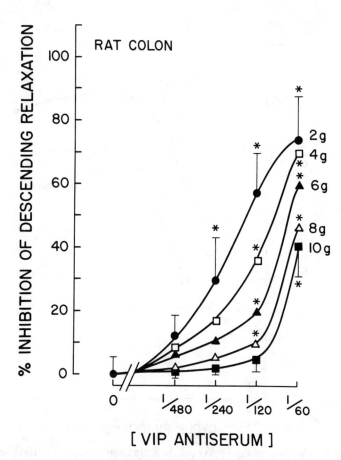

FIGURE 3. Concentration-response curves for the effect of various dilutions of VIP antiserum on descending relaxation in rat colonic segments. Each point represents percent inhibition of descending relaxation elicited by various grades of stretch (2-10 g). Values are means ± SEM. Asterisks denote significant inhibition of descending relaxation.

on smooth muscle cells. Recent studies indicate that somatostatin neurons influence peristaltic activity by modulating the activity of VIP neurons.[26] Somatostatin, like VIP, is released during descending relaxation only. Somatostatin antiserum inhibits selective descending relaxation as well as the concomitant release of VIP.[26] Exogenous somatostatin augments descending relaxation and induces a further increase in VIP release. Together, these results imply that somatostatin neurons act as facilitatory interneurons coupled to VIP neurons in descending pathways.

RESTRICTIVE INFLUENCE OF OPIOID NEURONS ON VIP NEURONS

The opioid antagonist, naloxone, causes an increase in descending relaxation and a decrease in ascending contraction suggesting that endogenous opioid peptides exert

TABLE 1. Effects of VIP Antiserum, VIP Antagonists, and an Activated Photoaffinity Analogue of ATP (benzoyl ATP) on Relaxation Induced by Exogenous ATP, Exogenous VIP, Neural Stimulation of Tenia Coli, and Gastric Fundus Strips, and by Orad Radial Stretch of Small Intestinal or Colonic segments[a]

	Stimulus				
			Field Stimulation		
	ATP	VIP	Tenia	Fundus	Descending Relaxation
VIP Antiserum	−	+	+	+	+
VIP Antagonists	NT	+	+	+	+
Benzoyl ATP	+	−	−	−	NT

[a] Results summarized from References 8, 9, 16, 24, and 25. + = inhibition; − = no inhibition; NT = not tested.

a modulatory influence on peristaltic activity.[27] Exogenous opioid agonists have opposite effects to those of naloxone. The effects of opioid agonists and antagonists are partly mediated by corresponding changes in VIP release. Naloxone enhances VIP release whereas [Met]enkephalin inhibits VIP release.[27] The results imply that opioid neurons exert a tonic restraint on VIP neurons. Opioid peptide release (measured as dynorphin immunoreactivity) decreases during the initial (i.e., descending relaxation) phase of peristalsis thereby eliminating the tonic restraint of opioid neurons on VIP release. Thus, the decrease in opioid neural activity and the increase in somatostatin neural activity act in concert to initiate and/or enhance the activity of VIP motor neurons responsible for descending relaxation.

REFERENCES

1. MAKHLOUF, G. M. 1982. Role of VIP in the function of the gut. In Vasoactive Intestinal Peptide. S. I. Said, Ed.: 425-446. Raven Press. New York.

2. MAKHLOUF, G. M. 1985. Enteric neuropeptides: Role in neuromuscular activity of the gut. Trends Pharmacol. Sci. **6**: 214-218.
3. MATON, P. N., V. E. SUTLIFF, Z-C. ZHOU, J. D. GARDNER & R. T. JENSEN. 1986. Gastroenterology **90**: 1537.
4. KITABGI, P. & J.-P. VINCENT. 1981. Neurotensin is a potent inhibitor of guinea pig colon contractile activity. Eur. J. Pharmacol. **74**: 311-318.
5. COSTA, M. & J. B. FURNESS. 1983. The origins, pathways and terminations of neurons with VIP-like immunoreactivity in the guinea pig small intestine. Neuroscience **8**: 665-676.
6. FURNESS, J. B., M. COSTA & J. H. WALSH. 1981. Evidence for and significance of the projection of VIP neurons from the myenteric plexus to the tenia coli in the guinea pig. Gastroenterology **80**: 1557.
7. BITAR, K. N. & G. M. MAKHLOUF. 1982. Relaxation of isolated gastric smooth muscle cells by vasoactive intestinal peptide. Science **216**: 531-533.
8. GRIDER, J. R., M. B. CABLE, S. I. SAID & G. M. MAKHLOUF. 1985. Vasoactive intestinal peptide (VIP) as neural mediator of gastric relaxation. Am. J. Physiol. **248**: G73-G78.
9. GRIDER, J. R., M. B. CABLE, K. N. BITAR, S. I. SAID & G. M. MAKHLOUF. 1985. Vasoactive intestinal peptide. Relaxant neurotransmitter in tenia coli of the guinea pig. Gastroenterology **89**: 36-42.
10. BIANCANI, P., J. H. WALSH & J. BEHAR. 1984. Vasoactive intestinal polypeptide. A neurotransmitter for lower esophageal sphincter relaxation. J. Clin. Invest. **73**: 963-967.
11. ANGEL, F. V., L. W. GO, P. F. SCHMALZ & J. H. SZURSZEWSKI. 1983. Vasoactive intestinal polypeptide. A putative neurotransmitter in the canine gastric muscularis mucosa. J. Physiol. London **341**: 641-645.
12. GRIDER, J. R. & G. M. MAKHLOUF. 1987. Suppression of inhibitory neural input to colonic circular muscle by opioid peptides. J. Pharmacol. Exp. Ther. **243**: 205-210.
13. GRIDER, J. R. & G. M. MAKHLOUF. 1985. Inhibition of VIP release by VIP-like peptides and apamin: Presynaptic regulation of neurotransmitter peptide release. Gastroenterology **88**: 1406.
14. BIANCANI, P., J. H. WALSH & J. BEHAR. 1985. Vasoactive intestinal peptide: A neurotransmitter for relaxation of the rabbit internal anal sphincter. Gastroenterology **89**: 867-874.
15. GOYAL, R. K., S. RATTAN & S. I. SAID. 1985. VIP as a possible neurotransmitter of noncholinergic, non-adrenergic inhibitory neurons. Nature **288**: 378-380.
16. GRIDER, J. R. & G. M. MAKHLOUF. 1986. Colonic peristaltic reflex: Identification of vasoactive intestinal peptide as mediator of descending relaxation. Am. J. Physiol. **251**: G40-G45.
17. COSTA, M. & J. B. FURNESS. 1976. The peristaltic reflex: An analysis of the nerve pathways and their pharmacology. Naunyn Schmiedebergs Arch. Pharmacol. **294**: 47-60.
18. FAHRENKRUG, J., T. BEK, J. M. LUNDBERG & T. HOKFELT. 1985. VIP and PHI in cat neurons: Co-localization but variable tissue content possibly due to differential processing. Reg. Peptides **12**: 21-34.
19. ITOH, N., K. OBATA, N. YANAIHARA & H. OKAMOTO. 1983. Human preprovasoactive intestinal polypeptide contains a novel PHI-27-like peptide, PHM-27. Nature **304**: 547-549.
20. BITAR, K. N. & R. T. JENSEN. 1983. Binding of [^{125}I]VIP to isolated gastric smooth muscle cells (Abstract). Gastroenterology **84**: 1107.
21. JAFFER, S. S., J. T. FARRAR, W. M. YAU & G. M. MAKHLOUF. 1974. Mode of action and interplay of vasoactive intestinal peptide (VIP), secretin and octapeptide of cholecystokinin on duodenal and ileal muscle in vitro. Gastroenterology **66**: 737.
22. WOOD, J. 1980. Intracellular study of effects of morphine on electrical activity of myenteric neurons in cat small intestine. Gastroenterology **79**: 1222-1230.
23. WOOD, J. 1972. Excitation of intestinal muscle by atropine, tetrodotoxin and xylocaine. Am. J. Physiol. **222**: 118-125.
24. GRIDER, J. R., J. RIVIER & G. M. MAKHLOUF. 1987. Evidence for VIP as transmitter of inhibitory motor neurons: Blockade of neurally mediated relaxation by VIP antagonists. Gastroenterology **92**: 1415.

25. GRIDER, J. R., J. RIVIER & G. M. MAKHLOUF. 1987. Identification of the transmitters regulating the peristaltic reflex in human intestine. Gastroenterology **92:** 1415.
26. GRIDER, J. R., A. ARIMURA & G. M. MAKHLOUF. 1987. Role of somatostatin neurons in intestinal peristalsis: Facilitatory interneurons in descending pathways. Am. J. Physiol. **253:** G434-438.
27. GRIDER, J. R. & G. M. MAKHLOUF. 1987. Role of opioid neurons in the regulation of intestinal peristalsis. Am. J. Physiol. **253:** G226-G231.

Role of Vasoactive Intestinal Peptide and Peptide Histidine Isoleucine in the Cerebral Circulation

LARS EDVINSSON [a]

Department of Internal Medicine
University of Lund
Lund, Sweden

JAMES McCULLOCH, PAUL A. T. KELLY, AND
URSULA I. TUOR

Wellcome Surgical Institute
University of Glasgow
Glasgow, Scotland

INTRODUCTION

A growing number of peptides have been isolated from both mammalian gut and brain, where they are thought to have neurotransmitter-neuromodulator actions. Among these vasoactive intestinal peptide (VIP)[1] exists in identical molecular forms in both intestinal and cerebral tissue. The heptacosapeptide, peptide histidine isoleucine amide, (PHI)-27, is a relatively recent addition to the list, having been isolated initially from porcine intestinal extract[2] and subsequently found also in the brain tissue of the same species.[3] Amino acid sequence analysis of PHI has revealed a considerable degree of structural homology with the glucagon-secretin family of peptides. There is approximately a 50% homology between the structure of the PHI and the VIP molecules. A lesser degree of homology is seen for the other peptides of this family. Studies aimed at elucidating peptidergic biosynthetic mechanisms have revealed that VIP is synthesized by cleavage of a larger precursor molecule, termed proVIP.[4] Analysis of the whole amino acid sequence of the primary translation product, termed prepro-VIP with about 170 amino acid residues,[5] revealed that this molecule contained not only the amino acid sequence of VIP, but also a sequence that closely resembled the PHI structure found in porcine tissues. Thus, the human homologue of PHI differs at two loci and has been termed PHM. In rat PHI differs from that initially described from porcine sources, again by two amino acids, although in this instance the terminal histidine and isoleucine residues remain the same.[6]

[a]Address for correspondence: Dr. Lars Edvinsson, M.D., Ph.D., Department of Internal Medicine, University Hospital, S-221 85 Lund, Sweden 046 - 10 10 00.

IMMUNOCYTOCHEMICAL LOCALIZATION OF
CEREBROVASCULAR VIP/PHI FIBERS

The presence of VIP/PHI-like immunoreactive fibers has been demonstrated in cerebrovascular tissues using specific antisera and indirect immunocytochemical procedures. Well-developed plexuses of perivascular nerve fibers containing VIP- and PHI-like immunoreaction products were identified at the adventitia-medial border in the walls of cortex pial arteries and in the major arteries at the base of the brain[7–10] (FIG. 1). The sequential incubation of the vessel preparations with PHI followed by VIP antisera revealed an almost precise topographic matching of PHI- and VIP-immunoreactive perivascular fibers[8] (FIG. 1). Although the VIP/PHI immunoreactivity was seen in all major cerebral arteries of the cat, those vessels arising from the rostral part of the circle of Willis (anterior and middle cerebral arteries) generally contained more VIP-immunoreactive fibers than those from the caudal portions (basilar and cerebellar arteries; FIG. 2). Indeed all of the evidence currently available points towards the coexistance of PHI with VIP in a single neuronal system innervating the cerebrovasculature.

The source of the perivascular VIP/PHI innervation of cerebral arteries is not clear. There is some evidence indicating that these peptides are contained within the cerebrovascular parasympathetic innervation derived from the sphenopalatine ganglion.[11,12] However, VIP-immunoreactive perikarya have in addition been observed within microganglia in the cavernous plexus and in the external rete of the cat; this could provide another source of perivascular VIP.[9] A possible innervation of penetrating arterioles by central neurons of the brain itself has been suggested; VIP-containing neocortical interneurons have been shown to make intimate contacts with intracortical blood vessels, as well as synapsing with other neurons.[13] Interestingly, there is a parallel here with the conditions pertaining in the periphery in that, in these cortical neurons, VIP coexists with acetylcholine.

CEREBROVASCULAR RESPONSIVENESS TO VIP/PHI

Considerable evidence is available describing dilatory actions of VIP upon cerebral vessels both in vitro[8,10,14–16] and in situ.[17–19] In appropriate intact animal preparations, these actions of VIP are manifested, as might be expected, as an increased cerebral blood flow.[18,20,21] Studies performed in vitro have shown that PHI may also elicit concentration-dependent vasodilatation of bovine and feline middle cerebral, and porcine basilar arteries preconcentrated with either prostaglandins or KCl, while other peptides with structural similarities, secretin, glucagon, and VIP fragments had no effect.[8,22] In cat arteries it was observed that 25 times more PHI was required to produce an equal dilatory response to that elicited by VIP[8] (FIG. 3). Although vessels responding maximally to either PHI or VIP were capable of further dilatation in response to papaverine, while the administration of PHI to vessels already dilated in response to VIP showed no further effect, and the reverse procedure (PHI followed by VIP) had very little effect. Thus, it appears that both PHI and VIP act upon cerebral smooth muscle at a common receptor site or via a common mechanism.

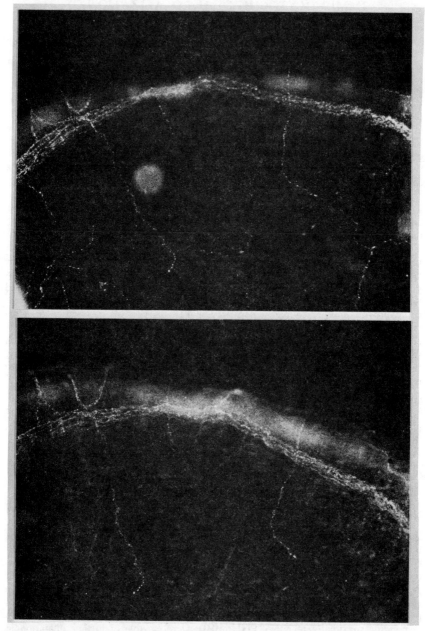

FIGURE 1. Immunocytochemical demonstration of perivascular PHI- (above) and VIP-containing (below) nerve fibers in the wall of a feline pial artery. Magnification ×300. (From Edvinsson & McCulloch[8]; reprinted with permission from *Regulatory Peptides*.)

VIP

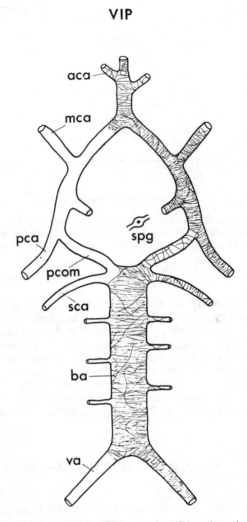

FIGURE 2. A schematic overview of the VIP innervation of the guinea pig cerebral circulation.

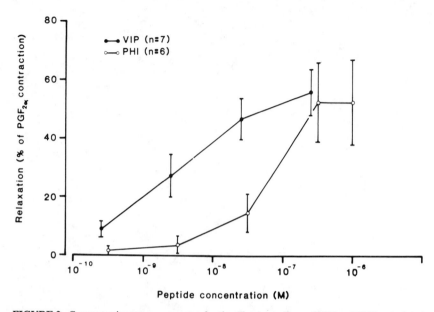

FIGURE 3. Concentration-response curves for the dilatatory effects of VIP and PHI on isolated cat middle cerebral arteries precontracted by the addition of 3×10^{-6} M of prostaglandin $F_{2\alpha}$. (From Edvinsson & McCulloch[8]; reprinted with permission from *Regulatory Peptides.*)

Microapplication of VIP or PHI into the perivascular space around cat pial arterioles *in situ* both produced vasodilatation and significant increases in arteriolar caliber.[8,18] The preinjection resting caliber of the arterioles investigated *in situ* had no measurable effect upon the magnitude of the response to PHI. However, the arterioles were almost 60-fold less sensitive to PHI than to VIP, although the maximal response to the two peptides was indistinguishable (FIG. 4). No significant effect of PHI was found upon pial veins. These results confirm the conclusion from *in vitro* studies that PHI, like VIP, if released from perivascular nerves, could induce vasodilatation and thereby contribute considerably to the control of cerebral blood flow.

BIOACTIVITY OF VIP AND PHI

The homologous amino acid sequences of VIP and PHI, particularly at the COOH-terminal region, may account for the remarkably similar biological profiles of the two peptides. Both VIP and PHI can stimulate adenylate cyclase activity in isolated cells and membrane preparations derived from a variety of tissues, for example, intestine, liver, fat, and stomach,[23] resulting in increased levels of cAMP. VIP has been found to be a potent vasodilator in, for example, mesenteric and cerebral arteries; in parallel with inducing dilatation the peptide activates vascular smooth muscle adenylate cyclase.[24,25] Furthermore, the response to VIP is unmodified by the removal of the

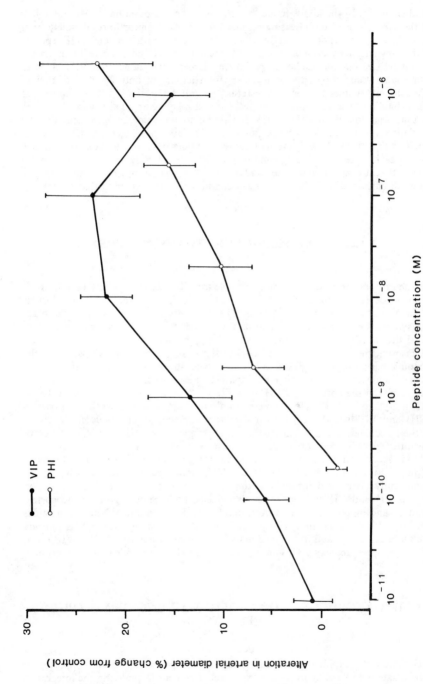

FIGURE 4. Dose-response curves for the dilatory effects of VIP and PHI on cat pial arterioles *in situ*. (From Edvinsson & McCulloch[8]; reprinted with permission from *Regulatory Peptides*.)

endothelium.[15,24] In the above tissues, no PHI-specific receptors have been identified, and the effects of PHI in increasing cellular cAMP levels appear to result solely from the binding of the peptide to VIP-preferring receptors. With iodinated VIP, specific VIP binding sites have been observed in the medial layers of bovine cerebral arteries.[26]

Competitive binding studies in peripheral tissues have shown that PHI binds to the available recognition sites with an apparent affinity of only 20-25% of that of VIP itself, but 10 times greater than secretin.[23] In contrast, PHI and VIP are equipotent in their binding to secretin-preferring receptors, displaying an affinity some 300 times less than secretin. With PHI and VIP binding to the same receptor and thereby stimulating the production of the putative secondary messenger cAMP, it is not surprising that the biological action of the two peptides described to date are identical. Differences in receptor binding affinity are reflected directly in the differences in potency that are apparent in the modulation of biological processes, although the maximum efficacy of PHI is, under most conditions, very similar to that of VIP.

VIP AND PHI AS NEUROTRANSMITTERS

A neurotransmitter-neuromodulatory role for VIP has been clearly established,[27] and evidence is accumulating that PHI has a similar neuronal function both in peripheral and central nervous systems. The discovery of a PHI-like peptide in rat brain synaptosomal preparations, and its Ca^{2+}-dependent release in response to K^+-evoked depolarization of rat cortical slices[28] is consistent with the hypothesis that PHI is stored in nerve endings and could play a role in neurotransmission. In the autonomic nervous system, PHI and VIP have been shown to coexist within the same neurons,[30] and stimulation of the parasympathetic nerves to the submandibular salivary gland results in the corelease of PHI and VIP, as well as of the classical neurotransmitter acetylcholine.[30] The closely related molecular structure and synthetic processes of PHI and VIP, together with their similar pharmacology and biological activity, and their occurrence in the same neurons, all suggest that PHI and VIP as neurotransmitter/neuromodulators should be considered conjointly.

Using specific antibodies it has been possible to map the distribution of endogenous PHI in porcine and rat brain.[31] Like VIP,[32] PHI-containing neurons are widely, though nonuniformly distributed throughout the brain. In most areas a strong correlation between PHI and VIP concentrations is evident, both being highest in neocortex, amygdala, and hippocampus. However, in a few regions the ratio of the two peptides differs significantly from unity, most notably in the cerebellum where PHI appears to be more abundant, and in the medulla where the reverse is true (PHI : VIP ratios 6.25 and 0.29, respectively). This has been thought to be due to differential processing.

2-DEOXYGLUCOSE METABOLIC MAPPING OF VIP/PHI EFFECTS

The autoradiographic 2-deoxyglucose technique[33] provides a unique opportunity to investigate the role of neurotransmitters, including neuropeptides, in the integrative activity of the brain.[34] The efferent pathways of the striatum to the globus pallidus,

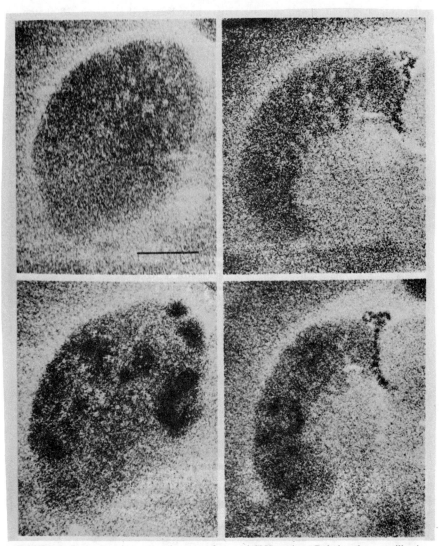

FIGURE 5. Representative autoradiograms of coronal CNS sections. Relative glucose utilization is approximately proportional to relative optical density. (**A**) Upper left: Caudate nucleus, ipsilateral and approximately 1 mm caudal to site of intrastriatal injection of CSF. Optical density (and hence glucose utilization) is fairly homogenous throughout the caudate nucleus. (**B**) Upper right: Caudate nucleus, ipsilateral and approximately 2.5 mm caudal to site of intrastriatal injection of CSF. Optical density is fairly homogenous throughout caudate nucleus. (**C**) Lower left: Caudate nucleus, ipsilateral and approximately 1 mm caudal to site of intrastriatal injection of VIP. Punctate areas of increased optical density interspersed with patches of relatively reduced optical density are present throughout the caudate nucleus. (**D**) Lower right: Caudate nucleus, ipsilateral and approximately 2.5 mm caudal to site of intrastriatal injection of VIP. Although punctate areas of increased density are present in the caudate nucleus and at this level, the regions of reduced glucose utilization are more widespread.

entopeduncular nucleus, and substantia nigra have been well characterized anatomically and pharmacologically, and have provided a particularly useful model within which to study the effects of classical neurotransmitters. Thus, intrastriatal microinjections of dopamine[35] or the GABA agonist, muscimol,[36] in the conscious rat elicit similar homogenous decreases in glucose use within the injected nucleus, and the effects of this are manifest in all primary striatal projection areas. In contrast, picomolar amounts of VIP produce spectacular heterogenous alterations in glucose use within the injected striatum with punctate areas of increased activity against a background of generalized decrease in glucose use[37] (FIG. 5). These discrete striatal effects appear to activate only one specific efferent pathway, so that altered glucose use is manifest in the substantia nigra pars compacta, the pallidal complex and lateral habenula (FIG. 6) while most other regions are unaltered (FIGS. 7 and 8). From preliminary studies it would appear that injection of similar concentrations of PHI produce less striking, but qualitatively similar effects both within the striatum and in the same efferent structures. Thus, it would appear that in common with other systems in the brain and periphery, PHI has an identical effect to that of VIP upon integrated functional activity of the basal ganglia, of which the striatum is a part. Injections of VIP (20 pmol) into the anterior cingulate cortex result in local increases in glucose utilization.[38] In addition, focal alterations in glucose use are in CNS regions that have known neuronal connections with the injected regions, for example, ipsilateral mediodorsal

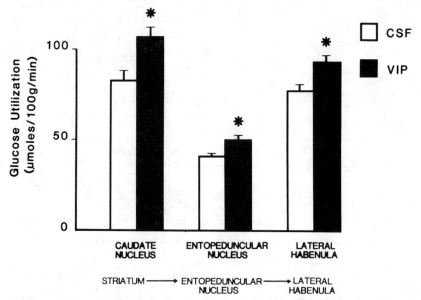

FIGURE 6. Effects of intrastriatal administration of VIP upon glucose use in three neuroanatomically connected brain areas ipsilateral to the injection. Unilateral injections of VIP (20 pmol) or artificial cerebrospinal fluid, CSF (2 μl) were made 10 minutes before the measurement of local cerebral glucose utilization in conscious rats. Glucose use was significantly elevated in the vicinity of the injection (caudate nucleus) in the entopeduncular nucleus (which receives striatal afferent nerve fibers) and in the lateral habenular nucleus (which receives fibers from the entopeduncular nucleus). *$p < 0.02$. Data are from McCulloch et al.[37]

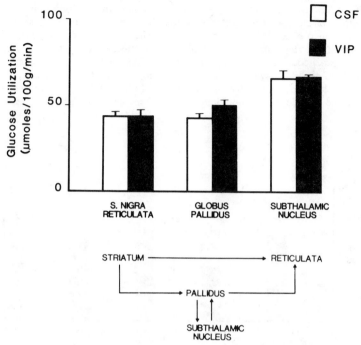

FIGURE 7. Effects of intrastriatal administration of VIP on glucose use in three neuroanatomically connected brain areas ipsilateral to the injection. Unilateral injections of VIP (20 pmol) or artificial cerebrospinal fluid, CSF (2 μl) were made 10 minutes before the measurement of local cerebral glucose utilization in conscious rats. Glucose use was not significantly altered by VIP in the striatal efferent circuit (anatomical connections are displayed diagrammatically). Data are from McCulloch *et al.*[37]

thalamus, ventral tegmental area, nucleus accumbens, caudate nucleus and contralateral cingulate cortex (FIG. 9). This provides further support for the possibility that VIP may modify the processing of afferent and efferent information in a cerebral cortical region.

VIP/PHI AND THE RELATIONSHIP BETWEEN LOCAL CEREBRAL BLOOD FLOW AND GLUCOSE USE

The vascular response to VIP and PHI described *in vitro* and *in situ* would, if transposed unaltered into the whole animal, result in increased cerebral perfusion through the dilated vessels. In suitable animal preparations, VIP has indeed been shown to increase blood flow,[18,20,21] and with its similarities in pharmacology, PHI may be expected to exert a similar effect. In general terms, the actions of VIP/PHI upon cerebral energy processes[39] would also provide a reinforcing metabolic drive to elicit vasodilatation.

When VIP and PHI are administered centrally into the striatum of conscious rats, the pattern of glucose utilization is very complex: There are small, punctate areas of increased glucose use, but there is also a more generalized reduction in the nucleus as a whole, and this more than cancels out the increases (FIG. 10). If blood flow of the striatum is coupled to metabolism as the only vasomotor effector system, then on the basis of the 2-deoxyglucose results one might predict that there would be no change in blood flow in the nucleus as a whole. If on the other hand a direct vascular effect of the peptides were to predominate, then one would expect an increased blood flow.

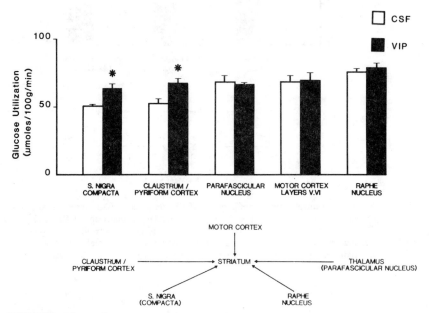

FIGURE 8. Effects of intrastriatal administration of VIP on glucose use in five ipsilateral regions that give rise to striatal afferent projections. Unilateral injections of VIP (20 pmol) of artificial cerebrospinal fluid, CSF (2 μg), were made 10 minutes before the measurement of local cerebral glucose utilization in conscious rats. Glucose use was significantly elevated in the pars compacta of the substantia nigra and pyriform cortex but not in the other areas. Data are from McCulloch et al.[37]

Using the same experimental model as that used for the 2-deoxyglucose studies but with the iodoantipyrine autoradiographic technique,[40] VIP and PHI were injected into the striatum and the effects upon blood flow measured. Intrastriatal injections of artificial CSF were found themselves to produce a 10-20% decrease in blood flow throughout the nucleus, even at quite considerable distances from the highly localized injection site (FIG. 10). At the injection site and slightly anterior, the injection of picomolar amounts of VIP produced a very variable effect upon blood flow. There was, however, a definite trend toward increase in flow, which in individual animals were quite marked, while both PHI and artificial CSF reduced the blood flow (FIG.

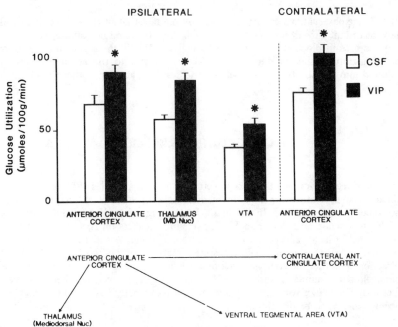

FIGURE 9. Effects of intracortical administration of VIP upon glucose use in four neuroanatomically connected brain areas. Unilateral injections of VIP (20 pmol) of artificial CSF (2 μl) were made into the anterior cingulate cortex 10 minutes before the measurement of local cerebral glucose utilization in conscious rats. Glucose use is significantly elevated in the vicinity of the injection site and in the three areas into which it projects, namely the ipsilateral mediodorsal thalamic nucleus, ipsilateral ventral tegmental area (VTA), and the contralateral anterior cingulate cortex. *$p < 0.02$. Data are from McCulloch and Kelly.[38]

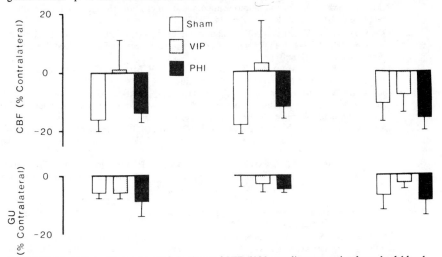

FIGURE 10. Effect of intrastriatal injections of VIP (200 pmol) upon striatal cerebral blood flow (CBF) and glucose use (GU) at three coronal levels of the caudate nucleus, namely anterior (left), midcaudate (center), and posterior (right histograms). VIP produces relative increases in cerebral blood flow in excess of alteration in glucose use. Data are from Tuor *et al.*[41]

10). These observations are strengthened by the fact that in the same animals, blood flow at distant sites in the nucleus, to which the VIP could not diffuse, never showed any increase in blood flow, and indeed seemed to follow the metabolic depression in both magnitude and direction (FIG. 10). In contrast to the actions of VIP, PHI injected into the striatum was never seen to result in anything other than a decrease in flow.[41]

CONCLUDING REMARKS

The direct actions of the two structurally related peptides, VIP and PHI, upon the cerebrovasculature appear to be mediated via the same receptor mechanisms and are qualitatively identical. In the intact brain of rat there is some indication, albeit slight, that while both VIP and PHI have similar effects on functional activity as it is reflected in local rates of glucose utilization, VIP may act directly upon the vessels to elicit an increase in blood flow despite metabolic factors working in the opposite direction. Whether the complete lack of any evidence that PHI is acting upon cerebral blood flow in a similar manner to VIP is purely a dose effect, or whether there is in fact a divergence of roles not apparent in any other body tissues where the peptides occur, remains to be determined.

REFERENCES

1. CARLQUIST, M., T. J. McDONALD, V. L. W. GO, D. BATAILLE, C. JOHANSSON & V. MUTT. 1982. Isolation and amino acid composition of human vasoactive intestinal polypeptide (VIP). Horm. Metab. Res. **14:** 28-29.
2. TATEMOTO, K. & V. MUTT. 1981. Isolation and characterization of the intestinal peptide porcine PHI (PHI-27), a new member of the glucagon-secretin family. Proc. Natl. Acad. Sci. USA **78:** 6603-6607.
3. TATEMOTO, K., M. CARLQUIST, T. J. McDONALD & V. MUTT. 1983. Isolation of a brain peptide identical to the intestinal PHI (peptide HI). FEBS Lett. **153:** 248-252.
4. OBATA, K., N. ITOH, H. OKAMOTO, C. YANAIHARA, N. YANAIHARA & T. SUZUKI. 1981. Identification and processing of biosynthetic precursors to vasoactive intestinal peptide in human neuroblasma cells. FEBS Lett. **136:** 123-126.
5. ITOH, N., K. OBATA, N. YANAIHARA & H. OKAMOTO. 1983. Human preprovasoactive polypeptide contains a novel PHI-27-like peptide, PHM-27. Nature (London) **304:** 547-549.
6. NISHIZAWA, M., Y. HAYAKAWA, N. YANAIHARA & H. OKAMOTO. 1985. Nucleotide sequence divergence and functional constraint in VIP precursor mRNA evolution between human and rat. FEBS Lett. **183:** 55-59.
7. EDVINSSON, L., J. FAHRENKRUG, J. HANKO, C. OWMAN, F. SUNDLER & R. UDDMAN. 1980. VIP (vasoactive intestinal polypeptide)-containing nerves of intracranial arteries in mammals. Cell. Tissue Res. **208:** 135-142.
8. EDVINSSON, L. & J. McCULLOCH. 1985. Distribution and vasomotor effects of peptide HI (PHI) in feline cerebral blood vessels in vitro and in situ. Regul. Peptides **10:** 345-356.
9. GIBBINS, I. L., J. E. BRAYDEN & J. A. BEVAN. 1984. Perivascular nerves with immunoreactivity to vasoactive intestinal polypeptide in cephalic arteries of the cat: Distribution, possible origins and functional implications. Neuroscience **13:** 1327-1346.

10. LARSSON, L.-I., L. EDVINSSON, J. FAHRENKRUG, R. HÅKANSON, C. OWMAN, O. SCHAF-FALITZKY DE MUCKADELL & F. SUNDLER. 1976. Immunohistochemical localization of vasodilatory peptide (VIP) in cerebrovascular nerves. Brain Res. **113:** 400-404.
11. HARA, H., G. S. HAMILL & D. M. JACOBOWITZ. 1985. Origin of cholinergic nerves to the rat major cerebral arteries: Coexistence with vasoactive intestinal polypeptide. Brain Res. Bull. **14:** 179-188.
12. WALTERS, B. B., S. A. GILLESPIE & M. A. MOSKOWITZ. 1986. Cerebrovascular projections from the sphenopalatine and otic ganglia to the middle cerebral artery of the cat. Stroke **17:** 488-494.
13. ECKENSTEIN, F. & R. W. BAUGHMAN. 1984. Two types of cholinergic innervation in cortex, one co-localized with vasoactive intestinal polypeptide. Nature (London) **309:** 153-155.
14. DUCKLES, S. P. & S. I. SAID. 1982. Vasoactive intestinal polypeptide as a neurotransmitter in the cerebral circulation. Eur. J. Pharmacol. **78:** 371-374.
15. LEE, T. J.-F., A. SAITO & I. BEREZIN. 1984. Vasoactive intestinal polypeptide-like substance: The potential transmitter for cerebral vasodilation. Science **224:** 898-901.
16. BEVAN, J. A., G. M. BUGA, M. A. MOSKOWITZ & S. I. SAID. 1986. *In vitro* evidence that vasoactive intestinal peptide is a transmitter of neuro-vasodilation in the head of the cat. Neuroscience **19:** 597-604.
17. EDVINSSON, L., J. MCCULLOCH & R. UDDMAN. 1982. Feline cerebral veins and arteries: Comparison of autonomic innervation and vasomotor responses. J. Physiol. **325:** 161-173.
18. MCCULLOCH, J. & L. EDVINSSON. 1980. Cerebral circulatory and metabolic effects of vasoactive intestinal polypeptide. Am. J. Physiol. **238:** H449-H456.
19. WEI, E. P., H. A. KONTOS & S. I. SAID. 1980. Mechanism of action of vasoactive intestinal polypeptide on cerebral arterioles. Am. J. Physiol. **239:** H765-H768.
20. HEISTAD, D. D., M. L. MARCUS, S. I. SAID & P. M. GROSS. 1980. Effect of acetylcholine and vasoactive intestinal peptide on cerebral blood flow. Am. J. Physiol. **239:** H73-H80.
21. WILSON, D. A., J. T. O'NEILL, S. I. SAID & R. J. TRAYSTMAN. 1981. Vasoactive intestinal polypeptide and the canine cerebral circulation. Circ. Res. **48:** 138-148.
22. SUZUKI, Y., D. MCMASTER, K. LEDERIS & O. P. RORSTAD. 1984. Characterization of the relaxant effects of vasoactive intestinal peptide (VIP) and PHI on isolated brain arteries. Brain Res. **322:** 9-16.
23. BATAILLE, D., C. GESPACH, M. LABURTHE, B. AMIRANOFF, K. TATEMOTO, N. VAUCLIN & V. MUTT. 1980. Porcine peptide having N-terminal histidine and C-terminal isoleucine amide (PHI). FEBS Lett. **114:** 240-242.
24. EDVINSSON, L., B. B. FREDHOLM, E. HAMEL, I. JANSEN & C. VERRECCHIA. 1985. Perivascular peptides relax cerebral arteries concomitant with stimulation of cyclic adenosine monophosphate accumulation or release of an endothelium-derived relaxing factor in the cat. Neurosci. Lett. **58:** 213-217.
25. GANZ, P., A. W. SANDROCK, S. C. LANDIS, J. LEOPOLD, M. A. GRIMBONE, JR. & R. W. ALEXANDER. 1986. Vasoactive intestinal peptide: Vasodilation and cyclic AMP generation. Am. J. Physiol. **250:** H755-H760.
26. POULIN, P., Y. SUZUKI, K. LEDERIS & O. P. RORSTAD. 1986. Autoradiographic localization of binding sites for vasoactive intestinal peptide (VIP) in bovine cerebral arteries. Brain Res. **381:** 382-384.
27. ROSTENE, W. H. 1984. Neurobiological and neuroendocrine functions of the vasoactive intestinal peptide (VIP). Prog. Neurobiol. **22:** 103-129.
28. KORCHAK, D. M., K. GYSLING & M. C. BEINFELD. 1985. The subcellular distribution of peptide histidine isoleucine amide-27-like peptides in rat brain and their release from rat cerebral cortical slices in vitro. J. Neurochem. **44:** 255-259.
29. LUNDBERG, J. M., J. FAHRENKRUG, T. HÖKFELT, C.-R. MARTLING, O. LARSSON, K. TATEMOTO & A. ÅNGGÅRD. 1984. Co-existence of peptide HI (PHI) and VIP in nerves regulating blood flow and bronchial smooth muscle tone in various mammals including man. Peptides **5:** 593-606.
30. LUNDBERG, J. M., J. FAHRENKRUG, O. LARSSON & A. ÅNGGÅRD. 1984. Corelease of vasoactive intestinal polypeptide and peptide histidine isoleucine in relation to atropine-resistant vasodilation in cat submandibular salivary gland. Neurosci. Lett. **52:** 37-42.

31. BEINFELD, M. C., D. M. KORCHAK, B. L. ROTH & T. L. O'DONOHUE. 1984. The distribution and chromatographic characterization of PHI (peptide histidine isoleucine amide)-27-like peptides in rat and porcine brain. J. Neurosci. **4:** 2681-2688.

32. BESSON, J., W. ROTSZTEJN, M. LABURTHE, J. EPELBAUM, A. BEAUDET, C. KORDON & G. ROSSELIN. 1979. Vasoactive intestinal peptide (VIP): Brain distribution, subcellular localization and effect of deafferentation of the hypothalamus in male rats. Brain Res. **165:** 79-85.

33. SOKOLOFF, L., M. REIVICH, C. KENNEDY, M. H. DES ROSIERS, C. S. PATLAK, K. D. PETTIGREW, O. SAKURADA & M. SHINOHARA. 1977. The [^{14}C]deoxyglucose method for the measurement of local cerebral glucose utilisation: Theory, procedure and normal values in the conscious and anaesthetised albino rat. J. Neurochem. **28:** 897-916.

34. MCCULLOCH, J. 1982. Mapping functional alterations in the CNS with [^{14}C]deoxyglucose. *In* Handbook of Psychopharmacology. L. L. Iversen, S. D. Iversen & S. H. Snyder, Eds. **15:** 321-410. Plenum Press. New York.

35. BROWN, L. L. & L. I. WOLFSON. 1983. A dopamine-sensitive striatal efferent system mapped with [^{14}C]deoxyglucose in the rat. Brain Res. **261:** 213-229.

36. KELLY, P. A. T. & J. MCCULLOCH. 1984. Extrastriatal circuits activated by intrastrial muscimol: A [^{14}C]2-deoxyglucose investigation. Brain Res. **292:** 357-366.

37. MCCULLOCH, J., P. A. T. KELLY, R. UDDMAN & L. EDVINSSON. 1983. Functional role for vasoactive intestinal polypeptide in the caudate nucleus: A 2-deoxy[^{14}C]glucose investigation. Proc. Natl. Acad. Sci. USA **80:** 1472-1476.

38. MCCULLOCH, J. & P. A. T. KELLY. 1983. A functional role for vasoactive intestinal polypeptide in anterior cingulate cortex. Nature **304:** 438-440.

39. MAGISTRETTI, P. J., J. H. MORRISON, W. J. SHOEMAKER, V. SAPIN & F. E. BLOOM. 1981. Vasoactive intestinal polypeptide induces glycogenolysis in mouse cortical slices: A possible regulatory mechanism for the local control of energy metabolism. Proc. Natl. Acad. Sci. USA **78:** 6535-6539.

40. SAKURADA, O., C. KENNEDY, J. JEHLE, J. D. BROWN, G. L. CARBIN & L. SOKOLOFF. 1978. Measurement of local cerebral blood flow with iodo[^{14}C]antipyrine. Am. J. Physiol. **234:** H59-H66.

41. TUOR, U. I., L. EDVINSSON, P. A. T. KELLY & J. MCCULLOCH. 1988. Effects of VIP and PHI on local cerebral blood flow: A comparative autoradiographic study. J. Cereb. Blood Flow Metab. In press.

Vasoactive Intestinal Polypeptide and the Reproductive System

JAN FAHRENKRUG,[a] BENT OTTESEN, AND
CONNIE PALLE

Department of Clinical Chemistry
Bispebjerg Hospital
Copenhagen, Denmark
and
Department of Gynaecology and Obstetrics
Hvidovre Hospital
Copenhagen, Denmark

It is now recognized that vasoactive intestinal polypeptide (VIP) plays an important role in the control of the reproductive system both at hypothalamic-hypophyseal level as well as locally in the genital organs. This report will be limited to dealing with the involvement of VIP as transmitter in the autonomic nervous control of functions in the male and female genital tracts. Secretion, motility, and blood flow are not solely controlled by cholinergic or adrenergic nerves. The demonstration of a number of biologically active peptides in nerves of the genital tract, among which VIP was the first to be shown,[1,2] led to studies of their possible neurotransmitter function.

LOCALIZATION AND DISTRIBUTION OF VIP AND PHM

The cellular localization of the two peptides VIP and PHM (peptide with NH_2-terminal histidine and COOH-terminal methionine), which apparently are derived from a common precursor, has been examined by immunocytochemistry and the concentration of immunoreactivity in the various regions quantified by radioimmunoassay of tissue extracts.[1-19]

In the female genital tract VIP-containing (VIPergic) nerve fibers have been demonstrated in all species examined, but the number of fibers display a considerable species variation. The following distribution pattern is, however, common: VIP is most abundant in the vagina, the cervix, and clitoris, less numerous in the uterine body and oviduct and rare or absent in the ovary. Locally a rich nerve supply is present around the natural sphincters, that is, the internal and external cervical os and isthmic part of the Fallopian tube. Clusters of VIP containing ganglionic cells are located in paracervical ganglia at the uterovaginal junction.[4,8] Transsection of the

---

[a] Address for correspondence: Jan Fahrenkrug, M.D., Ph.D., Department of Clinical Chemistry, Bispebjerg Hospital, DK-2400 Copenhagen NV, Denmark.

hypogastric nerves has no effect on the VIPergic nerve supply, while removal of paracervical ganglia considerably reduces the number of genital VIPergic nerve fibers, except for those in the ovary, which probably originate from the superior ovarian nerves.[20] Following transsection of the uterine cervix, VIPergic fibers disappear from the body of the uterus and the oviduct, while the nerves in the cervix below the lesion are unaffected.[4] The findings indicate that most VIPergic nerves in the female genital tract are intrinsic originating from local ganglia. This notion is supported by a recent study using combined retrograde tracing technique and immunocytochemistry.[21] Throughout the female genital tract the VIPergic fibers are associated with blood vessels, nonvascular smooth muscle, lining epithelium, and glands. In the ovary of some species, especially in the immature organ, VIPergic fibers seem to innervate the vasculature, the interstitial tissue and the cell layers of the developing follicles.[22] The distribution of PHM/PHI immunoreactive nerves are similar to the VIPergic, although they appear to be less abundant.[23,24]

VIP is present in the male genital tract of all the species examined.[13-19] The highest concentrations of VIP immunoreactivity occur in the corpus cavernosum and deep arteries of the penis. Besides innervating arteries and arterioles, the nonvascular smooth muscles, particularly the muscle of the corpus cavernosum and the corpus spongiosum, the prostate and seminal vesicle are supplied with VIPergic nerves. In the vas deferens a subepithelial plexus of VIPergic fibers are present in the muscular coat. Scattered neuronal cell bodies containing VIP occur within the proximal corpus cavernosum and more frequently in the interstitial tissue of the prostate. Studies in the rat indicate that the major source of the VIPergic innervation to the erectile tissue is VIP-containing cell bodies in the major pelvic ganglion.[17] Both in the male and female genital tract VIP is stored and released from large (100 nm) spherical dense-cored vesicles in the nerve terminals.[18]

EFFECTS OF VIP

Blood Flow

In the female genital tract, VIP induces a dose-related increase in vaginal as well as endometrial, myometrial, and total uterine blood flow.[25-31] In the uterine vascular bed, VIP seems on a molar basis to be more potent than other known vasodilators such as acetylcholine, bradykinin, prostaglandins, and estrogen.[25,28,31] On myometrial blood flow in rabbits, PHI and VIP produce identical vasodilatory responses.[32] VIP is also a potent vasodilator in the normal human placenta.[33] The investigations on uterine blood flow have been performed on animals with intact ovaries or on oophorectomized animals substituted with estrogen and progesterone. It is possible that the responsiveness of the vascular smooth cells to VIP depends on reproductive phase and pregnancy.[34] Thus, evidence for a relationship between sex steroid hormones and effect of VIP has been shown for nonvascular smooth muscle.[35] In the male genital tract VIP causes a dose-dependent relaxation of smooth muscle specimens in vitro.[14,15] By close intraarterial infusion in dogs VIP elicits a moderate erection and a penile vasodilatory response,[36] and in man intracavernous injection of VIP provokes penile erection (FIG. 1).[37]

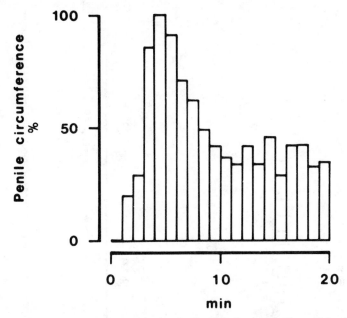

FIGURE 1. Effect of intracavernous injection (at 0 min) of vasoactive intestinal polypeptide (200 pmol) on penile erection in man, expressed as increase in penile circumference, measured with a strain gauge (full erection = 100%; flaccidity = 0%).

Nonvascular Smooth Muscle

In vitro VIP inhibits dose dependently both the mechanical and electrical activity in nonvascular smooth muscle preparations from any region in the female genital tract.[7,8,12,38–45] Both spontaneous as well as contractile activity induced by oxytocin, carbacholine, prostaglandin $F_{2\alpha}$, and substance P can be inhibited by VIP. Evidence exists that the relaxatory effect of VIP is direct on the smooth muscle cells via its own receptor since the VIP response is unaffected by adrenoceptor blocking agents, atropine and tetrodotoxin (a blocker of nerve transmission). Furthermore, specific and high-affinity binding sites for the peptide are present in membrane preparations of uterine smooth muscle.[46] From electrophysiological studies it is suggested that VIP acts on the calcium balance of the myometrial smooth muscle cells by accelerating sequestration and/or extrusion of calcium. Furthermore the peptide inhibits generator potential, causes hyperpolarization and increases membrane permeability to potassium.[42] Also *in vivo* VIP inhibits smooth muscle activity in the female genital tract as evidenced by a relaxation of spontaneous mechanical uterine contractions in non-pregnant human females after intravenous VIP administration.[30] In the male genital tract, the inhibitory effect of VIP on nonvascular smooth muscle has been demonstrated *in vitro* on specimens from vas deferens and urethra.[13,47,48] On human and rabbit smooth muscle strips, PHM/PHI displays an inhibition identical to that of VIP (FIG. 2),[32] but it remains to be clarified if the two peptides are working on a common receptor.

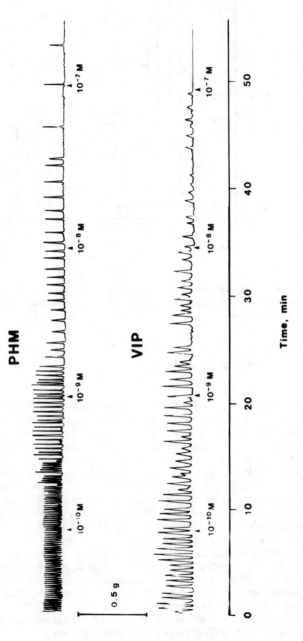

FIGURE 2. Effect of increasing doses of PHM (upper trace) and VIP (lower trace) on spontaneous contractions of smooth muscle strips from human Fallopian tube *in vitro*.

Secretion

Intravenous administration of VIP in nonpregnant women causes an increase in vaginal lubrication to a level that corresponds to the amounts produced on the vaginal surface during sexual self-stimulation to orgasm (FIG. 3). The increased fluid production on the vaginal surface is most likely due to transudation secondary to the VIP-induced vasodilation. Both *in vivo* (normal women) and *in vitro* exogenous VIP is able to elicit steroid hormone secretion from the ovary.[22,49] In the male dog, VIP itself has no effect on prostatic secretion but the peptide potentiates the secretory response to administration of pilocarpine and to electrical stimulation of the hypogastric nerves.[50]

RELEASE OF VIP

The release of VIP from the nerve terminals in the female genital tract has been examined in experimental animal by activating the autonomic nerve supply to the

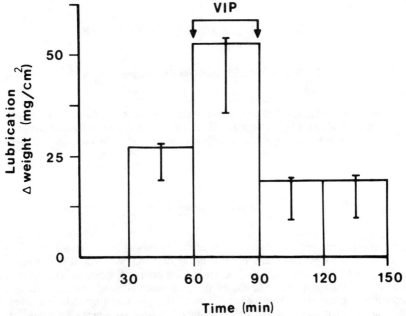

FIGURE 3. The effect of vasoactive intestinal polypeptide (900 pmol/kg $\times$ h i.v. during 30 min) on vaginal lubrication, that is, the amount of liquid produced on the surface of the vaginal wall measured during 30-minute periods by applying preweighed filter paper (diameter 12 mm) to the vaginal wall. The amount of liquid produced could be measured from the weight gain of the filter paper (diameter 12 mm). Figures are given as median weight gain and interquartile range of six normal women. A significant increase in vaginal lubrication was observed during the VIP infusion.

uterus and by electrical field nerve stimulation of smooth muscle strips *in vitro.*[51,52] In the basal state there is a small spontaneous release of VIP and efferent electrical stimulation of the parasympathetic nerve supply to the uterus (the pelvic nerves) causes a marked increase in the VIP release. The transmission of impulses from the pelvic nerve to the VIPergic neurons is blocked by the cholinergic nicotinic receptor blocker hexamethonium, suggesting that the VIPergic neurons are mostly postganglionic parasympathetic. The release of VIP, however, does not conform to the classical parasympathetic sequence of events, since it was unaffected by atropine and adrenoceptor blocking agents. A similar noncholinergic, nonadrenergic VIP release is induced by efferent electrical stimulation of the sympathetic nerve supplying the uterus (the hypogastric nerve), which is accompanied by an increase in uterovenous blood flow. Transmural electrical field stimulation induces a noncholinergic, nonadrenergic relaxation of smooth muscle strips *in vitro,* which is accompanied by a significant release of VIP (FIG. 4). The release is most likely of neuronal origin since tetrodotoxin, a blocker of nerve-impulse transmission, annuls both the electrically induced relaxation and the VIP release. In the male genital tract a VIP release is observed during electrical stimulation of the pelvic nerve in the dog and during visual sexual stimulation in man a VIP release accompanies penile erection.[36,37]

FUNCTIONAL SIGNIFICANCE OF VIP

Follicular Function and Ovarian Steroidogenesis

The demonstration of VIPergic nerve fibers close to follicles and in some species in the interstitial tissue indicates that VIP may participate in an autonomic regulation of ovarian function such as follicular rupture and steroid hormone secretion.

Ovum Transportation

The ovum reaches the proximal part of the ampule of the Fallopian tube within a few hours after ovulation and remains in the tube for two to three days before its rapid transit through the isthmus into the uterine cavity. A sphincter-like function is therefore attributed to the isthmus of the Fallopian tube and the existence of an unidentified neurotransmitter mediating noncholinergic, nonadrenergic relaxation of the smooth musculature in the Fallopian tube has been recognized for years.[53] The abundance of VIPergic nerve fibers in the Fallopian tube, especially in the isthmic part and the fact that VIP fulfills the criteria for neurotransmission in this area makes VIP the most likely candidate as the inhibitory transmitter.[7,41,54] Furthermore, the sensitivity of the isthmic sphincter to the relaxatory effect of VIP is increased in animals treated with estrogen and progesterone mimicking postovulatory concentrations in women.[35]

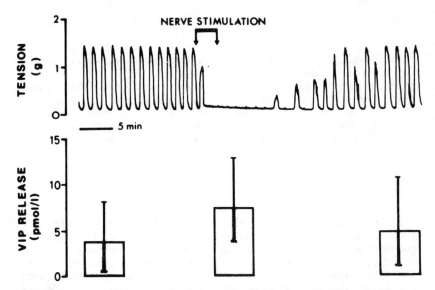

FIGURE 4. Isometric tension recordings from myometrial strip *in vitro*. Upper trace: Transmural electrical nerves stimulation (10 Hz, 2 msec, and 150 mA for a 3-min period) of feline myometrial preparations, abolishes the spontaneous contractions in the presence of α-β-adrenoceptor blocking agents and atropine. Lower trace: A significant release of VIP accompanied the smooth muscle relaxation. The figures are given as the median and ranges of eight experiments.

Uterine Motility and Blood Flow

As in the Fallopian tube, VIP seems to participate in the local nervous control of uterine muscle activity. VIP inhibits myometrial activity in nonpregnant women, both *in vivo* and *in vitro*, while the peptide has no effect on smooth muscle preparations from the uterine body at term, at which time the tissue VIP concentration is markedly reduced.[9,35,54] During pregnancy, however, VIP is still able to relax the uterine smooth muscle (Ottesen *et al.*, unpublished). The findings could suggest that VIP has a progesterone-like effect, keeping the uterine smooth muscle relaxed during pregnancy until the time of delivery. In accordance with this view, VIP antagonizes the uterine stimulatory effect of the two major initiators of labor: prostaglandin and oxytocin.[38,39] There does not seem to be any change in the VIPergic innervation of the uterine cervix during pregnancy.[55] Whether VIP participates in the relaxation and opening of the cervix during delivery remains to be established, but an increased VIP concentration in the circulation is observed at that period.[9] The existence of noncholinergic uterine vasodilation induced by nerve stimulation has been known for 20 years[56] and with our present knowledge VIP seems to be the unknown neurotransmitter. Whether VIP plays a role in the regulation of menstruation remains to be solved, but no menstruation-related changes in plasma VIP concentration in peripheral blood can be detected.[9]

Sexual Arousal

Sexual excitement is associated with an atropine-resistant increase in vaginal blood flow, vaginal lubrication, and intumescence of the clitoris.[57] VIP is most likely responsible for the changes observed during sexual arousal for the following reasons: there is a dense VIPergic innervation of the blood vessels and smooth musculature of the vagina and the clitoris; administration of VIP leads to increase in vaginal blood flow[30] and vaginal fluid production (FIG. 3); and during sexual stimulation in women VIP is released as demonstrated by a rise in systemic VIP concentration.[9]

Penile Erection

An essential part in the mechanism leading to erection is nonadrenergic, noncholinergic relaxation of vascular and cavernous smooth muscle.[58] VIP seems to fulfill several of the classical criteria to be a neurotransmitter in penile erection in man: it is present in nerve fibers with nerve endings around cavernous smooth muscle and blood vessels, mainly arteries and arterioles,[14,16,59] it is released when erection is induced (FIG. 5) and when applied exogenously it mimics the action of the endogenously released transmitter and displays identical pharmacological characteristics.[14,37,59,60]

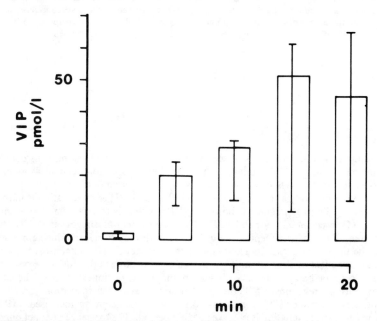

FIGURE 5. Concentration of vasoactive intestinal polypeptide (VIP) in corpus cavernosum at rest and during full erection or tumescence (figures are median and interquartile ranges of results obtained in 11 experiments in 8 men). Stimulation was started immediately after 0 min. Tumescence or erection was obtained after two to four minutes and was unchanged during the period of observation. The increase in concentration during erection and tumescence was significant.

VIPERGIC DYSFUNCTION

It is likely that dysfunction of the VIPergic nerves may be responsible for known disturbances in the function of the sexual organs. The evidence has been put forward that the number of VIPergic nerve fibers is decreased in penises from impotent men, especially in diabetics with neuropathy.[61,62] Whether this VIP depletion is the primary cause of impotence or the change is secondary remains to be established.

REFERENCES

1. LARSSON, L.-I., J. FAHRENKRUG & O. B. SCHAFFALITZKY DE MUCKADELL. 1977. Vasoactive intestinal polypeptide occurs in nerves of the female genitourinary tract. Science 197: 1374-1375.
2. LARSSON, L.-I., J. FAHRENKRUG & O. B. SHAFFALITZKY DE MUCKADELL. 1977. Occurrence of nerves containing vasoactive intestinal polypeptide immunoreactivity in the male genital tract. Life Sci. 21: 503-508.
3. ALM, P., J. ALUMETS, R. HÅKANSON & F. SUNDLER. 1977. Peptidergic (vasoactive intestinal peptide) nerves in the genitourinary tract. Neuroscience 2: 751-754.
4. ALM, P., J. ALUMETS, R. HÅKANSON, CH. OWMAN, N. O. SJÖBERG, F. SUNDLER & B. WALLES. 1980. Origin and distribution of VIP (vasoactive intestinal polypeptide)-nerves in the genito-urinary tract. Cell Tissue Res. 205: 337-347.
5. ALM, P., J. ALUMETS, R. HÅKANSON, G. HELM, CH. OWMAN, N.-O. SJÖBERG & F. SUNDLER. 1980. Vasoactive intestinal polypeptide nerves in the human female genital tract. Am. J. Obstet. Gynecol. 136: 349-351.
6. LUNDBERG, J. M., T. HÖKFELT, A. ÄNGGÅRD, K. UVNÄS-WALLENSTEN, S. BRIMIJOIN, E. BRODIN & J. FAHRENKRUG. 1980. Peripheral peptide neurons: Distribution, axonal transport, and some aspects on possible function. In Neural peptides and neuronal communication. E. Costa & M. Trabucchi, Eds.: 25-36. Raven Press. New York.
7. STRÖM, C., J. M. LUNDBERG, H. AHLMAN, A. DAHLSTRÖM, J. FAHRENKRUG & T. HÖKFELT. 1981. On the VIP-ergic innervation of the utero-tubal junctions. Acta Physiol. Scand. 111: 213-215.
8. OTTESEN, B., J.-J. LARSEN, J. FAHRENKRUG, M. STJERNQUIST & F. SUNDLER. 1981. Distribution and motor effect of VIP in female genital tract. Am. J. Physiol. 240: E32-E36.
9. OTTESEN, B., H. ULRICHSEN, J. FAHRENKRUG, J.-J. LARSEN, G. WAGNER, L. SCHIERUP & F. SØNDERGAARD. 1982. Vasoactive intestinal polypeptide and the female genital tract: Relationship to reproductive phase and delivery. Am. J. Obstet. Gynecol. 143: 414-420.
10. GOODNOUGH, J. E., T. M. O'DORISIO, C. I. FRIEDMAN & M. H. KIM. 1979. Vasoactive intestinal polypeptide in tissues of the human female reproductive tract. Am. J. Obstet. Gynecol. 134: 579-580.
11. LYNCH, E. M., J. WHARTON, M. G. BRYANT, S. R. BLOOM, J. M. POLAK & M. G. ELDER. 1980. The differential distribution of vasoactive intestinal polypeptide in the normal human female genital tract. Histochemistry 67: 169-177.
12. HELM, G., B. OTTESEN, J. FAHRENKRUG, J.-J. LARSEN, CH. OWMAN, N.-O. SJÖBERG, B. STOLBERG, F. SUNDLER & B. WALLES. 1981. Vasoactive intestinal polypeptide (VIP) in the human female reproductive tract: Distribution and motor effects. Biol. Reprod. 25: 227-234.
13. LARSEN, J.-J., B. OTTESEN, J. FAHRENKRUG & L. FAHRENKRUG. 1981. Vasoactive intestinal polypeptide (VIP) in the male genitourinary tract. Concentration and motor effect. Invest. Urol. 19: 211-213.
14. WILLIS, E. A., B. OTTESEN, G. WAGNER, F. SUNDLER & J. FAHRENKRUG. 1983. Vasoactive intestinal polypeptide (VIP) as a putative neurotransmitter in penile erection. Life Sci. 33: 383-391.

15. STEERS, W. D., J. MCCONNELL & G. S. BENSON. 1984. Anatomical localization and some pharmacological effects of vasoactive intestinal polypeptide in human and monkey corpus cavernosum. J. Urol. **132:** 1048-1053.

16. POLAK, J. M., J. GU, S. MINA & S. R. BLOOM. 1981. VIPergic nerves in the penis. Lancet **ii:** 217-219.

17. DAIL, W. G., M. A. MOLL & K. WEBER. 1983. Localization of vasoactive intestinal polypeptide in penile erectile tissue and in the major pelvic ganglion of the rat. Neuroscience **10:** 1379-1386.

18. GU, J., J. M. POLAK, L. PROBERT, K. N. ISLAM, P. H. MARANGOS, S. MINA, T. E. ADRIAN, G. O. MCGREGOR, D. J. O'SHAUGNESSY & S. R. BLOOM. 1983. Peptidergic innervation of the human male genital tract. J. Urol. **130:** 386-391.

19. GREENBERG, J., W. SCHUBERT, J. METZ, N. YANAIHARA & W.-G. FORSMANN. 1985. Studies of the guinea-pig epididymis. III. Innervation of epididymal segments. Cell Tissue Res. **239:** 395-404.

20. DEES, W. L., C. E. AHMED & S. R. OJEDA. 1986. Substance P- and vasoactive intestinal peptide-containing fibres reach the ovary by independent routes. Endocrinology **119:** 638-641.

21. GU, J., J. M. POLAK, H. C. SU, M. A. BLANK, J. F. B. MORRISON & S. R. BLOOM. 1984. Demonstration of paracervical ganglion origin for the vasoactive intestinal peptide-containing nerves of the rat uterus using retrograde tracing techniques combined with immunocytochemisry and denervation procedures. Neurosci. Lett. **51:** 377-382.

22. AHMED, C. E., W. L. DEES & S. R. OJEDA. 1986. The immature rat ovary is innervated by vasoactive intestinal peptide (VIP)-containing fibres and responds to VIP with steroid secretion. Endocrinology **118:** 1682-1689.

23. BLANK, M. A., J. GU, J. M. ALLEN, W. M. HUANG, Y. YIANGOU, J. CH'NG, G. LEWIS, M. G. ELDER, J. M. POLAK & S. R. BLOOM. 1986. The regional distribution of NPY-, PHM-, and VIP-containing nerves in the human female genital tract. Int. J. Fertil. **31:** 218-222.

24. FAHRENKRUG, J., T. BEK, J. M. LUNDBERG & T. HÖKFELT. 1985. VIP and PHI in cat neurons: Co-localization but variable tissue content possibly due to differential processing. Regul. Peptides **12:** 21-34.

25. OTTESEN, B. & J. FAHRENKRUG. 1981. Effect of vasoactive intestinal polypeptide (VIP) upon myometrial blood flow in non-pregnant rabbit. Acta Physiol. Scand. **112:** 195-201.

26. CARTER, A. M., N. EINER-JENSEN, J. FAHRENKRUG & B. OTTESEN. 1981. Increased myometrial blood flow evoked by vasoactive intestinal polypeptide in the non-pregnant goat. J. Physiol. **310:** 471-480.

27. OTTESEN, B. & N. EINER-JENSEN. 1984. Increased endometrial clearance of krypton-85 evoked by VIP in rabbits. Acta Physiol. Scand. **121:** 185-187.

28. OTTESEN, B., B. R. GRAM & J. FAHRENKRUG. 1983. Neuropeptides in the female genital tract: Effect on vascular and non-vascular smooth muscle. Peptides **4:** 387-392.

29. OTTESEN, B., N. EINER-JENSEN & A. M. CARTER. 1983. Vasoactive intestinal polypeptide and endometrial blood flow in goat. Animal Reprod. Sci. **6:** 217-222.

30. OTTESEN, B., T. GERSTENBERG, H. ULRICHSEN, T. MANTHORPE, J. FAHRENKRUG & G. WAGNER. 1983. Vasoactive intestinal polypeptide (VIP) increases vaginal blood flow and inhibits smooth muscle activity in women. Eur. J. Clin. Invest. **13:** 321-324.

31. CLARK, K. E., E. G. MILLS, S. J. STYS & A. E. SEEDS. 1981. Effects of vasoactive polypeptides on the uterine vasculature. Am. J. Obstet. Gynecol. **139:** 182-188.

32. BARDRUM, B., B. OTTESEN & J. FAHRENKRUG. 1986. Peptides PHI and VIP: Comparison between vascular and non-vascular smooth muscle effect in rabbit uterus. Am. J. Physiol. **251:** E48-E51.

33. MOURA, R. S. DE & P. G. WITHRINGTON. 1985. Vascular actions of VIP, substance P and neurotensin on the isolated perfused human fetal placenta. Contrib. Gynecol. Obstet. **13:** 174-175.

34. CLARK, K. E., J. E. AUSTIN & S. J. STYS. 1982. Effect of vasoactive intestinal polypeptide on uterine blood flow in pregnant ewes. Am. J. Obstet. Gynecol. **144:** 497-502.

35. OTTESEN, B., J.-J. LARSEN, P. STAUN-OLSEN, S. GAMMELTOFT & J. FAHRENKRUG. 1985. Influence of pregnancy and sex steroids on concentration, motor effect and receptor binding of VIP in the rabbit female genital tract. Regul. Peptides **11:** 83-92.

36. ANDERSSON, P.-O., S. R. BLOOM & S. MELLANDER. 1984. Haemodynamics of pelvic nerve induced penile erection in the dog: Possible mediation by vasoactive intestinal polypeptide. J. Physiol. (London) **350:** 209-224.
37. OTTESEN, B., G. WAGNER, R. VIRAQ & J. FAHRENKRUG. 1984. Penile erection: Possible role for vasoactive intestinal polypeptide as a neurotransmitter. Br. Med. J. **288:** 9-11.
38. OTTESEN, B., H. ULRICHSEN, G. WAGNER & J. FAHRENKRUG. 1979. Vasoactive intestinal polypeptide (VIP) inhibits oxytocin-induced activity of the rabbit myometrium. Acta Physiol. Scand. **107:** 285-287.
39. OTTESEN, B., G. WAGNER & J. FAHRENKRUG. 1980. Vasoactive intestinal polypeptide (VIP) inhibits prostaglandin- $F_{2\alpha}$-induced activity of the rabbit myometrium. Prostaglandins **19:** 427-435.
40. OTTESEN, B. 1981. Vasoactive intestinal polypeptide (VIP): Effect on rabbit uterine smooth muscle *in vivo* and *in vitro*. Acta Physiol. Scand. **113:** 193-199.
41. OTTESEN, B. 1983. Vasoactive intestinal polypeptide as a neurotransmitter in the female genital tract. Am. J. Obstet. Gynecol. **147:** 208-224.
42. BOLTON, T. B., R. J. LANG & B. OTTESEN. 1981. Mechanism of action of vasoactive intestinal polypeptide on myometrial smooth muscle of rabbit and guinea-pig. J. Physiol. (London) **318:** 41-56.
43. HELM, G., R. EKMAN, H. RYDHSTRÖM, N.-O. SJÖBERG & B. WALLES. 1985. Changes in oviductal VIP content induced by sex steroids and inhibitory effect of VIP on spontaneous oviductal contractility. Acta Physiol. Scand. **125:** 219-224.
44. FREDERICKS, C. M. & S. H. ASHTON. 1982. Effect of vasoactive intestinal polypeptide (VIP) on the *in vitro* and *in vivo* motility of the rabbit reproductive tract. Fertil. Steril. **37:** 845-850.
45. STJERNQUIST, M. & CH. OWMAN. 1984. Vasoactive intestinal polypeptide (VIP) inhibits neurally evoked smooth muscle activity of rat uterine cervix *in vitro*. Regul. Peptides **8:** 161-167.
46. OTTESEN, B., P. STAUN-OLSEN, S. GAMMELTOFT & J. FAHRENKRUG. 1982. Receptors for vasoactive intestinal polypeptide on crude smooth muscle membranes from porcine uterus. Endocrinology **110:** 2037-2043.
47. KASTIN, A. J., D. H. COY, A. V. SCHALLY & C. A. MEYERS. 1978. Activity of VIP, somatostatin and other peptides in the mouse vas deferens assay. Pharmacol. Biochem. Behav. **9:** 673-676.
48. KLARSKOV, P., T. GERSTENBERG & T. HALD. 1984. Vasoactive intestinal polypeptide influence on lower urinary tract smooth muscle from human and pig. J. Urol. **131:** 1000-1004.
49. OTTESEN, B., B. PEDERSEN, J. NIELSEN, D. DALGAARD & J. FAHRENKRUG. 1986. Effect of vasoactive intestinal polypeptide (VIP) on steroidogenesis in women. Regul. Peptides **16:** 299-304.
50. SMITH, E. R., T. B. MILLER, M. M. WILSON & M. C. APPEL. 1984. Effects of vasoactive intestinal peptide on canine prostatic contraction and secretion. Am. J. Physiol. **247:** R701-R708.
51. FAHRENKRUG, J. & B. OTTESEN. 1982. Nervous release of vasoactive intestinal polypeptide from the feline uterus: Pharmacological characteristics. J. Physiol. (London) **331:** 451-460.
52. HANSEN, B. R., B. OTTESEN & J. FAHRENKRUG. 1986. Neurotransmitter role of VIP in non-adrenergic relaxation of feline myometrium. Peptides **7:** 201-203.
53. LINDBLOM, B., B. LJUNG & L. HAMBERGER. 1979. Adrenergic and novel non-adrenergic neuronal mechanisms in the control of smooth muscle activity in the human oviduct. Acta Physiol. Scand. **196:** 215-220.
54. HELM, G., R. HÅKANSON, S. LEANDER, N.-O. SJÖBERG & B. SPORRONG. 1982. Neurogenic relaxation mediated by vasoactive intestinal polypeptide (VIP) in the isthmus of the human Fallopian tube. Regul. Peptides **3:** 145-153.
55. STJERNQUIST, M., P. ALM, R. EKMAN, C. OWMAN, N.-O. SJÖBERG & F. SUNDLER. 1985. Levels of neural vasoactive intestinal polypeptide in rat uterus are markedly changed in association with pregnancy as shown by immunocytochemistry and radioimmunoassay. Biol. Reprod. **33:** 157-163.

56. BELL, C. 1968. Dual vasoconstrictor and vasodilator innervation of the uterine arterial supply in the guinea pig. Circ. Res. **23:** 279-289.
57. LEVIN, R. H. 1980. The physiology of sexual function in women. Clin. Obstet. Gynecol. **7:** 213-252.
58. WAGNER, G. & G. S. BRINDLEY. 1980. The effect of atropine, alpha and beta blockers on human penile erection: A controlled pilot study. *In* Vasculogenic Impotence. Proceedings of the First International Conference on Corpus Cavernosum Revascularization. A. W. Zorgniotti & G. Rossi, Eds.: 77. Charles C. Thomas. Springfield, IL.
59. WILLIS, E., B. OTTESEN, J. FAHRENKRUG, F. SUNDLER & G. WAGNER. 1981. Vasoactive intestinal polypeptide as a possible neurotransmitter in penile erection. Acta Physiol. Scand. **113:** 545-547.
60. DIXSON, A. F., K. M. KENDRICK, M. A. BLANK & S. R. BLOOM. 1984. Effects of tactile and electrical stimuli upon release of vasoactive intestinal polypeptide in the mammalian penis. J. Endocrinol. **100:** 249-252.
61. GU, J., J. M. POLAK, M. LAZARIDES, R. MORGAN, J. P. PRYOR, P. J. MARANGOS, M. A. BLANK & S. R. BLOOM. 1984. Decrease of vasoactive intestinal polypeptide (VIP) in the penises from impotent men. Lancet **ii:** 315-318.
62. CROWE, R., J. LINCOLN, P. F. BLACKLONG, J. P. PRYOR, J. S. P. LUMLEY & G. BURNS-TOCK. 1983. A comparison between streptozotocin treated rats and man. Diabetes **32:** 1075-1077.

Vasoactive Intestinal Peptide in the Heart[a]

W. G. FORSSMANN,[b] J. TRIEPEL, C. DAFFNER, AND
CH. HEYM

Institute of Anatomy
University of Heidelberg
D-6900 Heidelberg
Federal Republic of Germany

P. CUEVAS

Departamento de Investigación
Servicio de Histología
Centro Ramón y Cajal
28034 Madrid, Spain

M. I. M. NOBLE

King Edward VII Hospital
Midhurst, West Sussex GU 29032
United Kingdom

N. YANAIHARA

College of Pharmacy
Shizuoka, Japan

INTRODUCTION

Among the neuropeptides exerting a neurotransmitter function on the autonomic nervous system and involved in the regulation of heart function and smooth vascular tone, vasoactive intestinal polypeptide (VIP)[1,2] and the related peptide histidine-isoleucine (PHI)[3] are of particular importance. These peptides are located in various

[a]Research on cardiac innervation was supported by the German Research Foundation, Grant SFB 320.

[b]Address for correspondence: Dr. W. G. Forssmann, Institute of Anatomy, University of Heidelberg, Im Neuenheimer Feld 307, D-6900 Heidelberg, Federal Republic of Germany.

functionally important regions of the heart, as well as in the perivascular nerve plexus of the coronary vessels.[4-9] The receptor distribution of these two neuropeptides in the cardiac tissue as well as in the different segments of the coronary vascular tree have also been described.[10] This paper reviews and updates knowledge of VIPergic cardiac innervation, including the superordinate extrinsic pathways containing VIP and/or PHI (FIG. 1), and discusses the functional relevance of VIP in the nervous regulation of the heart.

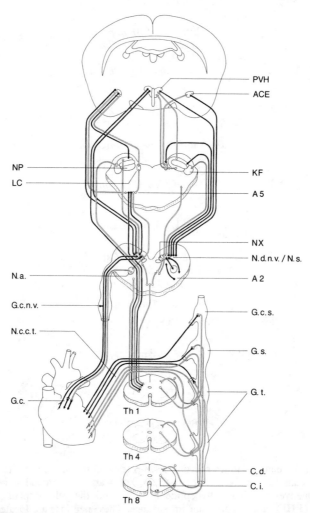

FIGURE 1. Schematic drawing of the neuronal elements involved in cardiac innervation. The relation of modulatory brain centers in the upper brainstem, that is, the diencephalon (PVH = periventricular hypothalamus, ACE = central amygdaloid complex) and the mesencephalon (NP = parabrachial nucleus, LC = locus ceruleus, KF = Koelliker-Fuse nucleus, A5 = A₅ region) to the primary medullary (NX, Ndnv, Ns = vagus-solitarius complex, Na = nucleus

MATERIALS AND METHODS

Immunohistochemistry

Tissue from perfusion-fixed laboratory animals was utilized. Fixation for light-microscopic immunohistochemistry was carried out following cannulation of the abdominal aorta and using a modified Bouin's fluid. The tissue was dehydrated, embedded in paraplast, and deparaffinized sections were incubated for VIP immunoreactivity (IR) and PHI-IR according to a modification of the PAP technique of Sternberger (see Forssmann *et al.*[11]). For electron microscopy, the fixation procedure was identical except for a formaldehyde-glutaraldehyde-picric-acid (FGP) fixative. Immunostaining was achieved by the protein-A-gold method after the embedding in LR-White.[12]

Electron Microscopy

For electron microscopy, conventional techniques were applied as described elsewhere.[13]

Cardiac Denervation

The experiments on cardiac denervation were performed on five dogs and eight rats. The dog hearts were denervated at the pericardial foldings, using the method of Donald *et al.*[14] Complete denervation was achieved according to physiological parameters.[14] Rat hearts were denervated using heterologous transplantation of hearts from donor animals into the abdominal cavity of receiver animals. The great cardiac blood vessels were connected to the abdominal aorta and the inferior vena cava. Only successfully transplanted hearts were investigated (i.e., those beating and with no macroscopic signs of infection or rejection). The dogs were perfusion-fixed after approximately three months. The rat hearts were analyzed one or two weeks after transplantation. For immunohistochemistry and electron microscopy, fixation was carried out retrogradely below the implant, beginning almost at the bifurcation of the aorta. The heart of the receiver animal was studied as a control.

---

amiguus, A_2 = lateral reticular formation) and spinal (Cd = dorsal column, Ci = intermediolateral substance) cardiac centers are depicted. The VIP-containing neuronal pathways are depicted as dense lines. The afferent and efferent connections between the heart and primary centers (Gcs = superior cervical ganglion, Gs = stellate ganglion, G = thoracic paravertebral ganglia, Gcnv = nodose ganglion of the vagus, Ncct = cervical and thoracic cardiac nerves, Gc = intracardiac ganglia) contain an important contribution of VIP neurons. Also the intracardiac intrinsic neurons exhibit a VIP-IR, but these constitute a minor portion of the intrinsic nerves. The exact percentage of VIPergic fibers and neurons involved in the cardiac innervation circuit is still unknown.

RESULTS AND DISCUSSION

Organization of Cardiac Innervation

The heart is supplied by four pathways of autonomic nerve fibers including vagal-efferent, sympathetic-efferent, vagal-afferent, and sympathetic-afferent. These pathways[15-27] are depicted with special emphasis on VIP perikarya and fibers in FIGURE 1 and TABLE 1: The vagal-efferent nerves contain perikarya within the nucleus dorsalis nervi vagi and the nucleus ambiguus of the medulla oblongata, and their neurites most likely join the vagus nerve in the intrinsic cardiac ganglia, where postganglionic fibers for the terminal effector nerves originate. The sympathetic perikarya for the efferent nerves are located in the columna intermedio-lateralis of the upper thoracic segments (Th1-Th8) of the medulla spinalis and course to the three upper thoracic ganglia of the sympathetic trunk. From there, the postganglionic neurons extend to the cardiac nerves, and the postganglionic neurites probably directly from the terminal efferent sympathetic innervation.

The afferent nerves from the heart run with the vagal as well as with sympathetic cardiac branches, ending in the medulla oblongata or in the medulla spinalis (FIG. 1).

TABLE 1. Distribution of VIP-IR in the Regions of the Nervous System Related to Cardiac Innervation[a]

Modulatory Brain Centers			Primary Centers			Periphery		
	perik	fib		perik	fib		perik	fib
PVH	+	++	NX	++++	+++	Gcnv	+++	+++
ACE	+++	+++	Ndvnv	++	+++	Gcs	+	+
NP	−	++	Ns	++	++	Gs	+	+
LC	−	+	A_2	−	+	Gt	+	+
KF	−	+	Na	+	+	Gc	++	+++
A_5	+	−	Cd	−	+++			
			Ci	−	+			

[a] Abbreviations: perik = perikarya; fib = fibers; all others as in FIGURE 1.

Immunohistochemistry of VIPergic Nerves in the Heart and the Coronary Vasculature

Immunohistochemically, VIP and PHI are localized in nerve fibers supplying different portions of the heart and the coronary vasculature (FIG. 2a, d, e, f). These fibers are also detected by ultrastructural immunocytochemistry using VIP antisera (see FIG. 4a). In general, the arterial branches of the coronary system contain a denser VIPergic innervation than the venous branches. There is a more pronounced vascular supply in the sinus- and atrioventricular nodes than in the surrounding myocardium.

Atrial Innervation

The atrial innervation exhibits a vascular and a nonvascular distribution of VIP-immunoreactive fibers that are mainly confined to the conductive system and to the endocrine heart (FIG. 2a). In the nonendocrine regions of the atria, few VIP-IR perikarya are observed along the myocardial cells and furthermore are closely apposed to the capillaries. These atrial fibers are similarly rare in both the right and left atrium.

Conductive System

A high density of VIP-IR fibers are observed in the sinus node (FIG. 2a) where a dense network of VIP fibers is seen closely apposed to the nodal cells. VIP innervation is observed adjacent to the AV node and the Purkinje-fiber system. However, it is less predominant than in the sinus node.

Endocrine Heart

The endocrine heart contains few VIP-IR fibers. Most of them are confined to the microvasculature of the endocrine heart, being located along the terminal arterioles (FIG. 2e).

Ventricular Myocardium

The ventricular myocardium rarely contains VIP-immunoreactive fibers. If present, these fibers course in the direction of capillaries (FIG. 2d, f). Most of the ventricular VIP innervation is seen surrounding the coronary vascular branches.

Large Vessels of the Heart

Moderate numbers of VIP-IR nerve fibers are located at the adventitia-media junction of the ascending aorta, the aortic arch, the pulmonary trunk, and the pulmonary veins. PHI-IR fibers occur infrequently. At the adventitia-media border of the caval veins, fibers showing VIP-IR and PHI-IR are found only sporadically. The peptidergic innervation of the superior caval vein appears to be more pronounced than that of the inferior caval vein. Small numbers of VIP-IR and PHI-IR fibers supply the vasa vasorum of the large vessels of the heart.

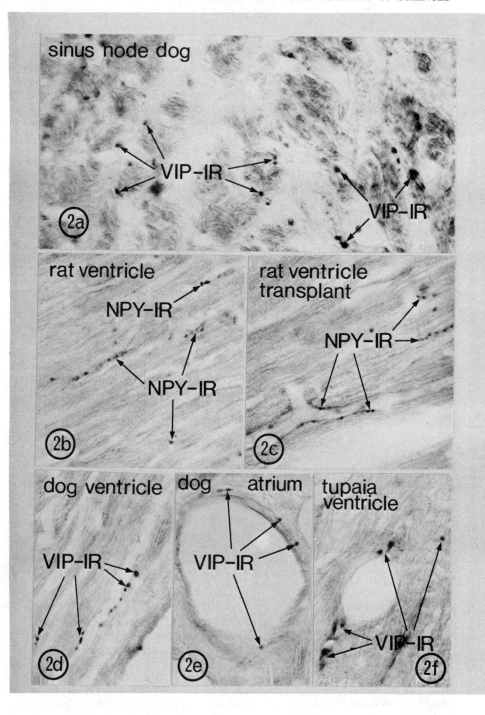

Main Branches of the Coronary Arteries

The extramural portions of the coronary arteries contain VIP- and PHI-ergic fibers in both the perivascular and the paravascular plexus. VIP-IR and PHI-IR fibers are present in the paravascular plexus in moderate numbers.

Intramural Arteries of the Atria and Ventricles

With respect to the intramural arterial portion of the coronary vasculature, VIP-IR and PHI-IR fibers are almost totally restricted to the atria.

Terminal Vasculature of Atria and Ventricles

The most evident neuropeptide innervating the small arteries and the arterioles of the atria is VIP (FIG. 2e, f). VIP-IR fibers occur within adjacent small atrial arteries and arterioles in a density exceeding that of VIP-IR nerves in the remaining segments of the coronary vasculature. Infrequently, VIP-IR fibers are in contact with the arterial segments of the terminal vasculature in the ventricles. The supply of small precapillary vessels with PHI-IR fibers is mainly restricted to the atria. VIP-IR and PHI-IR fibers are in obvious contact with capillaries. However, it is uncertain whether this contact is of functional importance, due to the fact that, in electron microscopy, VIP fibers seem to be polarized with their transmitter vesicles toward the adjacent myocardial cells. Both VIP and PHI supply the capillaries of the atria and the ventricles in similar densities. In the arterial portion of the terminal vasculature, VIP-IR fibers are also predominant in the postcapillary venules and veins.

Coronary Veins

VIP-IR nerve fibers occur only infrequently in the adventitia of the coronary veins.

◀ **FIGURE 2.** Immunohistochemical demonstration of VIP nerves in the heart. (**a**) The sinus node of the dog exhibits a rich VIP-IR innervation. Magnification × 800. (**b, c**) Ventricular nerves to the myocardial cells that contain NPY-IR in the rat are not affected by denervation when the heart is transplanted after 7 or 14 days; VIP nerves are reduced after denervation, however. Magnification × 500. (**c, d**) Two micrographs of a control dog heart showing myocardial VIP-IR nerves in the ventricle and atrial VIP-IR of nerves belonging to a small arteriolar blood vessel. Magnification × 600. (**f**) VIP-IR nerve fibers in a tupaia ventricle innervating the microvasculature and myocardial cells. Magnification × 600.

Intrinsic Ganglia

Within various diverse subepicardial regions, VIP-IR perikarya are regularly observed in all species investigated.[9] Additional VIP-IR perikarya are found within the tissue of the sinus node and infrequently in the interatrial septum. Furthermore, VIP-IR cell bodies occur adjacent to the entrance of the coronary sinus. At present, the existence of PHI-IR intracardiac ganglionic cells is still debated. According to our results on central and peripheral neurons, a coexistence is likely.[28,29]

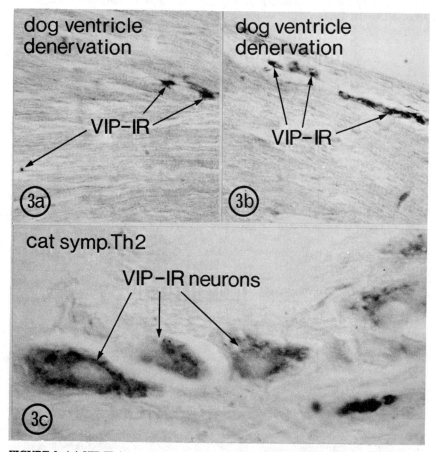

FIGURE 3. (a) VIP-IR innervation of canine ventricle after denervation. Note the VIP-IR in the perivascular plexus of a small arteriolar branch of the coronary vessels. Magnification ×600. (b) The dog ventricle also contains some VIP-IR nerves which are observed under the endocardium. Magnification × 600. (c) Cat sympathetic ganglion (Th2) exhibiting VIP-IR perikarya, which contribute to the extrinsic efferent cardiac innervation. Magnification × 640.

Effect of Heart Denervation on Cardiac Nerves and Subsequent Alteration of VIP-IR and PHI-IR

Further analysis of the intrinsic peptidergic system was carried out on mechanically denervated dog hearts and also on heterologously transplanted rat hearts. The dog hearts were denervated according to Donald *et al.*[14] Three months after denervation, electron microscopical studies revealed a moderately diminished number of nerve fibers in all regions of the heart. Most fibers, however, were in contact with the coronary vasculature. By means of immunohistochemistry, only VIP-IR (FIG. 3a, b) and NPY-IR (FIG. 2b, c) nerve fibers were unequivocally identified. In contrast to a significant decrease in VIP-IR, the myocardial innervation of NPY-IR nerves, analyzed for parallel controls, is not reduced after denervation (FIG. 2c). The remaining fibers represent projections of neurons located in the intracardiac ganglia exhibiting VIP-IR and NPY-IR. Ultrastructural immunohistochemistry reveals a characteristic population of dense-core-containing nerve endings or varicosities that react with VIP (FIG. 4a). This type of nerve fiber, however, is rarely encountered in hearts after denervation (FIGS. 4b, c and 5).

Extrinsic Cardiac Innervation by VIP

The origin of extrinsic preganglionic efferent VIP-IR fibers may be in the nucleus dorsalis nervi vagi, which, at least in the guinea-pig, is characterized by a high number of VIP-IR perikarya.[26,28] Since numerous VIP-IR perikarya occur in the cervical and thoracic paravertebral ganglia of different mammalian species,[18,19] sympathetic ganglia may constitute another source of efferent cardiac nerve fibers (FIG. 1). On the other hand, an afferent nature of VIP-IR fibers in the heart is conceivable since primary sensory neurons in the jugular and the nodose ganglion, as well as in the spinal ganglia, have been shown to contain VIP-IR.[16,17,21] Thus cardiac VIP-IR nerve fibers may originate from vagal or sympathetic efferents or may be of an afferent nature running within vagal or sympathetic nerves.

PHI and Extrinsic Cardiac Innervation

Immunohistochemical studies reveal that VIP- and PHI-IR may occur in identical neurons in several regions of the central nervous system as well as in the peripheral ganglia of various mammals, including man. The coexistence of these two neuropeptides was demonstrated for instance in perikarya of the nucleus dorsalis nervi vagi[28] and in those of the intestinal plexus.[28,29] Furthermore, striking similarities are obvious among the innervation patterns of VIP-IR and PHI-IR nerve fibers in the target cells of several organs[28] including the heart.[6,7] However, PHI-IR fibers are far less numerous than VIP-IR nerves. The coexistence of VIP-IR and PHI-IR in identical nerve fibers adjacent to coronary arteries in the atrium of the guinea pig has been illustrated.

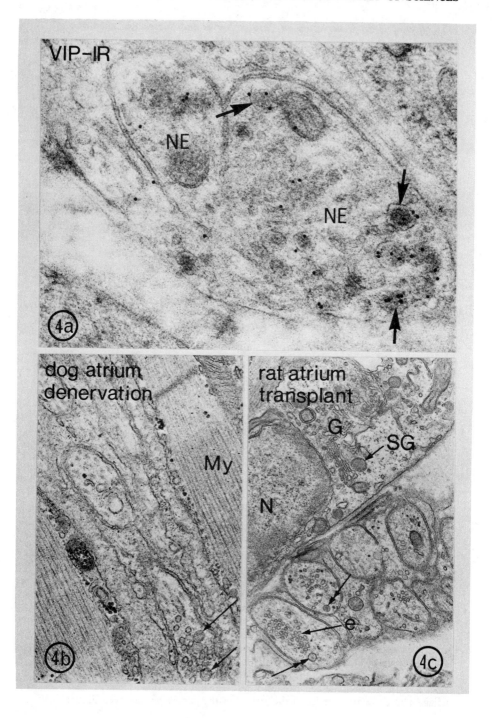

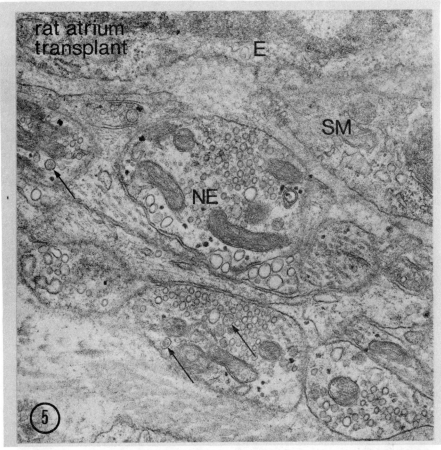

FIGURE 5. Perivascular nerves of a rat atrium seven days after transplantation. The persisting nerves exhibit a different ultrastructure than seen in VIPergic fibers (FIG. 4a). The dense-cored vesicles of the nerve endings (NE) are labeled (arrows). SM = smooth muscle cell; E = endothelium. Magnification × 35,000.

◀ **FIGURE 4.** (a) Electron microscopical demonstration of a VIP-IR nerve ending labeled by the immunogold method. Note the typical large dense-cored vesicles that are characterized by their size and by the membrane of the vesicle closely surrounding the core of the vesicle. Magnification × 60,000. (b) Dog atrial nerves after denervation still show the different vesicles in the varicosities, some of which look like those labeled in FIGURE 4a. Magnification × 30,000. (c) Rat endocrine heart (note the Golgi = G, secretory granules = SG, and nucleus = N of the myoendocrine cell) days after transplantation. The intrinsic nerves are still present and exhibit empty (= e) and dense-cored (double arrow) transmitter vesicles, few of which look like those labeled in FIGURE 4a. Magnification × 19,000.

Functional Implications of VIP and PHI in the Coronary Circulation

In the intact coronary circulation, the effects of VIP and PHI have been observed by several research groups. These investigations were carried out with isolated guinea-pig, rat, or rabbit hearts, and resulted in characteristic dose-dependent relaxation of coronary smooth muscle tone.[30-32] The effect of systemically applied VIP was studied in open-chest dogs.[32] These experiments revealed a vasodilatory action of VIP that was dose-dependent and remarkably preferential for the coronary vasculature when compared to the circulatory system as a whole. More recent studies using similar experimental models demonstrated that the coronary vasodilatory action of VIP is not endothelium-dependent (FIG. 6) and is probably due to a direct action of VIP on the smooth muscle membrane.[7,30,31] The effects of VIP on the coronary vasculature are thought to be mediated by interaction with receptors for VIP in the dog, monkey, and human hearts, and also with receptors for secretin in the rat heart.[33] Furthermore, the VIP, PHI, and secretin receptors are most likely coupled to a membrane adenylate cyclase.[34-36]

Isolated coronary arteries have been investigated by our research group,[7] and our results can be compared to those of Brum *et al.*,[31] who examined the effects of neuropeptides on isolated coronary arteries. VIP has been shown to relax ring preparations of the coronary circumflex artery after precontraction with prostaglandins.[31] We studied helical strips of isolated circumflex and anterior interventricular arteries of the pig precontracted with acetylcholine (FIG. 6). Application of increasing doses of VIP on the acetylcholine-pretreated coronary vessel smooth muscle resulted in a significant dilatation at a threshold of about $10^{-8}M$ VIP.

CONCLUSIONS

VIP plays an important role in the functional circuit involved in extrinsic cardiac innervation. Also intracardiac neurons may largely contribute to the intrinsic cardiac innervation although many other peptidergic nerves are found in the intracardiac plexus. The importance of VIP in central cardiovascular regulation is not yet fully understood because of the lack of studies in which VIP is applied to the specific cardiovascular modulatory or primary regulatory centers. However, immunohisto-chemical results suggest that VIP is strongly involved in cardiac functional circuits. In particular, the marked concentration of VIP in the vagal centers of the medulla oblongata and the presence of VIP in the branches of the vagal nerve and in the intracardiac plexus suggest that this peptidergic neurotransmitter plays an important role in the regulation of cardiac parameters.

One of the main cardiac functions of VIP is its marked influence on coronary circulation.[32] A dose-dependent relaxation of precontracted smooth muscle rings from porcine coronary arteries by both natural and synthetic VIP between 10^{-7} to 10^{-9} M has been documented. Our results confirm that this effect is not mediated by the endothelium. If VIP interacts with coronary artery smooth muscle independent of an intact endothelium, alterations of the intima in pathological processes would not alter the vasodilatory influence of this polypeptide. This is of great importance because an endothelial deficiency may result in an alteration of the coronary vascular tone in coronary diseases.

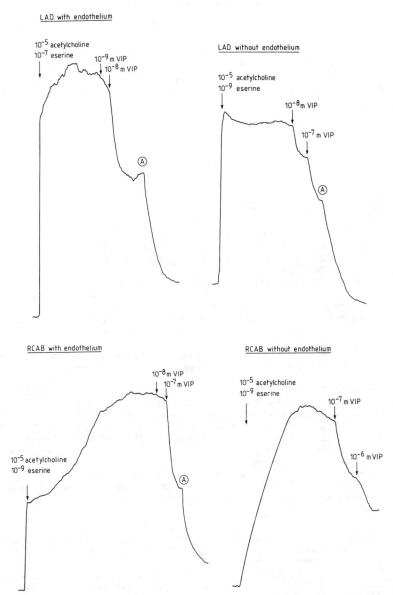

FIGURE 6. Effect of VIP on porcine coronary artery smooth muscle. The vasorelaxant effect of VIP is seen both in the left anterior descending branch (LAD) of the left coronary artery and the anterior segment of the right coronary artery (RCAB). Detachment of the endothelium does not abolish the vasorelaxant effect of VIP. The reduced responses in rings without endothelium may be due to the mechanical alteration when the endothelium is ripped off. A indicates change to organ bath solution without acetylcholine.

ACKNOWLEDGMENTS

The immunohistochemistry and electron microscopy was carried out by Ms. B. Brühl and Ms. B. Herbold to whom we are indebted. We also thank Ms. G. Sürig, Ms. R. Botz, Ms. J. Sis, and Dr. J. Greenberg for preparing the manuscript and for revising the English text. We are particularly grateful to Mr. R. Nonnenmacher who performed the graphic drawings.

REFERENCES

1. MUTT, V. & S. I. SAID. 1974. Structure of the porcine vasoactive intestinal octacosapeptide. Eur. J. Biochem. **42:** 581-589.
2. SAID, S. I. & V. MUTT. 1972. Isolation from porcine intestinal wall of a vasoactive octacosapeptide related to secretin and to glucagon. Eur. J. Biochem. **28:** 199-204.
3. TATEMOTO, K. & V. MUTT. 1981. Isolation and characterization of the intestinal peptide porcine PHI (PHI-27), a new member of the glucagon-secretin family. Proc. Natl. Acad. Sci. USA **78:** 6603-6607.
4. FORSSMANN, W. G., M. REINECKE & E. WEIHE. 1982. Cardiac innervation. *In* Systemic Role of Regulatory Peptides. S. R. Bloom, J. M. Polak, Eds: 329-349. Symposium. Oosterbeek, Netherlands. Schattauer Verlag. Stuttgart, Germany.
5. DELLA, N. G., R. E. PAPKA, J. B. FURNESS & M. COSTA. 1983. Vasoactive intestinal peptide-like immunoreactivity in nerves associated with the cardiovascular system of guinea-pigs. Neuroscience **9:** 605-619.
6. REINECKE, M. & W. G. FORSSMANN. 1984. Regulatory peptides (SP, NT, VIP, PHI, ENK) of autonomic nerves in the guinea pig heart. Clin. Exp.-Theor. Pract. **A6(**10&11**):** 1867-1871.
7. REINECKE, M. & W. G. FORSSMANN. 1987. Peptidergic innervation of the coronary vessels. *In* Progress in Peptides. G. Burnstock, Ed. In press.
8. WEIHE, E. & M. REINECKE. 1981. Peptidergic innervation of the mammalian sinus nodes: Vasoactive intestinal polypeptide, neurotensin, substance P. Neurosci. Lett. **26:** 283-288.
9. WEIHE, E., M. REINECKE & W. G. FORSSMANN. 1984. Distribution of vasoactive intestinal polypeptide-like immunoreactivity in the mammalian heart. Interrelation with neurotensin- and substance P-like immunoreactive nerves. Cell Tissue Res. **236:** 527-540.
10. CHRISTOPHE, J., M. WAELBROECK, P. CHATELAIN & P. ROBBERECHT. 1984. Heart receptors for VIP, PHI and secretin are able to activate adenylate cyclase and to mediate inotropic and chronotropic effects. Species variations and physiopathology. Peptides **5:** 341-353.
11. FORSSMANN, W. G., V. PICKEL, M. REINECKE, D. HOCK & J. METZ. 1981. Immunohistochemistry and immunocytochemistry of nervous tissue *In:* Techniques in Neuroanatomical Research. Ch. Heym & W. G. Forssmann, Eds.: 171-204. Springer. Berlin-Heidelberg-New York.
12. BENDAYAN, M. & M. ZOLLINGER. 1983. Ultrastructural localization of antigenic sites on osmium-fixed tissues applying the protein. A gold techniques method. J. Histochem. Cytochem. **31:** 101-109.
13. FORSSMANN, W. G. 1981. General methods in transmission electron microscopy of the nervous system. *In* Techniques in Neuroanatomical Research. Ch. Heym & W. G. Forssmann, Eds.: 21-39. Springer. Berlin-Heidelberg-New York.
14. DONALD, D. E. 1974. Myocardial performance after excision of the extrinsic cardiac nerves in the dog. Circ. Res. **34:** 417-424.
15. EIDEN, L. E., G. NILLAVER & M. PALKOVITS. 1982. Distribution of vasoactive intestinal polypeptide (VIP) in the rat brain stem nuclei. Brain Res. **231:** 472-477.

16. FUJI, K., E. SENBA, Y. UEDA & M. TOHYAMA. 1983. Vasoactive intestinal polypeptide (VIP)-containing neurons in the spinal cord of the rat and their projections. Neurosci. Lett. **37:** 51-55.

17. FUXE, K., T. HÖKFELT, S. I. SAID & V. MUTT. 1977. Vasoactive intestinal polypeptide and the nervous system: Immunohistochemical evidence for localization in central and peripheral neurons, particularly intracortical neurons of the cerebral cortex. Neurosci. Lett. **5:** 241-246.

18. HEYM, C., M. REINECKE, E. WEIHE & W. G. FORSSMANN. 1984. Dopamine-hydroxylase-, neurotensin-, substance-P, vasoactive intestinal polypeptide- and enkephalin-immunohistochemistry of paravertebral and prevertebral ganglia in the cat. Cell Tissue Res. **235:** 411-418.

19. HÖKFELT, T., L. G. ELFVIN, M. SCHULTZBERG, K. FUXE, S. I. SAID, V. MUTT & V. GOLDSTEIN. 1977. Immunohistochemical evidence of vasoactive intestinal polypeptide-containing neurones and nerve fibers in sympathetic ganglia. Neuroscience **2:** 885-896.

20. JEFTINIJA, S., K. MURASE, V. NEDELJKOV & M. RANDIC. 1982. Vasoactive intestinal and polypeptide excites mammalian dorsal horn neurons both *in vivo* and *in vitro*. Brain Res. **243:** 158-164.

21. KUO, D. C. *et al.* 1985. Vasoactive intestinal polypeptide identified in the thoracic dorsal root ganglia of the cat. Brain Res. **330:** 178-182.

22. LOREN, L., P. C. EMSON, J. FAHRENKRUG, A. BJÖRKLUND, J. ALUMETS, R. HAKANSON & F. SUNDLER. 1979. Distribution of vasoactive intestinal polypeptide in the rat and mouse brain. Neuroscience **4:** 1953-1976.

23. PALKOVITS, M., C. S. LERANTH, L. E. EIDEN, W. ROTSZTEJN & T. H. WILLIAMS. 1982. Intrinsic vasoactive intestinal polypeptide (VIP)-containing neurons in the baroreceptor nucleus of the solitary tract in rat. Brain Res. **244:** 351-355.

24. STOCK, G., M. SCHMELZ, M. M. KNUEPFER & W. G. FORSSMANN. 1984. Functional and anatomic aspects of central nervous cardiovascular regulation. *In* Current Topics in Neuroendocrinology 3. D. Ganten & D. Pfaff, Eds.: 1-30. Springer. Berlin-Heidelberg-New York.

25. ROBERTS, G. W., P. L. WOODHAMS, M. G. BRYANT, T. J. CROW, S. R. BLOOM & J. M. POLAK. 1980. VIP in the rat brain: Evidence for a major pathway linking the amygdala and hypothalamus via stria terminalis. Histochemistry **65:** 103-119.

26. TRIEPEL, J. 1982. Vasoactive intestinal polypeptide (VIP) in the medulla oblongata of the guinea pig. Neurosci. Lett. **29:** 73-78.

27. TRIEPEL, J. 1984. Immunhistochemische Untersuchungen zum Vorkommen von VIP- und PHI-IR Strukturen im zentralen und peripheren Nervensystem des Meerschweinchens. Habilitationsschrift. Fakultät für Naturwissenschaftliche Medizin. Universität Heidelberg. Heidelberg, FRG.

28. TRIEPEL, J., CH. HEYM & M. REINECKE. 1986. VIP- and PHI-immunoreactive neurons in the central nervous system. J. Autonom. Nerv. Syst. In press.

29. YANAIHARA, N., K. NOKIHARA, C. YANAIHARA, T. IWANAGA & T. FUJITA. 1983. Immunohistochemical demonstration of PHI and its co-existence with VIP in intestinal nerves of rat and pig. Arch. Histol. Jpn. **46:** 575-581.

30. BRUM, J. M., V. L. W. GO, P. M. VANHOUTTE & A. A. BOVE. 1985. Evidence for VIP-ergic control of coronary vasoregulation. Regul. Pept. Suppl. **3:** 37.

31. BRUM, J. M. *et al.* 1986. Action and localization of vasoactive intestinal peptide in the coronary circulation: Evidence for nonadrenergic, noncholinergic coronary regulation. J. Am. Coll. Cardiol. **7:** 406-413.

32. SMITHERMAN, T. C., H. SAKIO, A. M. GEUMEI, T. YOSHIDA, M. OYAMADA & S. I. SAID. 1982. Coronary vasodilator action of VIP. *In* Vasoactive Intestinal Peptide. S. I. Said, Ed.: 169-176. Raven Press. New York.

33. ROBBERECHT, P. & P. CHATELAIN. 1985. Effect of the peptides of the VIP family on the cardiovascular system. Regul. Pept. Suppl. **3:** 8.

34. LABURTHE, M., B. AMIRANOFF, N. BOIGE, C. ROUYER-FESSARD, K. TATEMOTO & L. MORODER. 1983. Interaction of GRF with VIP receptors and stimulation of adenylate cyclase in rat and human epithelial membranes. FEBS Lett. **159:** 89-92.

35. ROBBERECHT, P., L. GILLET, P. CHATELAIN, P. DE NEFF, J. C. CAMUS, M. VINCENT,

J. SASSARD & J. CHRISTOPHE. 1984. Specific decrease of secretin/VIP-stimulated adenylate cyclase in the heart from the Lyon strain of hypertensive rats. Peptides 5: 355-358.

36. TATON, G., P. CHATELAIN, M. DELHAYE, J. C. CAMUS, P. DE NEEF, M. WAELBROECK, K. TATEMOTO, P. ROBBERECHT & J. CHRISTOPHE. 1982. Vasoactive intestinal peptide (VIP) and peptide having N-terminal histidine and C-terminal isoleucine amide (PHI) stimulate adenylate cyclase activity in human heart membranes. Peptides 3: 897-900.

37. TRIEPEL, J., K. H. ELGER, I. KIEMLE, J. MADER, M. REINECKE, G. THIEKÖTTER, A. WEINDL & W. G. FORSSMANN. 1984. Neuropeptide in cardiovasculären Zentren. Verh. Anat. Ges. 78: 519-525.

38. TRIEPEL, J., J. METZ, D. MUNROE, S. LONDON, S. SWERIDUK & W. G. FORSSMANN. 1987. Vasoactive intestinal polypeptide immunoreactivity in the spinal cord of the guinea pig. Cell Tissue Res. In press.

Vasoactive Intestinal Peptide as a Coronary Vasodilator

THOMAS C. SMITHERMAN [a] AND
GREGORY J. DEHMER

*Veterans Administration Medical Center and
University of Texas Southwestern Medical Center
Dallas, Texas 75216*

SAMI I. SAID [b]

*University of Oklahoma Health Science Center and
Veterans Administration Medical Center
Oklahoma City, Oklahoma 73190*

INTRODUCTION

The source of the heart's energy is chiefly through oxidative pathways. Myocardial oxygen demand per unit weight exceeds those of all other organs and rapidly rises in response to stimuli that increase cardiac output. Oxygen delivery to the heart, in the basal state, is one of low flow and high extraction. Increased flow is the principal means of increasing oxygen delivery, and during physiologic stresses coronary flow may increase as much as fivefold. Regulation of the coronary circulation is complex and involves multiple factors, but the metabolic state of the myocardium is believed to be the major one. Local release of vasoactive substances and metabolites in response to hypoxia, leading to arteriolar dilation, probably plays the central role in coronary autoregulation.[1]

The large epicardial coronary vessels are conductance vessels, and in health usually contribute little to coronary vascular resistance. Angiographic observations indicate that these vessels are in a relaxed state at basal conditions. Intense vasoconstriction of normal epicardial coronary arteries may contribute substantially to coronary resistance. Lesser degrees of vasoconstriction of these vessels may contribute substantially to coronary resistance in the presence of atherosclerotic plaques. Inasmuch as there are several known endogenous constrictor agents that exert actions on these conductance vessels, it is reasonable to assume that there must also be means to provide stable vasodilator tone.[2]

[a] Address for correspondence: Thomas C. Smitherman, M.D., Cardiology Division (111A), VA Medical Center and University of Texas Southwestern Medical Center at Dallas, 4500 South Lancaster Road, Dallas, TX 75216.

[b] Current address: Department of Medicine, University of Illinois College of Medicine, P.O. Box 6998, Chicago, IL 60680.

The remarkable vasodilating properties of the vasoactive intestinal peptide (VIP) were responsible for its discovery, its name, and a bioassay for its presence. It has potent and diverse biological actions that include relaxation of smooth muscle at vascular and nonvascular sites. It is found in the central nervous system and in the peripheral nerves supplying many organs. Based on these findings, it has been postulated that a major physiological role for VIP is that of a local neurotransmitter, acting as a mediator of the nonadrenergic, noncholinergic inhibitory system, at least in some organs,[3] as one of several peptides in a peptidergic nervous system.[2-19]

These observations raise the possibility that VIP may be important in the regulation of coronary blood flow. In addressing this possibility, several questions are important:

1. Is VIP present in nerve terminals that innervate the coronary bed?
2. Is VIP a coronary vasodilator?
3. Is VIP released from coronary nerve terminals during physiological stimuli causing increased coronary flow?
4. Is coronary dilation with VIP mediated through other known coronary vasodilators such as prostacyclin or endothelium-derived relaxing factor?

INNERVATION OF THE CORONARY BED BY VIP-CONTAINING NERVE FIBERS

VIP-containing nerve fibers have been demonstrated microscopically in coronary arteries by immunochemical techniques in several mammalian species, although the innervation is not as dense as that found in arteries supplying the brain, gastrointestinal tract and the reproductive organs. Generally, the innervation appears to be greatest in the large coronary arteries, becoming less dense more distally in the coronary arterial vasculature. Nerve fibers immunoreactive to VIP were demonstrated in branches of coronary arteries, arterioles and to a lesser extent also at capillaries and venules in the hearts of monkeys, dogs, cats, and guinea pigs.[4] In a survey of nerve fibers immunoreactive to VIP in the cardiovascular system of guinea pigs, small coronary arteries were found to be sparsely (+) to moderately densely (+ +) supplied, but none were found associated with coronary veins.[6] In this grading scheme of 0 to + + + +, the densest supply of VIP-containing fibers—in the arteries to the gut, brain, and reproductive tract—was graded as + + +. An earlier report[7] on the absence of immunoreactive VIP in the coronary arteries of cats was probably falsely negative due to the technique of tissue-fixation that was used (personal communication, Dr. Frank Sundler).

Brum et al. measured by immunoassay the VIP content of extracts of canine aorta and segments from large epicardial coronary arteries.[2] VIP was present in all of the samples (TABLE 1). There were some differences in content from site to site. In segments of left anterior descending artery, but not of the circumflex arteries, there was a significant decrease in content more distally in the vessel. The importance of these site-to-site variations is not clear, but similar variations have been found with VIP in the cerebral circulation and with other neurotransmitter peptides in the coronary circulation. In these studies, the content of VIP was much higher in the epicardial vessels than in samples of ventricular myocardium, where the content was often below the sensitivity of the immunoassay.

The presence of VIP-containing nerve terminals in the heart is discussed in greater detail in this volume by Dr. Forssmann.

CORONARY VASODILATION IN RESPONSE TO VIP ADMINISTRATION

Intravenous VIP Administration

The intravenous infusion of VIP has consistently been found to cause coronary vasodilation. We infused VIP intravenously in dogs over a dose range of 0.25-5.0 μg/kg. This resulted in a sigmoidal-shaped dose-response increase in coronary blood flow, measured by electromagnetic flow probes, from 113% of the control value at the lowest dose to 268% of the control value at the highest dose.[8] There was a corresponding decline in coronary vascular resistance from 88% of the control value

TABLE 1. VIP Content of Aorta and Epicardial Coronary Artery Segments[a]

Tissue	VIP Content[b]
Aorta	5.46 ± 0.87
Right coronary artery	6.43 ± 1.22
Left anterior descending coronary artery	
Proximal	7.28 ± 1.65
Middle	3.74 ± 0.57
Distal	2.29 ± 0.53
Circumflex coronary artery	
Proximal	4.16 ± 1.52
Middle	4.58 ± 1.13
Distal	4.00 ± 0.81

[a] Data from Brum *et al.*[2]
[b] Results expressed in ng VIP/g tissue, mean ± SEM.

at the lowest dose to 34% of the control value at the highest dose (FIG. 1). Blintz and Charbon, in similar experiments, infused 1 to 1024 ng/kg intravenously in dogs and reported a 200% increase in coronary artery conductance.[9] Using radioactive microspheres, Unverferth and his associates demonstrated that a 10-minute intravenous infusion of 0.02 μg/kg/min and 0.05 μg/kg/min enhanced blood flow incrementally to both atria and both ventricles. The magnitude of the increased flow to left ventricular epicardium was slightly greater than that to the endocardium.[10] We reported that the intravenous infusion of VIP in men at two doses sufficient to raise mean plasma VIP levels from 45 pg/ml to 91 pg/ml and 180 pg/ml caused a 18% and a 32% increase, respectively, in coronary sinus blood flow and a 18% and a 33% decrease, respectively, in coronary vascular resistance.[11]

The coronary vasodilating effect of intravenous administration of VIP has always proved to be a prominent effect compared to changes in total flow and the flow to other organs. In our experiments with dogs, the increase in coronary blood flow was more than twice the increase in cardiac output (less coronary blood flow) as measured by an electromagnetic flow probe on the ascending aorta (TABLE 2).[8] In a similar work by Blintz and Charbon, the magnitude of the increase in coronary blood flow was exceeded only by that in the gastric and gastroduodenal arteries; it equaled that of the superior pancreatoduodenal artery and exceeded that of the common hepatic and vertebral arteries and total peripheral blood flow. They found no increase in flow in the inferior mesenteric, femoral, nor the renal arteries (TABLE 3).[9] Using radioactive microspheres, Unverferth *et al.*, in a survey of many organs, demonstrated significantly

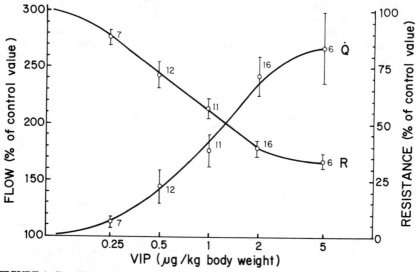

FIGURE 1. Dose(log)-response curve for the effects of VIP, 0.25–5 μg/kg of body weight, on coronary blood flow (Q) and resistance (R). The data are expressed as percent of the respective control values, which were obtained immediately before the given VIP infusion. The bars represent ± 1 SEM. The numbers beside each point represent the number of dogs studied at that dose.

increased flow only to the four cardiac chambers, esophagus, and pancreas (TABLE 4). These investigators also compared changes in coronary blood flow, cardiac output, and coronary and systemic vascular resistances in dogs given 0.1 μg/kg/min for 15 minutes. The changes in the coronary bed were somewhat greater in the coronary vasculature than in the systemic vasculature as a whole (TABLE 5).[10] In our experiments on the coronary vasodilator effects of the intravenous infusion of low to intermediate doses in men, we found that the coronary vasodilator effects were at least as potent as the effects on the total systemic vasculature and the pulmonary vasculature.[11] The mean value for the greatest decline in vasculature resistance observed in each patient, regardless of the infusion at which it occurred, was 33% in the coronary bed, 31% in the systemic bed, and 20% in the pulmonary bed.

TABLE 2. Coronary Blood Flow Versus Cardiac Output with VIP Infusion[a]

Dog#	Cardiac Output E/C (%)[b]	Coronary Blood Flow E/C (%)
A	113	320
B	115	255
C	144	196
D	120	327
E	175	338
Mean ± SEM	133 ± 12	287 ± 27

[a] Infusion concentration 2 μg/kg i.v.
[b] E/C = experimental/control.

TABLE 3. VIP Infusion and Blood Flow[a]

Artery	Change in Conductance (%)
Coronary (anterior descending)	+200
Gastric	+550
Sup. pancreatoduodenal	+200
Gastroduodenal	+220
Common hepatic	+60
Inferior	—[b]
Renal	—[b]
Femoral	—[b]
Vertebral	+100
Total peripheral	+45

[a] VIP, 1 to 1,024 ng/kg i.v., following a log scale at intervals of one minute (electromagnetic flow probes). Data from Blitz & Charbon.[9]
[b] No increase in flow.

TABLE 4. VIP Infusion and Blood Flow in Normal Dogs[a]

Increased Flow	No Change		Decreased Flow
All Cardiac Chambers	Stomach	Liver	Mid-brain
Esophagus	Duodenum	Spleen	Cerebellum
Pancreas	Jejenum	Cerebrum	
	Ileum	Eye	
	Colon		

[a] VIP, 0.02 and 0.05 μg/kg/min for 10 minutes each in six normal dogs (radioactive microspheres). Data from Unverferth *et al.*[10]

TABLE 5. VIP and Coronary Blood Flow[a]

	Control	VIP
CI (l/min/m²)	3.1 ± 0.5	4.8 ± 1.3[b]
CSBF (ml/min)	90 ± 25	159 ± 54[b]
CSBF/CO × 100	4.8 ± 1.8	5.6 ± 2.6
CVR (dyne-sec-cm⁻⁵/10³)	71 ± 16	36 ± 9[b]
SVR (dyne-sec-cm⁻⁵/10³)	3.4 ± 1.8	1.9 ± 1.0[b]

[a] Infusion (i.v.) 0.1 μg/kg/min × 15 minutes in six dogs. Mean ± SD. CI = cardiac index; CSBF = coronary sinus blood flow; CVR = coronary vascular resistance; SVR = systemic vascular resistance. Data from Unferth et al.[10]

[b] Statistically significant.

Direct Versus Indirect Coronary Vasodilator Effects of VIP

Interpretation of the coronary vasodilator effects of the intravenous infusion of VIP, however, is confounded by the influences on myocardial oxygen demand brought on by the hemodynamic effects of the administration of the peptide. All of the major determinants of myocardial oxygen demand, heart rate, myocardial wall tension development, and the contractile state of the heart, may be influenced by intravenous VIP. Heart rate increases, chiefly as a reflex response to vasodilation and the resulting decrease in blood pressure. The decrease in blood pressure reduces cardiac afterload and myocardial wall stress. VIP appears to have a weak positive inotropic effect.[10,20-21] In dogs[10] and man[11] intravenous VIP administration results in a small increase in myocardial oxygen consumption. In the work of Unferth et al.,[10] however, the percent of oxygen extracted from the canine coronaries decreased, suggesting that coronary flow increased out of proportion to the increase in oxygen demand (TABLE 6). Further confirmatory evidence for a direct effect was presented in the same work. These investigators measured tension developed by canine coronary artery strips over a range of potassium and VIP concentrations and demonstrated a relaxing effect of VIP, especially at the higher VIP and potassium concentrations.

The study of Brum et al.[2] provides further confirmation of a direct action of VIP on the canine coronary circulation. In this study 0.005, 0.05, and 0.1 μg/min of VIP were infused for 10 minutes directly into the left anterior descending coronary arteries

TABLE 6. VIP and Myocardial Energetics[a]

	Control	VIP
(A-Cs) O₂ (ml/l)	157 ± 19	132 ± 42[b]
MVO₂ (ml/min)	14.1 ± 3.9	19.8 ± 5.4[b]
Myo %O₂ Ext	86 ± 9	71 ± 22[b]

[a] Infusion (i.v.) 0.1 μg/kg/min × 15 minutes in six dogs. Mean ± SD. A-CS = aortic–coronary sinus; MVO₂ = myocardial oxygen consumption; MYO %O₂ Ext = % of available oxygen extracted by the myocardium. Data from Unferth et al.[10]

[b] Statistically significant.

of dogs. These low doses were chosen in order to chiefly assess changes in the caliber of large epicardial vessels in the absence of major peripheral vascular changes and in the absence of major increases in coronary blood flow. All segments of the artery, proximal, middle, and distal, showed significant cross-sectional increases during VIP infusions at the medium or higher dose level, ranging from 15.4-27.7% (equating to an increase in diameter of about 7-13%). The lowest and intermediate of the three doses of VIP did not change left coronary artery flow, measured by radioactive xenon washout. The highest of the three doses raised coronary flow, but only by 16%. There were no significant changes in heart rate or blood pressure at any of the VIP infusion doses. It is not possible to directly compare the magnitude of the exposure of the arterioles to VIP in this study and in our study of intravenous VIP infusion. Nevertheless, assuming that left anterior coronary artery flow was 2% of the cardiac output in these dogs, it is likely that the dose at the coronary arterioles was similar to that in our study with a single intravenous infusion of 0.25 μg/kg, the lowest dose. At that dose, we found a 13% increase in coronary flow. Therefore, these data of Brum *et al.* suggest that the vasodilator effects of infused VIP are more potent on the conductance (large epicardial) vessels than on the resistance vessels (arterioles). This effect is not a trivial one. It has been observed in humans undergoing coronary arteriography that drugs that have a marked coronary vasodilation effect, such as organic nitrates, increase the diameter of large epicardial vessels. The maximum increase in diameter is only about 25-50% (or an increase in cross-sectional area of about 50-125%).

RELEASE OF VIP DURING PHYSIOLOGIC STIMULI CAUSING INCREASED CORONARY FLOW

Release of VIP from coronary nerve endings during physiologic stimuli that cause increased blood flow has not yet been demonstrated. We measured the appearance of VIP in the coronary sinus during increased coronary blood flow induced by hypoxia.[8] We ventilated anesthetized, open-chest dogs with 100% oxygen, room air, and 8% oxygen. During 8% oxygen ventilation, coronary blood flow was 228% of that during room air ventilation. Neither VIP concentration in the coronary sinus, the gradient of VIP across the heart, nor total VIP release were significantly changed during the hypoxia-induced coronary vasodilation. Measurement of plasma values, however, may not be sensitive enough to detect release of VIP from nerve endings.

IS CORONARY DILATION WITH VIP MEDIATED THROUGH OTHER KNOWN CORONARY VASODILATORS?

For the most part, the vasodilator effects of VIP are not mediated by prostaglandins.[2] The vasodilator effect of VIP on pial arteries in cats, however, was shown to be dependent on prostacyclin.[22] This does not appear to be the case for coronary arteries. In men, we found that the coronary sinus concentration of the prostacyclin metabolite, 6-keto-prostaglandin $F_{1\alpha}$, was not elevated during coronary vasodilation induced by intravenous VIP. Furthermore, the vasodilator response to intravenous

VIP was not significantly reduced by the concurrent administration of cyclooxygenase inhibitors.[11]

The requirement for intact endothelium for the vasodilator effects of VIP depends upon the vascular site studied. VIP-induced relaxation of rat thoracic aorta is largely dependent upon the presence of intact endothelium, but the vasodilator effects of VIP at most other sites is independent of the presence of intact endothelium.[23] Brum *et al.* reported that the vasodilator action of VIP on canine coronary arteries was independent of intact endothelium.[12]

The relationship of the coronary vasodilator effects of VIP to serotonin is unclear. In mesenteric vessels, VIP was shown to be released by vessels exposed to serotonin.[24] In epicardial coronary vessels, the constrictor effect of serotonin was not blocked by VIP, neither was the vasodilator effect of serotonin on the resistance vessel enhanced by VIP.[2]

DOES VIP PLAY A ROLE IN REGULATION OF THE CORONARY CIRCULATION?

The results reviewed above can be briefly summarized as follows:

1. There is innervation of the coronary arteries by nerve terminals that contain VIP. These nerve terminals appear to be more densely located on the large epicardial vessels than on the arterioles and are absent on coronary veins.

2. VIP is a potent coronary vasodilator. The vasodilator effects are mediated both directly, by a relaxing effect on coronary conductance and resistance vessels, and indirectly, by an increase in myocardial oxygen demand. The effect on the conductance vessels may be more potent than the effect on the resistance vessels. Further work is needed to quantify the relative magnitudes of the direct and indirect effects and to determine the relative magnitudes of the direct effects on resistance and conductance vessels.

3. Release of VIP from coronary nerve endings during physiological stimuli that increase blood flow to the heart has not yet been demonstrated.

4. The coronary vasodilator effects of VIP do not appear to be mediated by prostaglandins, nor do they appear to be dependent on intact endothelium.

The currently available data are consistent with a possible role for VIP in regulation of coronary blood flow, both through changes in coronary vascular resistance and in maintenance of a relaxed state in the large epicardial arteries. Further work will be necessary to prove such a role.

The observations that innervation by VIP-containing nerve terminals is probably denser on the conductance than on the resistance vessels and that exogenously administered VIP may have a more potent effect on the conductance vessels than on the resistance vessels give rise to speculation about a role for VIP in maintaining the epicardial vessels in a relaxed state in health and disease. Because factors are present in the basal state that promote large coronary artery constriction, there are likely to be factors present to oppose these influences.[2] The remarkable but rare syndrome of intense epicardial coronary arterial spasm, variant or Prinzmetal's angina pectoris, is illustrative of the potential catastrophic consequences of the loss of normal vasodepressor tone, or excessive vasoconstrictor tone, that is insufficiently counterbalanced by vasodepressor tone. Less severe epicardial arterial constriction, near coronary atherosclerotic plaques, is a fairly common event and is important in the transient limitations in coronary blood flow that are thought to generally underlie the development of acute myocardial ischemia.[25] Whether VIP has any role in the regulation of coronary blood flow in such circumstances will need to be determined.

REFERENCES

1. ABBOUD, F. M., P. G. SCHMID, D. D. HEISTAD & A. L. MARK. 1976. Regulation of peripheral and coronary circulation. In Clinical Cardiovascular Physiology. H. J. Levine, Ed.: 143-205. Grune & Stratton. New York.
2. BRUM, J. M., A. A. BOVE, Q. SUFAN, W. REILLY & V. L. W. GO. 1986. Action and localization of vasoactive intestinal peptide in the coronary circulation: Evidence for nonadrenergic, noncholinergic coronary regulation. J. Am. Coll. Cardiol. 7: 406-413.
3. SAID, S. I. 1982. Vasodilator action of VIP: Introduction and general consideration. In Vasoactive Intestinal Peptide. S. I. Said, Ed.: 145-148. Raven Press. New York.
4. WEIHE, E. & M. REINECKE. 1981. Peptidergic innervation of the mammalian sinus nodes: Vasoactive intestinal polypeptide, neurotensin, substance P. Neurosci. Lett. 26: 283-288.
5. ROSSELIN, G., M. MALETTI, J. BESSON & W. ROSTENE. 1982. A new neuroregulator: The vasoactive intestinal peptide or VIP. Cell Endocrinol. 27: 243-262.
6. DELLA, N. G., R. E. PAPKA, J. B. FURNESS & M. COSTA. 1983. Vasoactive intestinal peptide-like immunoreactivity in nerves associated with the cardiovascular system of guinea-pigs. Neuroscience 9: 605-619.
7. UDDMAN, R., J. ALUMENTS, L. EDVINSSON, R. HAKANSON & F. SUNDLER. 1981. VIP nerve fibers around peripheral blood vessels. Acta. Physiol. Scand. 112: 65-70.
8. SMITHERMAN, T. C., H. SAKIO, A. M. GEUMEI, T. YOSHIDA, M. OYAMADA & S. I. SAID. 1982. Coronary vasodilator action of VIP. In Vasoactive Intestinal Peptide. S. I. Said, Ed.: 169-176. Raven Press. New York.
9. BLITZ, W. & G. A. CHARBON. 1983. Regional vascular influences of vasoactive intestinal polypeptide. Scand. J. Gastroenterol. 18: 755-763.
10. UNVERFERTH, D. V., T. M. O'DORISIO, W. W. MUIR III, J. WHITE, M. M. MILLER, R. L. HAMLIN & R. D. MAGORIEN. 1985. Effect of vasoactive intestinal polypeptide on the canine cardiovascular system. J. Lab. Clin. Med. 106: 542-550.
11. SMITHERMAN, T. C., S. I. SAID, G. J. KREJS & G. J. DEHMER. 1986. Coronary vasodilator action of vasoactive intestinal peptide in man. J. Am. Coll. Cardiol. 34: 212A.
12. BRUM, J. M., A. A. BOVE & P. VANHOUTTE. 1985. Participation of the endothelium in the vasodilator effects of vasoactive intestinal peptide and substance P in the coronary arteries. Circulation (Suppl. III, abstr.) III: 83.
13. BUCSICS, A., P. HOLZER & F. LEMBECK. 1983. The substance P content of peripheral tissues in several mammals. Peptides 4: 451-455.
14. HOKFELT, T., O. JOHANSSON, A. LJONGDAHL, J. M. LUNDBERG & M. SCHULTZBERG. 1980. Peptide neurons. Nature 184: 515-521.
15. POLAK, J. M. & S. R. BLOOM. 1983. Regulatory peptides: Key factors in the control of bodily functions. Br. Med. J. 283: 1451-1466.
16. SAID, S. I. 1983. Vasoactive peptides: State of the art review. Hypertension. 5(Suppl I): 17-26.
17. DUENWA, J. B., R. E. PAPKA, N. G. DELLA, M. COSTA & R. I. ESKAY. 1982. Substance P-like immunoreactivity in nerves associated with the vascular system of guinea-pigs. Neuroscience 7: 447-449.
18. FURNESS, J. B., M. COSTA, R. E. PAPKA, N. G. DELLA & R. MURPHY. 1984. Neuropeptides contained in peripheral cardiovascular nerves. Clin. Exp. Hyper. Theory Prac. A6: 91-106.
19. SAID, S. I. 1984. Vasoactive intestinal polypeptide (VIP): Current status. Peptides 5: 143-150.
20. KREJS, G. J., L. L. FRASE, F. A. GAFFNEY & C. G. BLOOMQVIST. 1983. VIP infusion and cardiovascular function in man. The Physiologist (abstr.) 26: A-81.

21. SAID, S. I., C. P. BOSCHER, J. A. SPATH & H. A. KONTOS. 1972. Positive inotropic action of newly isolated vasoactive intestinal peptide (VIP). Clin. Res. (Abstr.) **20:** 29.
22. WEI, E. P., H. A. KONTOS & S. I. SAID. 1980. Mechanisms of action of vasoactive intestinal polypeptide on cerebral arteries. Am. J. Physiol. **8:** H765-H768.
23. SATA, T., H. P. MISRA, E. KUBOTA & S. I. SAID. Vasoactive intestinal polypeptide relaxes pulmonary artery by an endothelium-independent mechanism. Peptides **7:** 225-227.
24. EKLUND, S., J. FAHRENKRUG & M. JODAL. 1980. Vasoactive intestinal polypeptide, 5-hydroxytryptamine and reflex hyperaemia in the small intestine of the cat. J. Physiol. **302:** 549-557.
25. SMITHERMAN, T. C. 1986. Unstable angina pectoris: The first half-century: Natural history, pathophysiology, and treatment. Am. J. Med. Sci. **292:** 395-406.

Neuroendocrine Significance of Vasoactive Intestinal Polypeptide[a]

SEYMOUR REICHLIN

Endocrine Division
New England Medical Center
and
Department of Medicine
Tufts University School of Medicine
Boston, Massachusetts 02111

Although VIP was isolated as early as 1970, the realization that it might play a role in neuroendocrine regulation has been relatively slow in coming, and even now there is not a complete understanding of its function. VIP (and its cosecreted peptide PHI (in hog and rat) and PHM (in man) appears to be important in the regulation of several pituitary functions through the tuberoinfundibular system and by exerting effects on somatostatin secretion by hypothalamus. This peptide may be important in the regulation of thyroid and ovarian function through a secretomotor mechanism. Comprehensive reviews by Besson *et al.*,[1] Nicosia *et al.*,[2] and Rostene[3] summarize this field up to 1984.

PITUITARY REGULATION

The most important function of VIP in anterior pituitary regulation appears to be as a prolactin-releasing factor. This section will review some recent work on the role of hypothalamic prolactin-releasing factors in normal PRL secretion, and will also present data on the intrinsic pituitary VIP-PRL regulatory system.

Under physiological circumstances prolactin (PRL) release occurs spontaneously during the early part of sleep, after suckling, and after certain kinds of stress.[4-7] The earliest hypothesis to be considered to explain stress-induced PRL release was that the secretion of a normally acting prolactin inhibitory factor responsible for the normal tonic-suppressive influence of the hypothalamus was disinhibited. The principal prolactin inhibitory factor is dopamine, a secretion of the arcuate-tuberoinfundibular complex,[4,5,7-10] but GABA,[11] and still other peptide PIFs have been described.[12,13]

An alternative view is that stress-induced PRL release is triggered by the release of a prolactin-releasing factor. One point in favor of this view is the finding that in rats in whom dopamine receptors have been blocked or all catecholamines depleted, the elevated PRL levels are raised even further by stress (FIG. 1).[14,15] Crude extracts of hypothalamic tissue stimulate PRL release (FIG. 2).[16] Based on bioassays of known

[a] Studies reported here were supported by United States Public Health Service Grant A16684.

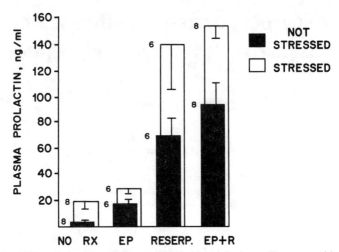

FIGURE 1. Effect of ether stress on serum PRL in reserpinized rats. Treatment with reserpine-depleted hypothalamic catecholamines, leading to disinhibition of the PIF effects of dopamine. Despite this depletion, stress still brought about an increase in PRL, indicating that the effect was not due to inhibition of dopamine or other catecholamine secretion. (From Valverde et al.[14] with permission.)

hypothalamic factors, there are several candidate PRFs. These include TRH,[17,18] VIP,[1-3,19,20] PHI,[21,22] oxytocin,[23] and less well-characterized factors in the neurohypophysis.[24]

The tuberoinfundibular TRH-, PHI-, and VIP-containing fibers arise in distinct populations of parvocellular neurons located in subdivisions of the paraventricular nucleus.[25,26] We have demonstrated that destruction of the paraventricular nucleus by electrolytic lesions blocks PRL release in response to 5-OH-tryptophan, ether, and restraint stress (FIGS. 3, 4, 5).[25,26] Because these lesions had no effect on GH secretion (known to be under control of the arcuate nucleus which is also the nucleus of origin of the tuberoinfundibular dopaminergic tract), we concluded that acute responses cannot be due to disinhibition of tonic dopamine secretion.

As first pointed out by Hokfelt and colleagues, the paraventricular nucleus is the site of origin of many of the neurons that subserve the acute ACTH response to stress.[25] The paraventricular nucleus contains cells of origin of the CRH neuronal projection to the median eminence.[27,28] Destruction of this nucleus markedly reduces the ACTH and/or corticosterone response to a variety of stresses.[29-32] The paraventricular nucleus can be looked upon as the final common neurohumoral pathway through which stress acts on the anterior pituitary. It is innervated by a large number of fibers projecting from other parts of the brain, mediated by an extraordinary variety of neurotransmitters[30,31] (TABLE 1). It appears likely that activation of these neurons is mediated by serotoninergic afferents. Treatment of rats with serotonin blockers abolishes stress-induced PRL release in the rat,[8,15] and the serotonin precursor 5-hydroxytryptophan stimulates PRL release[15,25]; this precursor is ineffective in animals whose paraventricular nuclei have been destroyed (FIG. 4).[26]

There is some uncertainty as to which of the several candidate PRFs localized in this region is responsible for the effects of the lesions. PHI is more readily demonstrated in median eminence then is VIP and both VIP and PHI are present in hypophysial-portal vessels,[33-38] and its concentration changes after administration of 5-OH-tryptophan[33] and prostaglandin D2,[37] two treatments that stimulate PRL release.

Another way to evaluate the role of VIP in regulating PRL release is to administer antisera directed against this peptide. Anti-VIP antiserum abolishes[39] or reduces[40-42] serotonergic and several stress-induced PRL responses (FIG. 6) and markedly reduces the PRL response to suckling (FIGS. 7, 8). Centrally administered anti-VIP blocks the PRL response to intraventricular injection of CCK.[43]

Although it seems most attractive to attribute the stress-increased release of PRL to VIP (and PHI/PHM), there are several unsettled problems with this hypothesis. Most important is the fact that the median eminence of the normal rat contains very few immunoreactive VIP nerve endings[44] and little immunoreactive VIP, which is in contrast to the plentiful distribution in the median eminence of the established releasing factors such as TRH and GHRH. However, during pregnancy (in the rat) the paraventricular VIP system becomes much more prominent.[45] In at least one study anti-VIP was only marginally effective as was anti-PHI in inhibiting PRL responses to ether stress but combined administration of both antisera markedly, but not completely,

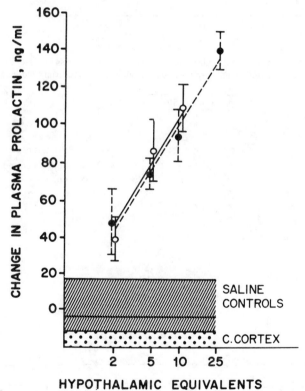

FIGURE 2. Effect of porcine hypothalamic extract on serum PRL in the rat. (From Valverde et al.[16] with permission.)

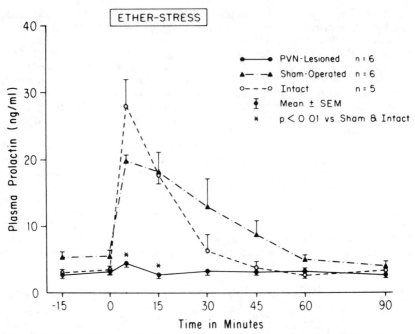

FIGURE 3. Effect of paraventricular nuclear lesions on ether stress-induced PRL release, indicating that this response is entirely mediated through the PV tuberoinfundibular system.

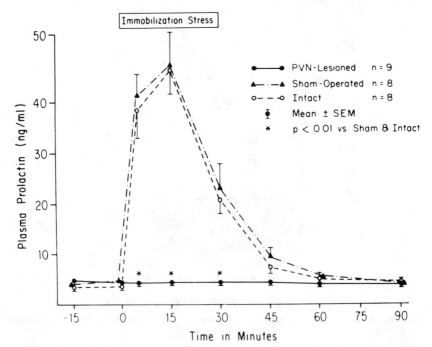

FIGURE 4. Effect of P-V lesions on restraint-induced PRL release. (From Minimitani *et al.*[25] with permission.)

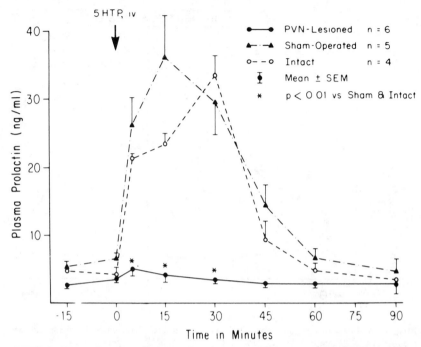

FIGURE 5. Effect of paraventricular nuclear lesions on PRL response to 5-OH-tryptophan, indicating the mediation of this pathway (From Minimitani et al.[25] with permission.)

reduced PRL response.[40] In the fowl, VIP and PHI are more plentiful in the median eminence and secretion of PRL is suppressed by anti-VIP.[46]

There is some evidence to support the view that a PRF distinct from VIP/PHI may be the mediator of suckling-induced PRL release. In our studies, doses of anti-VIP that completely blocked stress-induced responses merely delayed the onset of the PRL response to suckling but did not prevent the ultimate rise to the normal high levels, and hyperprolactinemia established during suckling was only partially reduced by anti-VIP.[39] The neural lobe may be the source of this regulator. Ben-Jonathan and her colleagues have shown that suckling-induced PRL release in the rat is completely abolished by neurolobectomy, that this procedure does not block stress-induced PRL

TABLE 1. Neuroactive Substances Identified in Paraventricular Nucleus[a]

Cell Bodies

oxytocin   vasopressin   somatostatin   dopamine   Met-enkephalin
Leu-enkephalin   neurotensin   dynorphin   substance P   glucagon
VIP   TRH   renin   CRH

Fibers

norepinephrine   epinephrine   serotonin   acetylcholine $ACTH_{1-39}$
β-endorphin α-MSH   GABA   LHRH   pancreatic polypeptide   bradykinin
prolactin   angiotensin II

[a] Modified from Swanson and Sawchenko.[31]

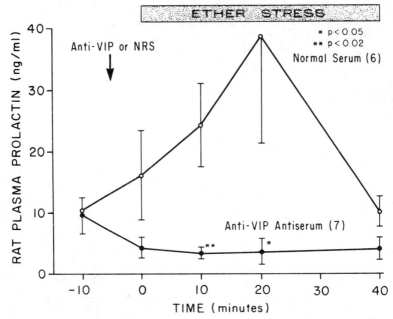

FIGURE 6. Effect of injection of anti-VIP antisera on stress-induced PRL release indicating the role of this system in PRL regulation. (From Abe et al.[39] with permission.)

release,[47] and that extracts of the neural lobe stimulate PRL release.[24] The means for extraction are such that they would not preserve oxytocin or VIP; preliminary data obtained by Dr. Karen Lam in our laboratory indicate that the extracts of Ben-Jonathan do not contain immunoreactive VIP (unpublished observations).

The role of VIP excess in bringing about hyperprolactinemia and prolactinoma should be considered. Indirect efforts to identify a role of VIP in causing hyperprolactinemia in man have been carried out by determining the pituitary response to VIP injections in normals and in patients with prolactinoma. In normals, several authors have convincingly shown that VIP stimulates acute release of PRL.[48–54] In contrast, almost all workers report that PRL responses to VIP in patients with prolactinomas are markedly reduced.[50–54] Unfortunately, no data exists to determine the effects of chronic infusion, or whether "down-regulation" occurs. When studied in vitro, adenomas show variable responsivity to injections of VIP (c.f. Conti et al.[50]). Conti and colleagues[50] have considered the possibility that the reduced response in hyperprolactinemic individuals is due to excess dopamine secretion (part of the negative feedback loop response). Indeed, dopamine agonists inhibit pituitary response to VIP.[50,52] However, administration of domperidone, a peripheral dopamine antagonist, to two such patients failed to reverse the blunted responses.[50]

An alternative (or complementary) hypothesis to explain the relationship between VIP and PRL secretion has been proposed by Hagen and colleagues.[55] Several workers had previously reported that extracts of the rat anterior pituitary contain VIP,[1,2,56] and Morel et al. stated that VIP was co-contained in lactotropes.[56] Hagen's group has shown that incubated pituitary fragments incorporate labeled amino acid into immunoprecipitable VIP, which can be released by K^+ depolarization,[57] and that exposure of dispersed pituitary cells in culture to anti-VIP antiserum reduces basal PRL release.[56] They propose that VIP may act as a paracrine regulator of PRL response. Denef previously had demonstrated that GnRH treatment of dispersed pituitary cells leads to the release of PRL, and that a gonadotropin-enriched preparation of pituitary cells contain this releasing activity.[58]

A relationship between pituitary VIP and prolactin secretion has also been proposed earlier by Maletti *et al.* who showed that estrogen treatment increased plasma PRL and pituitary VIP.[59] Adrenalectomy increases pituitary VIP content as well.[3]

Our group (Lam, Minimitani, Cacicedo, Lechan, Segerson, Stopa, and Reichlin, in preparation) have also been working on the pituitary VIP system and have made the following observations. Extracts of rat, human, and monkey pituitaries contain immunoreactive VIP and PHI/PHM. The immunoreactive VIP in rat pituitary has been found to behave identically to authentic VIP on exclusion chromatography (FIG. 9), and high-pressure liquid chromatography. In the normal rat, we have not been able to identify any cells containing VIP in the pituitary by immunohistochemical means, and only a few cells were identified in monkey and human glands. We found no nerve endings in the pituitary that stained positive for VIP.

Following the report of Morel *et al.*[56] that VIP is co-contained in lactotropes, we sought to determine whether the concentration of VIP and its secretion would vary in parallel with changes in PRL content and secretion under conditions of altered

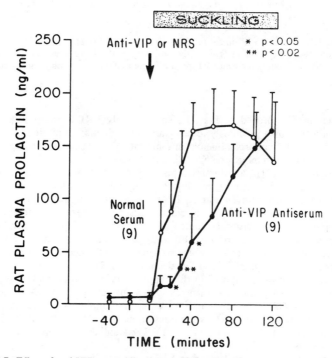

FIGURE 7. Effect of anti-VIP on suckling-induced PRL release. The onset is delayed, but final magnitude of response is achieved. These findings indicate that acute release of VIP plays a role in early release of PRL, but is not the entire mechanism of this response. (From Abe *et al.*[39] with permission.)

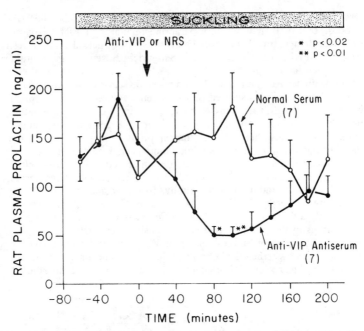

FIGURE 8. Effect of anti-VIP on serum PRL levels already elevated by suckling. Immuno-neutralization lowers the hormone level partly indicating that VIP is responsible at least in part for maintenance of suckling-induced PRL release. (From Abe *et al.*[39] with permission.)

PRL secretion. The procedure first chosen to modify PRL secretion was induced hypothyroidism, shown previously to bring about a reduction in pituitary PRL in the rat, associated with hypoprolactinemia in male rats[60,61] but either euprolactinemia or hyperprolactinemia in female rats.[62,63] Male and female rats weighing 50 g were treated with antithyroid drugs (propylthiouracil priming, followed by methimazole p.o.) and given replacement doses with T4, ranging from physiological to supraphysiological as judged by changes in serum T4 and TSH. At the time that animals were killed, after three weeks of treatment, the hypothyroid animals of both sexes were found to show a marked increase in the pituitary content of VIP, while supraphysiological doses of T4 suppressed pituitary levels of VIP (FIG. 10). In both sexes, pituitary PRL content was markedly decreased, but there was a striking sex difference in serum PRL levels, males showing low serum PRL, and females normal PRL levels (TABLE 2).

The high concentration of VIP in the hypothyroid pituitaries made it possible to identify the cells of origin of this hormone, to demonstrate VIP mRNA in these cells, and to carry out studies of regulation of secretion. Immunohistochemical examination revealed intense staining of secretory granules in many stellate cells distributed rather uniformly throughout the pituitary (FIG. 11). The staining was completely abolished by preabsorption with VIP.

These data clearly demonstrate that VIP is present in some pituitary cells, and that its concentration is regulated by thyroid hormone. Further, *in vitro* secretion studies indicate that dispersed cells from hypothyroid pituitaries release more VIP into the medium than do normal pituitary cells. Release is stimulated by TRH. This finding, taken together with the fact that thyrotropes are the only known pituitary cells that are stimulated by thyroid deficiency, suggests strongly that VIP is co-contained in thyrotropes but preliminary immunohistochemical study failed to show co-localization of TSH and VIP. To further document the autochthonous origin of VIP in these cells, we have utilized an antisense rat VIP mRNA "Riboprobe," to

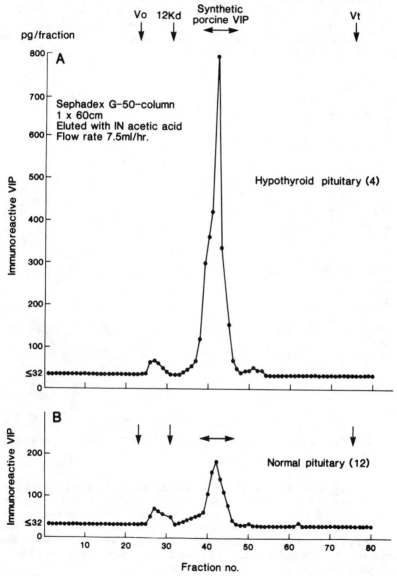

FIGURE 9. Extract of hypothyroid and euthyroid rat pituitary contains immunoreactive VIP with the chromatographic characteristics on Sephadex, G50 identical with porcine VIP. Note marked elevation in hypothyroidism. (From Lam *et al.*, in preparation.)

determine the presence of VIP mRNA in the pituitary. By liquid hybridization methods, VIP mRNA was shown to be present in the rat anterior pituitary; *in situ* hybridization (in collaboration with Drs. Hugh Wolfe and Edward Stopa) demonstrated the presence of many cells containing VIP mRNA. Further, the signal was much stronger in the pituitaries of hypothyroid animals than in the normal, and was reduced by hyperthyroidism. These studies unequivocally demonstrate that VIP arises within the pituitary, and that VIP gene expression is regulated by thyroxine. In this regard, it is worth noting that gene expression in thyrotropes, lactotropes, and somatotropes is also regulated by thyroid hormones, but only in thyrotropes has T4 deficiency been shown to be a stimulator of gene transcription.

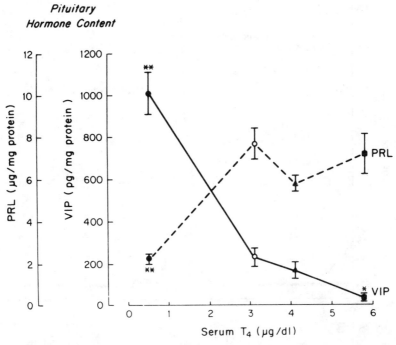

FIGURE 10. Reciprocal changes in pituitary PRL and VIP in hypothyroid pituitaries.

Several approaches have been taken to determine the role of endogenous VIP in PRL regulation. Following the suggestion of Hagen *et al.*,[55] we incubated dispersed pituitary cells and whole pituitary fragments, both from normal male rats in media to which anti-VIP antisera had been added. In contrast to the prior report of Hagen *et al.*, cells exposed to immune serum showed no decrease in basal PRL release compared to cells exposed to nonimmune serum, but we could demonstrate the effect in hypothyroid pituitaries.

We sought also to see some relevance of the endogenous VIP system to pathogenesis of human prolactinoma. In collaboration with Dr. Yogesh Dayal, six prolactinomas, eight chromophobe adenomas and one tumor immunopositive for TSH beta and LH

TABLE 2. Pituitary Concentrations of VIP and PRL, Hypothalamic Concentrations of VIP, and Serum Concentrations of PRL and TSH in Control and Hypothyroid Rats

Rat	(No.)	Pituitary VIP (pg/mg protein)	Hypothalamic VIP (pg/mg protein)	Pituitary PRL (μg/mg protein)	Serum PRL (ng/ml)	Serum TSH (ng/ml)
Male						
Control (12)		169.5 ± 20.3	597.4 ± 19.9	9.4 ± 1.0	28.9 ± 12.2	3.2 ± 0.5
Hypothyroid (12)		834.0 ± 82.2[a]	597.5 ± 27.8	2.3 ± 0.4[a]	7.4 ± 1.6[b]	31.8 ± 2.2[a]
Female						
Control (5)		103.1 ± 34.1	660.2 ± 62.3	18.6 ± 2.4	38.8 ± 14.3	2.3 ± 0.2
Hypothyroid (5)		771.6 ± 100.9[c]	561.0 ± 25.0	9.9 ± 0.8	41.4 ± 11.6	35.2 ± 2.4[a]

[a] $p < 0.0001$.
[b] $p < 0.01$.
[c] $p < 0.001$.

beta were examined using both anti-VIP and anti-PHI antisera. None of the tumors stained for these peptides. If the hypothyroidism-induced VIP secretion is important for regulation of human pituitary function, I would postulate that it is part of the mechanism by which hyperprolactinemia is brought about in hypothyroidism.

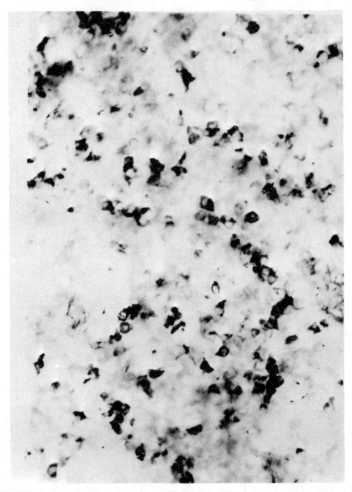

FIGURE 11. Immunohistochemical staining of IR-VIP in hypothyroid rat pituitary.

OTHER PITUITARY RESPONSES TO VIP

Central administration of VIP was shown by McCann's group to stimulate the secretion of GH and LH,[64] but subsequent studies suggested that this effect may be due to a central, rather than a direct, pituitary effect since in most studies VIP added directly to pituitary fragments did not release GH.[1,2,65]

VIP also stimulates the secretion of ACTH in both normal animals and in several cell lines.[1,2,65,66] In contrast to the situation in normals, patients with acromegaly release GH in response to VIP and their adenomas also release GH *in vitro* in response to addition of VIP.[52]

DIRECT SECRETOMOTOR EFFECTS OF VIP

Nerves innervating the rat ovary contain VIP and release this peptide upon stimulation.[67] The principal input is from the superior ovarian nerves. The functional significance of this innervation is suggested by the finding that VIP induces steroid secretion from prepubertal ovaries *in vitro*, induces aromatase activity in fetal ovaries, and induces the synthesis of the cholesterol side-chain cleavage enzyme complex in cultured ovarian granulosa cells.[68]

An analogous vasomotor control system has been postulated for the thyroid gland, because in both rat and mouse, nerve endings in the thyroid are immunoreactive for VIP and PHI.[69] However, although VIP stimulates regional blood flow, it has little or no effect on hormone secretion in rat and mouse.[70,71,72]

EFFECT OF VIP ON CORTICAL AND HYPOTHALAMIC SOMATOSTATIN SECRETION AND SYNTHESIS

VIP exerts stimulating effects on cerebral cortical metabolism[73,74] and appears in some systems to act as a neurotransmitter. Since VIPergic neurons are codistributed with somatostatinergic neurons, our group has studied the effects of VIP on somatostatin secretion. Somatostatin plays a significant role in the regulation of TSH and GH secretion. In previous studies using hypothalamic slices obtained from adult rats, VIP was reported by Epelbaum *et al.*[75] to inhibit somatostatin secretion, a finding that was compatible with the earlier report that intraventricular VIP stimulated GH release. However, Tapia-Arancibia and I found that VIP brought about an *increase* in somatostatin secretion from dispersed fetal cerebral cortical and hypothalamic cells,[76] as did Robbins and Landon.[77]

We initially attributed this effect to the stimulation by VIP of neuronal cAMP, since VIP has been shown to increase cortical cAMP, and indeed Tapia-Arancibia *et al.* have recently shown that cortical cells respond to VIP by an increase in cAMP.[78] However, an increase in neuronal cAMP cannot be the sole mechanism of this response since she and her colleagues found that forskolin, a post-receptor adenylate cyclase stimulator, does not stimulate the release of somatostatin in a pure neuronal culture but only does so in the presence of glia. On the other hand VIP is effective both in mixed cultures and in pure neuronal culture. The most attractive hypothesis to explain this finding is that another second messenger system is involved, perhaps the phosphatydyl inositol pathway that has been shown to be involved in the stimulation by VIP of the rat superior cervical ganglion.[79] The glial requirement suggests a mediator role for these cells.

In addition to stimulating the release of somatostatin from both cortical and diencephalic neurons in culture, VIP increases the concentration of mRNA coding for somatostatin (FIG. 12) a response that parallels exactly the dose response for secretion. In further studies of this phenomenon, Montminy et al. have shown that forskolin stimulation of somatostatin release from cortical cells is accompanied by an increase in somatostatin mRNA whereas K$^+$ depolarization does not stimulate mRNA formation.[80] These findings are interpreted to mean that VIP stimulates both secretion and synthesis by distinctly different mechanisms.

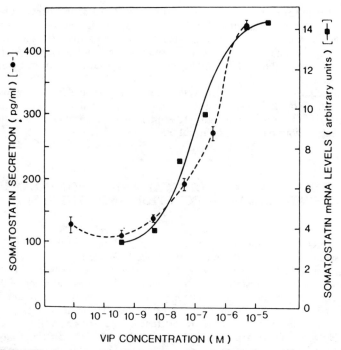

FIGURE 12. VIP releases somatostatin from incubated rat diencephalic cells in dispersed culture and in a parallel fashion stimulates the appearance of VIP mRNA.

Montminy et al. have extended these studies by transfecting the somatostatin gene into a fibroblast cell line and showing that somatostatin mRNA is increased in these cells by exposure to forskolin, and further they have identified a specific sequence in the gene that apparently is the responsive element.[80,81] Most recently, Montminy et al.[82] report the isolation of a soluble 42-kDa protein that binds to this sequence of the gene and is enhanced by exposure to forskolin. Presumably this is the intervening factor responsible for gene activation by factors such as VIP which stimulate the formation of cAMP.

SUMMARY

The new data reported here, and available in the literature, are interpreted to indicate that acute release of PRL in stress is probably mediated by secretion of VIP and PHI arising from a subpopulation of paraventricular cells in the tuberoinfundibular system, and that this secretion is under serotonergic control, presumably by way of the raphe nuclear projection to the hypothalamus. The acute PRL response to suckling response is only partially under VIP/PHI control, and may be regulated by an as yet unidentified neural lobe hormone. In addition to the hypothalamic component of PRL regulation, there is a well-defined population of VIP cells within the pituitary, representing the only known example of VIP expression outside of nerve cells. This population of VIP cells is exquisitely responsive to thyroid status, and in common with the thyrotrope cell, is activated by hypothyroidism. Since VIP secretion is enhanced in the hypothyroid pituitary, and VIP release is stimulated by TRH, it is reasonable to postulate that paracrine VIP secretion may play a role in the hyperprolactinemia that occurs in the hypothyroid human, although this is clearly not the case for the rat in whom hyperprolactinemia was not demonstrable. The role of VIP/PHI in human pituitary disease is unknown. We have been unable to identify any tumors that contain immunoreactive material using tissues prepared by standard methods. It may be that the demonstration of VIP/PHI is more demanding and will require better techniques for staining. The role of tuberoinfundibular VIP hypersecretion remains to be established but the evidence for stress-induced PRL hypersecretion in man encourages us to believe that at least some cases may be due to excessive hypothalamic activity. Additional potential neuroendocrine actions of VIP are in the secretomotor control of the ovary and thyroid, and in the regulation of somatostatin secretion and synthesis. In dispersed cell cultures (but not in whole hypothalamic slices from adult animals), VIP stimulates somatostatin secretion and independently stimulates the formation of somatostatin mRNA, an effect that can be duplicated in mixed cultures by treatment with forskolin, a postreceptor cAMP stimulator. In work carried out by Montminy and colleagues, the cAMP action has shown to be mediated by formation of a soluble protein that appears to activate the somatostatin gene promotor through interaction with a specific gene sequence.

REFERENCES

1. BESSON, J., W. Q. H. ROTSZDTEJN & D. BATAILLE. 1982. Involvement of VIP in neuroendocrine functions. *In* Vasoactive Intestinal Peptide. S. I. Said, Ed.: 253-262. Raven Press. New York.
2. NICOSIA, S., A. SPADA & G. GIANATTASIAW. 1982. Effects of vasoactive intestinal polypeptide on the pituitary gland. *In* Vasoactive Intestinal Peptide. S. I. Said, Ed.: 263-275. Raven Press. New York.
3. ROSTENE, W. H. Neurobiological and neuroendocrine functions of the vasoactive intestinal peptide (VIP). Prog. Neurobiol. **22:** 103-129.
4. MACLEOD, R. M. 1976. Regulation of prolactin secretion. *In* Frontiers in Neuroendocrinology. L. Martini & W. F. Ganong, Eds. **4:** 169-194. Raven Press. New York.
5. MARTIN, J. B. & S. REICHLIN. 1987. Clinical Neuroendocrinology. Second Edition.: 201-232. F. A. Davis. Philadelphia, Pa.
6. BOYD, A. E. & S. REICHLIN. 1978. Neural control of prolactin secretion in man. Psychoneuroendocrinology **3:** 113-130.

7. NEILL, J. D. 1980. Neuroendocrine regulation of prolactin secretion. *In* Frontiers in Neuroendocrinology. L. Martini & W. F. Ganong, Eds. **6:** 129-155. Raven Press. New York.

8. GANONG, W. F. 1984. Neurotransmitter mechanisms underlying stress responses. *In* Neuroendocrinology and Psychiatric Disorder. G. M. Brown, S. H. Koslow & S. Reichlin, Eds.: 133-144. Raven Press. New York.

9. GIBBS, D. M. & J. D. NEILL. 1978. Dopamine levels in hypophysial stalk blood in the rat are sufficient to inhibit prolactin secretion *in vivo*. Endocrinology **102:** 1895-1900.

10. DEMAREST, K. T., K. E. MOORE & G. D. RIEGLE. 1985. Acute restraint stress decreases tuberoinfundibular dopaminergic neuronal activity: Evidence for a different response in male versus female rats. Neuroendocrinology **41:** 504-510.

11. SCHALLY, A. V., T. W. REDDING, A. ARIMURA, A. DUPONT & G. L. LINTHICUM. 1977. Isolation of gamma-amino butyric acid from pig hypothalami and demonstration of its prolactin release-inhibiting (PIF) activity *in vivo* and *in vitro*. Endocrinology **100:** 681-691.

12. NICOLICS, K., A. J. MASON, E. SZONYI, J. RAMACHANDRAN & P. H. SEEBURG. 1985. A prolactin-inhibiting factor within the precursor for human gonadotropin-releasing hormone. Nature **316:** 511-517.

13. KHORRAM, O. & S. M. MCCANN. 1986. On the presence of a nondopaminergic, peptidergic prolactin release-inhibiting factor in hypothalamic extracts of infantile rats. Neuroendocrinology **44:** 65-69.

14. VALVERDE, R. C., V. CHIEFFO & S. REICHLIN. 1973. Failure of reserpine to block ether-induced release of prolactin: Physiological evidence that stress induced prolactin release is not caused by acute inhibition of PIF secretion. Life Sci. **12:** 327-335.

15. KRULICH, L. 1979. Central neurotransmitters and the secretion of prolactin, GH, LH, and TSH. Annu. Rev. Physiol. **41:** 603-615.

16. VALVERDE, C., V. CHIEFFO & S. REICHLIN. 1972. Prolactin releasing factor in porcine and rat hypothalamic tissue. Endocrinology **91:** 982-993.

17. SHEWARD, W. J., H. M. FRASER & G. FINK. 1985. Effects of immunoneutralization of thyrotrophin-releasing hormone on the release of thyrotrophin and prolactin during suckling or in response to electrical stimulation of the hypothalamus in the anaesthetized rat. J. Endocrinol. **106:** 113-119.

18. FINK, G., Y. KOCH & N. BENAROYA. 1983. TRH in hypophysial portal blood: Characteristics of release and relationship to thyrotropin and prolactin secretion. *In* Thyrotropin-Releasing Hormone. E. C. Griffiths & G. W. Bennett, Eds.: 127-143. Raven Press. New York.

19. FRAWLEY, L. S. & J. D. NEILL. 1981. Stimulation of prolactin secretion in rhesus monkeys by vasoactive intestinal polypeptide. Neuroendocrinology **33:** 79-83.

20. CHARPENTIER, G., J. P. BERCOVIA, P. JEDNAK, J. N. TALBOT, V. MUTT & G. ROSSELIN. 1982. VIP test in prolactinomas and in normal subjects. Biomedicine **36:** 105-107.

21. WERNER, S., A. L. HULTING, T. HOKFELT, P. ENEROTH, K. TATEMOTO, V. MUTT, L. MARODE & E. WUNSCH. 1983. Effect of peptide PHI-27 on prolactin release *in vitro*. Neuroendocrinology **37:** 476-478.

22. KAJI, H., K. CHIHARA, H. ABE, N. MINAMITANI, H. KODAMA, T. KITA, T. FUJITA & K. TATEMOTO. 1984. Stimulatory effect of peptide histidine isoleucine amide 1-27 on prolactin release in the rat. Life Sci. **35:** 641-647.

23. LUMPKIN, M. D., W. K. SAMSON & S. M. MCCANN. 1983. Hypothalamic and pituitary sites of action of oxytocin to alter prolactin secretion in the rat. Endocrinology **112:** 1711-1712.

24. ANDREWS, P. C., J. F. HYDE & N. BEN-JONATHAN. Fractionation by HPLC of prolactin-releasing factor (PRF) from rat and bovine posterior pituitaries. Program of the Endocrine Society. Indianapolis, IN. **631:** 179.

25. MINAMITANI, N., T. MINAMITANI, R. M. LECHAN, J. BOLLINGER-GRUBER & S. REICHLIN. 1987. Paraventricular nucleus mediates prolactin secretory responses to restraint stress, ether stress, and 5-hydroxy-L-tryptophan injection in the rat. Endocrinology **120:** 860-877.

26. HOKFELT, Y., J. FAHRENKRUG, K. TATEMOTO, V. MUTT, S. WERNER, A. L. HULTING, L. TERENIUS & K. J. CHANG. 1983. The PHI(PHI-27)/corticotropin-releasing factor/enkephalin immunoreactive hypothalamic neuron: Possible morphological basis for in-

tegrated control of prolactin, corticotropin, and growth hormone secretion. Proc. Natl. Acad. Sci. **80:** 895-898.

27. SWANSON, L. W., P. E. SAWCHENKO, J. RIVIER & W. W. VALE. 1983. Organization of ovine corticotropin-releasing factor immunoreactive cells and fibers in the rat brain: An immunohistochemical study. Neuroendocrinology **36:** 165-186.

28. HOKFELT, T., M. SCHULTZBERG, J. M. LUNDBERG, K. FUXE, V. MUTT, J. FAHRENKRUG & S. I. SAID. 1982. Distribution of vasoactive intestinal polypeptide in the central and peripheral nervous system as revealed by immunocytochemistry. *In* Vasoactive Intestinal Peptide. S. I. Said, Ed.: 65-86. Raven Press. New York.

29. BRUHN, T. O., P. M. PLOTSKY & W. W. VALE. 1984. Effect of paraventricular lesions on corticotropin-releasing factor (CRF)-like immunoreactivity in the stalk-median eminence: Studies on the adrenocorticotropin response to ether stress and exogenous CRF. Endocrinology **114:** 57-62.

30. SWANSON, L. W. & P. E. SAWCHENKO. 1980. Paraventricular nucleus: A site for the integration of neuroendocrine and automatic mechanisms. Neuroendocrinology **31:** 410-417.

31. SWANSON, L. W. & P. SAWCHENKO. 1983. Hypothalamic integration: Organization of the paraventricular and supraoptic nuclei. Annu. Rev. Neurosci. **6:** 269-324.

32. MINAMITANI, N., T. MINAMITANI, R. M. LECHAN, J. BOLLINGER-GRUBER & S. REICHLIN. Role of the paraventricular nucleus in the pituitary-adrenal responses to restraint stress, ether stress, and serotonergic stimulation by 5-HTP in conscious male rats. In preparation.

33. SHIMATSU, A., Y. KATO, N. MATSUSHITA, H. KATAKAMI, N. YANAIHARA & H. IMURA. 1982. Stimulation by serotonin of vasoactive intestinal polypeptide release into rat hypophysial portal blood. Endocrinology **111:** 338-340.

34. SAID, S. I. & J. C. PORTER. 1978. Vasoactive intestinal peptide release into hypophysial portal blood. Life. Sci. **24:** 227-230.

35. SHIMATSU, A., Y. KATO, T. INOUE, N. D. CHRISTOFIDES, S. R. BLOOM & H. IMURA. 1983. Peptide histidine isoleucine and vasoactive intestinal polypeptide-like immunoreactivity coexist in rat hypophysial portal blood. Neurosci. Lett. **43:** 259-262.

36. SHIMATSU, A., Y. KATO, N. MATSUSHITA, H. KATAKAMI, N. YANAIHARA & H. IMURA. 1981. Immunoreactive vasoactive intestinal polypeptide in rat hypophyseal-portal blood. Endocrinology **108:** 395-398.

37. SHIMATSU, A., Y. KATO, N. MATSUSHITA, H. OHTA, Y. KABAYAMA, N. YANAIHARA & H. IMURA. 1984. Prostaglandin D2 stimulates vasoactive intestinal polypeptide release into rat hypophysial portal blood. Peptides **5:** 395-398.

38. BRAR, A.K., G. FINK, M. MALETTI & W. ROSTENE. 1985. Vasoactive intestinal peptide in rat hypophysial portal blood: Effects of electrical stimulation of various brain areas, the oestrus cycle and anaesthetics. J. Endocrinol. **106:** 275-280.

39. ABE, H., D. ENGLER, M. E. MOLITCH, J. BOLLINGER-GRUBER & S. REICHLIN. 1985. Vasoactive intestinal peptide is a physiological mediator of prolactin release in the rat. Endocrinology **116:** 1383-1390.

40. KAJI, H., K. CHIHARA, H. ABE, T. KITA, Y. KASHIO, Y. OKIMURA & T. FUJITA. 1985. Effect of passive immunization with antisera to vasoactive intestinal polypeptide and peptide histidine isoleucine amide on 5-hydroxy-L-trytophan-induced prolactin release in rats. Endocrinology **117:** 1914-1919.

41. OHTA, H., Y. KATO, A. SHIMATSU, K. TOJO, Y. KABAYAMA, T. INOUE, N. YANAIHARA & H. IMURA. 1985. Inhibition by antiserum to vasoactive intestinal polypeptide (VIP) of prolactin secretion induced by serotonin in the rat. Eur. J. Pharmacol. **109:** 409-412.

42. KAJI, H., K. CHIHARA, T. KITA, Y. KASHIO, Y. OKIMURA & T. FUJITA. 1985. Administration of antisera to vasoactive intestinal polypeptide and peptide histidine isoleucine attenuates ether-induced prolactin secretion in rats. Neuroendocrinology **41:** 529-531.

43. TANIMOTO, K., T. TAMMINGA, N. CHASE & G. NILAVER. 1987. Intracerebroventricular injection of cholecystokinin octapeptide elevates plasma prolactin levels through stimulation of vasoactive intestinal polypeptide. Endocrinology **121:** 127-132.

44. LOREN, I., P. C. EMSON, J. FAHRENKRUG, A. BJORKLUND, J. ALUMETS, R. HAKANSON & F. SUNDLER. 1979. Distribution of vasoactive intestinal polypeptide in the rat and mouse brain. Neuroscience **4:** 1953-1976.

45. MEZEY, E. & J. Z. KISS. 1985. Vasoactive intestinal polypeptide containing neurons in the paraventricular nucleus may participate in regulating prolactin secretion. Proc. Natl. Acad. Sci. USA **82:** 245-247.
46. MACNAMEE, M. C., P. J. SHARP, R. W. LEA, R. J. STERLING & S. HARVEY. 1986. Evidence that vasoactive intestinal polypeptide is a physiological prolactin-releasing factor in the bantam hen. Gen. Comp. Endocrinol. **62:** 470-478.
47. MURAI, I. & N. BEN-JONATHAN. 1987. Posterior pituitary lobectomy abolishes the suckling-induced rise in prolactin (PRL) evidence for a PRL-releasing factor in the posterior pituitary. Endocrinology **121:** 205-211.
48. BATAILLE, D., J. N. TALBOT, C. MIHAUD, V. MUTT & G. ROSSELIN. 1981. Effect du peptide intestinal vasoactif (VIP) sur la secretion de prolactine chez l'homme. C. R. Acad. Sci. Paris **292:** 511-513.
49. CHARPENTIER, G., J. P. BERCOVICI, P. JEDNAK, J. N. TALBOT, V. MUTT & G. ROSSELIN. 1982. VIP test in prolactinomas and in normal subjects. Biomedicine **36:** 105-107.
50. CONTI, A., E. TOGNI, P. TRAVAGLINI, M. MURATORI & G. FAGLIA. 1987. Vasoactive intestinal polypeptide and dopamine: Effect on prolactin secretion in normal women and patients with microprolactinemia. Neuroendocrinology **46:** 241-245.
51. KAJI, H., K. CHIHARA, T. KITA, Y. KASHIO, Y. OKIMURA & T. FUJITA. 1985. Lack of plasma prolactin response to intravenously injected vasoactive intestinal polypeptide in patients with prolactin-secreting adenoma. Acta Endocrinol. Copenhagen **110:** 445-450.
52. KATO, Y., A. SHIMATSU, N. MATSUSHITA, H. OHTA & H. IMURA. 1984. Role of vasoactive intestinal polypeptide (VIP) in regulating the pituitary function in man. Peptides **5:** 389-394.
53. LIGHTMAN, S. L., R. J. UNWIN, K. GRAHAM, R. DIMALINE & G. McGARRICK. 1984. Vasoactive intestinal polypeptide stimulation of prolactin release and renin activity in normal man and patients with hyperprolactinemia: Effects of pretreatment with bromocriptine and dexamethasone. Eur. J. Clin. Invest. **14:** 444-448.
54. OTTESEN, B., A. N. ANDERSON, T. GERSTENBERG, H. ULRICHSEN, T. MANTHORPE & J. FAHRENKRUG. 1981. VIP stimulated prolactin release in women. Lancet ii: 696.
55. HAGEN, T. C., M. A. ARNAOUT, W. J. SCHERZER, D. R. MARTINSON & T. L. GARTHWAITE. 1986. Antisera to vasoactive intestinal polypeptide inhibit basal prolactin release from dispersed anterior pituitary cells. Neuroendocrinology **43:** 641-645.
56. MOREL, G., J. BESSON, G. ROSSELIN & P. M. DUBOIS. 1982. Ultrastructural evidence for endogenous vasoactive intestinal peptide-like immunoreactivity in the pituitary gland. Neuroendocrinology **34:** 85-89.
57. ARNAOUT, M. A., T. L. GARTHWAITE, D. R. MATINON & T. C. HAGEN. 1986. Vasoactive intestinal polypeptide is synthesized in anterior pituitary tissue. Endocrinology **119:** 2052.
58. DENEF, C. 1986. Paracrine interactions in the anterior pituitary. Clin. Endocrinol. Metab. **15:** 1-32.
59. MALETTI, M., W. H. ROTSZTEJN, L. CARR, H. SCHERRER, D. ROTTEN, C. KORDON & G. ROSSELIN. 1982. Interaction between estradiol and prolactin on vasoactive intestinal peptide concentrations in the hypothalamus and in the anterior pituitary of the female rat. Neurosci. Lett. **32:** 307.
60. DUNN, J. D., M. HESS & D. C. JOHNSON. 1976. Effect of thyroidectomy on rhythmic gonadotropin release. Proc. Soc. Exp. Biol. Med. **151:** 22.
61. JAHNKE, G., G. NICHOLSON, G. H. GREELEY, W. W. YOUNGBLOOD, A. J. PRANGE & J. KIZER. 1980. Studies on the neural mechanisms by which hypothyroidism decreases prolactin secretion in the rat. Brain Res. **191:** 429.
62. CAVE, W. T., J. D. DUNN & R. M. MACLEOD. 1977. Effects of altered thyroid states on mammary tumour growth and pituitary gland function in the rat. J. Natl. Inst. **59:** 993.
63. ROSE, D. P. & K. G. MOUNTJOY. 1983. Influence of thyroidectomy and prolactin suppression on the growth of N-nitrosomethylurea-induced mammary carcinomas. Cancer Res. **43:** 2588.
64. VIJAYAN, E., W. K. SAMSON, S. I. SAID & S. N. McCANN. 1979. Vasoactive intestinal peptide: Evidence for a hypothalamic site of action to release growth hormone, luteinizing hormone and prolactin in conscious ovariectomized rats. Endocrinology **104:** 53-57.
65. ROTSZTEJN, W. H., L. BENOIT, J. BESSON, G. BERAUD, M. T. BLUET-PAJOT, C. KORDON,

G. ROSSELIN & J. DUVAL. 1980. Effect of vasoactive intestinal peptide (VIP) on the release of adenohypophyseal hormones from purified cells obtained by unit gravity sedimentation. Neuroendocrinology 31: 282-286.
66. WESTENDORF, J. M. & A. SCHONBRUNN. 1985. Peptide specificity for stimulation of corticotropin secretion: Activation of overlapping pathways by the vasoactive intestinal peptide family and corticotropin-releasing factor. Endocrinology 116: 2528-2535.
67. DEES, W. L., C. E. AHMED & S. R. OJEDA. 1986. Substance P- and vasoactive intestinal peptide-containing fibers reach the ovary by independent routes. Endocrinology 119: 638-641.
68. TRZECIAK, W. H., C. E. AHMED, E. R. SIMPSON & S. T. OJEDA. Vasoactive intestinal peptide induces the synthesis of the cholesterol side-chain cleavage enzyme complex in cultured rat ovarian granulosa cells. Proc. Natl. Acad. Sci. USA 83: 7490-7494.
69. GRUNDITZ, T., R. HAKANSON, G. HEDGE, F. SUNDLER & R. UDDMAN. 1986. Peptide histidine isoleucine amide stimulates thyroid hormone secretion and coexists with vasoactive intestinal polypeptide in intrathyroid nerve fibers from laryngeal ganglia. Endocrinology 118: 783-90.
70. LAURBERG, P. 1986. VIP and hormone secretion from thyroidal follicular and C-cells. Horm. Metab. Res. 18: 230-233.
71. AHREN, B. 1985. Cholinergic and VIPergic effects on thyroid hormone secretion in the mouse. Peptides 6: 585-589.
72. HUFFMAN, L. & G. A. HEDGE. 1986. Effects of vasoactive intestinal peptide on thyroid blood flow and circulating thyroid hormone levels in the rat. Endocrinology 118: 550-7.
73. DESCHODT-LANCKMAN, D., P. ROBBERECT & J. CHRISTOPHE. 1977. Characterization of VIP-adenylate cyclase in guinea pig brain. FEBS Lett. 83: 76-80.
74. ETGEN, A. M. & E. T. Y. BROWING. 1983. Activators of cyclic adenosine 3', 5'-monophosphate accumulation in rat hippocampal slices: Action of vasoactive intestinal peptide (VIP). J. Neurosci. 3: 2487-2493.
75. EPELBAUM, J., L. TAPIA-ARANCIBIA, J. BESSON, W. ROTSZTEJN & C. KORDON. 1979. Vasoactive intestinal peptide inhibits release of somatostatin from hypothalamus in vitro. Eur. J. Pharmacol. 58: 493-495.
76. TAPIA-ARANCIBIA, L. & S. REICHLIN. 1985. Vasoactive intestinal peptide and PHI stimulate somatostatin release from rat cerebral cortical and diencephalic cells in dispersed culture. Brain Res. 336: 67-72.
77. ROBBINS, R. & R. M. LANDON. The effects of neurotensin, vasoactive intestinal polypeptide and other neuropeptides on the secretion of somatostatin from cerebral cortical cells. Brain Res. 332: 161-164.
78. TAPIA-ARANCIBIA, L., J. NATHANSON & S. REICHLIN. Adenylate cyclase activation of target cells is not the mechanism involved in vasoactive intestinal peptide (VIP)-stimulated somatostatin release from cortical and diencephalic neurons in primary culture. In preparation.
79. AUDIGIER, S., C. BARBERIS & S. JARD. 1986. Vasoactive intestinal polypeptide increases inositol phospholipid breakdown in the rat superior cervical ganglion. Brain Res. 376: 363-367.
80. MONTMINY, M. R., M. J. LOW, L. TAPIA-ARANCIBIA, S. REICHLIN, G. MANDEL & R. H. GOODMAN. 1986. Cyclic AMP regulates somatostatin mRNA accumulation in primary diencephalic cultures and in transfected fibroblast cells. J. Neurosci. 6: 1171-1186.
81. MONTMINY, M. R., K. A. SEVARINO, J. A. WAGNER, G. MANDEL & R. H. GOODMAN. 1986. Identification of a cyclic-AMP-responding element within the rat somatostatin gene. Proc. Natl. Acad. Sci. USA 18: 6682-6686.
82. MONTMINY, M. R. & L. M. BILEZIKJIAN. 1987. Binding of a nuclear protein to the cyclic-AMP response element of the somatostatin gene. Nature 328: 175-178.

Vasoactive Intestinal Peptide in the Lung

SAMI I. SAID[a]

University of Oklahoma Health Sciences Center and
Veterans Administration Medical Center
Oklahoma City, Oklahoma 73190

INTRODUCTION

The biological (vasodilator) activity of vasoactive intestinal peptide (VIP) was discovered in the lung[1,2] before the peptide was isolated and chemical identity characterized from intestine.[3-5] Although VIP levels in the lung as a whole are considerably lower than in brain or gut,[6] VIP is localized in key sites in the lung, has potent activities on its major functions, and appears to play an important role in pulmonary physiology and disease.

LOCALIZATION

The principal localization of VIP-containing neurons in the tracheobronchial tree is in the smooth muscle layer, around submucosal mucous and serous glands, and in the walls of pulmonary and bronchial arteries.[7-11] Immunoreactive VIP is also present in neuronal cell bodies forming microganglia that provide a source of intrinsic innervation of pulmonary structures.

Bronchial Smooth Muscle

VIP-containing nerve fibers are found in close association with the smooth muscle layer of airways from the trachea through the small bronchioles. In bronchi from cats and human subjects, VIP-containing nerve fibers come in close contact with and often penetrate into small fascicles of smooth muscle.

[a] Current address: Department of Medicine, University of Illinois, P.O. Box 6998, Chicago, IL 60680.

Bronchial Glands

The bronchial submucosal glands of cat, dog, and human airways are richly supplied with VIP-containing neurons. In human airways, VIP-containing nerve terminals are closely associated with secretory cells of submucosal gland acini: The nerves frequently encircle parts of the acinar units and are occasionally observed within the epithelial layer of the gland, but no VIP-containing fibers have been observed in airway epithelium.

Bronchial and Pulmonary Vessels

Like other systemic arteries, bronchial arteries receive a rich supply of VIP-containing nerve fibers, located predominantly at the medial-adventitial junction. Pulmonary arteries, too, are supplied with nerve fibers and nerve terminals containing immunoreactive VIP.[7-8]

Lamina Propria and Epithelium

An extensive network of VIP-containing nerve fibers and nerve terminals is present in the lamina propria. The close proximity of these fibers and terminals to the epithelial basement membrane explains how VIP that is released from nerve terminals within the lamina propria could influence epithelial cell function.

Bronchial Ganglia

Collections of nerve cell bodies, forming microganglia, are distributed along nerve bundles associated with extrapulmonary and larger intrapulmonary bronchi. VIP is present in many of the nerve cell bodies in these ganglia,[7,9] as well as in nerve terminals within the ganglia. The nerve fibers supplying pulmonary structures probably originate from the ganglion cell bodies.

Mast Cells

Immunocytochemical and radioimmunologic evidence suggests the presence of VIP in murine mast cells and its release with degranulation of these cells,[12] but the identity of VIP-like immunoreactivity in mast cells has yet to be established.

COLOCALIZATION WITH OTHER PEPTIDES AND
NEUROTRANSMITTERS

The coexistence of peptides and other neurotransmitters in the same neurons is now widely accepted.[13] Strong evidence suggests that VIP coexists with acetylcholine in many postganglionic cholinergic neurons supplying exocrine glands and blood vessels.[14-16] A recent ultrastructural immunocytochemical study of VIP in the airways[11] revealed VIP immunoreactivity in mixed populations of nerve terminals, some of which were of the "cholinergic type," with smaller (90-150 nm) vesicles, while others corresponded to the "p-type," containing numerous granular vesicles that are larger in diameter (120-210 nm) than those of cholinergic or adrenergic terminals.[17,18]

VIP may also be colocalized with other peptides. It coexists with peptide histidine-isoleucine (PHI),[19,20] a structurally homologous peptide having an NH_2-terminal histidine and a COOH-terminal isoleucine. Both peptides are synthesized from the same precursor molecule.[21] PHM, the human counterpart of PHI, has a COOH-terminal methionine residue. The distribution of PHI-containing nerve fibers in the airways is similar to, but less extensive than, that of VIP-containing fibers.[10,19,20] Immunocytochemical evidence suggests that VIP and substance P may be colocalized in some of the neurons that comprise bronchial ganglia and in nerve fibers distributed to bronchial smooth muscle, submucosal glands, and the lamina propria.[22] Other peptides that may coexist with VIP in the same neurons include vasopressin and certain opioid peptides.

ACTIONS ON AIRWAYS

VIP has potent effects on all major structural components of the airways. These actions include the following:

Airway Smooth Muscle

VIP relaxes airway smooth muscle both *in vitro* and *in vivo*. Thus, it relaxes isolated tracheal or bronchial segments from guinea pigs, rabbits, dogs, and humans and prevents or attenuates their contraction by a variety of constrictors, including histamine, $PGF_{2\alpha}$, kallikrein, leukotriene D_4, and neurokinin A (FIG. 1).[23-28] This action is long-lasting and is unaffected by blockade of adrenergic or cholinergic receptors or of cyclooxygenase activity.[24,29-31] Inhaled VIP protects against the bronchoconstriction induced by histamine or prostaglandin $F_{2\alpha}$ in dogs (FIG. 2),[32] and by histamine in guinea pigs.[33] Infused VIP reverses serotonin-induced bronchoconstriction in cats.[34] In human subjects, however, VIP has been found to be generally less effective in protecting against asthmatic or histamine-induced bronchoconstriction.[35-38]

Tracheobronchial Secretion

VIP stimulates water and ion transport in canine tracheal epithelium,[39] and stimulates the secretion of sulfated macromolecules by tracheal explants from ferrets[40] but, paradoxically, inhibits macromolecular secretion in human tracheal explants.[41]

Bronchial and Pulmonary Vessels

VIP dilates the vessels supplying the nose, upper airways,[42] and trachea and bronchi,[43] as well as pulmonary vessels.[44,45] As a pulmonary vasodilator, VIP is 50

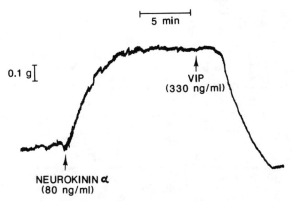

FIGURE 1. Contraction of guinea pig trachea by neurokinin A (80 ng/ml) was abruptly reversed by administration of VIP (330 ng/ml).

times as potent as prostacyclin (FIG. 3).[31] The pulmonary vasodilator action of VIP is independent of endothelium.[46]

Immunologic Release of Mediators

VIP has a moderate inhibitory effect on antigen-induced release of histamine from guinea pig lung.[47] Since VIP may normally be present in mast cells,[12] it may act as a natural modulator of mast cell function.

INTERACTIONS WITH OTHER NEUROPEPTIDES AND
NEUROTRANSMITTERS

Multiple interactions have been described between VIP and other neurotransmitters. Although most have been described in other tissues, similar interactions may exist in the regulation of respiratory function.

1. VIP always *coexists* and is *coreleased* with PHI (or PHM) and, in many neurons, also with acetylcholine.[14,19,20,48,49] Recent work suggests that VIP also coexists

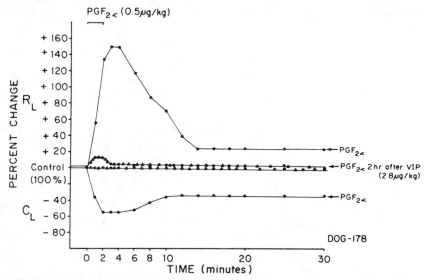

FIGURE 2. Protective effect of VIP aerosol against bronchoconstriction induced by challenge with histamine (32 μg/kg) (A) and PGF$_{2α}$ (0.5 μg/kg) (B) in anesthetized dog. Increase in lung resistance (R$_L$) and decrease in lung compliance (C$_L$), percent of control values, are plotted against time. Circles are values obtained with histamine or PGF$_{2α}$ alone, and triangles are those obtained after treatment with VIP (0.8 and 2.8 μg/kg) as shown.

with vasopressin in magnocellular hypothalamic neurons,[50] and with substance P in some neurons within the lung.[22]

2. VIP *enhances* the affinity of acetylcholine for muscarinic receptors and acetylcholine-induced secretion of saliva.[15] The blood flow-promoting effect of VIP in salivary glands is, in turn, potentiated by acetylcholine.[15] VIP *stimulates* the release of acetylcholine from myenteric neurons,[51] and induces depolarization and muscarinic excitation in sympathetic ganglionic synapses.[52]

3. VIP *release is stimulated by* cholinergic agonists,[53,54] by pretreatment with atropine,[55] and by dopaminergic agonists,[56] GABA antagonists,[54] and opiate antagonists.[54]

4. VIP *acts synergistically* with norepinephrine to stimulate cyclic AMP production in cerebral cortex,[57] and with ATP to relax gastric smooth muscle.[58]

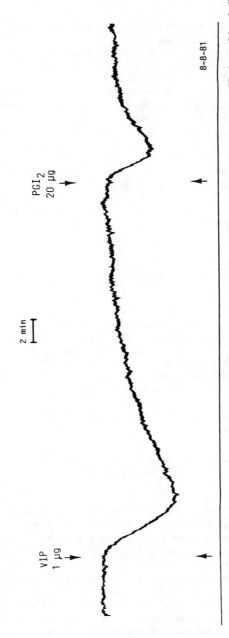

FIGURE 3. Tracing of relaxation of isolated strip of cat PA in response to VIP (1 µg) and PGI₂ (20 µg), given at arrows. Horizontal bar indicates two-minute duration.

RECEPTORS

Specific, high-affinity receptors for VIP have been identified in membrane preparations of rat, mouse, guinea pig, and human lungs and in human lung tumor cells.[59,60] These receptors have been localized immunocytochemically, by demonstration of the increased cAMP levels stimulated by the binding of VIP to its receptors,[59,61,62] in submucosal serous and mucous glands of the ferret,[63] and in ciliated and basal cells of tracheal epithelium of dog.[63] The use of autoradiographic techniques has confirmed the presence of VIP uptake sites in bronchial epithelium, submucosal glands, smooth muscle, and alveolar cells.[64–67] Autoradiographic uptake sites (and, presumably, receptors) of VIP are extensively distributed in dog bronchial epithelium and bronchial smooth muscle.[68] As in other cells and tissues,[73] the binding of VIP to airway sites is coupled to an adenylate cyclase. The resultant increase in cyclic AMP levels is believed to mediate the airway relaxation and other biological effects of the peptide.

VIP receptors in human and other mammalian lungs have recently been characterized using covalent cross-linking[70] and solubilization[70,71] techniques. The binding of VIP to its high-affinity receptors in the lung is rapid, reversible, and sensitive to the guanine nucleotide GTP.

MECHANISMS OF ACTION

The importance of cyclic AMP in mediating the actions of VIP is well documented, but cyclic AMP accumulation alone may not fully explain these actions. Thus, another relaxant of airway and pulmonary vascular smooth muscle, atrial natriuretic peptide, stimulates the intracellular accumulation of cyclic GMP, not cyclic AMP. The contribution of other intracellular second messengers, for example, cytosolic calcium,[73] protein kinase C, and inositol phospholipid turnover,[74,75] to the actions of VIP remain largely unexplored.

IMPORTANCE OF VASCULAR ENDOTHELIUM AND AIRWAY EPITHELIUM

The vasodilator or vasoconstrictor activity of several peptides and other pharmacologically active agents has recently been shown to depend on the presence of intact vascular endothelium.[76] Similar observations on airways suggest that tracheobronchial epithelium plays a correspondingly important role in airway responses to bronchoactive agents. In experiments on isolated strips of guinea pig trachea, removal of tracheal epithelium enhanced the contraction induced by acetylcholine and reduced the relaxation induced by VIP, as well as by norepinephrine and by sodium nitroprusside.[77,78] The manner in which airway epithelium can modify airway smooth muscle tone is still unknown. Just as vascular endothelium generates one or more smooth muscle-relaxant factor(s) (endothelium-derived relaxant factor[s]), so may tracheobronchial epithelium release one or more factors promoting airway relaxation (epithelium-derived relaxant factor[s]).

ENZYMATIC DEGRADATION

One fundamental feature of all neurotransmitters is their specific degradation or removal, at or near their target sites. Recently, the enzymatic inactivation of VIP has been examined. Use of various protease inhibitors[79] has provided indirect evidence for the enzymatic inactivation of VIP (and substance P)[80] in bronchial mucosa by an "enkephalinase": an enkephalinase inhibitor, phosphoramidon, potentiated the tracheal-relaxant activity of VIP[81] and slowed its enzymatic degradation by lung extracts.[82] A neutral metalloendopeptidase (or "enkephalinase") has recently been described in human lung tissue.[83] Other proteases may participate in the degradation of VIP in the lung.

VIP AS A REGULATOR OF LUNG FUNCTION

The presence of VIP in the smooth muscle layer of the tracheobronchial tree,[7] its potent relaxant activity on airway smooth muscle, and its binding to specific receptors on these cells, strongly suggest a physiological role for this peptide in regulating airway smooth muscle function.

Strong evidence suggests that VIP may be a transmitter of the nonadrenergic, noncholinergic component of the autonomic innervation of the lung.[84-86] Activities mediated by this system include relaxation of airways and pulmonary vessels, and secretion of bronchial water, chloride ion, and macromolecules.[68] In addition, VIP may modulate the release of mast-cell mediators of inflammation.[47]

Evidence that VIP is a likely transmitter of nonadrenergic relaxation of airway smooth muscle includes the following:

1. VIP fulfills the criteria of a neurotransmitter.[87,88]
2. VIP is present in the vagus nerve;[89] vagal electrical stimulation in the presence of cholinergic and adrenergic blockade causes bronchodilation.[90]
3. VIP mimics the electrophysiological changes in airway smooth muscle produced by nonadrenergic, noncholinergic nerve stimulation.[26,27]
4. Prolonged incubation of airway smooth muscle with VIP reduces subsequent relaxation by VIP (tachyphylaxis), and also reduces the magnitude of nonadrenergic, noncholinergic relaxation in cats[26] and in guinea pigs.[91]
5. VIP is released on transmural stimulation of guinea pig tracheal segments, in the presence of adrenergic and muscarinic cholinergic receptor blockade, and the release is in direct proportion to the relaxation of these segments.[92]
6. Both the VIP release cited above, and the associated tracheal relaxation, are markedly inhibited by blockade of neurotransmission with tetrodotoxin.[92]
7. The relaxation is also greatly reduced by preincubation of the tracheal segments with a specific VIP antiserum.[92]

A number of other observations, on the other hand, have been interpreted against VIP as the transmitter of nonadrenergic airway relaxation:

1. Immunoreactive VIP is present in the canine tracheobronchial tree, but the

nonadrenergic relaxant system is weak or absent in this species.[93] This apparent discrepancy may be explained by the less-intimate anatomic relationship between VIP-containing nerves and airway smooth muscle in dog airways, compared to those of cats or humans.[8]

2. Guinea pig tracheas that had been fully relaxed by application of VIP could be made to relax further with transmural (electrical field) stimulation.[94,95] This additional relaxation could be due to the release of PHI (or PHM), itself a potent relaxant of airways[96] from nerve terminals in the airways. Further, electrical field stimulation may, under certain conditions, induce direct (myogenic) relaxation, which persists after blockade of neurotransmission.[84]

3. The proteolytic enzyme α-chymotrypsin, which hydrolyzes VIP *in vitro*,[5] did not inhibit relaxation induced by electrical field stimulation.[97] This negative result may be explained by the failure of the enzyme to reach the sites of VIP release in sufficient concentrations to degrade the peptide.

4. Human airways exhibit a major component of nonadrenergic relaxation, but human asthmatics, at least in some studies, respond relatively weakly to VIP. The weaker-than-expected airway relaxation of human asthmatics to inhaled VIP may be due to inadequate access of the biologically active peptide to its receptors on airway smooth muscle, probably due to its inactivation by airway proteases (please see below). As mentioned earlier, VIP effectively relaxes isolated strips of human bronchi *in vitro*.[31]

VIP IN THE PATHOGENESIS OF LUNG DISEASE

On the basis of experimental and clinical observations, the hypothesis was advanced several years ago that decreased biological activity of VIP (resulting from deficiency of VIP neurons, impaired binding to its receptors, or the presence of an inhibitor or antibody) may contribute to the pathogenesis of two major diseases of the airways and lungs: cystic fibrosis and bronchial asthma.[92,98,99]

The possibility that cystic fibrosis may be causally related to a deficiency of VIP is based on the following lines of evidence: (a) VIP-containing nerves richly supply all exocrine organs,[15] the target organs in this disorder; (b) VIP influences all major exocrine function, stimulating water, intestinal and bronchial chloride, pancreatic bicarbonate, and macromolecular secretion, and increasing blood flow;[100] (c) VIP binds to specific receptors on exocrine glands, including salivary and sweat glands, bronchial glands, and exocrine pancreas.[69] Examined against some of the key manifestations of cystic fibrosis, notably the decreased Cl^- permeability in sweat gland ducts,[101] and respiratory epithelial cells,[102,103] the changes promoted by VIP, especially the stimulation of chloride secretion, are consistent with the view that VIP deficiency may help explain these manifestations.

This hypothesis has recently received experimental support. Normal sweat glands are well supplied by VIP-immunoreactive nerves, which richly innervate the acini and moderately innervate the ducts. In cystic fibrosis patients, on the other hand, VIP-innervation of sweat glands is significantly decreased around the acini and is virtually absent around the ducts.[104]

A similar hypothesis links the pathogenesis of bronchial asthma to a postulated lack of VIP innervation of airway smooth muscle.[92,98] This proposed link is based on (a) the evidence, presented above, that VIP may be the transmitter of nonadrenergic relaxation of airways; (b) the dominant, if not exclusive, role of this relaxant system in human airways,[86] and (c) the plausible speculation that a lack of nonadrenergic relaxation could explain the airway hyperreactivity of bronchial asthma.[92,105]

VIP IN THE TREATMENT OF LUNG DISEASE

Extensive data from experiments on isolated airway segments *in vitro* and on anesthetized and unanesthetized animals show that VIP can potently and effectively relax tracheobronchial smooth muscle and prevent or reduce the bronchoconstriction induced by histamine, serotonin, prostaglandin $F_{2\alpha}$, leukotriene D_4, and neurokinin A.[24,25,28,32–34] In addition to relaxing airway smooth muscle, VIP also inhibits the pulmonary release of histamine induced by antigen,[47] and of peptide leukotrienes induced by platelet-activating factor or by calcium ionophore.[106]

These properties of VIP, along with its normal presence in nerve fibers and nerve terminals in close proximity to airway smooth muscle, bronchial glands, and epithelium, and the presence of specific receptors for it on these sites, make it an excellent candidate as a "natural" therapeutic agent in bronchial asthma. The aerosol route is particularly attractive, as large doses of the peptide can be given with minimal systemic side effects.[32,38] Results to date of several trials of VIP aerosol in asthma have been variable but generally less favorable than expected from data obtained *in vitro* and in animals.[29,35,38] Possible reasons for lack of success in asthmatics include: (a) failure of aerosolized VIP to reach its airway smooth muscle receptors in sufficient concentrations, due to impediment by mucus; (b) degradation or inactivation of the peptide by peptidases in bronchial secretions or in bronchial epithelium (please see above); and (c) altered responsiveness of asthmatic airways to VIP. Attempts to improve the effectiveness of VIP aerosol in asthmatics are continuing, especially by adding appropriate anti-proteases to protect the peptide against enzymatic degradation.[81,82]

REFERENCES

1. SAID, S. I. 1967. Vasoactive substances in the lung. *In* Proceedings of the Tenth Aspen Emphysema Conference. June 7-10. Aspen, CO. U.S. Public Health Serv. Publication **1787:** 223-228.
2. SAID, S. I. & V. MUTT. 1969. Long acting vasodilator peptide from lung tissue. Nature **224:** 699-700.
3. SAID, S. I. & V. MUTT. 1970. Polypeptide with broad biological activity: Isolation from small intestine. Science **169:** 1217-1218.
4. SAID, S. I. & V. MUTT. 1972. Isolation from porcine intestinal wall of a vasoactive octacosapeptide related to secretin and to glucagon. Eur. J. Biochem. **28:** 199-204.
5. MUTT, V. & S. I. SAID. 1974. Structure of the porcine vasoactive intestinal octacosapeptide. Eur. J. Biochem. **42:** 581-589.
6. SAID, S. I. & R. N. ROSENBERG. 1976. Vasoactive intestinal polypeptide: Abundant immunoreactivity in neural cell lines and normal nervous tissues. Science **192:** 907-908.
7. DEY, R. D., W. A. SHANNON & S. I. SAID. 1981. Localization of VIP-immunoreactive nerves in airways and pulmonary vessels of dogs, cats and human subjects. Cell Tissue Res. **220:** 231-238.

8. DEY, R. D. & S. I. SAID. 1985. Lung peptides and the pulmonary circulation. *In* The Pulmonary Circulation and Acute Lung Injury. S. I. Said, Ed.: 101-122. Futura Publishing Co. New York.

9. UDDMAN, R., A. LUTS & F. SUNDLER. 1985. Nerves fibres containing peptide histidine isoleucine (PHI) in the respiratory tract. Arch. Otorhinolaryngol. **242:** 189-193.

10. UDDMAN, R. & F. SUNDLER. 1979. VIP nerves in human upper respiratory tract. Otorhinolaryngology **41:** 221-226.

11. LAITINEN, A., M. PARTANEN, A. HERVONEN, M. PELTO-HUIKKO & L. A. LAITINEN. 1985. VIP-like immunoreactive nerves in human respiratory tract. Histochemistry **82:** 313-319.

12. CUTZ, E., W. CHAN, N. S. TRACK, A. GOTH & S. I. SAID. 1978. Release of vasoactive intestinal polypeptide in mast cells by histamine liberators. Nature **275:** 661-662.

13. LUNDBERG, J. M. & T. HÖKFELT. 1983. Coexistence of peptides and classical neurotransmitters. Trends Neurosci. **6:** 325-333.

14. LUNDBERG, J. M., T. HÖKFELT, M. SCHULTZBERG, K. UVNÄS-WALLENSTEN, C. KOHLER & S. I. SAID. 1979. Occurrence of VIP-like immunoreactivity in certain cholinergic neurons of the cat: Evidence from combined immunohistochemistry and acetylcholinesterase staining. Neuroscience **4:** 1539-1559.

15. LUNDBERG, J. M., A. ÄNGGÅRD, J. FAHRENKRUG, T. HÖKFELT & V. MUTT. 1980. Vasoactive intestinal polypeptide in cholinergic neurons of exocrine glands: Functional significance of co-existing transmitters for vasodilation and secretion. Proc. Natl. Acad. Sci. USA **77:** 1651-1655.

16. LUNDBERG, J. M., A. ÄNGGÅRD, P. EMSON, J. FAHRENKRUG & T. HÖKFELT. 1981. VIP and cholinergic mechanisms in cat nasal mucosa: Studies on choline acetyltransferase and release of vasoactive intestinal peptide. Proc. Natl. Acad. Sci. USA **78:** 5255-5259.

17. BAUMGARTEN, H. G., A. F. HOLSTEIN & C. OWMAN. 1970. Auerbachs plexus of mammals and man: Electron microscopic identification of three different types of neuronal processes in myenteric ganglia of the large intestine from rhesus monkeys, guinea-pigs and man. J. Zellforsch. **106:** 376-397.

18. LARSSON, L. I. 1977. Ultrastructural localization of a new neuronal peptide (VIP). Histochemistry **54:** 173-176.

19. LUNDBERG, J. M., J. FAHRENKRUG, T. HÖKFELT, C.-R. MARTLING, O. LARSSON, K. TATEMOTO & A. ÄNGGÅRD. 1984. Co-existence of peptide HI (PHI) and VIP in nerves regulating blood flow and bronchial smooth muscle tone in various mammals including man. Peptides **5:** 593-606.

20. LUNDBERG, J. M., J. FAHRENKRUG, O. LARSSON & A. ÄNGGÅRD. 1984. Corelease of vasoactive intestinal polypeptide and peptide histidine isoleucine in relation to atropine-resistant vasodilation in cat submandibular salivary gland. Neurosci. Lett. **52:** 37-42.

21. ITOH, N., K. OBATA, N. YANAIHARA & H. OKAMOTO. 1983. Human prepro-vasoactive intestinal polypeptide contains a novel PHI-27-like peptide, PHM-27. Nature **304:** 547-549.

22. DEY, R. D., J. HOFFPAUIR & S. I. SAID. 1988. Co-localization of vasoactive intestinal peptide- and substance P-containing nerves in cat bronchi. Neuroscience **24:** 275-281.

23. PIPER, P. J., S. I. SAID & J. R. VANE. 1970. Effects on smooth muscle preparations of unidentified vasoactive peptides from intestine and lung. Nature **225:** 1144-1146.

24. SAID, S. I., S. KITAMURA, T. YOSHIDA, J. PRESKITT & L. D. HOLDEN. 1974. Humoral control of airways. Ann. N.Y. Acad. Sci. **221:** 103-114.

25. WASSERMAN, M. A., R. L. GRIFFIN & P. E. MALO. 1982. Comparative *in vitro* tracheal-relaxant effects of porcine and hen VIP. *In* Vasoactive Intestinal Peptide. S. I. Said, Ed.: 177-184. Raven Press. New York.

26. ITO, Y. & K. TAKEDA. 1982. Non-adrenergic inhibitory nerves and putative transmitters in the smooth muscle of cat trachea. J. Physiol. **330:** 497-511.

27. CAMERON, A. C., C. F. JOHNSON, C. T. KIRKPATRICK & M. C. A. KIRKPATRICK. 1983. The quest for the inhibitory neurotransmitter in bovine tracheal smooth muscle. Q. J. Exp. Physiol. **68:** 413-426.

28. HAMASAKI, Y., T. SAGA, M. MOJARAD & S. I. SAID. 1983b. VIP counteracts leukotriene D$_4$-induced contractions of guinea pig trachea, lung, and pulmonary artery. Trans. Assoc. Am. Physicians 96: 406-411.

29. ALTIERE, R. J. & L. DIAMOND. 1984. Comparison of vasoactive intestinal peptide and isoproterenol relaxant effects in isolated cat airways. J. Appl. Physiol. 56: 986.

30. HAND, J. M., R. B. LARAVUSO & J. A. WILL. 1984. Relaxation of isolated guinea pig trachea, bronchi and pulmonary arteries produced by vasoactive intestinal peptide (VIP). Eur. J. Pharmacol. 98: 279-284.

31. SAGA, T. & S. I. SAID. 1984. Vasoactive intestinal peptide relaxes isolated strips of human bronchus, pulmonary artery, and lung parenchyma. Trans. Assoc. Am. Physicians. 97: 304-310.

32. SAID, S. I., A. GEUMEI & N. HARA. 1982. Bronchodilator effect of VIP *in vivo:* Protection against bronchoconstriction induced by histamine or prostaglandin F$_{2\alpha}$. *In* Vasoactive Intestinal Peptide. S. I. Said, Ed.: 185-191. Raven Press. New York.

33. COX, C. P., M. R. LERNER, J. J. WELLS & S. I. SAID. 1983. Inhaled vasoactive intestinal peptide (VIP) prevents bronchoconstriction induced by inhaled histamine. Am. Rev. Respir. Dis. 127: 249.

34. DIAMOND, L., J. L. SZAREK, M. N. GILLESPIE & R. J. ALTIERE. 1983. *In vivo* bronchodilator activity of vasoactive intestinal peptide in the cat. Am. Rev. Respir. Dis. 128: 827-832.

35. MORICE, A. 1983. Vasoactive intestinal peptide causes bronchodilation and protects against bronchoconstriction in asthmatic subjects. Lancet. ii: 1225-1227.

36. MORICE, A. H., R. J. UNWIN & P. S. SEVER. 1984. Vasoactive intestinal peptide as a bronchodilator in asthmatic subjects. Peptides 5: 439-440.

37. BARNES, P. J. & C. M. S. DIXON. 1984. The effect of inhaled vasoactive intestinal peptide on bronchial reactivity to histamine in humans. Am. Rev. Respir. Dis. 130: 162-166.

38. MOJARAD, M., T. L. GRODE, C. P. COX, G. KIMMEL & S. I. SAID. 1985. Differential responses of human asthmatics to inhaled vasoactive intestinal peptide (VIP). Am. Rev. Resp. Dis. 131: 281A.

39. NATHANSON, I., J. H. WIDDICOMBE & P. J. BARNES. 1983. Effect of vasoactive intestinal peptide on ion transport across dog tracheal epithelium. J. Appl. Physiol. 55: 1844-1848.

40. PEATFIELD, A. C., P. J. BARNES, C. BRATCHER, J. A. NADEL & B. DAVIS. 1983. Vasoactive intestinal peptide stimulates tracheal submucosal gland secretion in ferret. Am. Rev. Respir. Dis. 128: 89-93.

41. COLES, S. J., S. I. SAID & L. M. REID. 1981. Inhibition by vasoactive intestinal peptide of glycoconjugate and lysozyme secretion by human airways *in vitro.* Am. Rev. Respir. Dis. 124: 531-536.

42. MALM, L., F. SUNDLER & R. UDDMAN. 1980. Effects of vasoactive intestinal polypeptide (VIP) on resistance and capacitance vessels in the nasal mucosa. Acta Otolaryngol. (Stockholm) 90: 304-308.

43. WIDDICOMBE, J., A. LAITINEN & L. A. LAITINEN. 1987. Effects of inflammatory and other mediators on airway vascular beds. Am. Rev. Respir. Dis. 135(Suppl.): S67-70.

44. HAMASAKI, Y., M. MOJARAD & S. I. SAID. 1983. Relaxant action of VIP on cat pulmonary artery: Comparison with acetylcholine, isoproterenol and prostaglandin E$_1$. J. Appl. Physiol. 54: 1607.

45. NANDIWADA, P. A., P. J. KADOWITZ, S. I. SAID, M. MOJARAD & A. L. HYMAN. 1985. Pulmonary vasodilator responses to vasoactive intestinal peptide in the cat. J. Appl. Physiol. 58: 1723-1728.

46. SATA, T., H. P. MISRA, E. KUBOTA & S. I. SAID. 1986. Vasoactive intestinal polypeptide relaxes pulmonary artery by an endothelium-independent mechanism. Peptides 7: 225-227.

47. UNDEM, B. J., E. C. DICK & C. K. BUCKNER. 1983. Inhibition by vasoactive intestinal peptide of antigen-induced histamine release from guinea-pig minced lung. Eur. J. Pharmacol. 88: 247-249.

48. ECKENSTEIN, F. & R. W. BAUGHMAN. 1984. Two types of cholinergic innervation in cortex, one co-localized with vasoactive intestinal polypeptide. Nature 309: 153-155.

49. LUNDBERG, J. M. 1981. Evidence for co-existence of vasoactive intestinal polypeptide (VIP) and acetylcholine in neurons of cat exocrine glands. Acta. Physiol. Scand. **496:** 1-57.

50. OKAMURA, H., S. MURAKAMI, K. FUKUI, K. UDA, K. KAWAMOTO, S. KAWASHIMA, N. YANAIHARA & Y. IBATA. 1986. Vasoactive intestinal peptide and peptide histidine isoleucine amide-like immunoreactivity colocalize with vasopressin-like immunoreactivity in the canine hypothalamo-neurohypophysial neuronal system. Neurosci. Lett. **69:** 227-232.

51. YAU, W., M. YOUTHER & P. VERDUN. 1985. A presynaptic site of action of substance P and vasoactive intestinal polypeptide on myenteric neurons. Brain Res. **330:** 382-385.

52. KAWATANI, M., M. RUTIGLIANO & W. C. DEGROAT. 1985. Depolarization and muscarinic excitation induced in a sympathetic ganglion by vasoactive intestinal polypeptide. Science **229:** 879-881.

53. BITAR, K. N., S. I. SAID, G. C. WEIR, B. SAFFOURI & G. M. MAKHLOUF. 1980. Neural release of vasoactive intestinal peptide from the gut. Gastroenterology **79:** 1288-1294.

54. WANG, J., T. YAKSH, G. HARTY & V. GO. 1986. Neurotransmitter modulation of VIP release from cat cerebral cortex. Am. J. Physiol. **250:** R104-R111.

55. HEDLUND, B., J. ABENS & T. BARTFAI. 1983. Vasoactive intestinal polypeptide and muscarinic receptors: Supersensitivity induced by long-term atropine treatment. Science **220:** 519-521.

56. UVNÄS-MOBERG, K., M. GOINY, B. POSLONCEC & L. BLOMQUIST. 1982. Increased levels of VIP (vasoactive intestinal polypeptide)-like immunoreactivity in peripheral venous blood in dogs following injections of apomorphine and bromocriptine. Do dopaminergic agents induce gastric relaxation and hypotension by a release of endogenous VIP? Acta. Physiol. Scand. **115:** 373-375.

57. MAGISTRETTI, P. J. & M. SCHORDERET. 1984. VIP and noradrenaline act synergistically to increase cyclic-AMP in cerebral cortex. Nature **308:** 208-282.

58. BITAR, K. N. & G. M. MAKHLOUF. 1982. Relaxation of isolated gastric smooth muscle cells by vasoactive intestinal peptide. Science **216:** 531-533.

59. ROBBERECHT, P., P. CHATELAIN, P. DE NEEF, J.-C. CAMUS, M. WAELBROECK & J. CHRISTOPHE. 1981. Presence of vasoactive intestinal peptide receptors coupled to adenylate cyclase in rat lung membranes. Biochim. Biophys. Acta **678:** 76-82.

60. TATON, G., M. DELHAYE, J.-C. CAMUS, P. DE NEEF, P. CHATELAIN, P. ROBBERECHT & J. CHRISTOPHE. 1981. Characterization of the VIP- and secretin-stimulated adenylate cyclase system from human lung. Pflugers Arch. **391:** 178-182.

61. FRANDSEN, E. K., G. A. KRISHNA & S. I. SAID. 1978. Vasoactive intestinal polypeptide promotes cyclic adenosine 3', 5'-monophosphate accumulation in guinea pig trachea. Br. J. Pharmacol. **62:** 367-369.

62. KITAMURA, S., Y. ISHIHARA & S. I. SAID. 1980. Effect of VIP, phenoxybenzamine and prednisolone on cyclic nucleotide content of isolated guinea-pig lung and trachea. Eur. J. Pharmacol. **67:** 219-223.

63. LAZARUS, S. C., C. B. BASBAUM, P. J. BARNES & W. M. GOLD. 1986. Mapping of VIP receptors by use of an immunocytochemical probe for the intracellular mediator cyclic AMP. Am. J. Physiol. **251:** C115-119.

64. BARNES, P. J. 1986. Neural control of human airways in health and disease. Am. Rev. Respir. Dis. **134:** 1289-1314.

65. CARSTAIRS, J. R. & P. J. BARNES. 1986. Visualization of vasoactive intestinal peptide receptors in human and guinea pig lung. J. Pharmacol. Exp. Ther. **239:** 249-255.

66. LEROUX, P., H. VAUDRY, A. FOURNIER, S. ST.-PIERRE & G. PELLETIER. 1984. Characterization and localization of vasoactive intestinal peptide receptors in the rat lung. Endocrinology **114:** 1506-1512.

67. LEYS, K., A. MORICE, A. HUGHES, M. SCHACHTER & P. SEVER. 1986. Autoradiographic visualization of VIP receptors in human lung. FEBS Lett. **199:** 198-202.

68. SAID, S. I. & R. D. DEY. 1988. VIP in the airways. *In* The Airways: Neural Control in Health and Disease. M. A. Kaliner & P. Barnes, Eds.: 395-416. *In* Lung Biology in Health and Disease. C. Lenfant, Exec. Ed. Marcel Dekker. New York.

69. AMIRANOFF, B. & G. ROSSELIN. 1982. VIP receptors and control of cyclic AMP production. *In* Vasoactive Intestinal Peptide. S. I. Said, Ed.: 307-322. Raven Press. New York.

70. DICKINSON, K. E. J., M. SCHACHTER, C. M. M. MILES, D. H. COY & P. S. SEVER. 1986. Characterization of vasoactive intestinal peptide (VIP) receptors in mammalian lung. Peptides **7:** 791-900.
71. PAUL, S. & S. I. SAID. 1986. Solubilization of active receptors for VIP from guinea pig lung. Peptides **7:** 147-149.
72. PAUL, S. & S. I. SAID. Characterization of receptors for vasoactive intestinal peptide solubilized from the lung. J. Biol. Chem. **262:** 158-162.
73. HASSID, A. 1986. Atriopeptin II decreases cytosolic free Ca in cultured vascular smooth muscle cells. Am. J. Physiol. **251:** C681-C686.
74. BERRIDGE, M. J. & R. F. IRVINE. 1984. Inositol trisphosphate, a novel second messenger in cellular signal transduction. Nature **312:** 315-321.
75. KIKKAWA, U. & Y. NISHIZUKA. 1986. The role of protein kinase C in transmembrane signalling. Ann. Rev. Cell Biol. **2:** 149-178.
76. FURCHGOTT, R. F. 1983. Role of endothelium in responses of vascular smooth muscle. Circ. Res. **53:** 557-573.
77. CHOU, J. & S. I. SAID. 1987. Removal of epithelium attenuates airway relaxation and enhances constriction. Fed. Proc. **46:** 659.
78. FLAVAHAN, N. A., L. L. AARHUS, T. J. RIMELE & P. M. VANHOUTTE. 1985. Respiratory epithelium inhibits bronchial smooth muscle tone. J. Appl. Physiol. **58:** 834-838.
79. SCHWARTZ, J.-C., J. COSTENTIN & J.-M. LECOMTE. 1985. Pharmacology of enkephalinase inhibitors. Trends Pharmacol. Sci. **6:** 472-476.
80. BORSON, D. B., R. CORRALES, S. VARSANO, M. GOLD, N. VIRO, G. CAUGHEY, J. RAMACHANDRAN & J. A. NADEL. 1987. Enkephalinase inhibitors potentiate substance P-induced secretion of $^{35}SO_4$-macromolecules from ferret trachea. Exp. Lung Res. **12:** 21-36.
81. LIU, L. W., T. SATA, E. KUBOTA, S. PAUL & S. I. SAID. 1987. Airway relaxant effect of vasoactive intestinal peptide (VIP): Selective potentiation by phosphoramidon, an enkephalinase inhibitor. Am. Rev. Resp. Dis. **135:** A86.
82. LIU, L. W., T. SATA, E. KUBOTA, S. PAUL, T. IWANAGA, H. FODA & S. I. SAID. VIP is enzymatically degraded in the trachea, probably by an enkephalinase. Unpublished paper presented at the conference Vasoactive Intestinal Peptide and Related Peptides held in New York, N.Y. March 2-4, 1987.
83. JOHNSON, A. R., J. ASHTON, W. W. SCHULZ & E. G. ERDÖS. 1985. Neutral metalloendopeptidase in human lung tissue and cultured cells. Am. Rev. Respir. Dis. **132:** 564-568.
84. COBURN, R. F. & T. TOMITA. 1973. Evidence for nonadrenergic inhibitory nerves in guinea pig trachealis muscle. Am. J. Physiol. **224:** 1072-1080.
85. RICHARDSON, J. 1985. Neurotransmitters and their role in pulmonary physiology. Recent Results Cancer Res. **99:** 29-33.
86. RICHARDSON, J. & J. BELAND. 1976. Nonadrenergic inhibitory nervous system in human airways. J. Appl. Physiol. **41:** 764-771.
87. GIACHETTI, A., S. I. SAID, R. C. REYNOLDS & F. C. KONIGES. 1977. Vasoactive intestinal polypeptide (VIP) in brain: Localization in, and release from, isolated nerve terminals. Proc. Natl. Acad. Sci. **74:** 3424-3428.
88. SAID, S. I., A. GIACHETTI & S. NICOSIA. 1980. VIP: Possible functions as a neural peptide. *In* Neural Peptides and Neuronal Communication. E. Costa & M. Trabucchi, Eds.: 75-82. Raven Press. New York.
89. LUNDBERG, J. M., T. HÖKFELT, G. NILSSON, L. TERENIUS, J. REHFELD, R. ELDE & S. I. SAID. 1978. Peptide neurons in the vagus, splanchnic, and sciatic nerves. Acta Physiol. Scand. **104:** 499-501.
90. IRVIN, C. G., R. BOILEAU, J. TREMBLAY, R. R. MARTIN & P. T. MACKLEM. 1980. Bronchodilation: Noncholinergic, nonadrenergic mediation demonstrated *in vivo* in the cat. Science **207:** 791-792.
91. VENUGOPALAN, G. S., S. I. SAID & J. M. DRAZEN. 1984. Effect of vasoactive intestinal peptide on vagally mediated tracheal pouch relaxation. Resp. Physiol. **56:** 205-216.
92. MATSUZAKI, Y., Y. HAMASAKI & S. I. SAID. 1980. Vasoactive intestinal peptide: A possible transmitter of non-adrenergic relaxation of guinea pig airways. Science **210:** 1252-1253.
93. RUSSELL, J. A. 1980. Nonadrenergic inhibitory innervation in canine airways. J. Appl. Physiol. **48:** 16-22.

94. KARLSSON, J. A. & C. G. A. PERSSON. 1983. Evidence against vasoactive intestinal polypeptide (VIP) as a dilator and in favour of substance P as a constrictor in airway neurogenic responses. Br. J. Pharmacol. **79:** 634-636.

95. KARLSSON, J. A. & C. G. A. PERSSON. 1984. Neither vasoactive intestinal peptide (VIP) nor purine derivatives may mediate nonadrenergic tracheal inhibition. Acta. Physiol. Scand. **122:** 589-598.

96. PALMER, J. B., F. M. C. CUSS & P. J. BARNES. 1986. VIP and PHM and their role in nonadrenergic inhibitory responses in isolated human airways. J. Appl. Physiol. **61:** 1322-1328.

97. DIAMOND, L. & R. A. ALTIERE. 1988. *In* Airway nonadrenergic noncholinergic inhibitory nervous system. The Airways: Neural Control in Health and Disease. M. A. Kaliner & P. Barnes, Eds.: 343-394. *In* Lung Biology in Health and Disease. C. Lenfant, Exec. Ed. Marcel Dekker. New York.

98. SAID, S. I. 1982. Vasoactive peptides in the lung, with special reference to vasoactive intestinal peptide. Exp. Lung. Res. **3:** 343-348.

99. SAID, S. I. 1987. Influence of neuropeptides on airway smooth muscle. Am. Rev. Respir. Dis. **136**(Suppl.): 552-58.

100. SAID, S. I. 1986. Vasoactive intestinal peptide: A brief review. J. Endocrinol. Invest. **9:** 191-200.

101. QUINTON, P. M. & J. BIJMAN. 1983. Higher bioelectrical potentials due to decreased chloride absorption in the sweat glands of patients with cystic fibrosis. N. Engl. J. Med. **308:** 1185-1189.

102. FRIZZELL, R. A., G. RECHKEMMER & R. L. SHOEMAKER. 1986. Altered regulation of airway epithelial cell chloride channels in cystic fibrosis. Science **233:** 558-560.

103. WIDDICOMBE, J. H., M. J. WELSH & W. E. FINKBEINER. Cystic fibrosis decreases the apical membrane chloride permeability of monolayers cultured from cells of tracheal epithelium. Proc. Natl. Acad. Sci. USA **82:** 6167-6171.

104. HEINZ-ERIAN, P., R. D. DEY & S. I. SAID. 1985. Deficient vasoactive intestinal peptide innervation in sweat glands of cystic fibrosis patients. Science **229:** 1407-1408.

105. RICHARDSON, J. B. 1979. Nerve supply to the lungs. Am. Rev. Respir. Dis. **119:** 785-802.

106. DI MARZO, V., J. R. TIPPINS & H. R. MORRIS. 1986. The effect of vasoactive intestinal peptide and calcitonin gene-related peptide on peptidoleukotriene release from platelet activating factor stimulated rat lungs and ionophore stimulated guinea pig lungs. Biochem. Int. **13:** 933-942.

Vasoactive Intestinal Peptide and Renin Secretion[a]

JAMES P. PORTER

Department of Physiology
University of Louisville
Louisville, Kentucky 40292

WILLIAM F. GANONG

Department of Physiology
University of California
San Francisco, California 94143

INTRODUCTION

The renin-angiotensin system plays a major role in maintaining fluid and electrolyte homeostasis. In addition, this hormonal system has been implicated in the development and maintenance of several forms of hypertension. The regulation of renin secretion from the kidney is complex and involves a number of intra- and extrarenal mechanisms. We have been interested for a number of years in the possibility that vasoactive intestinal peptide (VIP) is another agent that contributes to the control of renin release. This hypothesis arose from a chance observation made while investigating the effects of intravenous VIP on pituitary hormone secretion in anesthetized dogs. Subsequent investigations by us and others have clearly established VIP as a renin-releasing factor.[1-3] In the pages that follow, we will review the evidence that links VIP with renin secretion and discuss possible situations where the peptide might play a role as a physiological regulator of renin release.

THE RENIN ANGIOTENSIN SYSTEM

Renin is a protein hormone that is secreted into the circulation by the juxtaglomerular cells of the kidney. Once in the blood, renin acts on a circulating $\alpha2$ globulin, angiotensinogen, to produce the decapeptide, angiotensin I. As angiotensin I passes through the lungs it is converted to the octapeptide, angiotensin II (AII) by converting enzyme. AII has a number of important actions that help regulate fluid and salt

[a] This work was supported in part by United States Public Health Service Grant #HL-29714 and the Smokeless Tobacco Research Council.

balance and arterial pressure. It promotes sodium and water retention by increasing the release of aldosterone and vasopressin and by stimulating drinking behavior.[4,5] AII is a potent vasoconstrictor and can also increase arterial pressure by an action in the brain.[6] It is interesting that in many cases the effects of AII are opposite to those of VIP, that is, VIP is a vasodilator and tends to produce loss of fluid and electrolytes.[7,8] VIP's increase in renin secretion might be thought of as activation of a compensatory feedback mechanism.

CONTROL OF RENIN SECRETION

The control of renin secretion is complex.[9] FIGURE 1 illustrates three primary regulatory mechanisms that are active within the kidney. A specialized region at the beginning of the distal convoluted tubule known as the macula densa comes in contact with the renin-secreting juxtaglomerular cells. A decreased concentration of NaCl in the tubular fluid at this point results in increased renin secretion.[10] A decreased delivery of Cl^- to the macula densa cells appears to be the actual excitatory stimulus.[11] Renin secretion is also controlled by an intrarenal baroreceptor mechanism. A decrease in renal perfusion pressure produces less stretch on the juxtaglomerular cells and induces renin secretion.[12] The juxtaglomerular cells are innervated by sympathetic nerves and release of norepinephrine by these neurons is known to increase renin release.[13] This effect is mediated by a β-adrenergic mechanism.[14] Increased renal sympathetic activity could be generated from important integrating sites in the brain[15] or could result indirectly from reflexes. A decrease in blood volume or systemic arterial pressure is known to reflexively increase renal nerve activity and increase renin secretion.[16,17] Circulating catecholamines can also gain access to these receptors and induce renin release.[18] Several other humoral agents are also known to act within the kidney to affect renin secretion. AII and vasopressin exert an inhibitory effect and the prostaglandins appear to increase renin release.[19,20]

If VIP is a renin-releasing factor, where does it fit into the scheme outlined above? Experiments aimed at determining the mechanism for the effect of VIP on renin secretion will need to take into account possible actions of the peptide to alter renal perfusion pressure, renal handling of NaCl, and reflex control of renal nerves. In the discussion that follows, we will outline evidence that suggests that VIP may not act through any of these mechanisms but instead may produce its effect on renin secretion by a direct action on the juxtaglomerular cells.

EFFECT OF VIP ON RENIN SECRETION RATE

In preliminary studies aimed at determining the effect of intravenous VIP on adrenocorticotropic hormone, we made the chance observation that the peptide also produced an increase in PRA.[21] This increase occurred even if the drop in renal perfusion pressure was experimentally prevented. An increase in PRA could reflect an increased renin secretion, but it could also come about by changes in the metabolism of renin or other components in the renin-angiotensin cascade.

Thus, our very early investigations were aimed at determining if VIP did indeed increase renin secretion rate.[1] Those experiments were performed in anesthetized dogs instrumented with an electromagnetic flow probe on one renal artery. VIP was infused directly into the renal artery, and plasma for determination of plasma renin activity (PRA) was simultaneously collected from the renal vein and femoral artery. The renin secretion rate was calculated by multiplying the renal venous-arterial difference in PRA by the renal plasma flow. Our initial experiments showed clearly that the increase in PRA was indeed due to an increased renin secretion rate (FIG. 2).

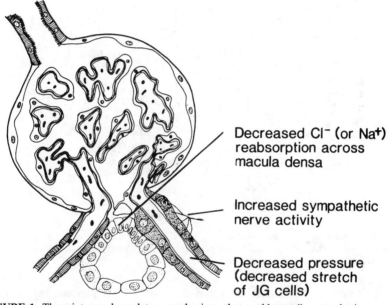

Decreased Cl⁻ (or Na⁺) reabsorption across macula densa

Increased sympathetic nerve activity

Decreased pressure (decreased stretch of JG cells)

FIGURE 1. Three intrarenal regulatory mechanisms that could contribute to the increase in renin secretion produced by VIP. (Modified from W. F. Ganong. Review of Medical Physiology, 13th Edition. Lange Medical Publications. Los Altos, CA.)

EFFECT OF VIP: EXTRARENAL OR INTRARENAL?

In other experiments, we sought to determine whether VIP could exert its effect on renin secretion by acting directly within the kidney.[1] Experiments were performed in pentobarbital-anesthetized dogs. The dose-response to intravenous VIP was compared to the response produced by similar doses administered directly into the renal artery. We found that a 15-minute intravenous infusion of VIP at a rate of 3.3 ng/kg/min increased circulating levels of VIP by 28% but had no effect on plasma renin activity (PRA). Higher doses (13 and 33 ng/kg/min) produced significant increases

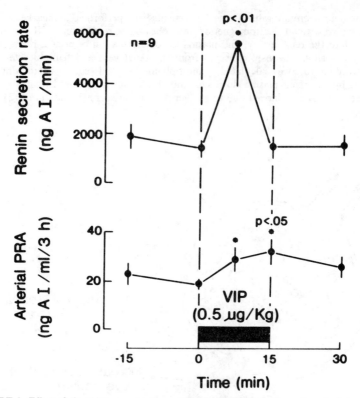

FIGURE 2. Effect of direct intrarenal infusion of VIP on renin secretion rate and plasma renin activity (PRA). The infusion rate (0.5 μg/kg for 15 min) corresponds to 33 ng/kg/min. (Reproduced by permission from Porter & Ganong.[21])

in PRA (FIG. 3). The higher doses also decreased arterial pressure, but in these experiments, renal perfusion pressure was held constant so that changes in systemic pressure were not detected by the kidneys. When VIP was infused directly into the renal artery at the lowest dose (3.3 ng/kg/min), PRA was significantly increased (FIG. 4). These data suggest that the increase in PRA produced by the intrarenal infusion of VIP was due to an action of the peptide within the kidney and not due to a peripheral effect. These data also give us an idea of how much VIP the kidney must "see" to respond with increased renin release. With intravenous infusions, significant effects on PRA were observed when plasma levels of VIP increased from a baseline of 33 pmole/liter to 75 pmole/liter. The direct intrarenal infusion with the lowest dose (3.3 ng/kg/min) increased renal venous levels of VIP to 87 pmole/liter. These data suggest that any stimulus that increases plasma VIP by approximately 2.5-fold might also be expected to increase release of renin.

EFFECT OF VIP: MACULA DENSA MECHANISM?

The data presented above suggest that VIP can act directly on the kidney to increase renin release. Since renal perfusion pressure was not allowed to change, the intrarenal baroreceptor mechanism probably was not responsible for the increase. VIP is known to have profound effects on electrolyte transport in the gut.[8] Could the effects of this peptide on renin release be due to changes in delivery of NaCl to the macula densa? We tested this possibility in a separate group of anesthetized dogs by determining the effect of intrarenal VIP on renal functions. In this group of hydropenic dogs, we found that VIP produced a significant increase in renal blood flow and GFR (TABLE 1). Urine flow and sodium and potassium excretion tended to increase, but the effect was not statistically significant. Since a decrease in Na excretion would be expected in cases where the macula densa mechanism is activated, these data suggest that the increase in renin secretion with VIP occurred through some other mechanism. It should be noted that there are conflicting reports concerning the effect of VIP on renal functions. Using an isolated perfused rat kidney, Rosa et al.[22] reported a significant increase in Na and K excretion with VIP, although in their preparation, renal flow and GFR did not change. On the other hand, in conscious rabbits, urine flow

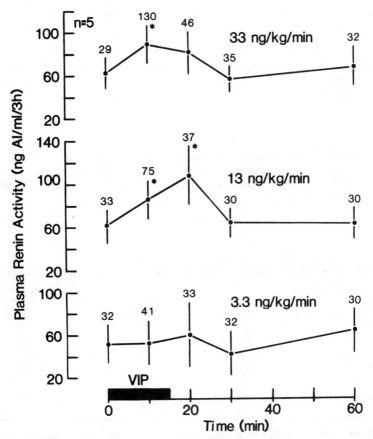

FIGURE 3. Effect of intravenous infusions of VIP on plasma renin activity. All three infusion rates were given to each dog in the same order (3.3, then 13, then 33 ng/kg/min). Mean arterial plasma concentrations of VIP are indicated above the standard error bar for each point; *$p <$ 0.05.

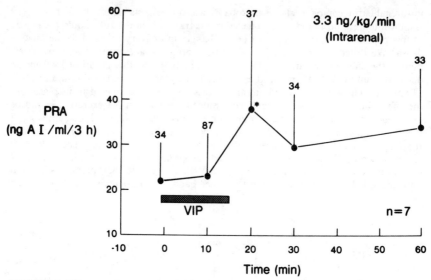

FIGURE 4. Effect on plasma renin activity (PRA) of intrarenal infusion of VIP at a rate of 3.3 ng/kg min. Mean renal venous concentrations of VIP are indicated above the standard error bar of each point; *$p < 0.05$.

decreased while sodium excretion increased,[3] and in humans VIP induced decreases in both urine flow and sodium excretion.[23] Clearly some of these differences are due to the method of administration (intrarenal versus intravenous) and presence or absence of anesthesia.

TABLE 1. Effect of Intrarenal Infusion of VIP on Renal Function[a]

Measure of Function	Control	Infusion	Recovery
Creatinine clearance (ml/min)	20 ± 7	29 ± 7[b]	31 ± 10
Renal blood flow (ml/min)	221 ± 34	281 ± 42[b]	254 ± 40
Urine flow (ml/min)	0.40 ± 0.14	0.65 ± 0.27	0.47 ± 0.20
Sodium excretion (μEq/min)	60 ± 20	107 ± 43	70 ± 28

[a] Values are means ± SE, $n = 7$. Urine was collected from the ureter of the infused kidney for 15-minute periods before, during, and after the infusion of VIP. VIP introduced at a rate of 33 ng/kg/min. Modified with permission from Porter et al.[1]
[b] $p < 0.05$ compared to control.

EFFECT OF VIP: *In Vitro*

Our experiments using whole animals suggested that VIP was not increasing renin secretion by any of the known intrarenal regulatory mechanisms. This led us to consider the possibility that VIP exerted its effect directly on the juxtaglomerular cells. This possibility was tested using an *in vitro* isolated glomerular preparation where the intrarenal baroreceptor and macula densa mechanisms are presumably absent.[2] Glo-

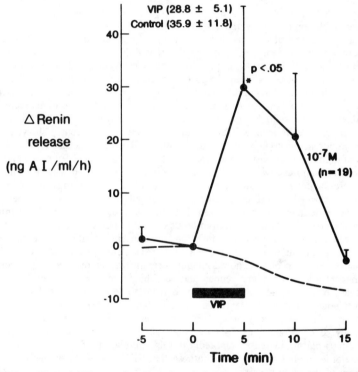

FIGURE 5. Effect of VIP on renin release from isolated superfused glomeruli. Absolute renin concentrations of time 0 samples for VIP- and vehicle-superfused glomeruli are shown in upper left portion of figure. VIP at doses of 10^{-8} and 10^{-9} M also produced a significant increase in renin release; however, 10^{-10} M was not effective. (Reproduced with permission from Porter *et al.*[2])

meruli were isolated from rat kidneys using a series of filters with smaller and smaller openings. The glomeruli, which included some cells that secreted renin, were placed in glass chambers and superfused with a modified Krebs solution. The effect of adding isoproterenol or VIP to the superfusion fluid on renin release was compared. We found that VIP increased renin release from these glomeruli in a dose-related manner (FIG. 5). Isoproterenol was also effective as predicted, a test used to establish the viability of the preparation. Since these glomeruli are presumably denervated and devoid of other mechanisms for regulating renin release, these *in vitro* data suggest that VIP can act directly on the juxtaglomerular cells to stimulate secretion of renin.

PHYSIOLOGICAL ROLE FOR VIP

Our search for a physiological role for VIP in the regulation of renin secretion was hampered somewhat by the unavailability of specific antagonists for the VIP receptor. Given the ubiquitous distribution of VIP in neurons of the central and peripheral nervous system, we hypothesized that VIP in renal nerves might be involved in stimulating renin secretion in situations that clearly involved renal sympathetic activation. There were conflicting reports concerning the existence of VIP in renal nerves. Hokfelt *et al.*[24] reported sparse VIP-ergic innervation of the kidney in the guinea pig, but two other groups reported the absence of VIP immunoreactivity in the kidney.[25,26] We could not demonstrate VIPergic neurons in the dog kidney even though ganglion cells from salivary tissue processed simultaneously showed strong VIP immunoreactivity (unpublished observation). Recently, Barajas *et al.*[27] showed VIP-containing neurons near blood vessels and tubules in kidneys from rats and dogs. However, immunoreactivity could not be conclusively associated with afferent arterioles where the juxtaglomerular cells occur. It seems likely that if these renin-secreting cells are innervated by VIP-containing neurons at all, it is only a sparse innervation.

In vivo experiments in anesthetized dogs support this suggestion. We stimulated the renal nerves directly and measured levels of VIP in renal venous plasma.[28] If VIP was indeed released during the stimulation, the concentration of the peptide in the renal venous effluent would be expected to increase. Lundberg *et al.*[29] showed that electrical stimulation of the chorda-lingual nerve in the cat resulted in an increased VIP concentration in salivary venous plasma. This increase was presumably due to "spillover" of the peptide that was released from VIPergic synapses. In our hands, electrical stimulation of the renal nerves increased renal venous PRA as expected, but had no effect on renal venous VIP.[28] Spillover of neurotransmitter can occur in the kidney, since Oliver *et al.*[30] showed that the concentration of norepinephrine in renal venous plasma increased markedly during stimulation of the renal nerves. Our data, therefore, do not support the hypothesis that VIP is released from neurons during activation of the renal nerves.

If VIP does not act as a neurotransmitter to affect renin secretion, the possibility that the peptide acts as a humoral regulator still remained. VIP is normally found in the plasma, and there are stimuli that are known to increase circulating levels of the peptide. In fact, stimuli such as endotoxemia and neostigmine administration can elevate plasma VIP to levels that would be expected to stimulate renin secretion.[31,32] Of course, circulating VIP is also elevated markedly in certain pathological conditions.[33]

We chose to investigate the possibility for a humoral role for VIP using two approaches. We initially looked at two potent stimuli for renin secretion to determine if plasma levels of VIP increased along with the increase in renin release. In a second approach, we raised plasma levels of endogenous VIP using neostigmine and measured PRA to see if it increased along with the VIP.

EFFECT OF HEMORRHAGE

Four conscious dogs, previously instrumented with indwelling femoral arterial catheters, were subjected to four different levels of hemorrhage. At least three days were allowed to pass between each hemorrhage treatment. Blood for determination of PRA and VIP was collected before and at 15, 30, 45, and 60 minutes after the end of the hemorrhage. In these animals, PRA increased as expected in a manner that was directly related to the volume of blood removed. On the other hand, plasma levels of VIP did not change during any of the hemorrhage treatments.[28] These data suggest that it is highly unlikely that circulating VIP contributes to the increase in PRA induced by hemorrhage.

TABLE 2. Effect of 14 Days of Dietary Sodium Restriction[a]

Day	Sodium Intake (mEq/day)	Sodium Excretion (mEq/day)	Plasma Renin Activity (ngAl/ml/3h)	Plasma VIP (pmole/liter)
−2	28.6 ± 3.7	29.3 ± 3.0	4.1 ± 1.0	33 ± 2
0	0–1.5	30.1 ± 34	3.4 ± 0.8	38 ± 3
1	0–1.5	9.0 ± 3.8[b]	5.2 ± 1.7	33 ± 6
3	0–1.5	3.2 ± 1.0[b]	5.5 ± 1.2	34 ± 6
5	0–1.5	1.9 ± 0.5[b]	8.2 ± 2.7[b]	38 ± 5
7	0–1.5	1.7 ± 0.7[b]	8.6 ± 1.3[b]	33 ± 4
9	0–1.5	1.5 ± 0.6[b]	5.2 ± 0.9	26 ± 2
11	0–1.5	1.4 ± 0.7[b]	7.4 ± 1.5[b]	27 ± 2
14	0–1.5	0.9 ± 0.4[b]	8.0 ± 0.9[b]	32 ± 3

[a] Modified with permission from Porter et al.[28]
[b] $p < 0.05$ compared to day 0.

EFFECT OF DIETARY SODIUM RESTRICTION

Six dogs were fed a low-salt diet for 14 days. Urine was collected in metabolic cages and sodium and potassium excretion was calculated throughout the experiment. Blood samples were collected via venous puncture every two to three days for measurement of VIP and PRA. All dogs showed a marked decrease in sodium excretion during the low-salt diet and PRA increased as expected by the fifth day.[28] Plasma VIP levels, however, did not change (TABLE 2). Here again, a humoral role for VIP in the renin response to salt restriction is unlikely.

EFFECT OF NEOSTIGMINE

Neostigmine is an agent that interferes with the enzymatic breakdown of acetylcholine in synapses. In the presence of neostigmine, acetylcholine is allowed to remain in the synapse longer and hence produce prolonged activation of postsynaptic neurons. Sympathetic and parasympathetic ganglia that involve cholinergic synapses will thus be activated as well as parasympathetic synapses at end organs. Ebeid et al.[32] showed that neostigmine produced a marked increase in circulating VIP. This VIP presumably represented spillover of peptide released from nerve terminals, with neurons in the gut making a large contribution.[32,34]

We gave neostigmine to anesthetized dogs and simultaneously measured plasma levels of VIP and PRA. As might be expected, the neostigmine produced an increase in systemic arterial pressure, so renal perfusion pressure was held constant in these experiments. Plasma VIP was elevated by the neostigmine to levels that we would predict are sufficient to increase renin release. As shown in FIGURE 6, PRA did indeed

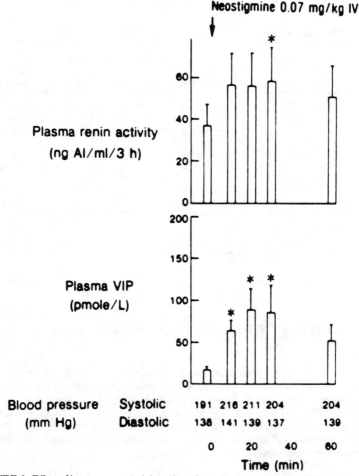

FIGURE 6. Effect of intravenous administration of neostigmine on plasma renin activity, plasma VIP, and arterial pressure; $*p < 0.05$. (Reproduced with permission from Porter et al.[28])

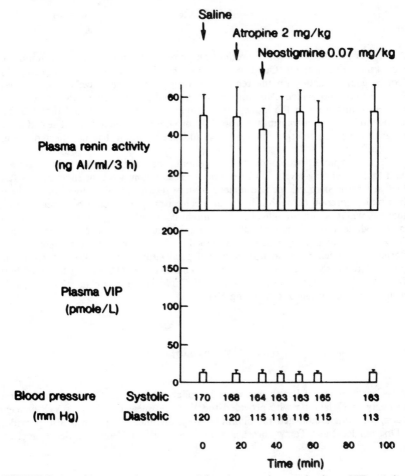

FIGURE 7. Atropine pretreatment prevented the subsequent increase in plasma VIP and plasma renin activity expected with intravenous neostigmine.

increase after neostigmine administration. Obviously, neostigmine could produce a generalized sympathetic activation that would be expected to increase PRA through a neural mechanism without having to invoke a VIP-dependent effect. However, when neural influences were eliminated with either β-adrenergic blockade or renal denervation, the increase in VIP and PRA still occurred.[28] These data strongly suggest that the increased levels of circulating VIP produced by neostigmine were able to stimulate renin secretion. However, the evidence is clearly correlative and not definitive.

In a recent experiment, we used atropine to block the increase in plasma VIP produced by neostigmine. Atropine is a muscarinic receptor antagonist that has also been shown to block the effects of cholinesterase inhibitors on autonomic ganglia.[35] Intravenous atropine (2 mg/kg) completely prevented the increase in VIP and MAP expected with subsequent administration of neostigmine (FIG. 7). Interestingly, the increase in PRA with neostigmine was also prevented. These data strongly support our suggestion that the increase in renin release with neostimine is due to the elevation in plasma VIP.

SUMMARY

VIP has now been shown to produce an increase in renin release in a number of species, including humans. Our work suggests that VIP is capable of producing this effect by a direct action on the renin-secreting juxtaglomerular cells of the kidney. We have found no evidence to support the possibility that VIP produces this effect as a neurotransmitter in the kidney. In this regard, it should be noted that VIP has been identified as a cotransmitter primarily in cholinergic neurons.[36] The kidney is thought to lack cholinergic innervation,[37] and acetylcholine has no effect on renin secretion.[38]

We have explored two conditions where renin secretion is known to increase and found that circulating levels of VIP did not increase along with the increase in PRA. Thus, at least in hemorrhage and dietary sodium restriction, VIP does not appear to affect renin secretion through a humoral mechanism. There could be other untested situations where a humoral effect of VIP might come into play since we have shown that the whole animal is capable of increasing plasma VIP to levels that affect renin release. Studies employing recently developed VIP antagonists have the potential to determine in which physiological or pathological situations VIP contributes to the control of renin secretion. For example, in endotoxic shock, plasma levels of both VIP and PRA are significantly elevated.[31,39] Could the increase in PRA be partly dependent on an action of circulating VIP?

ACKNOWLEDGMENTS

The work reported herein was done in collaboration with Dr. Sami Said of the University of Oklahoma who provided the VIP and measured plasma VIP concentrations with his established radioimmunoassay. Significant input was also provided by Drs. Ian Reid and Terry Thrasher of the University of California, San Francisco.

REFERENCES

1. PORTER, J. P., I. A. REID, S. I. SAID & W. F. GANONG. 1983. Am. J. Physiol. **234:** F306-F310.
2. PORTER, J. P., S. I. SAID & W. F. GANONG. 1984. Neuroendocrinology **36:** 404-408.
3. DIMALINE, R., W. S. PEART & R. J. UNWIN. 1983. J. Physiol. (London) **344:** 379-388.
4. DAVIS, J. O. 1974. The renin/angiotensin system in the control of aldosterone secretion. *In* Angiotensin. I. H. Page & F. M. Bampus, Eds.: 322-336. Springer. New York.
5. REID, I. A., V. L. BROOKS, C. D. RUDOLPH & L. C. KEIL. 1982. Am. J. Physiol. **243:** R82-R91.
6. SEVERS, W. B. & A. E. DANIELS-SEVERS. 1973. Pharmacol. Rev. **25:** 415-449.
7. KREJS, G. J. 1982. Effect of VIP infusion on water and electrolyte transport in the human intestine. *In* Vasoactive Intestinal Peptide. S. I. Said, Ed.: 193-200. Raven Press. New York.
8. SAID, S. I. & V. MUTT. 1970. Science **169:** 1217-1218.
9. DAVIS, J. O. & R. H. FREEMAN. 1976. Physiol. Rev. **56:** 1-56.
10. VANDER, A. J. & R. MILLER. 1964. Am. J. Physiol. **207:** 537-545.

ENTATION

ATION

11. KOTCHEN, T. A., J. H. GALLA & R. G. LUKE. 1978. Kidney Int. **13:** 201-208.
12. TOBIAN, L., A. TOMBOULIAN & J. JANECEK. 1959. J. Clin. Invest. **38:** 605-610.
13. LAGRANGE, R. G., G. H. SLOOP & H. E. SCHMID. 1973. Circ. Res. **33:** 704-712.
14. TAHER, M. S., L. G. MCLAIN, K. M. MCDONALD & R. W. SCHRIER. 1976. J. Clin. Invest. **57:** 459-465.
15. BROSNIHAN, K. B. & C. M. FERRARIO. 1984. Central regulation of renin release. *In* Hypertension and the Brain. G. P. Guthrie, Jr. & I. A. Kotchen, Eds.: 83-112. Futura Publishing Co. Mt. Kisco, NY.
16. AMMONS, W. S., A. L. SANTIESTEBAN, S. KOYAMA & J. W. MANNING. 1980. Am. J. Physiol. **239:** H342-H348.
17. THAMES, M. D., O. M. JARECKI & D. E. DONALD. 1978. Circ. Res. **42:** 237-245.
18. JOHNSON, J. A., J. O. DAVIS, F. R. T. WITTY. 1971. Circ. Res. **29:** 646-653.
19. VANDER, A. J. & G. W. GEELHOED. 1965. Proc. Soc. Exp. Biol. Med. **120:** 399-403.
20. BOLGER, P. M., G. M. EISNER, P. W. RAMWELL & L. M. SLOTKOFF. 1976. Nature **259:** 244-245.
21. PORTER, J. P. & W. F. GANONG. 1982. Relation of vasoactive intestinal polypeptide to renin secretion. *In* Vasoactive Intestinal Peptide. S. I. Said, Ed.: 285-305. Raven Press. New York.
22. ROSA, R. M., P. SILVA, J. S. STOFF & F. H. EPSTEIN. 1985. Am. J. Physiol. **249:** E494-E497.
23. CALAM, J., R. DIMALINE, W. S. PEART, J. SINGH & R. J. UNWIN. 1983. J. Physiol. (London) **345:** 469-475.
24. HOKFELT, T., M. SCHULTZBERG, R. ELDE, G. NILSSON, L. TERENIUS, S. SAID & M. GOLDSTEIN. 1978. Acta Pharmacol. Toxicol. (Copenhagen) **43**(Suppl. II): 79-89.
25. ALM, P., J. ALUMETS, R. HAKASON, CH. OWMAN, N-O. SJOBERG, F. SUNDLER & B. WALLES. 1980. Cell Tissue Res. **205:** 337-347.
26. LARSSON, L. I., J. FAHRENKRUG & O. B. SCHAFFALITZKY DE MUCKADELL. 1977. Science **197:** 1374-1375.
27. BARAJAS, L., K. N. SOKOLSKI & J. LECHAGO. 1983. Neurosci. Lett. **43:** 263-269.
28. PORTER, J. P., T. N. THRASHER, S. I. SAID & W. F. GANONG. 1985. Am. J. Physiol. **249:** F84-F89.
29. LUNDBERG, J. M., A. ANGGARD, J. FAHRENKRUG, T. HOKFELT & V. MUTT. 1980. Proc. Natl. Acad. Sci. USA **77:** 1651-1655.
30. OLIVER, J. A., J. PINTO, R. R. SCIACCA & P. J. CANNON. 1980. Am. J. Physiol. **239:** F371-F377.
31. FREUND, H., A. M. EBEID & J. E. FISCHER. 1981. Surg. Gynocol. Obstet. **152:** 604-606.
32. EBEID, A. M., R. ATTIA, P. SUNDARAM & J. E. FISCHER. 1979. Am. J. Surg. **137:** 123-127.
33. SAID, S. I. & G. R. FALOONA. 1975. N. Engl. J. Med. **293:** 155-160.
34. SAKIO, H., Y. MATSUZAKI & S. I. SAID. 1978. Clin. Res. (Abstract) **26:** 665A.
35. VOLLE, R. L. 1969. Ann. Rev. Pharmacol. **9:** 35-146.
36. LUNDBERG, J. M., T. HOKFELT, M. SCHULTZBERG, K. URANAS-WALLENSTEN, C. KOHLER & S. I. SAID. 1979. Neuroscience **4:** 1539-1559.
37. DIBONA, G. F. 1982. Rev. Physiol. Biochem. Pharmacol. **94:** 75-181.
38. ABE, Y., T. OKAHARA, T. KISHIMOTO, K. YAMAMOTA & J. UEDA. 1973. Am. J. Physiol. **225:** 319-323.
39. SCHALLER, M. D., B. WAEBER, J. NUSSBERGER & H. R. BRUNNER. 1985. Am. J. Physiol. **249:** H1086-H1092.

The Role of Vasoactive Intestinal Peptide and Other Neuropeptides in the Regulation of the Immune Response *in Vitro* and *in Vivo*

ANDRZEJ M. STANISZ, RAFFAELE SCICCHITANO,
AND JOHN BIENENSTOCK

Department of Pathology
Intestinal Diseases Research Unit
McMaster University
Hamilton, Ontario, L8N 3Z5, Canada

INTRODUCTION

A substantial body of evidence exists to suggest that neuropeptides, including vasoactive intestinal peptide (VIP), can modulate immune responses and that they may play an important role in inflammatory disease states.[1] For example, it was shown that VIP is found in increased amounts in the intestinal tissue of patients with Crohn's disease, an inflammatory bowel disease that is associated with severe immunological dysfunction.[2] A similar association between elevated neuropeptide levels and immune abnormalities was found in cystic fibrosis patients.[1]

Most of our observations on the effects of neuropeptides on immunity have been based on *in vitro* studies. Vasoactive intestinal peptide in physiological doses inhibited lymphocyte proliferation.[3,4] The activity of so called "natural killer" cells is also affected by VIP, although there is some controversy regarding this, possibly due to differences in methodologies used.[5,6] Very little is known about their effects *in vivo*. There is evidence, however, that they may have an immunoregulatory role *in vivo*. Vasoactive intestinal peptide appears to play an important role in determining the selective migration of murine T lymphocytes into the intestine.[7] Specific receptors for VIP are present on human[8] and murine lymphocytes,[9] the majority of them on T lymphocytes with an equal distribution among T helper and T suppressor cells. A single class of receptor with dissociation constant in the nanomolar range, which is within the concentration that gives the most pronounced physiological effects, has been described on lymphocytes and lymphoblastic cell lines.[9,10]

Vasoactive intestinal peptide is said to be present in mucosal mast cells[11] and polymorphonuclear leukocytes[12] as well as in neurons and their endings[13] leaving the question of its origin and local synthesis by cells of the immune system as yet unanswered.

Vasoactive intestinal peptide can influence immunity in both direct and indirect ways. Its indirect effects include relaxation of vascular smooth muscle and subsequent vasodilatation at sites of inflammation, modulation of lymphocyte traffic and stimulation of mediator release from mast cells.[1] Secondly VIP can act directly on cells of the immune system often via specific receptors modulating their proliferative responses as in the case of lymphocytes or release of mediators as mentioned above for mast cells. The direct receptor-mediated effect on lymphocytes was shown to be secondary to activation of membrane adenylate cyclase and selective phosphorylation of a specific protein.[14] In this report we will review some of our own observations concerning the effects of VIP on immune responses and compare them to those of other neuropeptides. We have been particularly interested in substance P (SP) and somatostatin (SOM) since these substances, similar to VIP, are found in high concentrations in mucosal tissues where they are thought to act primarily as neurotransmitters, although there is increasing evidence that they act as local immunomodulators. In addition to its effect on immunity, SOM is also a potent inhibitor of VIP synthesis and SP has many physiological actions that appear antagonistic to those of VIP.[1]

LYMPHOCYTE PROLIFERATION

Vasoactive intestinal peptide significantly inhibited *in vitro* concanavalin A (ConA) induced murine splenic and Peyer's patch lymphocyte proliferation (as measured by the incorporation of [^{3}H]thymidine) when cells were incubated with this peptide for 72 hours. This effect was particularly pronounced in the dose range 10^{-7} to $10^{-9} M$. Under identical culture conditions, SOM also had an inhibitory effect. In contrast SP significantly enhanced cell proliferation (FIG. 1).

However, when cells were incubated with neuropeptides for periods less than 24 hours, we were able to demonstrate a dual effect in that SP also caused significant inhibition in cell proliferation of both Peyer's patch (FIG. 2) and splenic lymphocytes. Somatostatin and VIP were always inhibitory and the maximal inhibitory effect was seen after four to six hours' incubation. Other workers, however, have shown that SOM and VIP may also have this dual effect.[15,16]

IMMUNOGLOBULIN SYNTHESIS

The effect of VIP on *in vitro* ConA-induced immunoglobulin synthesis was more complex. Firstly, it appeared to be isotype specific: IgA synthesis was most affected, IgM synthesis less so and IgG synthesis remained virtually unchanged. Secondly its effect was organ specific, that is, it was dependent on the source of lymphocytes. For all the neuropeptides the effects were dose-dependent and optimal in the concentration range 10^{-7} to $10^{-9} M$. FIGURE 3 is a summary of the effects at $10^{-8} M$. For example VIP increased IgM synthesis in Peyer's patch lymphocyte cultures (70%, $p < 0.01$) and increased IgA synthesis by splenic cells (30%, $p < 0.05$). In contrast IgA synthesis by Peyer's patch lymphocytes was significantly inhibited (70%, $p < 0.01$). Somatostatin was always inhibitory particularly for IgA synthesis, whereas SP significantly enhanced IgA synthesis by lymphocytes from spleen (30%, $p < 0.05$) and particularly Peyer's patches (300%, $p < 0.001$).

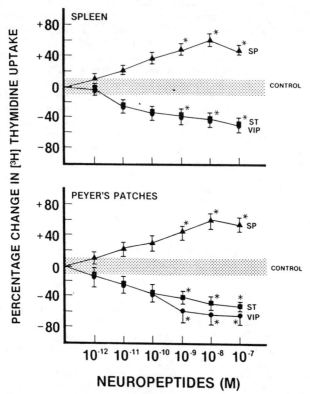

FIGURE 1. The dose-dependent effect of neuropeptides on ConA-induced cell proliferation. Murine spleens and Peyer's patches were aseptically removed and lymphocytes obtained by mechanical dispersion followed by sedimentation over fetal bovine serum. Cells were resuspended in medium (RPMI 1640), buffered with HEPES (10 mM; pH 7.4) and supplemented with L-glutamine, gentamicin (0.05 mg/ml), 10% heat-inactivated fetal calf serum, 2-mercaptoethanol ($2 \times 10^{-5} M$, and 1 μg/ml ConA (referred to as complete medium). Cells were cultured in 96-well, flat-bottomed plates (2.5×10^5 cells/0.2 ml/well) with or without various neuropeptides for 24 hours in an atmosphere of 7% CO_2 : 93% air at 37°C. [^{3}H]thymidine (specific activity 6.7 nmol; 0.5 μCi/well/50 μl) was then added and incubation continued for a further 24 hours. Data are expressed as percent change in [^{3}H]thymidine uptake as compared to controls (no neuropeptides added).

EFFECT OF *IN VIVO* ADMINISTRATION OF NEUROPEPTIDES

Neuropeptides VIP, SP, and SOM were administered continuously *in vivo* by means of miniosmotic pumps (ALZA, Palo Alto, CA) implanted subcutaneously. Mice received approximately 12 μl/day of neuropeptides (starting concentration of 10^{-4} M) for seven days. Cells from Peyer's patches were tested immediately after removal using the reverse hemolytic plaque assay to quantitate isotype-specific plaque-forming cells (PFC), and after 24 hours and seven days in culture with ConA to assess cell proliferation and immunoglobulin synthesis (both PFC and total immunoglobulin concentration in culture supernatants as tested by radioimmunoassay).

Substance P had dramatic enhancing effects on cell proliferation after 24 hours and seven days in culture in the absence of further exposure to this peptide (FIG. 4). Immunoglobulin synthesis was also increased and this effect was particularly evident for IgA (FIG. 5). Serum SP levels in animals treated with this peptide were increased three- to fivefold compared to control animals (saline infusion). Somatostatin, which is an inhibitory neuropeptide *in vitro,* also enhanced cell proliferation and immunoglobulin synthesis when administered *in vivo.* This suggests either that at this dose SOM is a potent enhancer, once again demonstrating the dual actions of neuropeptides or that the observed effect of SOM on immune responses *in vivo* is an indirect one possibly related to its effects on hormone secretion or cells with a regulatory function for lymphocytes. In contrast to the *in vivo* effects of SOM and SP our preliminary data failed to show any significant effects of VIP on cell proliferation or immunoglobulin synthesis. This is not to say that we believe VIP is not an immunomodulating substance *in vivo.* The lack of effect probably reflects an inadequate dose of VIP.

In summary, the effect of administration of SP *in vivo* was similar to its effects when lymphocytes are exposed to this peptide *in vitro.*[4] However, SOM *in vivo* enhanced cell proliferation and immunoglobulin synthesis, whereas VIP appeared to have little if any effect. It is likely that SP administered *in vivo* is acting in a similar fashion to

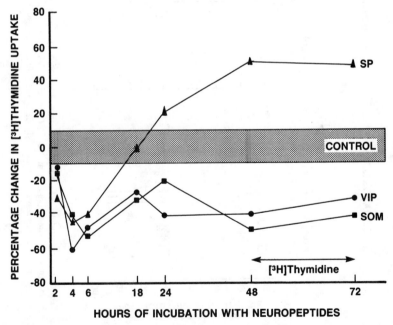

FIGURE 2. The time-dependent effect of neuropeptides on ConA-induced Peyer's patch lymphocyte proliferation. Cells were incubated in complete medium with neuropeptides ($10^{-8} M$) for the times indicated on the abscissa. After extensive washing cells were resuspended in complete medium without neuropeptides and incubation continued for a total of 72 hours. For the last 24 hours of incubation [^{3}H]thymidine was added. Culture conditions and calculation of data as described in FIGURE 1.

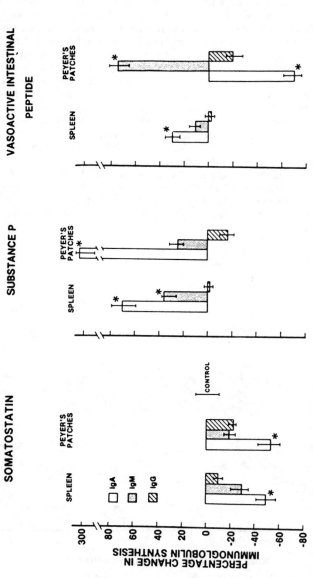

FIGURE 3. The effect of neuropeptides on ConA-induced immunoglobulin synthesis. Cells (2.5×10^6/ml; total volume 2 ml) in 24-well plates were cultured in complete medium with neuropeptides at 10^{-8} M for seven days. Immunoglobulin concentration in culture supernatants was measured by solid-phase inhibition-type radioimmunoassay as previously described.[4] Data expressed as percent change compared to control.

that *in vitro*. Vasoactive intestinal peptide and SOM *in vivo,* however, could be acting indirectly through their actions on accessory cells with a regulatory function on lymphocytes or through stimulation or inhibition of hormone secretion.

We therefore provide evidence that the neuropeptides SOM, SP, and VIP can significantly alter immune responses *in vitro* and that SOM and SP also modulate immunity *in vivo.* These effects are probably mediated by binding to specific surface membrane receptors for neuropeptides on lymphocytes or other immunocompetent cells. Such receptors for VIP on murine lymphocytes have been described.[9] Similarly SP receptors have been reported to be present on human peripheral blood T cells[17] and the human B lymphoblastic cell line IM-9.[18] Somatostatin receptors were described

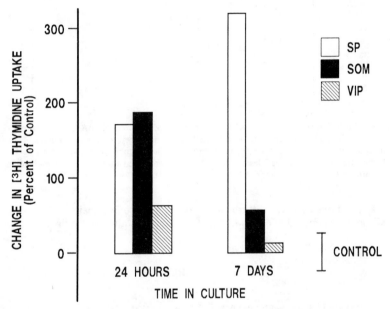

FIGURE 4. The effect of neuropeptides administered *in vivo* on ConA-induced Peyer's patch lymphocyte proliferation. Cells were obtained from mice that had received a continuous infusion of saline or various neuropeptides for seven days. Cells were cultured in complete medium for 24 hours or seven days and [³H]thymidine was added immediately or for the last 24 hours of culture, respectively. Data expressed as percent change compared to control.

on human monocytes and lymphocytes.[19] We have recently reported that murine splenic and Peyer's patch lymphocytes express surface membrane SP receptors,[20] and we have preliminary evidence that they also express SOM receptors. It is interesting to note that we found that lymphocytes from Peyer's patch had three to five times more SP receptors per cell when compared to splenic cells. This finding may in fact help us to understand why Peyer's patch lymphocytes are preferentially affected by neuropeptides.

We believe that various neuropeptides and presumably the nervous system are involved in immune-regulation, and it is important to realize that *in vivo* they probably act in conjunction in the homeostasis of the immune system. Therefore, diseases or

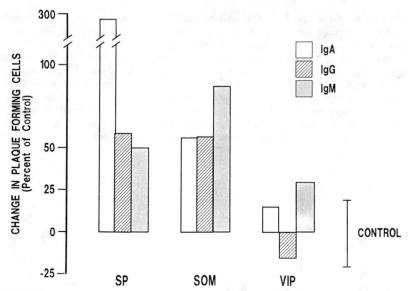

FIGURE 5. The effect of neuropeptides administered *in vivo* on ConA-induced immunoglobulin synthesis by Peyer's patch lymphocytes. Cells, from neuropeptide-treated animals, were cultured in complete medium for seven days. Isotype-specific plaques were quantitated by the reverse hemolytic plaque assay as described.[21] Data are presented as the percent change in plaque-forming cell numbers compared to controls.

manipulations that will disturb their natural balance and their levels, in addition to all the physiological effects, will also be reflected in altered immunity.

REFERENCES

1. PAYAN, D. G., J. P. MCGILLIS & E. J. GOETZL. 1986. Neuroimmunology. Adv. Immunol. **39:** 299-323.
2. BISHOP, A. E., J. M. POLAK, M. G. BRYANT, S. R. BLOOM & S. HAMILTON. 1980. Abnormalities of vasoactive intestinal polypeptide-containing nerves in Crohn's disease. Gastroenterology **79:** 853-860.
3. OTTAWAY, C. A., C. BERNAERTS, B. CHAN & G. R. GREENBERG. 1983. Specific binding of vasoactive intestinal peptide to human circulating mononuclear cells. Can. J. Physiol. Pharmacol. **61:** 664-671.
4. STANISZ, A. M., D. BEFUS & J. BIENENSTOCK. 1986. Differential effects of vasoactive intestinal peptide, substance P and somatostatin on immunoglobulin synthesis and proliferation by lymphocytes from Peyer's patches, mesenteric lymph nodes, and spleen. J. Immunol. **132:** 152-156.
5. ROLA-PLESZCZYNSKI, M., D. BOLDUE & S. ST-PIERRE. 1985. The effects of vasoactive intestinal peptide on human natural killer cell function. J. Immunol. **135:** 2569-2573.
6. KRCO, C. J., A. GORES & V. L. W. GO. 1986. Gastrointestinal regulatory peptides modulate *in vitro* immune reactions of mouse lymphoid cells. Clin. Immunol. Immunopathol. **39:** 308-318.
7. OTTAWAY, C. A. 1984. *In vitro* alteration of receptors for vasoactive intestinal peptide changes the *in vivo* localization of mouse T cells. J. Exp. Med. **160:** 1054-1069.

8. DANEK, A., M. S. O'DORISIO, T. M. O'DORISIO & J. M. GEORGE. 1983. Specific binding sites for vasoactive intestinal peptide on nonadherent peripheral blood lymphocytes. J. Immunol. **131:** 1173-1177.
9. OTTAWAY, C. A. & G. R. GREENBERG. 1984. Interaction of vasoactive intestinal peptide with mouse lymphocytes: Specific binding and the modulation of mitogen responses. J. Immunol. **132:** 417-423.
10. BEED, E. A., M. S. O'DORISIO, T. M. O'DORISIO & T. S. GAGINELLA. 1983. Demonstration of a functional receptor for vasoactive intestinal polypeptide on Molt 4b T lymphoblasts. Reg. Peptides **6:** 1-12.
11. CUTZ, E., W. CHAN, N. S. TRACK, A. GOTH & S. I. SAID. 1978. Release of vasoactive intestinal polypeptide in mast cells by histamine liberators. Nature **275:** 661-662.
12. O'DORISIO, M. S., T. M. O'DORISIO, S. CATLAND & S. BALCERZAK. 1980. Vasoactive intestinal polypeptide as a biochemical marker for polymorphonuclear leukocytes. J. Lab. Clin. Med. **96:** 666-672.
13. PEARSE, A. G. E., J. M. POLAK & S. R. BLOOM. 1977. The newer gut hormones. Cellular sources, physiology, pathology, and clinical aspects. Gastroenterology **72:** 746-761.
14. O'DORISIO, S. M., N. S. HERMINA, T. M. O'DORISIO & S. P. BALCERZAK. 1981. Vasoactive intestinal polypeptide modulation of lymphocyte adenylate cyclase. J. Immunol. **127:** 2551-2554.
15. PAWLIKOWSKI, M., H. STEPIEN, J. KUNERT-RADEK & A. V. SCHALLY. 1985. Effect of somatostatin on the proliferation of mouse spleen lymphocytes *in vitro*. Biochem. Biophys. Res. Com. **129:** 52-55.
16. NORDLIND, K. & V. MUTT. 1986. Influence of beta-endorphin, somatostatin, substance P and vasoactive intestinal peptide on the proliferative response of human peripheral blood T lymphocytes to mercuric chloride. Int. Arch. Allergy Appl. Immun. **80:** 326-328.
17. PAYAN, D. G., D. R. BREWSTER, A. MISSIRIAN-BASTIAN & E. J. GOETZL. 1984. Substance P recognition by a subset of human T lymphocytes. J. Clin. Invest. **74:** 1532-1539.
18. PAYAN, D. G., D. R. BREWSTER & E. J. GOETZL. 1984. Stereospecific receptors for substance P on cultured human IM-9 lymphoblasts. J. Immunol. **133:** 3260-3264.
19. BHATHENA, S. J., J. LOVIE, G. P. SCHECHTER, R. S. REDMAN, L. WAHL & L. RECANT. 1981. Identification of human mononuclear leukocytes bearing receptors for somatostatin and glucagon. Diabetes **30:** 127-131.
20. STANISZ, A. M., R. SCICCHITANO, P. DAZIN, J. BIENENSTOCK & D. G. PAYAN. Distribution of substance P receptors on murine spleen and Peyer's patch T and B cells. J. Immunol. **139:** 749-754.
21. GRONOWICZ, E. A., A. COUTINHO & F. MELCHERS. 1976. A plaque assay for all cells secreting Ig of a given type or class. Eur. J. Immunol. **6:** 588-590.

Vasoactive Intestinal Peptide as a Modulator of Lymphocyte and Immune Function[a]

C. A. OTTAWAY[b]

Department of Medicine
St. Michael's Hospital
University of Toronto
Toronto, Ontario, Canada

INTRODUCTION

Immunoregulatory mechanisms are crucial to our understanding of immunology.[1] Although it has been established that many aspects of the control of immune responses are exerted through mechanisms that are entirely autonomous to the immune system, it is now clear that a variety of potentially important regulatory relationships may exist between the immune and nervous systems in the intact animal.[2,3] A direct means by which signals arising in the nervous system may influence immunological responses in particular tissues is through the ability of lymphoid cells to recognize and respond to neuropeptides. Several features suggest that neuropeptide-mediated immunoregulation may be especially relevant to the intestine.

First, the intestine is both a very richly innervated and an extensively lymphoid tissue (FIG. 1). Neuropeptide-containing nerves, which are found throughout the body, are present within a minority of the nerves of the extrinsic innervation[4] (vagus and splanchnic nerves) of the gut, but are especially abundant within the nerves serving the intestinal submucosa and mucosa.[5,6] Large numbers of lymphoid cells are found within the epithelial layer of the intestine (intraepithelial lymphocytes), within the lamina propria, and in the aggregated lymphoid tissues such as the Peyer's patches.[7] Although a complete picture of the peptidergic-innervation of the lymphoid aggregates of the intestine is not yet available, the extensive ramification of peptidergic nerves within the mucosa suggests that close proximity of neural structures to lymphoid cells within the lamina propria and the intraepithelial layer may be readily achieved.

Second, a number of neuropeptides that are found in the intestine have been implicated as potential immunoregulators. These include substance P,[8-10] somatostatin,[9-10] and VIP. The concept that VIP, one of the most abundant neuropeptides in the gut,[6,11] may function as an immunoregulatory molecule has been suggested by many different lines of investigation from a number of laboratories.

The purpose of this chapter is to examine some of the major lines of evidence for

[a] Grant support was received from the Medical Research Council.

[b] Address for correspondence: Dr. C. A. Ottaway, Room 6360 Medical Sciences Building, University of Toronto, 1 King's College Circle, Toronto, Ontario, Canada M5S 1A8.

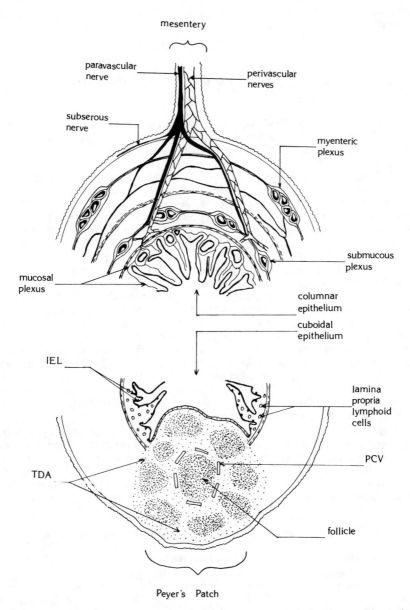

FIGURE 1. Diagram illustrating the enteric neural and immunological structures. The top half (after Furness and Costa[11]) shows the distribution of nerves and plexuses in a section of the intestine. The bottom half illustrates features of the lymphoid intestine. (IEL, intraepithelial lymphocytes; TDA, thymus-dependent areas of the internodular regions where T cells predominate; PCV, specialized postcapillary venules that serve as the point of entry of blood-borne lymphocytes into Peyer's patches). The neural and lymphoid elements are shown separately only for convenience.

this concept, and to present some of the approaches that are being used in this laboratory.

SPECIFIC RECEPTORS FOR VIP ON LYMPHOID CELLS

The specific binding of radiolabeled VIP to human blood lymphoid cells has been reported now by a number of different workers (TABLE 1). Features of these reports are of interest both because of areas of agreement and because of areas in which they disagree.

Although these studies used different media, various conditions of pH, ionic strength, and temperature, a variety of definitions of specific versus nonspecific binding, different means for the radioiodination of the peptide, and even VIP of different sources (i.e., native, synthetic, or derivatized VIP), they all indicate binding properties for the high-affinity specific binding sites on peripheral blood mononuclear cells that are remarkably similar (TABLE 1). Furthermore, these studies all suggest that this high-affinity binding of VIP has the kinetics, temperature dependence, reversibility, saturability, and marked molecular specificity for VIP as a competitor compared to peptides that are homologous to VIP that one would expect for a cell surface receptor.

In contrast, there is much less agreement regarding the presence or properties of low-affinity sites for VIP on human lymphoid cells (TABLE 1). Scatchard analyses of the inhibition of tracer binding have suggested two classes of VIP binding sites in some studies, but not in others (TABLE 1). A practical point may contribute to some of these discrepancies in that those studies that suggest multiple classes of binding sites have employed definitions of noninhibitable or nonspecific binding using substantially higher concentrations of unlabeled VIP $(1-10 \ \mu M)$[12,15,16] than those that have not $(0.05-0.1 \ \mu M)$.[13,14] A more important feature may be that the binding properties of particular cell populations within the peripheral blood mononuclear (PBM) preparations may in fact be heterogeneous.

Several observations suggest that there are differences in the VIP binding properties of subpopulations of human lymphoid cells, but there is no general agreement, as yet, as to which specific subpopulations express high-affinity VIP receptors (TABLE 2). For example, Wiik and coworkers enriched for monocytes from PBM using a centrifugation method[15] and found a high affinity and capacity for VIP binding, but Calvo et al.[16] were unable to detect specific binding of VIP to monocytes enriched by

TABLE 1. Specific Receptors for VIP Identified on Human Lymphoid Cells[a]

| High-Affinity | | Low-Affinity | | |
K_D	Sites/Cell	K_D	Sites/Cell	Reference
2.4	4800	250	10,800	Guerrero et al.[12]
4.7	1700	not detected		Danek et al.[15]
2.4	2040	not detected		Ottaway et al.[14]
2.2	4800	140	19,800	Wiik et al.[15]
1.1	2760	800	480,000	Calvo et al.[16]

[a] Results are the mean values found in that particular study. The dissociation constant K_D is expressed in units of $10^{-10} \ M$ VIP.

TABLE 2. High-Affinity Specific Receptors for VIP Identified on Human Blood Lymphoid Cell Subpopulations[a]

Fraction Studied	K_D	Sites/Cell	Reference
T enriched	4.7	1700	Danek et al.[13]
T enriched	not detected		Calvo et al.[16]
T depleted	2.0	3000	Calvo et al.[16]
T enriched	2.0	2800	Lay et al.[17]
T depleted	4.3	1400	Lay et al.[17]
Monocytes	2.5	9600	Wiik et al.[15]
Monocytes	not detected		Calvo et al.[16]
LGL enriched	3.9	2400	Lay et al.[17]
B enriched	4.7	600	Lay et al.[17]

[a] Results are the mean values found in that particular study. The K_D is expressed in units of $10^{-10}\,M$ VIP.

adherence separation methods. It is possible that monocytes isolated by these different approaches differ in their state of activation.

Other important disagreements also exist. Danek and coworkers identified high-affinity receptors on preparations that consisted predominantly of T cells prepared by nylon wool filtration of PBM.[13] In contrast, Calvo et al.[16] fractionated PBM using rosetting with sheep erythrocytes into T-enriched and T-depleted populations and could only detect specific binding within the T-depleted population (TABLE 2). My colleagues and I have used a similar rosetting fractionation strategy[17] and found that specific binding could be measured in both populations, but that the affinity and the binding capacity for VIP was approximately twofold higher in the T-enriched than in the T-depleted fraction (TABLE 2).

Calvo and his coworkers postulated that B cells and large granular lymphocytes (LGL), a minority population of PBM that support natural killer (NK) cell activity, that might be isolated with T cells by filtration methods may be the only subpopulations that express high-affinity receptors.[16] In our studies,[17] we further fractionated T-depleted populations into B-cell-enriched and LGL-enriched fractions using percoll density gradient centrifugation. We found differences in the specific binding of VIP in these populations, but the affinity of the binding was less than that found with T-enriched preparations (TABLE 2).

The diversity of these findings may relate, at least in part, to the difficulties inherent in obtaining purified preparations of subpopulations of lymphocytes by physical methods. They also emphasize, however, that studies of the binding of a radiolabeled peptide to cell populations yield parameters that reflect the number-averaged behavior of the cells studied, and that the interpretation of these results is difficult if heterogeneity exists in the binding of the peptide to different cell types. The extent to which particular types of lymphoid cells participate in the binding of VIP has important functional implications, however, and other means for determining the ability of cells of particular immunological phenotypes to recognize VIP will be needed before a complete picture is available.

In this regard, it is noteworthy that specific binding of VIP has been found with the MOLT-4b cell line.[18] This is a malignant T cell line, originally from a patient with acute lymphoblastic leukemia, and its binding properties ($K_D = 73 \times 10^{-10}\,M$, receptor density approximately 15,000/cell[18]) differ substantially from those found with circulating lymphocytes of healthy subjects (TABLES 1, 2), supporting the idea that VIP recognition capabilities may be heterogeneous among lymphoid cell populations. The interaction of this cell line with VIP has been very elegantly exploited by O'Dorisio and her colleagues, and has permitted studies in which radiolabeled VIP has been specifically cross-linked to a 47,000-dalton surface protein of intact MOLT-4b cells.[19] This protein is presumably an integral part of the VIP receptor of these cells, and strongly supports the reality of VIP receptors on lymphoid cells. Furthermore, it is expected that this work may soon yield a specific antibody that could be used to probe the structure and function of the VIP receptor, and to determine whether the VIP receptor of this cell line is similar to or different from those on normal lymphoid cells.

In parallel with our studies of the differential binding of radiolabeled VIP to different PBM fractions (TABLE 2), we have investigated the binding of fluorescent polystyrene beads that had been covalently coated with VIP to single lymphoid cells that were colabeled with fluorescent antibodies directed to specific surface determinants.[17] We found that the VIP-coated beads bound to the surface of individual lymphocytes and inhibited the specific binding of [^{125}I]VIP to the cell suspensions in a dose-dependent manner. Even at saturation, however, when the specific binding of radiolabeled VIP was completely blocked, only a minority of the cells in suspension displayed binding of the beads. Using dual-label flow cytometry to analyze for the presence of beads and surface markers, we found that only one-third of T cells expressing the CD3, CD4, or CD8 determinants actually participated in the binding of the VIP-coated beads. We also found the ability to bind the VIP-coated beads among two important minority populations of PBM. Within the various PBM fractions, there was a consistent minority population (approximately 15%) of B cells, and a regular proportion (about 30%) of LGL that expressed the CD16 surface determinant, which is a phenotypic feature of cells displaying NK cell activity, that also bound the beads.[17] Taken together with the observations of differences in the VIP-binding parameters of different PBM fractions (TABLE 2), these observations support the notion that the ability to recognize VIP is markedly heterogeneous. There appear to be major differences in the VIP recognition capabilities between major subpopulations of circulating lymphocytes, and heterogeneity even within given subpopulations.

High-affinity specific receptors for VIP have also been identified on lymphoid cells of both mice and rats. The binding capacity for VIP, determined by analyses of tracer

TABLE 3. High-Affinity Specific Receptors for VIP Identified on Lymphocytes of Experimental Animals[a]

Source of Cells	K_D	Sites/Cell
Mice[20]		
Subcutaneous lymph node	2.0	2760
Mesenteric lymph node	2.2	2150
Spleen	2.2	880
Peyer's patch	2.4	490
Thymus	1.9	150
Rats[21]		
Blood	0.5	1560
Spleen	1.0	2760
Thymus	not detected	

[a] Results are the mean values for that study. K_D is expressed as 10^{-10} M VIP.

TABLE 4. The Effect of Selective Killing of Lymphocytes on the Specific Binding of VIP to MLN[a]

Determinant	Percent Cells Killed	Percent Inhibition of Binding
Thy-1.2	53 (3)	91 (7)
Lyt-1.2	39 (3)	76 (6)
L3T4	36 (5)	59 (3)
Lyt-2.2	24 (6)	3 (9)

[a] Mesenteric lymph node lymphocytes (MLN) were treated with monoclonal antibodies to the determinants shown in the presence of complement, and the specific binding of [^{125}I]VIP to the treated cells was measured. The results are the means (SD) of three experiments with each condition.

dilution studies, varies with the tissue source of the lymphocytes in both these animals (TABLE 3), and once again focuses interest on the question of heterogeneity. We have shown previously that, for mice, enrichment of lymph node lymphocytes for T cells enhances the observed VIP binding, and that the distribution of VIP-binding capacity expressed by lymphocyte suspensions obtained from different secondary lymphoid organs is positively correlated with the proportion of T cells within the preparations.[20]

We have also explored the heterogeneity of the murine cellular distribution of VIP binding properties using a different strategy,[22] namely the effect of complement-mediated cytotoxicity permitted by antibodies directed to distinct cell surface determinants of murine cells on the ability of mesenteric lymph node (MLN) cells to bind VIP (TABLE 4). Antibodies to mouse T-cell antigens such as Thy-1, Lyt-1, and Lyt-2 have been used extensively to characterize T-cell subpopulations and their functions. Treatment of MLN with complement alone, or antibodies to Thy-1, Lyt-1, or Lyt-2 in the absence of complement, had no effect on the amount of VIP specifically bound by the cells. But when MLN were treated with anti-Thy-1 plus complement, more than 90% of the specific binding of VIP by the cells was eliminated even though only about 50% of the cells were killed (TABLE 4). High densities of the Thy-1 antigen are expressed by all T cells,[23] and thus this effect is consistent with the view that T cells predominantly account for the specific VIP binding expressed by MLN.

In contrast, the Lyt-2 antigen (a homologue to the human CD8 determinant) is expressed by only a minority of mature murine T cells,[23] and, although cytoxicity directed by antisera to this marker killed a proportion of MLN, this treatment did not affect the amount of VIP specifically bound to the cells (TABLE 4). Treatment of MLN with anti-Lyt-1 plus complement, however, eliminated approximately 75% of the specific binding of VIP while killing about one-third of the cells. It is known that Lyt-1 antigen can be detected on virtually all T (i.e., Thy-1 bearing) cells, but is expressed with higher density on T cells that do not bear the Lyt-2 determinant,[23] and cells that express Lyt-1 but not Lyt-2 are more easily killed by anti-Lyt-1-directed cytotoxicity.[23] The discrepancy between the effects of anti-Lyt-1- and anti-Lyt-2-mediated killing on VIP binding imply that a large proportion of the VIP specifically bound by T cells is on Lyt-2 cells.

Another important subpopulation of mature T cells is those cells that express the L3T4 (homologue of the human CD4) determinant. T cells that express this antigen account for helper-inducer activities in many assays and are restricted to class II major histocompatibility (MHC) reactivity,[24] whereas those expressing Lyt-2 predominantly act as suppressor-cytotoxic cells and are restricted to class I MHC recognition.[25] Cytotoxic treatment in the presence of anti-L3T4-disrupted specific VIP binding more effectively than anti-Lyt-2 treatment, but had less effect than either Lyt-1- or Thy-1-targeted cell killing (TABLE 4).

Thus, VIP recognition ability is not uniformly expressed by all T cells, even within a single tissue source such as MLN. Interestingly, however, in mice and rats the immature T cell population of the thymus has been found to have extremely low or undetectable levels of specific VIP binding (TABLE 3). This dichotomy between the VIP binding properties of mature T cells and thymocytes raises the question of where and how VIP receptor expression is acquired by T cells during their development. It is noteworthy that VIP-like immunoreactive nerve profiles have been identified deep within the thymic cortex of the rat,[26] and if VIP receptor expression develops during thymic maturation, it may do so only late in intrathymic development.

Overall, it appears that, for both humans and mice, VIP receptors are better expressed by T cells than non-T cells. In both species there appears to be substantial heterogeneity in the expression of VIP receptors by major phenotypic subsets of T cells, and, at least in humans, heterogeneity of VIP receptor expression has been identified in other important minority populations of lymphocytes such as B cells and LGL. This apparently discontinuous distribution of VIP receptors within the lymphocyte repertoire suggests that interactions of lymphocytes with VIP might be able to exert diverse and yet selective effects on the immune function of the lymphocytes that recognize the neuropeptide.

EFFECTS OF VIP ON LYMPHOID CELL FUNCTION

Similar to the functional VIP receptors that have been identified on a variety of nonlymphoid tissues,[27] the binding of VIP to its receptors on lymphoid cells appears to be immediately coupled to intracellular mechanisms via the production of cAMP. Many workers have demonstrated the rapid accumulation of intracellular cAMP in human PBM populations in response to VIP,[12,14,16] and the same is true for MOLT-4b[18] and murine lymphoid cells (Ottaway, unpublished observations).

Very early on in the development of investigations aimed at VIP as an immunoregulator, O'Dorisio and her colleagues[28] showed that VIP was a potent stimulator of adenylate cyclase activation in preparations of PBM, T-enriched PBM, and MOLT-4b lymphoblasts. These observations, together with the repeated identification of lymphoid cell, high-affinity VIP receptors, and the demonstration of VIP-mediated activation of cAMP-dependent protein kinases in both PBM[29] and MOLT-4b cells,[30] suggest that VIP receptor-bearing lymphoid cells contain the metabolic machinery that would permit major intracellular effects in response to the peptide.

Indeed, the presence of VIP in a variety of standardized immunological assays

TABLE 5. Effects of VIP on Human Blood Lymphoid Cells

1. Activation of adenylate cyclase.[28]
2. Activation of cAMP-dependent protein kinases.[29,30]
3. Modulation of NK cell activity.[31,32]
4. Modulation of mitogen-stimulated immunoglobulin production.[32]
5. Modulation of T cell proliferative responses.[33]

TABLE 6. Effects of VIP on Lymphoid Cells of Experimental Animals

1. Modulation of T cell mitogen-stimulated proliferation.[20,34,35]
2. Modulation of mitogen-stimulated immunoglobulin production.[34]
3. Modulation of mixed lymphocyte reactions.[35]
4. Exposure of T cells to VIP modulates the expression of VIP receptors.[36]
5. Modulation of VIP receptors on T cells decreases the rate of migration of the cells into Peyer's patches and mesenteric lymph nodes *in vivo*.[36,37]
6. Direct infusion of VIP modulates the traffic of lymphocytes through lymph nodes *in vivo*.[38]

has been shown to modulate a diversity of functions of human and murine lymphocytes (TABLES 5, 6). The molar potency and the specificity of VIP as a modulator in these assays has been largely consistent with the VIP binding characteristics that have been identified in the receptor studies, suggesting that these effects are most likely mediated directly by receptor occupancy. The cellular mechanisms that are being controlled, however, are not yet entirely clear.

For example, the effect of VIP on NK cell activity is,[31,32] at least initially, explicable by the recognition that some LGL can bind the peptide.[17] But the extent to which the modulatory effect of VIP on this activity reflects changes in the activation of the NK cell, the release of killing factors, or interactions of the NK cell with the target cell are not known.

The mechanism of the observed effects of VIP on immunoglobulin production in mitogen-stimulated cultures[32,34] may also be complex. Stanisz *et al.*[34] have shown that the degree of modulation exerted by VIP differs both with the isotype of immunoglobulin examined and the tissue source of the lymphocytes. The extent to which these effects are due to direct effects on VIP receptor-bearing B cells, as opposed to regulation of B cell function exerted by receptor-bearing T cells or other mechanisms, is at present an open question. The resolution of these questions, however, is important if we are to more fully understand the ways in which VIP functions as a regulator of immune processes.

Many aspects of the autonomous control of immune responses depend upon two major features: regulation (positive and negative) mediated by interactions between different subpopulations of lymphocytes, especially T cells, and the activation of other cells by signals from inducer subpopulations of cells.[1] One signal that plays a fundamental role in the regulation of T-cell responses is the lymphokine interleukin-2 (IL2, T-cell growth factor).[39] Recent work in this laboratory has examined the effect of VIP on the production of IL2 by murine MLN during stimulation by the mitogen ConA.[22] Supernatants were harvested from ConA-stimulated cultures at different times after activation, and their ability to support the growth of the IL2-dependent HT-2 cell line was examined. The supernatants from cultures stimulated in the presence of VIP were much less able to support the growth of the IL2-dependent cells (TABLE 7), and the effect of VIP on this activity was dose-dependent (TABLE 8). Because the responder cells were found not to have the ability to specifically bind VIP, and because the addition of VIP to the responder cells had no effect on their response to directly administered IL2,[22] it was concluded that the exposure of the initial MLN cultures to VIP had modulated their production of the interleukin. The production of IL2 by ConA-stimulated murine cell cultures has been shown by others to depend almost entirely on the activity of L3T4+, Lyt2-ve T cells.[40,41] Thus, the effect of VIP on IL2 production is most easily interpreted as a direct effect of the peptide on the L3T4+ VIP receptor-bearing lymphocytes (TABLE 4).

TABLE 7. The Effect of VIP on the IL-2 Activity of Mitogen-Stimulated Lymphocyte Cultures[a]

Time Harvested	No VIP in Culture	10^{-7} M VIP in Culture
24 h	122.4 (11.4)	44.9 (4.8)
48 h	115.3 (7.4)	76.7 (2.9)
96 h	61.5 (5.8)	37.4 (9.2)

[a] Murine mesenteric lymph node lymphocytes were stimulated with the mitogen ConA in the presence or absence of VIP and the culture supernatants were harvested at the times shown. These supernatants were tested for their ability to support the growth of IL-2-dependent HT2 cells. The results represent the means (SD) of triplicate measures of three experiments for each condition in which the uptake of [^{3}H]thymidine by the HT 2 cells (cpm $\times$ 10^{-3}/well) was measured.

The ability of VIP to regulate the production of this interleukin is important for two reasons. First, it places VIP-mediated immunoregulation directly within the realm of the major "autonomous" immunoregulatory mechanisms. Second, it suggests that functional regulatory effects of the peptide can be transduced into more remote effects on cells that may not themselves have the ability to recognize the peptide.

In addition to its effects on diverse immune responses, VIP may also play an important regulatory role in the *in vivo* migration of lymphocytes. The migration of lymphocytes from one tissue to another facilitates the initiation and the propagation of immune responses and is an important process in the immunological integrity of the intestine.[42] Moore[38] has shown, in sheep, that the acute infusion of VIP into the afferent lymphatic of cannulated lymph nodes dramatically decreased the output of lymphocytes from the node. In mice, we have obtained evidence (FIG. 2) that implicates local interactions of VIP receptor-bearing lymphocytes with VIP in the regulation of T-cell migration from the blood into Peyer's patches and mesenteric lymph nodes.

Briefly, we found that exposure of T cells to VIP produced a dose-dependent decrease in the density of VIP receptors expressed by the cells.[36] Furthermore, this experimental alteration of the numbers of VIP receptors on the cells affected their migration *in vivo*, such that T cells with reduced numbers of receptors for VIP localized less well, after intravenous transfer, in Peyer's patches and mesenteric nodes than

TABLE 8. The Effect of Varying Doses of VIP on IL-2 Activity[a]

Molar VIP Concentration	HT 2 Proliferation ([^{3}H]thymidine, cpm $\times$ 10^{-3}/well)
0	129.7 (4.3)
10^{-10}	123.5 (13.4)
10^{-9}	96.8 (9.9)
10^{-8}	86.4 (9.3)
10^{-7}	79.9 (7.7)
10^{-6}	60.6 (6.5)

[a] Mesenteric lymph node lymphocytes were stimulated with ConA for 48 hours in the presence of various concentrations of VIP. The supernatants were harvested and assayed for their ability to support the growth of HT 2 cells. The results are the means (SD) for three experiments at each condition.

VIP RECEPTORS AND LYMPHOCYTE MIGRATION

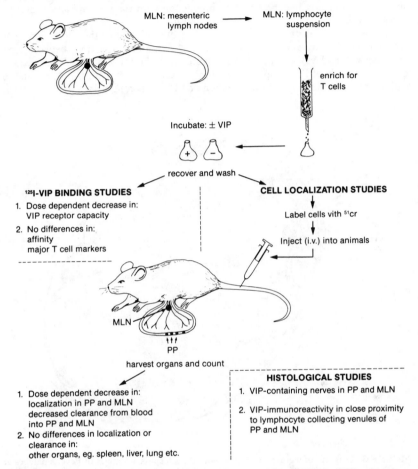

FIGURE 2. Overview of the evidence implicating the recognition of VIP by VIP receptors on T cells as a regulatory process in T-cell migration in mice. The key findings are discussed in the text and in detail in Ottaway[36,37] and Ottaway et al.[51] (MLN, mesenteric lymph node; PP, Peyer's patches.)

cells with greater numbers of VIP receptors.[36] This altered migration was selective for those tissues, and in kinetic studies it was found that this effect was due to a decrease in the rate of clearance of the receptor-depleted cells from the blood into those tissues.[36,37]

The entry of blood-borne lymphocytes into tissues such as Peyer's patches and lymph nodes is a very dynamic process that depends upon the rapid and efficient adherence of lymphocytes to specialized endothelial cells in the postcapillary venules of these tissues.[43] It has been clearly established that the adherence of lymphocytes to this endothelium is mediated by complementary surface components of the lymphocytes and the specialized endothelial cells,[44–50] and that lymphocytes express distinct surface determinants that permit their interaction with the postcapillary venular endothelium of either Peyer's patches or lymph nodes.[45,50]

It was postulated, therefore, that the effect of alteration of the expression of VIP receptors on the migration of T cells was a reflection of interactions between locally available VIP and VIP receptor-bearing lymphocytes in the vicinity of the specialized collecting vessels of Peyer's patches and mesenteric nodes.[36,37] With this in mind, my colleagues and I examined the localization of VIP-containing nerves in mouse Peyer's

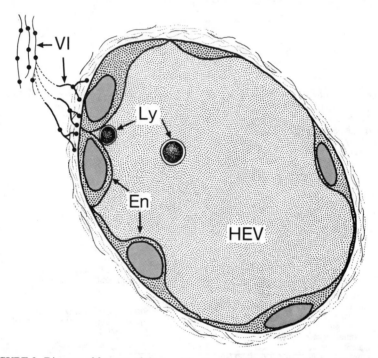

FIGURE 3. Diagram of features of the specialized postcapillary venules of Peyer's patches and mesenteric lymph nodes. These vessels are the site of lymphocyte migration from the blood into these lymphoid tissues. The endothelial cells (En) are polygonal in form, and lymphocyte (Ly) attachment to these cells is rapid and efficient *in vivo*[43] and depends upon mutual recognition determinants on both cells.[44–50] VIP-like immunoreactivity (VI) has been identified in nerves, and in proximity to the basal aspects of the endothelial cells.[51] This probably provides a local source of VIP that facilitates the migration of VIP receptor-bearing T cells *in vivo*.[36,37]

patches and mesenteric nodes and found nerve fibers containing VIP-like immunoreactivity in these tissues.[51] Furthermore, VIP positivity was found in very close proximity to the specialized postcapillary collecting venules of these tissues.[51] These observations, in combination with the effects of VIP receptor manipulation on lymphocyte migration, support the concept that local interactions between VIP and lymphocytes are possible *in vivo* at the site where this migration process occurs, and that this would permit the regulation of the accumulation of VIP-recognizing cells in these lymphoid tissues. This relationship is illustrated in FIGURE 3.

The cellular mechanisms involved are not yet clear, but VIP receptor occupancy during the initial stages of migration from the blood may activate the cells and may make them more motile. Alternatively, recognition of VIP could lead to alterations in the expression or presentation of the cell surface determinants that participate in the adherence of cells to, or their transposition across, the endothelium. These questions will have to be pursued with further investigations, but the evidence implicating VIP as a regulator of both the local deployment and the local activity of lymphocytes suggests that this neuropeptide may be a major signal linking the nervous and immune systems in the intact animal.

CONCLUSION

The data discussed in this chapter indicate that VIP has all the properties required for it to be considered as an important immunoregulatory molecule. The evolution of this concept has been quite rapid, but the identification of receptors for VIP on particular populations of lymphoid cells and the demonstrated capacity of VIP to modulate a variety of immune activities, now provide a firm molecular and cellular framework within which further developments can occur. Because of the specialized nature of the enteric nervous system, and the local immune system of the gut and other mucosae, the concept of neuropeptide-mediated immunoregulation by VIP may be especially important as a model for examining the influence of neurophysiological events on the gastrointestinal immune system.

Examination of this model may lead to new understanding of the physiology of the immune system, and may provide new insights into human disease states. For example, abnormalities of VIP-containing nerves have been identified in the intestine of patients with Crohn's disease.[48-50] Furthermore, a great variety of immunological disturbances also appear to occur in Crohn's disease. Currently, the weight of immunological observations in Crohn's disease is consistent with the hypothesis that there is a diffuse impairment of local immunoregulation in the affected intestine.[55,56] A central problem is that in the absence of knowledge concerning the ways in which immunoregulation is locally controlled in the intestine, the significance of these observations is obscure.

In my view, future advances in this area will depend upon the following:

1. Further characterization of the structure, function and cellular distribution of VIP receptors on defined subpopulations of lymphoid cells, including those lymphocytes from intestinal tissues.
2. Dissection and delineation of the mechanisms by which VIP receptor occupancy are transduced into alterations in the expression of immune processes by lymphocytes.
3. The elaboration of new strategies for examining the effects of VIP and VIP-containing neurons on immune responses *in vivo* and mucosal immune responses in particular, and extension of these strategies to disease states.

Investigations along these lines will not necessarily be easy, but I think that they will be productive, and future developments in these areas are likely to lead to important new ideas both about this neuropeptide and about immunoregulation.

ACKNOWLEDGMENTS

I am grateful to my colleagues Drs. S. Asa, G. Greenberg, T. Lay, and D. Lewis for their contributions and to Mrs. R. Lindo for her expert technical help and for her artistic rendering of FIGURE 1.

REFERENCES

4. GREEN, D. R., P. M. FLOOD & R. K. GERSHON. 1983. Immunoregulatory T cell pathways. Ann. Rev. Immunol. **1:** 439-463.
5. GOETZL, E. J., Ed. 1985. Neuromodulation of immunity and hypersensitivity. J. Immunol. **135**(suppl):739s-862s.
6. GUEILLEMIN, R., M. COHN & T. MELNECHUK, Eds. 1985. Neural Modulation of Immunity. Raven Press. New York.
7. LUNDBERG, J. M., T. HOKFELT, G. NILSSON, L. TERENIUS, J. REHFELD, R. ELDE & S. I. SAID. 1978. Peptide neurons in the vagus, splanchnic and sciatic nerves. Acta Physiol. Scand. **104:** 499-506.
8. COSTA, M., J. B. FURNESS, R. BUFFA & S. I. SAID. 1980. Distribution of enteric nerve cell bodies and axons showing immunoreactivity for vasoactive intestinal polypeptides in the guinea-pig intestine. Neurosciences **5:** 587-596.
9. SCHULTZBERG, M., T. HOKFELT, G. NILSSON, L. TERENIUS, J. REHFELD, M. BROWN, R. ELDE, M. GOLDSTEIN & S. I. SAID. 1980. Distribution of peptide- and catecholamine-containing neurons in the gastrointestinal tract of the rat and guinea-pig: Immunohistochemical studies with antisera to substance P, vasoactive intestinal polypeptide, enkephalins, somatostatin, gastrin/cholecystokinin, neurotensin and dopamine beta-hydroxylase. Neurosciences **5:** 689-744.
10. OTTAWAY, C. A., M. ROSE & D. M. V. PARROTT. 1979. The gut as an immunological system. *In* International Review of Physiology, Gastrointestinal Physiology III, Vol 19. R. K. Crane, Ed. University Park Press. Baltimore, MD.
11. PAYAN, D. G., D. R. BREWSTER, A. MISSIRIAN-BASTIAN & E. J. GOETZL. 1984. Substance P recognition by a subset of human T lymphocytes. J. Clin. Invest. **74:** 1532-1539.
12. PAYAN, D. G. & E. J. GOETZL. 1985. Modulation of lymphocyte function by sensory neuropeptides. J. Immunol. **135**(Suppl): 783s-786s.
13. PAYAN, D. G., J. P. MCGILLIS & E. J. GOETZL. 1986. Neuroimmunology. Adv. Immunol. **39:** 299-323.
14. FURNESS, J. B. & M. COSTA. 1980. Types of nerves in the enteric nervous system. Neurosciences **5:** 1-20.
15. GUERRERO, J. M., J. C. PRIETO, F. L. ELORZA, R. RAMIREZ & R. GOBERNA. 1981. Interactions of vasoactive intestinal peptide with human blood mononuclear cells. Mol. Cell Endocrinol. **21:** 151-160.
16. DANEK, A., M. S. O'DORISIO, T. M. O'DORISIO & J. M. GEORGE. 1983. Specific binding sites for vasoactive intestinal polypeptide on nonadherent peripheral blood lymphocytes. J. Immunol. **131:** 1173-1177.
17. OTTAWAY, C. A., C. BERNAERTS, B. CHAN & G. R. GREENBERG. 1983. Specific binding of vasoactive intestinal peptide to human circulating mononuclear cells. Can. J. Physiol. Pharmacol. **61:** 664-671.
18. WIIK, P., P. K. OPSTAD & A. BOYUM. 1985. Binding of vasoactive intestinal polypeptide by human blood monocytes: Demonstration of specific binding sites. Regul. Peptides **12:** 145-153.
19. CALVO, J. R., J. M. GUERRERO, P. MOLINERO, R. BLASCO & R. GOBERNA. 1986. Interaction of vasoactive intestinal peptide with human blood lymphocytes: Specific binding and cyclic AMP production. Gen. Pharmacol. **17:** 185-189.

20. LAY, T. E., G. R. GREENBERG & C. A. OTTAWAY. 1988. Heterogeneity of vasoactive intestinal peptide binding to subsets of human circulating lymphocytes. Submitted.
21. BEED, E. A., M. S. O'DORISIO, T. M. O'DORISIO & T. S. GAGINELLA. 1983. Demonstration of a functional receptor for vasoactive intestinal polypeptide on Molt-4b T lymphoblasts. Regul. Peptides 6: 1-8.
22. WOOD, C. L. & M. S. O'DORISIO. 1985. Covalent cross-linking of vasoactive intestinal polypeptide to its receptors on intact human lymphoblasts. J. Biol. Chem. 260: 1243-1247.
23. OTTAWAY, C. A. & G. R. GREENBERG. 1984. Interaction of vasoactive intestinal peptide with mouse lymphocytes: Specific binding and modulation of mitogen responses. J. Immunol. 132: 417-423.
24. CALVO, J. R., P. MOLINERO, J. JIMENEZ, R. GOBERNA & J. M. GUERRERO. 1986. Interaction of vasoactive intestinal peptide with rat lymphoid cells. Peptides 7: 177-181.
25. OTTAWAY, C. A. 1987. Selective effects of vasoactive intestinal peptide on the mitogenic response of murine T cells. Immunology 62: 291-297.
26. LEDBETTER, J. A., R. V. ROUSE, H. S. MICKLEM & L. A. HERZENBERG. 1980. T cell subsets defined by the expression of Lyt-1,2,3 and Thy-1 antigens. J. Exp. Med. 152: 280-295.
27. DIALYNAS, D. P., D. B. WILDE, P. MARRACK, A. PIERRES, K. WALL, W. HAVRAN, G. OTTEN, M. LOKEN, M. PIERRES, J. KAPPLER & F. W. FITCH. 1983. Characterization of the murine antigenic determinant designated L3T4a, recognized by monoclonal antibody GK1.5: Expression of L3T4 by functional T cell clones appears to correlate primarily with class II MHC antigen-reactivity. Immunol. Rev. 74: 29-57.
28. SWAIN, S. L. 1981. Significance of Lyt phenotypes: Lyt-2 antibodies block the activity of T cells that recognize class I MHC antigens regardless of their function. Proc. Natl. Acad. Sci. USA 78: 7101-7110.
29. FELTEN, D. L., S. Y. FELTEN, S. L. CARLSON, J. A. OLSCHOWKA & S. LIVNAT. 1985. Noradrenergic and peptidergic innervation of lymphoid tissues. J. Immunol. 135(Suppl): 755s-765s.
30. SAID, S. I. 1984. Vasoactive intestinal polypeptide: Current status. Peptides 5: 143-150.
31. O'DORISIO, M. S., N. S. HERMINA, T. M. O'DORISIO & P. BALCERZAK. 1981. Vasoactive intestinal polypeptide modulation of lymphocyte adenylate cyclase. J. Immunol. 127: 2551-2556.
32. GUERRERO, J. M., J. C. PRIETO, J. R. CALVO & R. GOBERNA. 1984. Activation of cyclic AMP-dependent protein kinase by VIP in blood mononuclear cells. Peptides 5: 371-373.
33. O'DORISIO, M. S., C. L. WOOD, G. D. WENGER & L. M. VASALO. 1985. Cyclic AMP dependent protein kinase in MOLT 4B lymphoblasts: Identification by photoaffinity labeling and activation in intact cells by VIP and PHI. J. Immunol. 134: 4078-4085.
34. ROLA-PLESZCZYNSKI, M., D. BOLDUC & S. ST-PIERRE. 1985. The effects of vasoactive intestinal peptide on human natural killer cell function. J. Immunol. 135: 350-354.
35. DREW, P. A. & D. J. C. SHEARMAN. 1985. Vasoactive intestinal peptide: A neurotransmitter which reduces human NK cell activity and increases Ig synthesis. Aust. J. Exp. Biol. Med. Sci. 63: 313-318.
36. NORDLIND, K. & V. MUTT. 1986. Influence of beta-endorphin, somatostatin, substance P and VIP on the proliferative response of human peripheral blood T cells to mercuric chloride. Int. Archs. Allergy Appl. Immunol. 80: 326-328.
37. STANISZ, A. M., D. BEFUS & J. BIENENSTOCK. 1986. Differential effects of vasoactive intestinal peptide, substance P and somatostatin on immunoglobulin synthesis and proliferation by lymphocytes from Peyer's patches, mesenteric lymph nodes and spleen. J. Immunol. 136: 152-156.
38. KROC, C. J., A. GORES & V. L. GO 1986. Gastrointestinal regulatory peptides modulate in vitro immune reactions of mouse lymphoid cells. Clin. Immunol. Immunopath. 39: 308-318.
39. OTTAWAY, C. A. 1984. In vitro alteration of receptors for vasoactive intestinal peptide changes the in vivo localization of mouse T cells. J. Exp. Med. 160: 1054-1069.
40. OTTAWAY, C. A. 1985. Evidence for local neuromodulation of T cell migration in vivo. Adv. Exp. Med. Biol. 186: 637-645.
41. MOORE, T. C. 1984. Modification of lymphocyte traffic by vasoactive neurotransmitter substances. Immunology 52: 511-518.

42. SMITH, K. A. 1984. Interleukin 2. Ann. Rev. Immunol. **2:** 319-333.

43. MILLER, R. A. 1983. IL2 production by mitogen stimulated T cell subsets: Helper precursors are predominantly Lyt-2. J. Immunol. **131:** 2864-2871.

44. MALEK, T. R., J. A. SCHMIDT & E. M. SHEVACK. 1985. The murine IL2 receptor: Cellular requirements for the induction of IL2 receptor expression on T cell subpopulations. J. Immunol. **134:** 2405-2412.

45. OTTAWAY, C. A. 1986. Lymphoid cell migration to the intestine in health and disease. *In* Gut Defenses in Clinical Practice. M. Losowsky & R. Heatley, Eds.: 48-66. Churchill Livingstone. Edinburgh, Scotland.

46. BJERKNES, M., H. CHENG & C. A. OTTAWAY. 1986. Dynamics of lymphocyte-endothelial interactions *in vivo*. Science **231:** 402-405.

47. CHIN, Y. H., G. D. CAREY & J. J. WOODRUFF. 1982. Lymphocyte recognition of lymph node high endothelium: IV Cell surface structures mediating entry into lymph nodes. J. Immunol. **129:** 1911-1917.

48. GALLATIN, W. M., I. L. WEISMANN & E. C. BUTCHER. 1983. A cell surface molecule involved in the organ specific homing of lymphocytes. Nature (London) **304:** 30-35.

49. STOOLMAN, L. M., T. S. TENEFORDE & S. D. ROSEN. 1984. Phosphomannosyl receptors may participate in the adhesive interaction between lymphocytes and high endothelial venules. J. Cell Biol. **99:** 1535-1541.

50. CHIN, Y. H., R. RASMUSSEN, A. CAKIROGLU GOKHAN & J. J. WOODRUFF. 1984. Lymphocyte recognition of lymph node high endothelium: VI Evidence of distinct structures mediating binding to high endothelial cells of lymph nodes and Peyer's patches. J. Immunol. **133:** 2961-2968.

51. ROSEN, S. D., M. S. SINGER, T. A. YEDNOCK & L. M. STOOLMAN. 1985. Involvement of sialic acid on endothelial cells in organ-specific lymphocyte recirculation. Science **228:** 1005-1009.

52. RASMUSSEN, R. A., Y. H. CHIN & J. J. WOODRUFF. 1985. Lymphocyte recognition of lymph node high endothelium. VII Cell surface proteins involved in adhesion defined by monoclonal anti-HEBF (A.11) antibody. J. Immunol. **135:** 19-24.

53. CHIN, Y. H., R. RASMUSSEN, J. J. WOODRUFF & T. G. EASTON. 1986. A monoclonal anti-HEBF$_{pp}$ antibody with specificity for lymphocyte surface molecules mediating adhesion to Peyer's patches high endothelium of the rat. J. Immunol. **136:** 2556-2561.

54. OTTAWAY, C. A., D. L. LEWIS & S. L. ASA. 1987. Vasoactive intestinal peptide-containing nerves in Peyer's patches. Brain Behav. Immunol. **1:** 148-158.

55. BISHOP, A. E., J. M. POLAK, M. G. BRYANT, S. R. BLOOM & S. HAMILTON. 1980. Abnormalities of vasoactive intestinal polypeptide-containing nerves in Crohn's disease. Gastroenterology **79:** 853-860.

56. SJOLUND, K., O. B. SCHAFFALITZKY DE MUCKADELL, J. FAHRENKRUG, R. HAKANSON, B. G. PETERSON & F. SUNDLER. 1983. Peptide-containing nerve fibers in the gut wall in Crohn's disease. Gut **24:** 724-733.

57. O'MORAIN, C., A. E. BISHOP, G. P. McGREGOR, A. J. LEVI, S. R. BLOOM, J. M. POLAK & T. J. PETERS. 1984. Vasoactive intestinal peptide concentrations and immunocyto-chemical studies in rectal biopsies from patients with inflammatory bowel disease. Gut **25:** 57-61.

58. JANOWITZ, H. D. & D. B. SACHAR. 1982. Inflammatory bowel disease. Adv. Intern. Med. **27:** 205-246.

59. STRICKLAND, R. G. & D. P. JEWELL. 1983. Immunoregulatory mechanisms in nonspecific inflammatory bowel disease. Ann. Rev. Med. **34:** 195-204.

Effect of Vasoactive Intestinal Peptide in Man

GUENTER J. KREJS[a]

Department of Internal Medicine
Karl-Franzens-University School of Medicine
Graz, Austria

The concepts and understanding of the physiological role of VIP have undergone considerable changes in the past 20 years. Although VIP was discovered by Said as a vasoactive substance,[1-3] it was viewed as a candidate gastrointestinal hormone by the late Morton Grossman.[4] When in 1976, the peptide was demonstrated in neurons of the central and peripheral nervous system, it soon became apparent that the major function of VIP was that of a neurotransmitter.[5-8] Plasma concentration of VIP in healthy subjects is low. Since it has not been possible to demonstrate a hormonal role of VIP, circulating VIP is considered a "neuronal overflow phenomenon." Circulating VIP concentration is high in patients with pancreatic cholera syndrome in which the peptide is produced and released by a tumor (Verner-Morrison syndrome, watery diarrhea, hypokalemia, hypochlorhydria syndrome).[9] These patients suffer from large-volume secretory diarrhea, hypokalemia, acidosis, and volume depletion.

Until recently a controversy existed whether VIP was the true mediator of the pancreatic cholera syndrome.[10,11] This controversy was due to the fact that not all patients with pancreatic islet cell tumor and watery diarrhea had elevated plasma VIP levels, that some healthy subjects were reported to have high plasma VIP levels, and because islet cell tumors often produce several peptides, a yet unidentified peptide might be the true mediator. Therefore, experiments were carried out in our laboratory to mimic pancreatic cholera syndrome by VIP infusion in healthy subjects.

INTESTINAL PERFUSION EXPERIMENTS

The triple-lumen tube technique was used to study intestinal water and electrolyte transport in healthy subjects.[12,13] During steady-state conditions, a plasma-like electrolyte solution was perfused in 30-cm segments of jejunum or ileum or the entire colon. Polyethylene glycol was used as a nonabsorbable volume marker. Net water and ion movement across the mucosa is calculated from the perfusion rate and the change in concentration of the nonabsorbable marker and the respective solute ac-

[a] Address for correspondence: Guenter J. Krejs, M.D., Professor and Chairman, Department of Internal Medicine, Karl-Franzens-Universität Graz, Auenbruggerplatz 15, A-8036 Graz, Austria.

cording to standard marker perfusion equations. Intestinal perfusion was carried out during a control period (saline intravenously) and VIP infusion (100, 200, and 400 pmol/kg/h). When VIP was infused at a rate of 400 pmol/kg/h, plasma concentration in the healthy subjects rose to levels observed in patients with pancreatic cholera syndrome (FIG. 1).

VIP infusion abolished water absorption in the jejunum, ileum, and colon (FIG. 2).[14] The effect of VIP was dose-dependent. The relationship between plasma VIP concentration and net water movement is shown in FIGURE 3 with net secretion

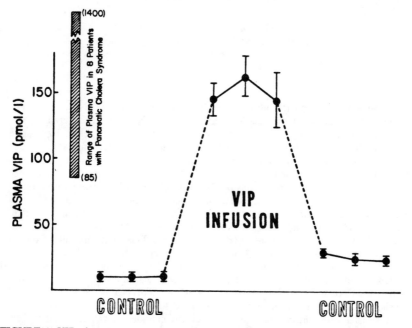

FIGURE 1. VIP plasma concentration in six healthy subjects before, during, and after VIP infusion. Measurements within the test and control periods are 30 minutes apart, and 45 minutes of equilibration lie between the test period and the control periods. VIP rose from about 10 to 150 pmol/l and lay well within the range of VIP levels observed in patients with VIPoma (hatched bar). (Radioimmunoassay results of Drs. J. Fahrenkrug and O. B. Schaffalitzsky de Muckadell, Copenhagen, Denmark.)

occurring in several subjects. While water and sodium absorption were abolished, chloride was secreted (FIG. 4). Chloride secretion was active since it occurred against an electrical and chemical gradient.

PROLONGED VIP INFUSION

In five healthy subjects VIP was infused for 10 hours (400 pmol/kg/h) following a breakfast (and without intubation). The rise in plasma VIP concentration during

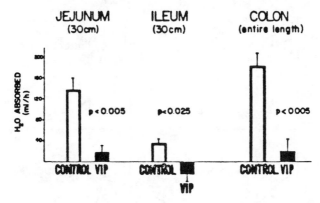

FIGURE 2. Net water movement in the jejunum ($n = 6$), ileum ($n = 10$), and colon ($n = 8$) during control period and VIP infusion. VIP abolished water absorption in all three areas tested.

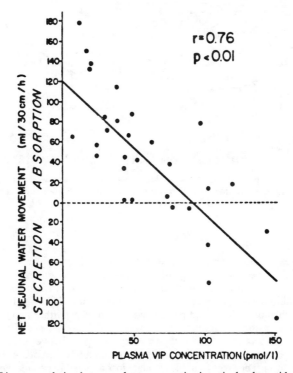

FIGURE 3. Linear correlation between plasma vasoactive intestinal polypeptide (VIP) concentration and net water movement in 30-cm jejunal test segments from 30 healthy volunteers. VIP was infused at rates of 100, 200, or 400 pmol per kilogram of body weight per hour. Data are taken from two previous studies published four years apart. Plasma VIP values were calculated using a mean standard curve. Fluid secretion is observed at high VIP plasma concentrations.

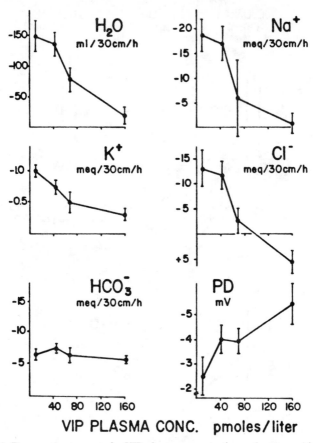

FIGURE 4. Dose-response curves for VIP plasma concentration and water and ion movement and PD in the jejunal test segment of six healthy volunteers (Radioimmunoassay of Drs. J. Fahrenkrug and O. B. Schaffalitzky de Muckadell, Copenhagen, Denmark.)

the 10-hour experiment is shown in FIGURE 5.[15] VIP plasma concentration was well within the range seen in patients with pancreatic cholera syndrome. Plasma VIP concentration continued to rise throughout the experiment, a response that may have been due to inhibition of plasma peptidases by aprotinine, which was infused together with VIP. Each subject developed profuse watery diarrhea within two to six hours of infusion and mean stool weight in 10 hours was 2441 ± 600 g (mean ± SEM; TABLE 1). Stool analysis was consistent with secretory diarrhea. Between the first and last stool, there were significant increases in fecal sodium and bicarbonate concentrations and pH (TABLE 1). The large fecal bicarbonate loss induced hyperchloremic metabolic acidosis. (Serum chloride increased from 107 ± 1 to 118 ± 3 mEq/l, and serum bicarbonate decreased from 24 ± 2 to 18 ± 3 mEq/l during 10 hours of VIP infusion.) These experiments showed that pancreatic cholera syndrome can be mimicked by 10-hour VIP infusion in healthy subjects who developed secretory diarrhea and hyperchloremic metabolic acidosis. VIP has convincingly been shown to be the major mediator of the watery diarrhea in pancreatic cholera syndrome.

CARDIOVASCULAR EFFECTS

Some patients with VIPomas have cardiovascular disturbances such as flushing and hypotension. During VIP infusion for the above-described intestinal perfusion experiments, we regularly observed flushing in all subjects and therefore wished to investigate the cardiovascular effects of VIP, which was originally discovered as a vasoactive peptide by Dr. Said.

We made serial measurements of heart rate, blood pressure, cardiac output, and forearm blood flow in six healthy subjects during constant VIP infusion (400 pmol/kg/h for 100 min). VIP infusion reduced total peripheral resistance by 30% and increased forearm blood flow by 270%. Diastolic and mean arterial pressure fell due to a decrease in peripheral resistance. Echocardiograms during the infusion demonstrated increased fractional shortening associated with decreased afterload. Contrac-

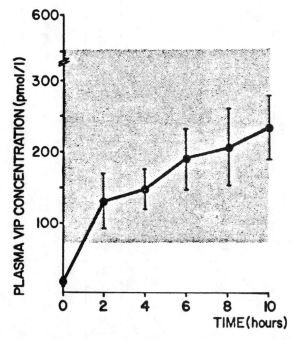

FIGURE 5. Plasma VIP concentration during 10-hour infusion of VIP. Points are mean ± SEM of five subjects. After a rapid rise in VIP concentration during the first two hours, there was a statistically significant rise in VIP between two and 10 hours ($p < 0.005$). The shaded area represents the range observed in 27 patients with pancreatic cholera syndrome, 68-556 pmol/l.

TABLE 1. Stool Analysis[a]

Experiment	Weight	Na⁺	K⁺ (mEq/1)	Cl⁻	HCO₃⁻	Osmolality (mosm/kg)	Osmotic G$_{ap}$[b]	pH
Control[c] (24 h before)	93 ± 37	—	—	—	—	—	—	—
First Exp. stool	617 ± 145	109 ± 7	38 ± 5	50 ± 6	37 ± 9	308 ± 13	15 ± 15	7.2 ± 0.1
Final Exp. stool	470 ± 150	128 ± 7	24 ± 6	62 ± 12	68 ± 9	294 ± 4	−11 ± 5	8.2 ± 0.2
Total Exp. stool (10 h)	2441 ± 600	122 ± 4	33 ± 5	55 ± 7	52 ± 7	305 ± 6	2 ± 7	7.6 ± 0.1
14 h post-infusion[d]	20 ± 20	—	—	—	—	—	—	—
Control[c] (24 h after)	158 ± 48	—	—	—	—	—	—	—
Probability (first vs final stool)	n.s.	< 0.02	n.s.	n.s.	< 0.001	n.s.	n.s.	< 0.025

[a] Numbers are mean ± SEM of five subjects.
[b] Osmotic gap: difference between measured osmolality and 2 × (Na + K concentrations).
[c] Control stools from the 24-hour days before and after the day of the experiment were solid and could not be analyzed. Normal 24-hour stool weight: < 200-250 g.
[d] This 14-hour stool volume completes the 24-hour day of the experiment; it was too solid to analyze.

tibility, defined as the relationship between end systolic stress and shortening fraction, was increased. These findings demonstrate potent vasodilator and inotropic actions of VIP.

REFERENCES

1. SAID, S. I. & V. MUTT. 1970. Potent peripheral and splanchnic vasodilator peptide from normal gut. Nature 225: 863-864.
2. SAID, S. I. & V. MUTT. 1970. Polypeptide with broad biological activity: Isolation from small intestine. Science 169: 1217-1218.
3. SAID, S. I. & V. MUTT. 1972. Isolation from porcine-intestinal wall of a vasoactive octacosapeptide related to secretin and glucagon. Eur. J. Biochem. 28: 199-204.
4. GROSSMAN, M. 1972. Candidate hormones of the gut. Gastroenterology 67: 730-755.
5. PEARSE, A. G. E. 1976. Peptides in brain and intestine. Nature 262: 92-94.
6. FAHRENKRUG, J. 1979. Vasoactive intestinal polypeptide: Measurement, distribution and putative neurotransmitter function. Digestion 19: 149-169.
7. SAID, S. I. 1979. Vasoactive intestinal polypeptide (VIP) as a neural peptide. In Gut peptides, Secretion, Function and Clinical Aspects. A. Miyoshi & M. Grossman, Eds.: 268-273. Elsevier-North Holland Biomedical Press. Amsterdam-New York-Oxford.
8. BRYANT, M. G., J. M. POLAK, I. MODLIN, S. R. BLOOM, R. H. ALBUQUERQUE & A. G. E. PEARSE. 1976. Possible dual role for vasoactive intestinal peptide as gastrointestinal hormone and neurotransmitter substance. Lancet 1: 991-993.
9. PRIEST, W. M. & M. K. ALEXANDER. 1957. Islet-cell tumor of the pancreas with peptic ulceration, diarrhea, and hypokalaemia. Lancet 2: 1145.
10. UNWIN, R. J., J. CALAM & W. S. PEART. 1982. VIPoma and watery diarrhea. New Engl. J. Med. 307: 377-378.
11. GINSBERG, A. L. 1978. The VIP controversy. Stephen R. Bloom vs. Jerry D. Gardner. Dig. Dis. 23: 370-376.
12. KREJS, G. J., J. S. FORDTRAN, S. R. BLOOM, J. FAHRENKRUG, O. B. SCHAFFALITZKY DE MUCKADELL, J. E. FISCHER, C. S. HUMPHREY, T. M. O'DORISIO, S. I. SAID, J. H. WALSH & A. A. SHULKES. 1980. Effect of VIP infusion on water and ion transport in the human jejunum. Gastroenterology 78: 722-727.
13. KREJS, G. J. 1981. Peptidergic control of intestinal secretion—Studies in man. In Gut Hormones. S. R. Bloom & J. M. Polak, Eds. Vol. 2: 516-520. Churchill Livingstone. Edinburgh, Scotland.
14. KREJS, G. J. 1982. Effect of VIP infusion on water and electrolyte transport in the human intestine. In Vasoactive Intestinal Peptide. S. I. Said, Ed.: 193-200. Raven Press. New York.
15. KANE, M. G., T. M. O'DORISIO & G. J. KREJS. Intravenous VIP infusion causes secretory diarrhea in man. 1983. New Engl. J. Med. 309: 1482-1485.

The Morphology and Neuroendocrine Profile of Pancreatic Epithelial VIPomas and Extrapancreatic, VIP-Producing, Neurogenic Tumors[a]

ENRICO SOLCIA,[b] CARLO CAPELLA, AND
CRISTINA RIVA

Department of Pathology
University of Pavia
Pavia, Italy

GUIDO RINDI AND JULIA M. POLAK

Department of Histochemistry
Royal Postgraduate Medical School
London, United Kingdom

Vasoactive intestinal peptide (VIP)-producing pancreatic endocrine tumors are a well-established cause of the watery diarrhea, hypokalemia, and anachlorhydria (WDHA) syndrome.[1-3] However, VIP-producing diarrheogenic tumors of various types, from epithelial endocrine to neurogenic tumors, have also been reported in the jejunum, adrenals, retroperitoneum, mediastinum, lung, and thyroid.[2,4-6] Moreover, peptides other than VIP, such as peptide histidine-methionine (PHM),[7] pancreatic polypeptide (PP),[8] neurotensin,[9] and calcitonin,[10] as well as prostaglandins,[11] have been implicated in the genesis of the syndrome, thus raising the possibility that it may encompass different clinicopathologic entities.

In this paper the histologic, histochemical, and ultrastructural patterns of 37 VIP-producing tumors associated with the WDHA syndrome (VIPomas) have been reinvestigated in an effort to identify distinct morphologic and functional profiles, to be correlated with the polymorphism of clinicopathologic and hormonal findings. For comparison, six VIP-producing tumors unassociated with the syndrome have also been studied.

[a]This work was supported in part by grants from the Italian National Research Council (Special Projects on Oncology and Biomedical Technologies; Gastroenterology Group) and Health and Education Ministry.

[b]Address for correspondence: E. Solcia, Department of Human Pathology, University of Pavia, Via Forlanini 16, I-27100 Pavia, Italy.

MATERIALS AND METHODS

Twenty-nine (28 pancreatic and one jejunal) of the 32 VIPomas investigated in a previous study[6] have been restudied, together with four new pancreatic VIPomas, three ganglioneuroblastomas (one retroperitoneal and two mediastinic) and a mixed ganglioneuroma-pheochromocytoma, all associated with the WDHA syndrome, as well as six VIP-producing nondiarrheogenic tumors (two pancreatic endocrine tumors, two adrenal ganglioneuromas and two adrenal pheochromocytomas). The histologic structure, immunohistochemical reactivity, and ultrastructural patterns of primary or metastatic tumor tissue were investigated as reported previously.[6]

VIP, glucagon, serotonin, enkephalin, neurotensin, α-chain of human chorionic gonadotropin (α-hCG), PP, somatostatin, insulin, PHI/PHM, growth hormone releasing hormone (GRH), neuropeptide Y (NPY), neuron-specific enolase (NSE), chromogranin A, and synaptophysin (P38 protein) antibodies were obtained as reported in previous papers.[6,7,12,13] Cytokeratin A, S-100, and α_1-antitrypsin antibodies were from Ortho Diagnostic Systems (Milan, Italy) and microtubule-associated protein (MAP2) antibodies from Sclavo (Siena, Italy). Immunofluorescence, immunoperoxidase and avidin-biotin immunohistochemical tests were applied to paraffin sections of tumor tissue using pertinent specificity tests.[6,12]

RESULTS

The 34 pancreatic tumors and the jejunal case showed histologic patterns of epithelial endocrine tumors, with three main structural patterns: solid, trabecular, and tubulo-acinar in order of decreasing frequency. No obvious difference between metastatic (21 cases) and nonmetastatic, or diarrheogenic and nondiarrheogenic, tumors was observed. Immunohistochemical tests showed reactivity of tumor cells for the following general markers of epithelial endocrine cells: NSE (23 reactive cases out of 24 investigated), cytokeratin A (8 out of 13; FIG. 1), synaptophysin (14/15), chromogranin A (9/20), and α_1-antitrypsin (5/15). No consistent staining of tumor cells was obtained with antibodies against serotonin (20 tumors tested), MAP2 (13 tumors), and S-100 protein (20 tumors). Among neuroendocrine peptides, VIP (27 reactive tumors out of 31 tested; of the four unreactive cases, two showed high VIP content in tumor extracts and all had high VIP levels in blood as well as the WDHA syndrome), PHM/PHI (13 out of 23), GRH (9/18), PP (16/30), insulin (5/29), neurotensin (2/11), glucagon (3/29), somatostatin (4/27), and Met-enkephalin (1/12) were found to be immunoreactive (FIGS. 2-4; TABLE 1).

Ultrastructurally, the epithelial nature of all the tumors investigated (23 cases) was confirmed and variable amounts of secretory granules were observed. In three tumors numerous well-granulated endocrine cells with abundant rough endoplasmic reticulum, often forming parallel cisternae filled with secretory material, were found (FIG. 5). Their granules were of variable shape (round to ovoid, angular, pear-shaped or comma-shaped), size (from 150 to 250 nm of mean diameter) and density (from moderate to fairly high), thus closely resembling those of PP cells in normal human pancreas, with special reference to F-type cells forming PP-rich irregular islets of the posterior head.[14]

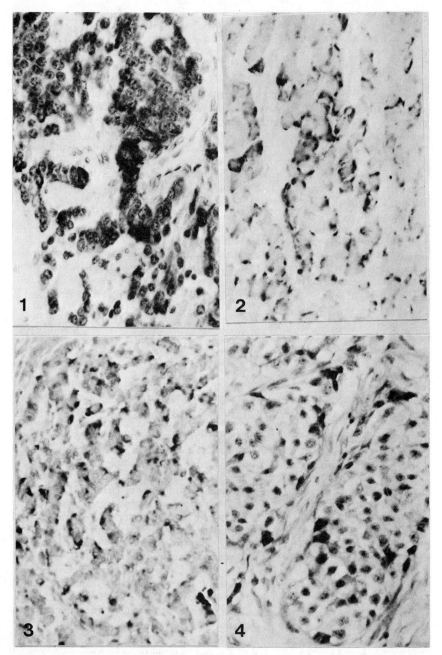

FIGURES 1 to 4. Pancreatic VIPomas immunostained with (**1**) cytokeratin A (magnification × 350); (**2**) VIP (magnification × 250); (**3**) PP (magnification × 350); and (**4**) GRH (magnification × 350) antibodies. Avidin-biotin technique; hematoxylin counterstain.

TABLE 1. Immunohistochemical Profile of Pancreatic and Neurogenic VIPomas

Tumors	VIP	PHM	NSE	P38	Chromogranin A	Somatostatin, Enkephalin, or Neurotensin
Pancreatic	27/31	13/23	22/23	14/15	9/20	6/28
Neurogenic[a]	7/7	6/7	6/6	5/5	4/7	4/7

Tumors	Cytokeratin A	PP	GRH	α-hCG	Insulin or Glucagon	NPY	MAP2
Pancreatic	8/13	16/29	9/18	13/27	7/28	0/13	0/13
Neurogenic[a]	0/6	0/6	0/5	0/5	0/5	4/6	4/5

[a] Five ganglioneuromas or ganglioneuroblastomas; two pheochromocytomas.

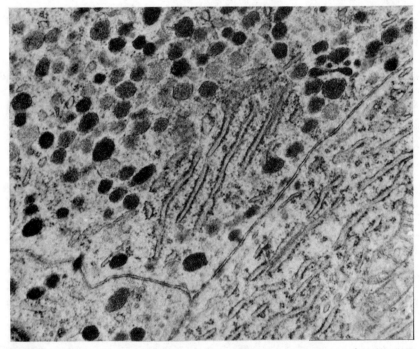

FIGURE 5. Pancreatic endocrine tumor with abundant PP-immunoreactive cells, rare VIP-immunoreactive cells and the WDHA syndrome. Note F-type secretory granules and well-developed rough endoplasmic reticulum forming parallel cisternae. Magnification × 28,000.

The three tumors showed a fairly prominent trabecular structure, often made up of a single layer of tall, columnar cells, sometimes forming tubules or microacini. In two of the three cases (both arising in the head, one corresponding to the case published by Lundqvist et al.[15] and the other to case 20 of Greider et al.[16]), the PP cell nature of the majority of tumor cells was confirmed immunohistochemically.

The remaining tumors were mostly composed of poorly granulated or agranular cells with well-developed endoplasmic reticulum and Golgi complex (poorly granulated "active" cells). A few agranular cells with poorly developed organelles (stem cells) and well-granulated cells (well-differentiated endocrine cells) were also found to be scattered in the tumor growth. Most secretory granules were round and small (120-190 nm); among which two subpopulations were identified in some tumors: (1) smaller (120-160 nm), thin-haloed granules containing a moderately dense core (FIG. 6), shown to react with VIP antibodies in an electron immunocytochemical test,[6] and (2) slightly larger (140-190), more solid granules reacting with anti-PP antibodies.[6] In addition, larger granules resembling more or less those of glucagon, neurotensin, somatostatin, or insulin cells were observed in occasional cells of individual tumors.

A population of small (40-50 nm), round to ovoid, empty vesicles resembling synaptophysin-reactive small, clear vesicles of nerves and neuroendocrine cells,[13] was observed in many tumors, either scattered in the cytoplasm or forming small collections, sometimes near to the cell membrane (FIG. 6).

Elongated, electron-dense bodies of peculiar morphology, apparently arising from deposition of highly osmiophilic material into tubules of the endoplasmic reticulum, were also observed in 17 of 25 tumors investigated ultrastructurally (FIG. 7). They were more prominent in two tumors whose cells showed very few or no secretory granules, abundant, fairly large mitochondria, extensively developed tubules of smooth

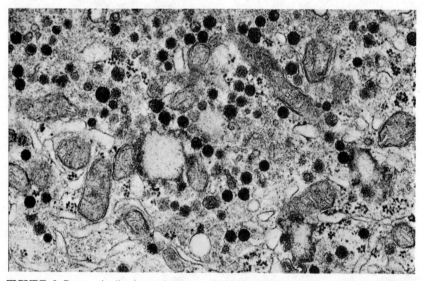

FIGURE 6. Pancreatic diarrheogenic tumor with fairly numerous VIP- and no PP-immunoreactive cells. Note round, thin-haloed secretory granules and a few small clear vesicles. Magnification × 28,000.

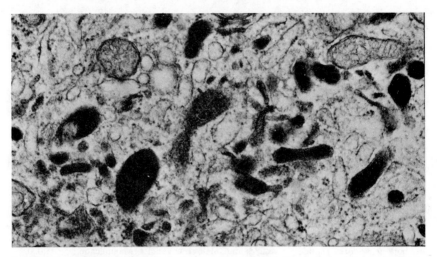

FIGURE 7. Elongated osmiophilic bodies, apparently arising from tubules of endoplasmic reticulum, in a pancreatic VIPoma. Magnification × 35,000.

endoplasmic reticulum and scattered small clear vesicles in a clear cytoplasm. Under light microscopy these two tumors were characterized by their reactivity for α_1-antitrypsin and unreactivity for most "neuroendocrine" markers, with the only exceptions being synaptophysin antibodies and VIP/PHM antibodies, staining a few tumor cells. Thus, the osmiophilic bodies seem to lack the usual components of endocrine granules, including hormonal peptides, monoamines and chromogranins, while they may contain α_1-antitrypsin.

Microlumina, which were especially abundant in two cases and scattered in 12 cases, were mostly formed by agranular or poorly granular cells with clear cytoplasm, abundant smooth reticulum, juxtaluminal pinocytotic-like vesicles, and elongated, thin microvilli lacking the long cytoplasmic rootlets of large pancreatic ducts, while resembling closely the microvilli of intralobular ductules. No, or only scanty, immunoreactivity for endocrine markers was observed in the tubulo-acinar areas.

All the diarrheogenic and nondiarrheogenic ganglioneuromas or ganglioneuroblastomas showed well-developed ganglion cells, axons, nerve fibers, and Schwann-like cells; in addition, neuroblastic foci were found in ganglioneuroblastomas. Ultrastructural investigation confirmed the presence of neurons and axons, showing small clear vesicles, dense-cored granules, neurofilaments and microtubules, admixed with Schwann cells (FIG. 8). Pheochromocytomas showed epithelial cells storing fairly large, osmiophilic, solid to vesicular granules and forming solid alveoli or trabeculae. No tubular structures with luminal differentiation of bordering cells (microvilli, pinocytotic-like vesicles, junctional complexes, etc.) of the type found in pancreatic VIPomas has been observed in these tumors.

Immunohistochemically, VIP, PHM/PHI, NPY, enkephalin, somatostatin, NSE, MAP2, and synaptophysin were more or less widely represented in nerve cell bodies and fibers as well as in pheochromocytes. S-100 protein was detected in Schwann cells. No reactivity was obtained with PP, GRH, and cytokeratin-A antibodies (FIG. 9).

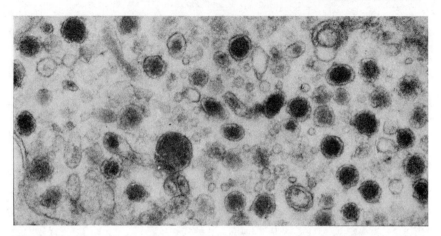

FIGURE 8. Nerve ending in a diarrheogenic ganglioneuroma-pheochromocytoma tumor, showing both dense-cored peptidergic vesicles and small clear vesicles. Magnification × 45,000.

DISCUSSION

Taken as a whole our histologic, histochemical, and ultrastructural findings support the interpretation of pancreatic and intestinal VIPomas as epithelial endocrine tumors of endodermal origin. The occurrence of ductular components, lack of histological and ultrastructural patterns of neurogenic tumors, expression of cytokeratin-A immunoreactivity, failure to express microtubule-associated protein, production of peptide hormones, such as PP, GRH, insulin, and glucagon, regularly found in pancreatic endocrine tumors but not in peripheral neurogenic tumors, are all in keeping with this interpretation.[17,18]

Neuron-specific enolase, chromogranins, somatostatin, neurotensin, dense-cored granules storing peptides and chromogranins, as well as synaptophysin and small clear vesicles, should be considered as "neuroendocrine" markers common to both neuroectodermal (neuronal or paraganglionic) cells and epithelial endocrine cells of endodermal origin, such as those forming the gastroenteropancreatic endocrine system.[19] The production by pancreatic and intestinal tumors of VIP and PHM (normally found only in neuroectodermal cells of mammals,[20] although VIP seems to occur in intestinal endocrine cells of lower vertebrates[21]) may be attributed to the increased plasticity shown by tumor cell lines in their process of differentiation. In fact, epithelial endocrine cells undergoing neoplastic transformation have been found to increase their spectrum of morphofunctional expression to include some "neurogenic" markers, as for instance the neurofilament 68K protein,[18,22] normally lacking in corresponding nontumor cells.

The lack of any tumor growth in 20% of patients with the WDHA syndrome reported in the literature,[23] the finding of pancreatic endocrine hyperplasia (sometimes VIP-immunoreactive and coupled with increased VIP levels in serum) in a number of such patients, and the disappearance of the syndrome after pancreatectomy[5,23] raise the possibility that some endocrine cell line normally occurring in the human pancreas may be involved in the genesis of pancreatic VIPomas. The frequent presence in such tumors of PP-producing cells,[6,8,24] the increased PP levels found in serum of as many as 77% of patients,[3] the occasional finding of both PP and VIP immunoreactivities in the same tumor cell[25] as well as the occurrence of tumor cells with ultrastructural features intermediate between those of PP cells and VIP-immunoreactive cells, suggest that a cell line somewhat akin to pancreatic PP cells is involved.

Although VIP seems lacking in normal PP cells, these cells store a peptide reacting with some antisera directed against GRH,[26] a known VIP-like peptide. Our demonstration of GRH immunoreactivity in seven out of 10 PP-producing pancreatic VIPomas also supports an involvement of the PP cell line or, more likely, of some pluripotent ductular stem cell somewhat committed to differentiation along the PP/GRH cell line, though frequently switching to "inappropriate" VIP/PHM peptide expression. This interpretation would also explain the occasional presence of ductules in pancreatic VIPomas as well as the frequent finding of ductular hyperplasia intimately admixed with endocrine hyperplasia in nontumor pancreas of WDHA patients, with or without associated tumor.[5,23] Alternatively, the ductular-centroacinar hyperplasia of nontumor pancreas might be secondary to VIP-induced functional overstimulation.

From a revision of our cases and those collected by Morrison,[23] it appears that 52% of 102 pancreatic tumors (mean diameter around 4.5 cm) associated with the WDHA syndrome proved malignant, mostly with metastases to liver and regional lymph nodes. The exact behavior of some of the remaining tumors remained uncertain, due to equivocal histologic findings and/or lack of follow-up, thus suggesting that potentially malignant growths represent a consistent majority of such tumors. Both malignancy rates and tumor size of pancreatic VIPomas resemble those of another type of "inappropriate" endocrine tumor arising in the pancreas, the gastrin-producing tumor, while differing sharply from those of insulinomas, most of which are known to be benign and of small (1 or 2 cm) size.[17]

In conclusion, VIP-producing diarrheogenic endocrine tumors of the pancreas and intestine, despite their pleomorphic morphology and secretory activity, represent a distinct clinico-pathologic entity, likely due to tumor growth of a transformed epithelial

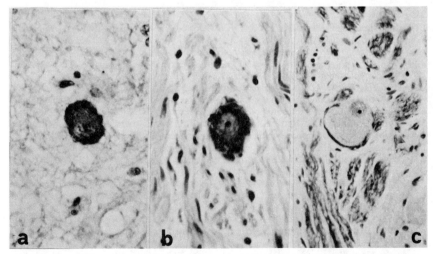

FIGURE 9. VIP (a) and MAP2 (b) immunoreactive neurons and S-100 (c) reactive Schwann cells in the ganglioneuromatous component of a diarrheogenic ganglioneuroblastoma. Avidin-biotin technique; hematoxylin stain. Magnification × 350 for a and b; × 250 for c.

cell line genetically related with pancreatic PP cells and clearly separated from neurogenic cell lines forming VIP-producing ganglioneuroblastomas, ganglioneuromas and pheochromocytomas.

SUMMARY

The histology, histochemistry, and ultrastructure of 43 VIP-producing tumors (34 from the pancreas, one jejunal, six retroperitoneal and two mediastinic), 37 of which were associated with the WDHA syndrome, have been investigated on paraffin sections of primary or metastatic tumor tissue. The pancreatic and jejunal tumors showed all structural and secretory patterns of epithelial endocrine tumors, including expression of cytokeratin, neuroendocrine markers like neuron-specific enolase, chromogranins and synaptophysin, peptides like VIP, PHM, GRH, PP, insulin, neurotensin, glucagon, somatostatin and enkephalin, secretory granules, small clear vesicles, peculiar osmiophilic bodies, and occasional formation of tubules or microacini with specialized luminal surfaces.

All the remaining tumors were neurogenic, showing either neurons and nerve fibers together with Schwann cells (ganglioneuromas and ganglioneuroblastomas) or endocrine cells (pheochromocytomas) reacting with VIP, PHM, NPY, enkephalin, somatostatin, neuron-specific enolase, synaptophysin, and MAP2 (but not cytokeratin, PP, or GRH) antibodies. A possible origin of pancreatic VIPomas from transformed pancreatic PP cells or ductular stem cells partially committed to differentiation along the PP cell line is suggested.

REFERENCES

1. BLOOM, S. R., J. M. POLAK & A. G. E. PEARSE. 1973. Vasoactive intestinal peptide and watery-diarrhea syndrome. Lancet 2: 14-16.
2. SAID, S. I. & G. R. FALOONA. 1975. Elevated plasma and tissue levels of vasoactive intestinal polypeptide in the watery-diarrhea syndrome due to pancreatic, bronchogenic and other tumors. N. Engl. J. Med. 293: 155-160.
3. LONG, R. G., M. G. BRYANT, S. I. MITCHELL, T. E. ADRIAN, J. M. POLAK & S. R. BLOOM. 1981. Clinicopathological study of pancreatic and ganglioneuroblastoma tumours secreting vasoactive intestinal polypeptide (VIPomas). Br. Med. J. 282: 1767-1771.
4. SWIFT, P. G. F., S. R. BLOOM & F. HARRY. 1975. Watery diarrhea and ganglioneuroma with secretion of vasoactive intestinal peptide. Arch. Dis. Child 50: 896-899.
5. MENDELSOHN, G. 1982. Vasoactive intestinal polypeptide (VIP) and the spectrum of tumors producing the watery diarrhea syndrome. Progr. Surg. Pathol. 4: 199-216.
6. CAPELLA, C., J. M. POLAK, R. BUFFA, F. J. TAPIA, PH. HEITZ, S. R. BLOOM & E. SOLCIA. 1983. Morphological patterns and diagnostic criteria of VIP-producing endocrine tumors. A histological, histochemical, ultrastructural, and biochemical study of 32 cases. Cancer 52: 1860-1874.
7. YIANGOU, Y., S. J. WILLIAMS, A. E. BISHOP, J. M. POLAK & S. R. BLOOM. 1987. Peptide histidine-methionine immunoreactivity in plasma and tissue from patients with vasoactive intestinal peptide-secreting tumors and watery diarrhea syndrome. J. Clin. Endocr. Metab. 64: 131-139.
8. LARSSON, L-I., T. W. SCHWARTZ, G. LUNDQVIST, R. E. CHANCE, F. SUNDLER, J. F. REHFELD, L. GRIMELIUS, J. FAHRENKRUG, O. B. SCHAFFALITZKY DE MUCKADELL &

N. Moon. 1976. Occurrence of human pancreatic polypeptide in pancreatic endocrine tumors. Am. J. Pathol. **85:** 675-684.

9. Feurle, G. E., V. Helmstaedter, K. Tischbirek, R. Carraway, W. F. Forssman, D. Grube & H. Roher. 1981. A multihormonal tumor of the pancreas producing neurotensin. Dig. Dis. Sci. **26:** 1121-1133.

10. Öberg, K., L. Lööf, H. Boström, L. Grimelius, J. Fahrenkrug & G. Lundqvist. 1981. Hypersecretion of calcitonin in patients with the Verner-Morrison syndrome. Scand. J. Gastroenterol. **16:** 135-144.

11. Jaffe, B. M., D. F. Kopen, K. de Schryver-Kecskemeti, R. L. Gingerich & M. Greider. 1977. Indomethacin-responsive pancreatic cholera. N. Engl. J. Med. **297:** 817-821.

12. Rindi, G., R. Buffa, F. Sessa, O. Tortora & E. Solcia. 1986. Chromogranin A, B and C immunoreactivities of mammalian endocrine cells. Distribution, distinction from costored hormones/prohormones and relationship with the argyrophil component of secretory granules. Histochemistry **85:** 19-28.

13. Navone, F., R. Jahn, G. di Gioia, H. Stukenbrok, P. Greengard & P. de Camilli. 1986. Protein P38: An integral membrane protein specific for small clear vesicles of neurons and neuroendocrine cells. J. Cell. Biol. **103:** 2511-2527.

14. Fiocca, R., F. Sessa, P. Tenti, L. Usellini, C. Capella, M. M. T. O'Have & E. Solcia. 1983. Pancreatic polypeptide (PP) cells in the PP-rich lobe of the human pancreas are identified ultrastructurally and immunocytochemically as F cells. Histochemistry **77:** 511-523.

15. Lundqvist, G., U. Krause, L-I. Larsson, L. Grimelius, O. B. Schaffalitzky de Muckadell, J. Fahrenkrug, M. Johnson & R. E. Chance. 1978. A pancreatic-polypeptide-producing tumor associated with the WDHA syndrome. Scand. J. Gastroenterol. **13:** 715-718.

16. Greider, M. H., J. Rosai & J. E. McGuigan. 1974. The human pancreatic islet cells and their tumors. Cancer **33:** 1423-1443.

17. Solcia, E., C. Capella, R. Buffa, P. Tenti, G. Rindi & M. Cornaggia. 1986. Antigenic markers of neuroendocrine tumors: Their diagnostic and prognostic value. *In* New Concepts in Neoplasia as Applied to Diagnostic Pathology. C. M. Fenoglio, R. S. Weinstein & N. Kaufman, Eds.: 242-261. Williams and Wilkins. Baltimore, MD.

18. Wiedenmann, B., W. W. Franke, C. Kuhn, R. Moll & V. E. Gould. 1986. Synaptophysin. A marker protein for neuroendocrine cells and neoplasms. Proc. Natl. Acad. Sci. USA **83:** 3500-3504.

19. Ayer-Le Lievre, C. & J. Fontaine-Perus. 1982. The neural crest: Its relations with APUD and paraneuron concepts. Arch. Histol. Jpn. **45:** 409-427.

20. Larsson, L-I., J. M. Polak, R. Buffa, F. Sundler & E. Solcia. 1979. On the immunocytochemical localization of the vasoactive intestinal polypeptide. J. Histochem. Cytochem. **27:** 936-938.

21. Reinecke, M., P. Schluter, N. Yanaihara & W. G. Forsmann. 1981. VIP-immunoreactivity in enteric nerves and endocrine cells of the vertebrate gut. Peptides 2(Suppl.2): 149-156.

22. Miettinen, M., V.-L. Lehto, D. Dahl & I. Virtanen. 1985. Varying expression of cytokeratin and neurofilaments in neuroendocrine tumors of human gastrointestinal tract. Lab. Invest. **52:** 429-436.

23. Morrison, A. B. 1978. Islet cell tumors and the diarrheogenic syndrome. *In* The Pancreas. P. J. Fitzgerald & A. B. Morrison, Eds.: 185-207. IAP Monograph. Williams and Wilkins. Baltimore, MD.

24. Welbourn, R. B., J. M. Polak, S. R. Bloom, A. G. E. Pearse & R. B. Galland. 1978. Apudomas of the pancreas. *In* Gut Hormones. S. R. Bloom, Ed.: 561-569. Churchill Livingstone. Edinburgh, Scotland.

25. Kameya, T., M. Tsmuraya, Y. Shimosato, K. Abe & N. Yanaihara. 1982. Demonstration of multiple hormone production by single cells in neoplasia. H. Histochem. Cytochem. **30:** 554.

26. Bosman, F. T., C. van Assche, A. C. N. Kruseman, S. Jackson & P. J. Lowry. 1984. Growth hormone releasing factor (GRF) immunoreactivity in human and rat gastrointestinal tract and pancreas. J. Histochem. Cytochem. **32:** 1139-1144.

Vasoactive Intestinal Peptide Secreting Tumors

Pathophysiological and Clinical Correlations

S. R. BLOOM,[a] Y. YIANGOU, AND J. M. POLAK

Departments of Medicine and Histochemistry
Royal Postgraduate Medical School
Hammersmith Hospital
London W12 OHS, United Kingdom

In 1958 Verner and Morrison described two cases of severe watery diarrhea, associated with noninsulin-secreting islet cell adenomas of the pancreas.[1] It was assumed that the tumor released a hormone that resulted in the watery diarrhea, and in 1973 this was demonstrated to be the newly discovered regulatory vasoactive intestinal peptide (VIP).[2,3] Subsequently it was demonstrated that two main types of tumor, pancreatic endocrine tumors and ganglioneuroblastomas, secreted large quantities of VIP and thus were associated with a watery diarrhea syndrome.[4] Indeed in a series of 62 patients with watery diarrhea associated with elevated circulating plasma VIP concentrations, there were 52 cases of pancreatic tumor and ten cases of glanglioneuro-blastoma.[5] It was established that in animals and man, exogenous VIP infusions produced not only a striking inhibition of jejunal and colonic water and electrolyte absorption, but also a net secretion into the intestine and even secretory diarrhea.[6,7,8] Thus it was assumed that VIP was the main mediator of the watery diarrhea and the term "VIPomas" became popular to describe these tumors. Subsequently porcine peptide histidine isoleucine (PHI) was isolated from the pig intestine and shown to have sequence similarities with VIP and the rest of the secretin-glucagon family.[9] Radioimmunoassay data of PHI tissue distribution demonstrated a startlingly close correlation with that of VIP, leading to the hypothesis that the two might be cosynthesized.[10] When the messenger RNA was isolated, a precursor protein of 170 amino acid residues was deduced and PHI was found to occupy amino acid positions 81-107, while VIP occupied positions 125-152 (FIG. 1).[11,12] Since in man the terminal amino acid was not isoleucine but methionine, the term PHM was used for the human form of PHI. Both PHI and PHM stimulate intestinal juice production[13,14] (Calam, Yiangou, and Bloom, unpublished observations). Since the clearance rate of PHI is slower than that of VIP,[15] it is unclear which of these two peptides is the more important in the watery diarrhea syndrome, and therefore whether the term "VIPoma" is still appropriate.

[a] Address for correspondence: Professor S. R. Bloom, Department of Medicine, Royal Postgraduate Medical School, Hammersmith Hospital, Du Cane Road, London W12 OHS, UK.

HUMAN PREPRO-VIP/PHM

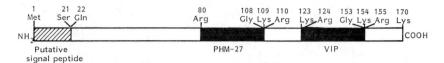

FIGURE 1. Schematic representation of the 170 amino acid precursor encoding PHM and VIP.

More recently the story has got more complicated: The main form of PHM in the nose, stomach, and genitalia (FIG. 2) is of larger molecular size than PHM itself.[16,17] Since this was found to be the case in all species examined (rat, guinea pig, cat, pig, and man), it was assumed that "big PHM" was also phylogenetically ancient.[16] Characterization by region-specific antibodies, in particular to preproVIP amino acid sequence 111 to 122 (the spacer peptide between PHM and VIP sequences) suggested that big PHM was COOH-terminally extended. This was unexpected, as the presence of a single arginine at the NH_2-terminus of PHM in preproVIP had led to suggestions that this might be the point of noncleavage in the production of a big form. It has subsequently been demonstrated that VIP-producing tumors usually secrete considerable quantities of big PHM (FIG. 3A and B).[18] Thus plasma levels of big PHM were considerably higher than those of PHM, which in turn were usually higher than those of VIP (FIG. 4). Assuming that the production rate of big PHM does not exceed that of VIP, it seems probable that the clearance rate of big PHM is relatively slow. Subsequently we have been able to purify big PHM from a human tumor (FIGS. 5 and 6) and using fast-atom bombardment (FAB) mapping[19–22] were able to show a molecular weight of 4547 (FIG. 7) corresponding to the sequence of preproVIP 81-122.

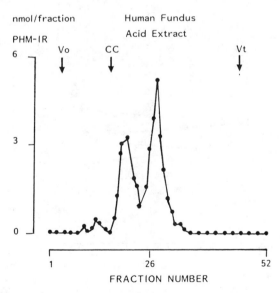

FIGURE 2. Representative Sephadex G-50 profile of an acid extract of human stomach measured by an NH_2-terminus-directed PHM antibody.

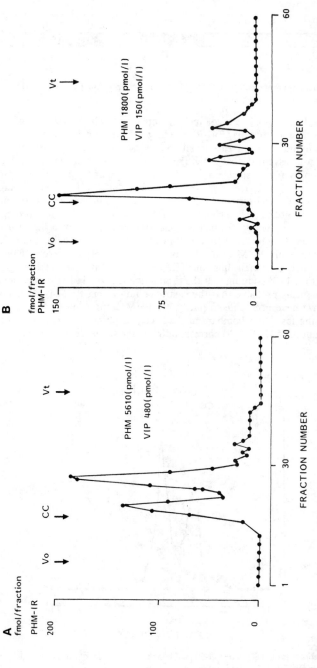

FIGURE 3. (A,B) Sephadex G-50 profile of plasma from two patients with VIP-producing tumors and watery diarrhea, with corresponding PHM and VIP plasma levels.

This peptide was designated PHV-42. We have subsequently synthesized it and demonstrated that it is biologically active with a similar spectrum to PHM but increased biological activity in certain systems. In view of its specific distribution, it would appear to have a distinct physiological role separate from that of VIP and PHM.

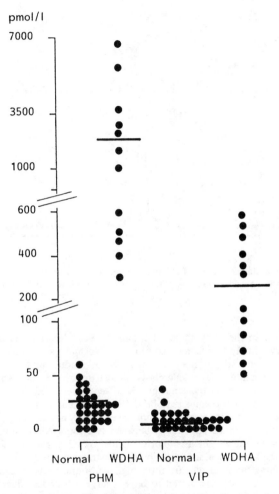

FIGURE 4. Comparison of VIP and PHM plasma levels in normals and patients with WDHA. Horizontal line represents the median of each group.

CLINICAL FEATURES OF THE SYNDROME

The single most striking clinical feature of the syndrome associated with a tumor and high circulating concentrations of peptides from the preproVIP family is severe

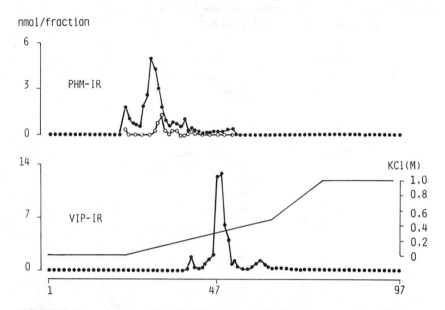

FIGURE 5. Ion-exchange profiles of PHM (top) and VIP-like immunoreactivity (IR) from a ganglioneuroblastoma acid extract. Both the NH_2-terminal-IR ● and "PHM-specific" IR ○ are shown (top).

watery diarrhea. In the early stages of tumor growth, the diarrhea is usually inter-mittent, but eventually it becomes continuous. Normal gastroenterological investi-gation, including endoscopy, mucosal biopsy, X-ray studies, and stool culture fail to reveal any abnormalities. Hypokalemia is almost invariable and can be sufficiently severe to lead to temporary quadraplegia. Kraft et al. reported the average length of symptoms before clinical diagnosis to be three years,[23] but this was before the intro-duction of VIP assays. However, this time interval was not strikingly different from our own observation in 62 patients of between two months and four years.[5] Other features are significant weight loss (not explained by dehydration), abdominal colic, and flushing attacks. Clinical investigation demonstrates normal or low acid secretion, thus distinguishing the syndrome from the high acid-induced diarrhea of gastrinomas. In surgery patients have been noted to have a large, distended, flaccid gall bladder and a high pancreatic juice production rate, both pharmacological effects of VIP.[23]

Diagnosis is usually made by measurement of plasma VIP concentrations. It is noteworthy that VIP has two double-basic amino acid residues in its sequence (14 and 15, 20 and 21) thus making it extremely susceptible to proteolytic enzyme deg-radation. Samples of blood must therefore be collected with the enzyme inhibitor aprotinin (Trasylol) and the plasma rapidly separated and deep frozen. Fortunately basal plasma VIP concentrations in healthy people are quite low,[24] and in our assay a cut-off limit of 30 pmol/1 has been established. Concentrations in the plasma of patients with symptoms from VIP-producing tumors are usually above 60 pmol/1.[5] Diagnosis by measurement of plasma PHM and PHV-42 (big PHM) may be easier as these moieties circulate in higher concentrations and appear to be more stable, but at present there is insufficient clinical experience to justify their routine use. It is noteworthy that elevated VIP concentrations are not found with infective diarrhea, purgative addiction, medullary carcinoma of the thyroid, small cell carcinoma of the bronchus, or the carcinoid syndrome. Thus a single elevated plasma VIP concentration in an ambulatory patient has a low incidence of false positive or negative error. Extremely ill patients, for example, patients in shock or with renal failure, may also have raised VIP-like immunoreactivity. Rarely, asymptomatic healthy persons are found with elevated high-molecular-weight VIP, presumably due to an error in their posttranslational enzymic processing resulting in small quantities of high-molecular-weight VIP that is slowly cleared from the bloodstream. These patients do not have elevated PHM immunoreactivity with our current assay. Plasma VIP concentrations are not only useful for diagnosis but also for monitoring therapy, as VIP concentrations return to normal after successful cytotoxic therapy. Many of the pancreatic VIPomas produce other pancreatic regulatory peptides. For example, approximately 75% of these tumors also produce pancreatic polypeptide (PP) and have fasting PP levels above the upper limit of normal (300 pmol/l).[25] Since the normal pancreatic PP cell is under positive vagal stimulation, the administration of atropine results in a dramatic fall in plasma PP concentrations in healthy subjects. This is not seen with tumor-produced PP and therefore offers an additional diagnostic test.[26] Neurotensin is also frequently coproduced by VIPomas,[27] and this may further stimulate the production of diarrhea.[28–29] Other biochemical features in the syndrome include the frequent finding

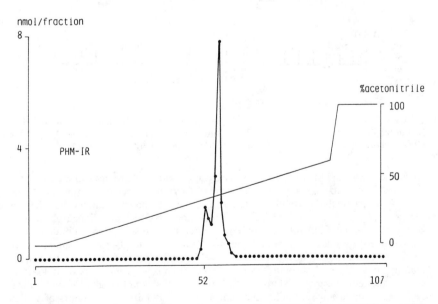

FIGURE 6. Reverse-phase liquid chromatography profile of NH_2-terminal PHM immunoreactivity of peak fractions (from FIG. 5, top).

of acidosis, hypophosphatemia, hyperglycemia, and hypercalcemia, all explainable by the known actions of VIP.

TREATMENT

The optimal treatment for tumors secreting prepro-VIP products is complete surgical removal. The tumor must first be localized and the most useful techniques

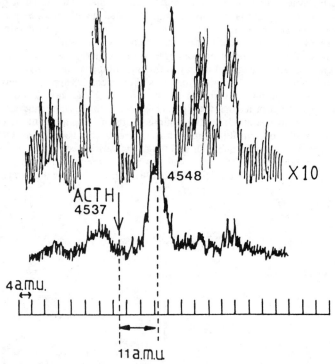

FIGURE 7. FAB-MS spectrum of PHV-42 (peak from FIG. 6). Synthetic human ACTH$_{1-39}$ (Peninsula Laboratories, m/z value 4537) was run separately, and used as reference to calibrate a mass marker to determine the m/z value of PHV-42 accurately.

are CT scanning and highly selective arteriography with background subtraction. Both are capable of showing a pancreatic primary and liver secondary tumors. NMR scanning is particularly useful for detecting hepatic secondary tumors, but there is less experience with pancreatic primary tumors. Localization of ganglioneuroblastomas is theoretically more difficult as they have a much wider distribution. In practice they are frequently physically large and therefore more obvious. Isotopic scanning techniques and ultrasound rarely add useful additional information. Selective venous sampling to look for a hot spot of hormone production is particularly useful in locating any ganglioneuroblastoma. Transhepatic portal venous sampling gives poor localization, has a significant morbidity and mortality, and requires many hours of skilled application by an experienced radiologist. It is therefore a procedure of last resort. If complete surgical removal is not possible, then tumor debulking may well allow useful palliation as the patient's symptoms are usually entirely due to the high level of hormonally active peptides. Reduction of these gives symptomatic relief. Similarly ischemic shrinkage of hepatic secondaries by hepatic artery embolization is a useful palliative, particularly as it can be done under local anesthetic. This procedure is successful (where hepatic artery ligation was not) because small emboli are first introduced into the peripheral arteries and successively larger emboli injected until the whole arteriol tree is blocked allowing little possibility of anastomotic channels to form.

The cytotoxic agent, streptozotocin, is dramatically effective and remissions may last many years. The main toxicity of streptozotocin is renal failure and extreme caution should be used when treating patients with renal impairment. The first sign of renal toxicity is proteinuria and a regime that allows a gap of one or two days between the multiple injections of a course to allow measurement of the 24-hour urine protein output offers maximum safety. A commonly used dose is 0.5 g/meter^2 on alternate days for ten days, repeated every other month. 5-Fluorouracil is less effective, but since its toxicity (bone marrow) has a different spectrum, it can usefully be administered additionally to streptozotocin.[30-31] Recently Ericsson *et al.* reported an excellent effect of interferon treatment in a series of seven VIPoma patients.[32] Our own experience with two patients treated with interferon was less good: We noted no remission and a high incidence of side effects.[33] Symptomatic relief has been obtained in individual patients (unrepeatably) with indomethacin,[34] lithium,[35] metoclopramide,[36] and trifluoperazine.[37] In contrast long-acting somatostatin has proved most useful.[38-39] An octapeptide, SMS 201-995 (Octreotide, Sandoz) lasts for up to eight hours after subcutaneous injection and can be administered at home by the patient using similar techniques to those used for insulin administration. Remission of symptoms lasting over a year can be achieved,[40] and tumor shrinkage has even been reported.[41] It is likely that somatostatin acts both on the tumor to inhibit peptide production and also directly on the enterocytes of the intestine to inhibit watery secretion. Recently SMS 201-995 has been shown to be active by mouth.[42] As a treatment of last resort, high-dose steroids induce a temporary remission.

In conclusion, the tumor syndrome originally described by Verner and Morrison is now extremely well defined. From the scientific viewpoint this "experiment of nature" has yielded both useful information on the chronic systemic effects in man of the VIP family of peptides and has also been of assistance in the isolation of the messenger RNA and peptide products of prepro-VIP. The recent identification of PHV-42 has opened up the question of which peptide product is mainly responsible for the diarrhea and other symptoms of the clinical tumor syndrome.

REFERENCES

1. VERNER, J. V. & A. B. MORRISON. 1958. Islet cell tumor and a syndrome of refractory watery diarrhea and hypokalaemia. Am. J. Med. **25:** 374-380.
2. SAID, S. I. & V. MUTT. 1970. Polypeptide with broad biological activity: Isolation from small intestine. Science **169:** 1217-1218.
3. BLOOM, S. R., J. M. POLAK & A. G. E. PEARSE. 1973. Vasoactive intestinal peptide and watery diarrhea syndrome. Lancet **2:** 14-16.
4. BLOOM, S. R. & J. M. POLAK. 1982. VIPomas. *In* Vasoactive Intestinal Peptides. S. I. Said, Ed.: 457-468. Raven Press. New York.
5. LONG, R. G., M. G. BRYANT, S. J. MITCHELL, T. E. ADRIAN, J. M. POLAK & S. R.

BLOOM. 1981. Clinicopathological study of pancreatic and ganglioneuroblastoma tumors secreting vasoactive intestinal polypeptide (VIPomas). Br. Med. J. **282:** 1767-1771.

6. MODLIN, I. M., S. R. BLOOM & S. J. MITCHELL. 1978. Experimental evidence for vasoactive intestinal peptide as the cause of the watery diarrhea syndrome. Gastroenterology **75:** 1051-1054.

7. KREJS, G. J., J. S. FORDTRAN & S. R. BLOOM. 1980. Effect of VIP infusion on water and ion transport in the human jejunum. Gastroenterology **78:** 722-727.

8. KREJS, G. J. 1980. Effect of VIP infusion on water and ion transport in the human large intestine. Gastroenterology **78:** 1200.

9. TATEMOTO, K. & V. MUTT. 1981. Isolation and characterization of a novel intestinal peptide, porcine PHI (PHI-27), a new member of the glucagon-secretin family. Proc. Natl. Acad. Sci. USA **78:** 6603.

10. CHRISTOFIDES, N. D., Y. YIANGOU, M. A. BLANK, K. TATEMOTO, J. M. POLAK & S. R. BLOOM. 1982. Are peptide histidine isoleucine and vasoactive intestinal peptide co-synthesised in the same pro-hormone? Lancet **2:** 1398.

11. ITOH, N., K. OBATA, N. YANAIHARA & H. OKAMOTO. 1983. Human prepro-vasoactive intestinal polypeptide contains a novel PHI-27-like peptide PHM-27. Nature **304:** 547.

12. BLOOM, S. R., N. D. CHRISTOFIDES, J. DELAMARTER, G. BUELL, E. KAWASHIMA & J. M. POLAK. 1983. Diarrhea in VIPoma patients associated with co-secretion of a second active peptide, PHI, explained by a single coding gene. Lancet **2:** 1163.

13. ANAGNOSTIDES, A. A., N. D. CHRISTOFIDES, K. TATEMOTO, V. S. CHADWICK & S. R. BLOOM. 1984. Peptide histidine isoleucine: A secretagogue in human jejunum. Gut **25:** 381-385.

14. MORIARTY, K. J., J. E. HEGARTY, K. TATEMOTO, V. MUTT, N. D. CHRISTOFIDES, S. R. BLOOM & J. R. WOOD. 1984. Effect of peptide histidine isoleucine on water and electrolyte transport in the human jejunum. Gut **25:** 624-628.

15. ALLEN, J. M., N. D. CHRISTOFIDES, G. GORNACZ, K. TATEMOTO, J. H. BARON & S. R. BLOOM. 1983. Infusion of a novel peptide, PHI, in man. Pharmacokinetics and effect on gastric secretion. Experientia **39:** 1129-1131.

16. YIANGOU, Y., F. REQUEJO, J. M. POLAK & S. R. BLOOM. 1986. Characterization of a novel prepro-VIP derived peptide. Biochem. Biophys. Res. Commun. **139:** 1142-1149.

17. YIANGOU, Y., N. D. CHRISTOFIDES, M. A. BLANK, N. YANAIHARA, K. TATEMOTO, A. E. BISHOP, J. M. POLAK & S. R. BLOOM. 1985. Molecular forms of peptide histidine isoleucine-like immunoreactivity in the gastrointestinal tract. Nonequimolar levels of peptide histidine isoleucine and vasoactive intestinal peptide in the stomach explained by the presence of a big peptide histidine isoleucine-like molecule. Gastroenterology **89:** 516-524.

18. YIANGOU, Y., S. J. WILLIAMS, A. E. BISHOP, J. M. POLAK & S. R. BLOOM. 1987. Peptide histidine-methionine immunoreactivity in plasma and tissue from patients with vasoactive intestinal peptide-secreting tumors and the watery diarrhea syndrome. J. Clin. Endocrinol. Metab. **64:** 131-139.

19. MORRIS, H. R. 1980. Biomolecular structure determination by mass spectrometry. Nature **286:** 447-452.

20. MORRIS, H. R. & M. PANICO. 1981. Fast atom bombardment: A new mass spectrometric method for peptide sequence analysis. Biochem. Biophys. Res. Commun. **101:** 623-631.

21. MORRIS, H. R., M. PANICO, A. KARPLUS, P. E. LLOYD & B. RINIKER. 1982. Elucidation by FAB-MS of the structure of a new cardiactive peptide from Aplysia. Nature **300:** 643-645.

22. MORRIS, H. R., M. PANICO, T. ETIENNE, J. TIPPINS, S. I. GIRGIS & I. MACINTYRE. 1984. Isolation and characterization of human calcitonin gene-related peptide. Nature **308:** 746-748.

23. KRAFT, A. R., R. K. TOMPKINS & R. ZOLLINGER. 1970. Recognition and management of the diarrhea syndrome caused by non beta islet cell tumors of the pancreas. Am. J. Surg. **119:** 163-170.

24. MITCHELL, S. J. & S. R. BLOOM. 1978. Measurement of fasting and postprandial plasma VIP in man. Gut **19:** 1043-1048.

25. POLAK, J. M., S. R. BLOOM, T. E. ADRIAN, P. HEIGHTS, M. G. BRYANT & A. G. E.

PEARSE. 1976. Pancreatic polypeptide in insulinomas, gastrinomas, VIPomas and glucagonomas. Lancet I: 328-330.

26. ADRIAN, T. E., L. O. UTTENTHAL, S. J. WILLIAMS & S. R. BLOOM. 1986. Secretion of pancreatic polypeptide in patients with pancreatic endocrine tumors. N. Engl. J. Med. **315:** 287-291.

27. BLACKBURN, A. M., M. G. BRYANT, T. E. ADRIAN & S. R. BLOOM. 1981. Pancreatic tumors produce neurotensin. J. Clin. Endocrinol. Metab. **52:** 820-822.

28. MITCHENERE, P., T. E. ADRIAN, R. M. KIRK & S. R. BLOOM. 1981. Effect of gut regulatory peptides on intestinal luminal fluid in the rat. Life Sci. **29:** 1563-1570.

29. CALAM, J., R. UNWIN & W. S. PEART. 1983. Neurotensin stimulates defaecation. Lancet **1:** 737-738.

30. KAHN, C. R., A. G. LEVY, J. D. GARDNER, J. V. MILLER, P. GORDON & P. S. SCHEIN. 1975. Pancreatic cholera: Beneficial effects of treatment with streptozotocin. N. Engl. J. Med. **292:** 941-945.

31. MOERTAL, C. G., J. A. HANLEY & L. A. JOHNSON. 1980. Streptozotocin alone compared with streptozotocin plus 5-fluorouracil in the treatment of advanced islet-cell carcinoma. N. Engl. J. Med. **303:** 1189-1194.

32. ERICSSON, B., K. OBERG, G. ALLEN *et al.* 1986. Treatment of malignant endocrine pancreatic tumors with human leucocyte interferon. Lancet **2:** 1307-1308.

33. ANDERSON, J. V. & S. R. BLOOM. 1987. Treatment of malignant endocrine pancreatic tumors with human leucocyte interferon. Lancet **1:** 97.

34. JAFFE, B. M., D. F. KOPEN, K. DE SCHRYVER-KECSKEMETI, R. L. GINGERICH & M. GREIDER. 1977. Indomethacin-responsive pancreatic cholera. N. Engl. J. Med. **197:** 817-821.

35. PANDOL, S. J., L. Y. KORMAN, D. M. MCCARTHY & J. D. GARDNER. 1980. Beneficial effect of oral lithium carbonate in the treatment of pancreatic cholera syndrome. N. Engl. J. Med. **302:** 1403-1404.

36. LONG, R. G., M. G. BRYANT, P. M. YUILLE, J. M. POLAK & S. R. BLOOM. 1981. Mixed pancreatic apudoma with symptoms of excess vasoactive intestinal polypeptide and insulin: Improvement of diarrhea with metoclopramide. Gut **22:** 505-511.

37. DONOWITZ, M., G. ELTA, S. R. BLOOM & L. NATHANSON. 1980. Trifluoperazine reversal of secretory diarrhea in pancreatic cholera. Ann. Intern. Med. **93:** 283-285.

38. LONG, R. G., A. J. BARNES, T. E. ADRIAN, C. N. MALLINSON, M. R. BROWN, W. VALE, N. D. CHRISTOFIDES & S. R. BLOOM. 1979. Suppression of pancreatic endocrine tumor secretion by long-acting somatostatin analogue. Lancet **2:** 764-767.

39. WOOD, S. M., M. E. KRAENZLIN, T. E. ADRIAN & S. R. BLOOM. 1985. Treatment of patients with pancreatic endocrine tumors using a new long-acting somatostatin analogue symptomatic and peptide responses. Gut **26:** 438-444.

40. CH'NG, J. L. C., J. V. ANDERSON, S. J. WILLIAMS, D. H. CARR & S. R. BLOOM. 1986. Remission of symptoms during long term treatment of metastatic pancreatic endocrine tumors with long acting somatostatin analogue. Br. Med. J. **292:** 981-982.

41. KRAENZLIN, M. E., J. L. C. CH'NG, S. M. WOOD, D. H. CARR & S. R. BLOOM. 1984. Long-term treatment of a VIPoma with somatostatin analogue resulting in remission of symptoms and possible shrinkage of metastases. Gastroenterology **88:** 185-187.

42. WILLIAMS, G., J. A. BALL, J. M. BURRIN, G. F. JOPLIN & S. R. BLOOM. 1986. Effective and lasting growth-hormone suppression in active acromegaly with oral administration of somatostatin analogue SMS 201-995. Lancet **II:** 774-777.

Somatostatin and Analogues in the Treatment of VIPoma

T. M. O'DORISIO,[a] T. S. GAGINELLA, H. S.
MEKHJIAN, B. RAO, AND M. S. O'DORISIO

Department of Internal Medicine and Pediatrics
The Ohio State University
College of Medicine
Columbus, Ohio 43210

Precedent for natural peptide therapy began with the use of insulin in the treatment of insulin-dependent diabetes mellitus in 1922.[1] More recently, we have witnessed the use of interferon, interleukin-2, and tumor necrosis factor (TNF), all naturally occurring peptides in man. Most recently, the novel long-acting analogue of natural somatostatin has become available on a compassionate need basis for refractory, symptomatic endocrine tumors of the gastroenteropancreatic (GEP) axis. $SMS_{201-995}$ (Sandostatin) is a long-acting analogue of the naturally occurring somatostatin$_{1-14}$.[2] Its clinical and therapeutic impact in gut endocrinology and tumors of the GEP system is rapidly being recognized.[3,4] The rationale for both the development and clinical use of a somatostatin analogue has been best demonstrated in the management of the VIPoma–watery diarrhea syndrome (WDS).[5,6]

Somatostatin was initially isolated, sequenced, and synthesized by Brazeau and colleagues in 1973.[7] Another form of a naturally occurring somatostatin is somatostatin-28. These two forms of somatostatin are localized in the hypothalamus, pancreas, stomach, and intestinal tract. The potential regulatory importance of these two natural forms of somatostatin has been recently reviewed.[8] Since somatostatin's discovery, much has been learned regarding its regulatory function. It is indeed a hormone in the classic sense, as it modulates inhibition of growth hormone via the hypothalamo-pituitary portal circulation. Further, because of its unique location in the pancreatic islet cell and in peptidergic nerve fibers, somatostatin is suggested to have an important role as both a paracrine and neurocrine substance.[9] In addition to its well-known growth hormone inhibition properties, somatostatin inhibits the release or action of thyrotropin, insulin, glucagon, secretin, gastrin, cholecystokinin, gastric inhibitory polypeptide (GIP), pancreatic polypeptide, neurotensin, and motilin. Its nonendocrine actions include inhibition of gastric acid secretion and gastric emptying, pancreatic bicarbonate and enzyme release, gall bladder contraction, and splanchnic blood flow. Further, it attenuates intestinal motility. Both the endocrine and nonendocrine effects of somatostatin have been recently reviewed.[9,10] It is of interest that in addition to its inhibitory action on VIP (discussed below), somatostatin has been shown to release VIP in brain cells by a cyclic AMP-mediated pathway.[9]

[a] Address for correspondence: T. M. O'Dorisio, M.D., Room N-1123, Doan Hall, The OSU Hospitals, 410 W. 10th Ave., Columbus, OH 43210-1228.

In 1958, Verner and Morrison described two patients with pancreatic tumors associated with fulminant secretory diarrhea.[11] It was appreciated early on that the mechanism of this secretory diarrhea was different than the diarrhea described in patients with gastrinoma, the Zollinger-Ellison (ZE) syndrome.[12] In the patients with ZE syndrome and hyperacid secretion, nasogastric suction relieved the diarrhea, but nasogastric suction had no effect on the secretory diarrhea of the Verner-Morrison syndrome. Although a number of peptides including GIP and secretin were incriminated as mediators of the secretory diarrhea, none fit the pathophysiologic observations of the syndrome, namely, secretory diarrhea, hypochlorhydria, hypokalemia, hypochloremic metabolic acidosis, and flushing. It was not until the isolation and description of vasoactive intestinal peptide (VIP) by Said and Mutt in 1970[13] that the possibility of a peptide-mediated cause of the Verner-Morrison syndrome could be seriously considered. In 1973, VIP was found to be elevated in both tumor and plasma of patients with WDS.[14] However, VIP was not immediately accepted as a major mediator of WDS or Verner-Morrison syndrome. This was due, in part, to the fact that the regulating function of VIP was not that of a true hormone such as gastrin, secretin, or GIP; rather, it more closely resembled a neuromodulating substance that was very difficult to demonstrate *in vivo*.

In 1978 Mitchel, Bloom, and Modlin demonstrated that chronic VIP infusion mimicking plasma levels observed in WDS patients was associated with clinical diarrhea in pigs.[15] Shortly thereafter, we were able to demonstrate that high-dose, short-term VIP infusion causes intestinal fluid secretion in an *in vivo* rat model.[16] The definitive causal association between VIP and intestinal secretion in humans was demonstrated by Cain and associates in 1983.[17] They found that chronic VIP infusion in normal humans (mimicking plasma levels observed in patients with VIPoma/WDS) resulted in a secretory diarrhea state. It is now well accepted that VIP is the major mediator of the Verner-Morrison or watery diarrhea syndrome.

Native somatostatin inhibits the effects of a number of hormones. However, the role of somatostatin as an antagonist of the normal or pathophysiologic action of VIP is less well delineated. For our purposes, we will consider the somatostatin analogue $SMS_{201-995}$ to have virtually the same properties as native somatostatin in terms of the mechanism through which it inhibits VIP-mediated intestinal secretion. Precedent for native somatostatin having an antagonistic effect on VIPoma/WDS was first noted in 1982 by Ruskone and colleagues.[18] They demonstrated that intravenous infusion of native somatostatin (500 μg/hr) in a patient with VIPoma/WDS caused a decrease of both ileal fluid flow and circulating plasma VIP levels. More recently, it has been shown that treatment with $SMS_{201-995}$ resulted in a dramatic improvement in patients with symptomatic watery diarrhea.[5,6,19,20]

Whether or not the beneficial effects of the somatostatin analogue in patients with VIPoma-WDS is due solely to inhibition of the release of VIP from its tumor site[6] and/or inhibition of the action of VIP on its target organ (intestinal epithelial cells) remains to be clarified. However, a number of studies point to a direct common action of native somatostatin and its synthetic analogue. In studies by Maton *et al.*,[5] Benson *et al.*,[20] and Edwards and colleagues,[21] $SMS_{201-995}$ prolonged inhibition of intestinal secretion even though plasma VIP concentrations remained at elevated levels associated with WDS.[17] It is assumed that the plasma VIP in these studies was the biologically active form of the peptide. However, a later report by Maton and colleagues of a patient with VIPoma/WDS treated for three months with $SMS_{201-995}$ suggested that conversion of VIP to an inactive form during drug therapy may have occurred.[22] Thus it appears reasonable to assume that at least part of the action of native somatostatin or $SMS_{201-995}$ is to interfere with VIP stimulation of the secretory process at the intestinal epithelial cell level. In broader terms, one might consider the effects of

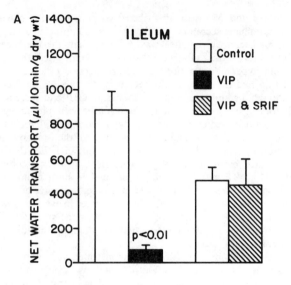

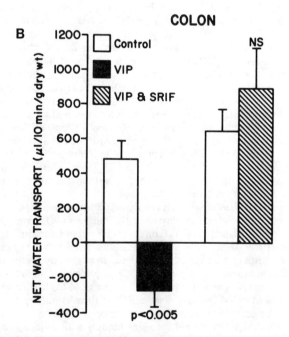

FIGURE 1. Panel **A** illustrates the inhibitory effect of VIP (14.3 μg/kg/hr, i.v.) on rat ileal water transport in the absence and presence (43 μg/kg/hr, i.v.) of somatostatin (SRIF). Panel **B** illustrates the effects of VIP with and without SRIF (same doses as ileum) in the colon. The bars represent mean ($\pm$ standard error) for six to eight separate animals.

somatostatin on motility. A slowing of motility might be envisioned as allowing more contact time with the mucosa, resulting in enhanced absorption of fluid and electrolytes throughout the gastrointestinal tract. This type of an effect would be much like that originally postulated for the opiates, which were thought to inhibit transit through the bowel thus allowing more contact time for absorption. Somatostatin may have effects on intestinal motility in part due to inhibition of the release of acetylcholine within the myenteric plexes.[23] Whether such an effect occurs in man is not known, nor is it likely that an inhibition of transit could completely explain the dramatic therapeutic effects of $SMS_{201-995}$ in patients with the massive fluid secretion that occurs in WDS. However, just as the opiates have been shown to enhance mucosal electrolyte absorption independent of effects on motility, we believe that $SMS_{201-995}$ also exerts direct effects on the mucosa.

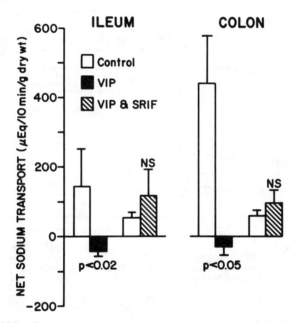

FIGURE 2. Net sodium transport in the rat ileum and colon in response to VIP in the absence and presence of SRIF (doses as in FIG. 1) means (± standard error), six to eight animals.

That VIP is a potent intestinal secretagogue has been established for more than a decade.[15,17] Active secretion of chloride has been observed in experimental animals and man after the administration of VIP. Furthermore, the effect of VIP appears to be directly upon the epithelial cells because it occurs *in vitro* and VIP receptors (linked to adenylate cyclase) exist on mammalian epithelial cell basal-lateral membranes. The high concentrations of VIP within enteric neurons, in close proximity to the epithelial cells, also suggests a possible role of VIP as a neuromodulator.[22] For a more detailed discussion of the effects of and the mechanism of action of VIP as an intestinal secretagogue, the reader is referred to a previous review.[25]

Somatostatin inhibits VIP-induced secretion and cyclic AMP accumulation in the rat colon.[26] The secretion of fluid in the rat jejunum is inhibited by somatostatin.[27] In the rat ileum, somatostatin enhances net chloride absorption as the result of enhance-

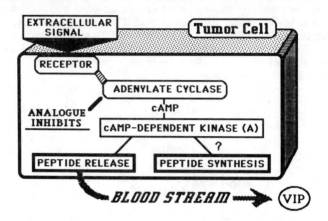

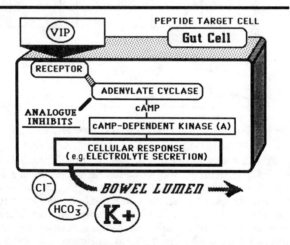

FIGURE 3. Panel **A** demonstrates a hypothetical mechanism whereby the somatostatin analogue $SMS_{201-995}$ (and somatostatin) acts on adenylate cyclase to alter the synthesis or release of VIP from a peptide-containing tumor. Panel **B** illustrates a mechanism by which $SMS_{201-995}$ may inhibit adenylate cyclase, post-recognition site (VIP receptor), thereby reducing electrolyte secretion by intestinal epithelial cells; inhibition of cAMP stimulation of protein kinase may also occur.

ment of mucosa-to-serosal chloride flux and simultaneous inhibition of secrosal-to-mucosal flux.[28] We have demonstrated that somatostatin reverses the secretory effects of VIP in ileal and colonic perfusion experiments in the rat (FIGS. 1 and 2). When VIP (14.3 μg/kg/hr) and somatostatin (42 μg/kg/hr) were infused simultaneously through separate jugular veins, VIP produced its characteristic inhibitory response in the ileum and induced secretion in the colon;[16] somatostatin significantly reversed these effects. These experiments further demonstrate functional antagonism by somatostatin of the VIP effect. However, they do not target the locus of action of the antagonism.

VIP receptors are present on rat intestinal epithelial cells.[29,30] Binding sites for somatostatin in cytosolic fractions of rabbit intestinal mucosa have been identified but these sites did not appear to cross-react with VIP.[31] Although we have not done studies to determine competition of somatostatin or SMS$_{201-995}$ for VIP binding sites on gut mucosal cells, we have obtained evidence for such a direct interaction on lymphocytes. Using lymphoblasts, we found that somatostatin inhibits the stimulatory effect of VIP on adenylate cyclase.[32] Whether this effect occurs in intestinal cells and at the G$_i$ or G$_s$ subunits or at the regulatory subunit (receptor binding site) remains to be elucidated. Perhaps studies with pertussis toxin, which uncouples the somatostatin receptors from adenylate cyclase,[33] may be helpful in this regard.

VIP induces intestinal secretion through the adenylate cyclase-cyclic AMP pathway, and it appears that somatostatin and SMS$_{201-995}$ probably act on the intestinal cell adenylate cyclase system to directly antagonize intestinal secretion. FIGURE 3A and B offers a schema that illustrates the possible antagonistic action of SMS$_{201-995}$ at both the peptide-containing tumor (in this case VIPoma) and on the target organ of the tumor peptide (in this case the secreting gut cell). As recently suggested, if peptide synthesis and release are coupled, it is quite possible that somatostatin and SMS$_{201-995}$ may modulate peptide synthesis at the tumor cell level and thus prevent release from the tumor of biologically active peptide. This may explain the observations of Maton *et al.*[22] and the dramatic diminution in plasma VIP levels in patients treated with SMS$_{201-995}$.[5,6,19,20]

REFERENCES

1. FORSHAM, P. H. 1982. Milestones in the 60-year history of insulin (1922-1982). Diabetes Care **5:** 1-3.
2. BAUER, W., U. BRINER, W. DOEPFNER *et al.* 1982. SMS 201-995. A very potent and selective octapeptide analogue of somatostatin with prolonged action. Life Sci. **31:** 1133-1140.
3. O'DORISIO, T. M., Guest Ed. 1986. Neuroendocrine disorders of the gastroenteropancreatic system. Am. J. Med. **81(6B):** 1-101.
4. KREJS, G. J., Guest Ed. 1987. Gut endocrine tumors. Am. J. Med. **82(5B):** 1-99.
5. MATON, P. H., T. M. O'DORISIO, B. A. HOWE *et al.* 1985. Effect of a long-acting somatostatin analogue (201-995) in a patient with pancreatic cholera. N. Engl. J. Med. **312:** 17-21.
6. SANTANGELO, W. C., T. M. O'DORISIO, J. G. KIM *et al.* 1985. Pancreatic cholera syndrome: Effect of a synthetic somatostatin analog on intestinal water and ion transport. Ann. Int. Med. **103:** 363-367.
7. BRAZEAU, P., W. L. VALE, R. BURGESS, H. LING *et al.* 1973. Hypothalamic polypeptide that inhibits the secretion of immunoreactive pituitary growth hormone. Science **179:** 77-79.

8. BRAZEAU, P. 1986. Somatostatin: A peptide with unexpected physiologic activities. Am. J. Med. **81(6B):** 8-13.
9. REICHLEN, S. 1986. Somatostatin: Historical aspects. Scand. J. Gastroenterol. **21:** 1-10.
10. SCHUSDZIARRA, V. & R. SCHMID. 1986. Physiological and pathophysiological aspects of somatostatin. Scand. J. Gastroenterol. **21:** 29-41.
11. VERNER, J. V. & A. B. MORRISON 1958. Islet cell tumor and a syndrome of refractory watery diarrhea and hypokalemia. Am. J. Med. **25:** 374-380.
12. ZOLLINGER, R. M. & E. H. ELLISON. 1955. Primary peptic ulcerations of the jejunum associated with islet cell tumors of the pancreas. Ann. Surg. **142:** 709-723.
13. SAID, S. I. & V. MUTT. 1970. Polypeptide with broad biological activity: Isolation from small intestine. Science **169:** 1217-1218.
14. BLOOM, S. R., J. M. POLAK & H. G. E. PEARSE. 1973. Vasoactive intestinal peptide and watery diarrhea syndrome. Lancet **2:** 14-16.
15. MODLIN, I. M., S. R. BLOOM & S. J. MITCHELL. 1978. Experimental evidence for vasoactive intestinal peptide as the cause of the watery diarrhoea syndrome. Gastroenterology **75:** 1051-1054.
16. WU, Z. C., T. M. O'DORISIO, S. CATALAND, H. S. MEKHJIAN & T. S. GAGINELLA. 1979. Effects of pancreatic polypeptide and vasoactive intestinal peptide on rat ileal and colonic water and electrolyte transport *in vivo.* Dig. Dis. Sci. **24:** 625-630.
17. KANE, M. G., T. M. O'DORISIO & G. J. KREJS. 1983. Production of secretory diarrhea by intravenous infusions of vasoactive intestinal polypeptide. N. Engl. J. Med. **309:** 1482-1485.
18. RUSKONE, A., E. RENE, J. CHOYVIALLE *et al.* 1982. Effect of somatostatin on diarrhea and on small intestinal water and electrolyte transport in a patient with pancreatic cholera. Dig. Dis. Sci. **27:** 459-466.
19. KRAENZLIN, M. E., J. L. C. CH'NG, S. M. WOOD, D. H. CARR & S. R. BLOOM. 1985. Long-term treatment of VIPoma with somatostatin analogue resulting in remission of symptoms and possible shrinkage of metastasis. Gastroenterology **88:** 185-187.
20. BENSON, G. D., T. M. O'DORISIO, E. C. ELLISON, E. A. WOLTERING & A. B. MORRISON. 1986. Control of watery diarrhea syndrome in a patient with a vasoactive intestinal peptide-secreting tumour, using SMS 201-995 and dexamethasone. Scand. J. Gastroenterol. **21(119):** 170-176.
21. EDWARD, C. A., P. A. CONN, N. W. READ & C. D. HOLDSWORTH. 1986. The effect of somatostatin analogue SMS 201-995 on fluid and electrolyte transport in a patient with secretory diarrhea. Scand. J. Gastroenterol. **21:** 259-261.
22. MATON, P. N., T. M. O'DORISIO, M. S. O'DORISIO *et al.* 1986. Successful therapy of pancreatic cholera with the long-acting somatostatin analogue SMS 201-995. Relation between plasma concentrations of drug and clinical and biochemical responses. Scand. J. Gastroenterol. **21(119):** 181-186.
23. TEITELBAUM, D. H., T. M. O'DORISIO, W. E. PERKINS & T. S. GAGINELLA. 1984. Somatostatin modulation of peptide-induced acetylcholine release in guinea pig ileum. Am. J. Physiol. **246:** G509-G514.
24. GAGINELLA, T. S. & T. M. O'DORISIO. 1979. Vasoactive intestinal polypeptide: Neuromodulator of intestinal secretion. *In* Mechanisms of Intestinal Secretion: 231-247. Allen R. Liss Inc. New York.
25. GAGINELLA, T. S., K. A. HUBEL & T. M. O'DORISIO. 1982. Effects of vasoactive intestinal peptide on intestinal chloride secretion. *In* Vasoactive Intestinal Peptide. Sami I. Said, Ed.: 211-222. Raven Press. New York.
26. CARTER, R. F., K. N. BITAR, A. M. ZFASS & G. M. MAKHLOUF. 1978. Inhibition of VIP-stimulated intestinal secretion and cyclic AMP production by somatostatin in the rat. Gastroenterology **74:** 726-730.
27. DHARMSATHAPHORN, K., R. S. SHERWIN & J. W. DOBBINS. 1980. Somatostatin inhibits fluid secretion in the rat jejunum. Gastroenterology **79:** 1554-1557.
28. DHARMSATHAPHORN, K., H. J. BINDER & J. W. DOBBINS. 1980. Somatostatin stimulates sodium and chloride absorption in the rabbit ileum. Gastroenterology **78:** 1559-1565.
29. AMIRANOFF, B., M. LABURTHE & G. ROSSELIN. 1980. Characterization of specific binding

sites for vasoactive intestinal peptide in rat intestinal epithelial cell membrane. Biochem. Biophys. Acta **627:** 215-224.

30. LABURTHE, M., J. C. PRIETO, B. AMIRANOFF *et al.* 1979. Interaction of vasoactive intestinal peptide with isolated intestinal cells from rat. Eur. J. Biochem. **96:** 239-248.

31. LOPEZ-RUIZ, M. P., E. ARILLA, L. GONZALES-GUIJANO & J. C. PRIETO. 1985. Somatostatin binding sites in cytosolic fractions of rabbit intestinal mucosa: Distribution throughout the intestinal tract. Comp. Biochem. Physiol. **81B:** 1041-1044.

32. O'DORISIO, M. S., N. S. HERMINS, T. M. O'DORISIO & S. P. BALCERZAK. 1981. Vasoactive intestinal polypeptide modulation of lymphocyte adenylate cyclase. J. Immunol. **127:** 2551-2554.

33. REISENE, T., ZHANG YAN-LING & R. SEKURA. 1985. Pertussis toxin treatment blocks the inhibition of somatostatin and increases the stimulation by forskolin of cyclic AMP accumulation and adreno-corticotropin secretion from mouse anterior pituitary tumor cells. J. Pharm. Exp. Ther. **232:** 275-282.

Vasoactive Intestinal Peptide in Sepsis and Shock

ARTHUR REVHAUG,[a] IDAR LYGREN, TROND G.
JENSSEN, KARL-E. GIERCKSKY, AND
PER G. BURHOL

Departments of Surgery and Internal Medicine
Tromsø University Hospital
Tromsø, Norway

The response to trauma, hypovolemia, septicemia, and circulatory collapse depends on a complex interaction between the nervous and humoral systems.[1-3] Recent investigations have demonstrated several neurotransmitters in both the central and peripheral nervous systems. Accordingly, their possible physiological actions may be responsible for widespread responses in the organism.

Vasoactive intestinal polypeptide (VIP) is a 28 amino acid residue peptide originally isolated from porcine intestine by Said and Mutt[4] and subsequently recognized as a neurotransmitter substance. Neurons containing VIP-like immunoreactivity have been demonstrated in the central nervous system, lung, and genitourinary tract, as well as in several other organs.[5-7]

The studies of Lillehei and Fine in the sixties suggested the GI tract to be of great importance in the development of irreversible shock. However, uncertainty has been reported with regard to the eventually important substances that might be released from the GI tract in shock.[8-10]

Among other characteristics of the GI tract is the fact that it represents an impressive hormonal organ. Large amounts of VIP-containing neurons are located in the gastrointestinal tract. VIP, which harbors potent vasodilatory effects, could be one of the connections between the classical neural and hormonal systems. In order to evaluate the possible role of VIP in sepsis and shock in general, we have tried to elucidate if—and eventually how—VIP is involved in shock states.

METHODS: EXPERIMENTAL STUDIES

Large blood volume, easy cardiovascular monitoring, and the fact that our VIP-RIA is based on original porcine material make a porcine experimental model a suitable large-animal model for shock studies.

[a]Address for correspondence: Arthur Revhaug, M.D., Ph.D., Department of Surgery, 9012 Tromsø University Hospital, Tromsø, Norway.

Animal Models

Anesthetized piglets were used to study the possible involvement of VIP in shock of different origins. After an overnight fast with free access to water, the animals are studied in inhalation anesthesia (halothane, N_2O, and oxygen). In this model, aortic blood pressure (BP), cardiac output (CO), pulmonary artery pressure (PA), left ventricular contractility (dp/dt), EKG, and diuresis are regularly measured.[11,12]

Blood samples may be drawn from different vessels like the superior caval, portal, and internal jugular veins as well as from the descending aorta. Hematological, chemical, and acid-base determinations are done using standard techniques.[11-13]

Endotoxin Studies

E. coli endotoxin (1 mg/kg body weight, lipopolysaccharide B, *E. coli* 026:B6, Difco, Michigan, U.S.A.) was administered intravenously over a two-hour period. With this dose, the animals developed a sublethal endotoxin shock.

In order to further evaluate the release mechanisms of VIP in endotoxinemia, in addition to the twenty animals used to determine cardiovascular, cellular, and changes in plasma VIP levels, another group ($n = 6$) of animals was studied in the same way after removal of the stomach and entire intestine.

Hemorrhagic Shock

Different kinds of hemorrhagic shock have been investigated. In one group of animals ($n = 12$), an external hemorrhagic shock was induced by rapid bleeding from the femoral artery. The systolic aortic pressure (BP) was lowered from a normal level to a level between 50 and 60 mm Hg during a 15-minute period. After the initial rapid bleeding, BP was maintained at 50-60 mm Hg for another 60 minutes by repeated smaller bleedings. Then 75 minutes after initiating the hemorrhage, the entire shed blood volume, which had been collected in standard blood bags, was reinfused into the superior caval vein over a 30-minute period. Six of the animals were used as controls.

A very peculiar, but clinically commonly seen hemorrhage, during which the bleeding takes place into the stomach or duodenum (upper gastroduodenal hemorrhage), was mimicked in different groups of animals. In one group ($n = 6$), a hemorrhagic shock identical in magnitude to the one described above, was studied by infusing the blood directly into the upper part of the duodenum. In a cross-over model ($n = 12$), paired animals were studied, one bleeding into the duodenum of the other, thus one group of animals only received blood into the duodenum. The effects of warm blood into the gut without the effects of any circulatory derangements could thereby be evaluated.[13,14]

Cardiodepressive Shock

A porcine model of cardiodepressive shock was developed to enable discrimination between a general low-flow state and an endotoxin reaction. Infusion of the tricyclic antidepressive agent nortryptiline 15 mg/kg body weight resulted in a severe shock state. To ensure whether or not this agent influenced on the capability of the animal to produce an adequate VIP response, endotoxin was administered to animals pretreated with nortryptiline.[15,16]

VIP in Anuria

Because any shock or low-flow state is followed regularly by severe impairment of renal function and oliguria, plasma VIP was studied in four animals in which both renal pedicles were acutely occluded, thereby inducing acute anuria.

Human Sepsis

Plasma VIP levels from peripheral blood in patients with severe bacterial pulmonary, abdominal, or urinary tract infections have been determined. The patients presented symptoms and signs of suffering from serious sepsis. Severe impairment of cardiovascular, renal, and metabolic functions were present when the blood samples were drawn. Positive blood cultures were later demonstrated in all septic patients. All patients recovered from their sepsis.

A corresponding group of noninfectious patients in good health was used for control measurements.

Assay of VIP in Plasma and Gel Permeation Chromatography

Plasma levels of VIP were determined using a radioimmunoassay previously described.[17] This assay had a detection limit of 0.8 pmol/l, within assay precision of 7.8%, and between assay precision of 13.1%. The final dilution of the antiserum to bind 50% of 0.9 fmol ^{125}I-labeled VIP was 1 : 250,000. No cross-reactivity is found with secretin, gastrin, glucagon, and insulin.

Plasma from animals stimulated with *E. coli* endotoxin was subjected to standard gel permeation chromatography procedures.

RESULTS

Endotoxin Studies

The animals developed a profound, but reversible state of shock with an increase in pulmonary artery pressure, a decrease in aortic blood pressure, cardiac output, and

TABLE 1. Cardiovascular Parameters in Endotoxinemia[a,b]

Parameter		0	1	Time (h) 2	3	6
Systolic aortic pressure, mm Hg	Endotoxin	100 ± 5	65 ± 8[c]	54 ± 8[c]	63 ± 5[c]	73 ± 12
	Controls	101 ± 2	98 ± 2	93 ± 4	96 ± 2	95 ± 2
Cardiac output liters/min	Endotoxin	5.1 ± 0.8	4.1 ± 0.6	2.8 ± 0.4[c]	2.6 ± 0.5[c]	2.3 ± 0.5[c]
	Controls	4.3 ± 0.5	4.1 ± 0.4	3.6 ± 0.5	3.8 ± 0.5	3.6 ± 1.3
Total peripheral resistance, mm Hg/1/min	Endotoxin	17.0 ± 3.2	10.2 ± 4.3[c]	13.8 ± 1.8[c]	16.4 ± 3.9	21.9 ± 3.6
	Controls	17.6 ± 1.8	18.3 ± 2.3	19.8 ± 3.3	18.9 ± 2.6	21.3 ± 2.0

[a] Endotoxin perfusion took place over a two-hour period, starting at time zero.
[b] Results are mean ± SD values.
[c] Significantly different from control animals ($p < 0.01$).

total peripheral resistance (TABLE 1). Infusion of endotoxin led to a significant rise in plasma VIP levels within 30 minutes after the infusion started. Peak values representing some 20-fold increase were seen near the end of the infusion. The differences between the aortal and caval and internal jugular veins were not significant. The increase in portal VIP levels was significantly higher than the one in the systemic levels ($p < 0.01$). The peak values of plasma VIP corresponded to the phase in which the reduction in systolic blood pressure and total peripheral resistance was most accentuated. Systemic levels of plasma VIP did not normalize until 24 hours after the shock period (FIG. 1).

When the same dose of endotoxin was infused into animals in which the gastrointestinal tract had been surgically removed, no increase in plasma VIP levels could be demonstrated (FIG. 2). The gel permeation study demonstrated that *E. coli* endotoxin-stimulated plasma VIP eluted from the Sephadex G-50 fine column in two peaks, the first corresponding to the void volume, and the second to the elution volume for ^{125}I-labeled VIP (FIG. 3).

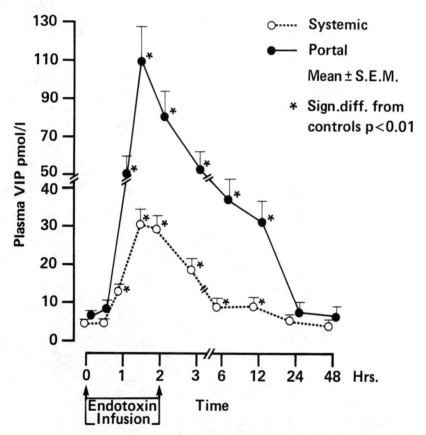

FIGURE 1. Plasma VIP levels in portal and caval veins following *E. coli* endotoxinemia in pigs ($n = 20$). Values are mean ± SD. In six control animals no change from basal levels could be measured (data not shown).

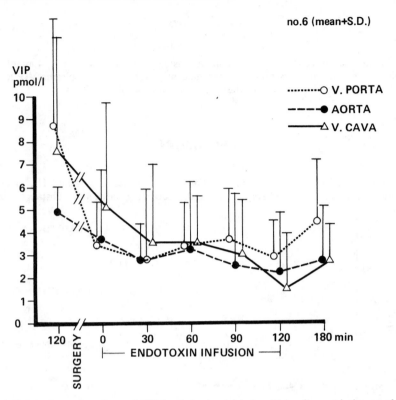

FIGURE 2. Systemic and portal VIP levels in six piglets in which, after surgical removal of the entire stomach and intestine, *E. coli* endotoxin was infused (1mg/kg BW). Values are mean ± SD.

Hemorrhage

No change in plasma VIP levels could be demonstrated in external hemorrhage, neither in the systemic nor portal circulation. When the hemorrhage was into the duodenum, a significant rise in the portal circulation was demonstrated. Infusion of blood into the duodenum without any circulatory derangement produced a similar significant short-lived rise in portal-VIP levels (FIG. 4).

Cardiodepressive Shock and Anuria

Cardiodepressive shock and anuria did not produce any change in plasma VIP levels.

Sepsis in Humans

In the healthy controls, the peripheral plasma VIP levels were 3 + 1 pmol/l, whereas the septic patients presented a significantly higher systemic plasma VIP level 24 ± 3.5 (SE), (p < 0.01) than the nonseptic patients (TABLE 2).

DISCUSSION

Several vasoactive agents (e.g., catecholamines, angiotensins II and III, prostaglandins, histamine, and others) are naturally occurring vasoactive substances that

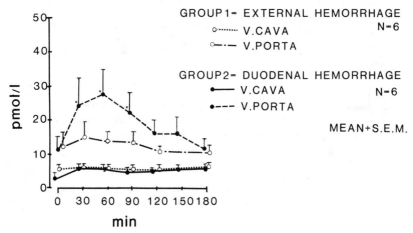

FIGURE 3. Systemic and portal plasma VIP levels in external (n = 6) and intraduodenal hemorrhage (n = 6) in pigs. Values are mean ± SE.

may contribute to the pathogenesis of shock.[1–3,18] Some of these substances have effects on the circulation throughout the organism while others may influence regional blood flow (e.g., angiotensin causes a shift in renal blood flow).

Endotoxin infusion produced an increase in plasma levels of a peptide with a VIP-like immunoreactivity. Gel permeation chromatography studies strongly indicate that the measured VIP-like immunoreactivity indeed is VIP. The highest levels measured corresponded to the hemodynamically most compromised state. The intestine seems to be the source of VIP during sepsis since the levels demonstrated in the portal vein were by far the highest. Also, the removal of the gastrointestinal tract abolished the VIP increase in plasma after endotoxin stimulation.

A specific endotoxin release of VIP may be assumed, as no increase in plasma VIP levels was observed in other low-flow states except in the septic state. Additionally, in a series of experiments, the installation into the duodenum of *E. coli* endotoxin did not induce any increase in plasma VIP levels (unpublished data). Thus, it may be concluded that endotoxin must be present in the circulation or in the tissue fluids before a release takes place.

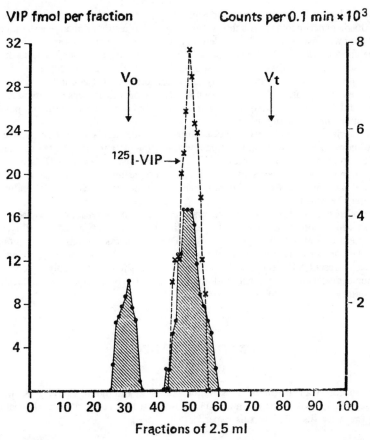

FIGURE 4. Elution diagram of immunoreactive plasma VIP in experimentally induced *E. coli* endotoxin shock in pigs (shaded area, ●——●) from a Sephadex G-50 Fine column (16 × 980 mm) calibrated with ^{125}I-labeled human serum albumin to indicate the void volume (V_o), ^{125}I-labeled VIP to indicate the elution volume for porcine VIP (x-----x) and ^{125}I to indicate the total mobile phase (V_t). Fractions of 2.5 ml were collected. Flow rate 15 ml/hr.

TABLE 2. Plasma VIP Levels in Normal and Septic Patients[a]

Subjects	Plasma VIP
Septic patients ($n = 7$)	24 ± 3.5 pmol/1[b]
Nonseptic patients ($n = 12$)	3 ± 1 pmol/1

[a] Results are mean ± SE.
[b] $p < 0.01$.

The modest and short-lived portal plasma VIP increase in the upper gastrointestinal hemorrhagic experiments is probably a "meal effect" as a similar change was observed when blood was installed into the duodenum in the absence of circulatory derangement.

The elevated plasma VIP levels in peripheral blood from human subjects during a severe sepsis confirm that this is a response that may also be of importance in man.

VIP has been demonstrated to play an important role in the control of vascular tone of several organs.[18] Therefore, vascular actions of VIP in sepsis seem probable. The amount of VIP measured in plasma can hardly be correlated with the possible impact upon the target organ.

The mechanism for the VIP release during endotoxinemia is, to our knowledge, yet not known. Exposure of cholera toxin on the feline intestine is reported to increase the VIP production from the intestine.[19] As no increased release of VIP is observed in other hypotensions except septic-endotoxin hypotension, the hypotension in shock in general does not seem to be the main release stimulator. Thus, a direct endotoxin action may be postulated.

The release of VIP in septic shock may represent an overreacting defense mechanism in which potentially beneficial effects like increased cardiac contractility, coronary artery dilatation, and lipo- and glycogenolytic effects no longer are contained within the compensated physiological response. The fact that circulating phagocytic blood cells present VIP receptors,[20,21] and that the VIP content in polymorpho- and mononuclear cells increases during endotoxinemia[22] could be of importance in localized inflammatory tissue.

ACKNOWLEDGMENTS

The authors want to thank O. K. Andersen, T. I. Lundgren, E. Berg, K. Myhr, J. Hansen, N. Vassvik, J. A. Reitan, and O. J. Østgaard for cooperation and assistance during the work discussed in this paper.

REFERENCES

1. MacLean, L. D. 1981. Shock, cause and management of circulatory collapse. *In* Textbook of Surgery. D. C. Sabiston, Ed.: 58. W. B. Saunders. Philadelphia, PA.
2. Shires, T. G., P. C. Camizaro & C. J. Carrico. 1984. Shock. *In* Principles of Surgery. 4th Edition. S. J. Schwartz, Ed.: 45. McGraw-Hill, Inc. New York.
3. Gann, D. S. & M. P. Lilly. 1983. Neuroendocrine response to trauma. World J. Surg. 7: 101.
4. Said, S. I. & V. Mutt. 1972. Isolation from porcine-intestinal wall of a vasoactive octacosapeptide related to secretin and to glucagon. Eur. J. Biochem. 28: 199-204.
5. Alm, P., J. Amulets, R. Håkonson & F. Sundler. 1977. Peptidergic (vasoactive intestinal peptide) nerves in the genitourinary tract. Neuroscience 2: 751-754.
6. Polak, J. & S. R. Bloom. 1979. The hormones of the gastrointestinal tract. *In* Scientific Basis of Gastroenterology. Churchill Livingstone. New York.
7. Robberecht, P., P. Chatelain, P. de Neef, J. C. Camus, M. Waelbroeck & J. Cristophe. 1981. Presence of vasoactive intestinal peptide receptors coupled to adenylate cyclase in rat lung membranes. Biochim. Biophys. Acta 678: 76-82.
8. Lillehei, R. C. 1957. The intestinal factor in irreversible hemorrhagic shock. Surgery 42: 1043.

9. LILLEHEI, R. C., J. K. LONGBEAM, J. H. BLOCH *et al.* 1964. The nature of irreversible shock: Experimental and clinical observations. Ann. Surg. **160:** 682.
10. FINE, J. & P. GUEVAS. 1974. Role of endotoxin and complement in shock. N. Engl. J. Med. **290:** 860.
11. REVHAUG, A., I. LYGREN, T. I. LUNDGREN *et al.* 1985. Increased plasma levels of vasoactive intestinal polypeptide in pigs during endotoxinaemia. Eur. Surg. Res. **17:** 75-82.
12. REVHAUG, A., I. LYGREN, T. I. LUNDGREN *et al.* 1984. Release of gastrointestinal peptides during *E. coli* endotoxinaemia. Acta Chir. Scand. **150:** 535-539.
13. REVHAUG, A. 1985. Gastrointestinal peptides in low flow states. Ph.D. thesis. Tromsø University. Tromsø, Norway.
14. REVHAUG, A., I. LYGREN, T. I. LUNDGREN *et al.* 1985. Changes in plasma levels of gastrointestinal peptides during hemorrhagic shock in pigs. Acta Chir. Scand.
15. REVHAUG, A., I. LYGREN, T. I. LUNDGREN *et al.* 1985. Release of gastrointestinal hormones in cardiopressive shock. Acta Anaesthesiol. Scand. **29.**
16. RUDORFER, M. W. 1982. Cardiovascular changes and plasma drug levels after amitryptiline overdose. J. Toxicol.-Clin. Toxicol. **19:** 67.
17. BURHOL, P. G., I. LYGREN, H. WALDUM *et al.* 1978. Radioimmunoassay of vasoactive intestinal polypeptide in plasma. Scand. J. Gastroenterol. **13:** 807-813.
18. LEFER, A. F. 1982. Vascular mediators in ischemia and shock. *In* Pathophysiology of Shock, Anoxia, and Ischmemia. R. A. Cowley & B. J. Trump, Eds. Williams & Wilkins. Baltimore, MD.
19. BLITZ, W. & G. A. CHARBON. 1983. Regional vascular influences of vasoactive intestinal polypeptide. Scand. J. Gastroenterol. **18:** 755.
20. CASSUTO, J., J. FAHRENKRUG, M. JODAL, R. TUTLE & O. LUNDGREN. 1981. Release of vasoactive intestinal polypeptide from the cat small intestine exposed to cholera toxin. Gut **22:** 958-963.
21. GUERRERO, J. M., J. C. PRIETO, F. L. ELORZA, R. RAMIREZ & R. GOBERNA. 1981. Interaction of vasoactive intestinal peptide with human blood mononuclear cells. Mol. Cell. Endocrinol. **21:** 151-160.
22. O'DORISIO, M. S., A. DANEK, T. M. O'DORISIO, J. M. GEORGE & S. P. BALCERZAK. 1981. Specific vasoactive intestinal peptide (VIP) binding to t lymphocytes. Clin. Res. **20:** No. 4.
23. REVHAUG, A., I. LYGREN, O. ANDERSEN, P. G. BURHOL & K-E. GIERCKSKY. 1983. Vasoactive intestinal polypeptide (VIP) in leucocytes. Scand. J. Clin. Lab. Invest. **43:** (Suppl. 164): 68.

Dysfunction of the Gastrointestinal Tract

Vasoactive Intestinal Peptide in Peristalsis and Sphincter Function

P. BIANCANI,[a,b] M. C. BEINFELD,[c] D. H. COY,[d] C. HILLEMEIER,[b] J. H. WALSH,[e] AND J. BEHAR [b]

[b] Division of Biological and Medical Sciences
Rhode Island Hospital
Brown University
Providence, Rhode Island 02902

[c] St. Louis University
St. Louis, Missouri

[d] Tulane University
New Orleans, Louisiana

[e] University of California at Los Angeles
Los Angeles, California

INTRODUCTION

Vasoactive intestinal peptide (VIP) is present in the esophagus, lower esophageal sphincter (LES), and internal anal sphincter. These organs relax in response to electrical stimulation, which is mediated by nonadrenergic, noncholinergic intrinsic inhibitory neurons as it is blocked by the neuropoison tetrodotoxin, but not by adrenergic, cholinergic, or other antagonists. They also relax in response to VIP, acting directly on myogenic receptors, since VIP-induced relaxation is not affected by tetrodotoxin (TTX). Both the relaxation induced by exogenous VIP and by stimulation of the inhibitory neurons can be blocked by incubation in highly specific antisera, and by VIP receptor antagonists. These findings are consistent with VIP being a (but not necessarily the only) neurotransmitter responsible for the descending inhibition associated with the peristaltic reflex in the gut. Dysfunction of VIP-mediated inhibitory reflex may be associated with esophageal spasm and dysphagia, achalasia, and Hirschprung disease, and a reduced VIPergic innervation has been demonstrated in some of these conditions.

[a] Address for correspondence: Piero Biancani, Ph.D., Gastrointestinal Motility Research Laboratory, 5SWP, Rhode Island Hospital, 593 Eddy Street, Providence, RI 02902.

Porcine peptide histidine isoleucine (PHI) may be a second inhibitory neurotransmitter, at least in the LES. Its precise role in peristalsis and in motility disfunction has not yet been established.

PHYSIOLOGICAL BASIS FOR VIP AS A NEUROTRANSMITTER IN THE GASTROINTESTINAL TRACT

Enteric Inhibitory Neurons in the Gut

Inhibitory neurons contained in the gut wall, and part of the enteric division of the autonomic nervous system, are responsible for a descending wave of inhibition that precedes peristaltic contraction.

Their existence has been known since the turn of the century. Langley first described stomach relaxation in response to vagal stimulation in 1898;[1] Bayliss and Starling (1899-1901)[2-4] described descending relaxation in the intestine, which persisted when the intestine was extrinsically denervated by resecting vagal and mesenteric fibers; and Langley and Magnus (1904) reported that this reflex was maintained *in vitro,* in the absence of any extrinsic innervation.[5]

In intervening years additional information has been acquired about the nature and function of these neurons. There is abundant evidence that these neurons are nonadrenergic, noncholinergic, and in most of the gastrointestinal tract, are postganglionic neurons of preganglionic cholinergic nerves. Several excellent reviews are available on this topic.[6-8] Only recently, however, we have begun to understand something about the nature of the neurotransmitter or neurotransmitters for these neurons.

We will discuss available evidence to support the role of VIP as an inhibitory neurotransmitter for these neurons in the esophagus,[9] lower esophageal sphincter,[10,11] and internal anal sphincter.[12] VIP involvement has also been demonstrated in the stomach[13] and colon.[14] In some parts of the gut, namely in the LES, PHI may be a second neurotransmitter.[15] The role of PHI in other portions of the gut is as yet undetermined.

Role of Enteric Inhibitory Neurons

The role of these neurons is to relax the circular muscle in order to facilitate passage of the bolus, and to allow those organs that act as reservoirs to expand and hold material. FIGURE 1 shows that the *in vitro* internal anal sphincter exhibits spontaneous high resting tone and relaxes in response to neural stimulation. The relaxation is neurally mediated as it is abolished by tetrodotoxin. It is, however, not affected by adrenergic or cholinergic blockers, nor by a variety of other receptor antagonists.[16,17] The lower esophageal sphincter behaves similarly[8] and so does the body of the esophagus, if its tone is elevated by the presence of bethanechol, thereby making it possible to visualize the effect of stimulation of inhibitory neurons. If inhibitory neurons are damaged, one may expect difficulty in bolus propulsion and in sphincter relaxation. Conversely, when these difficulties are experienced it is reasonable

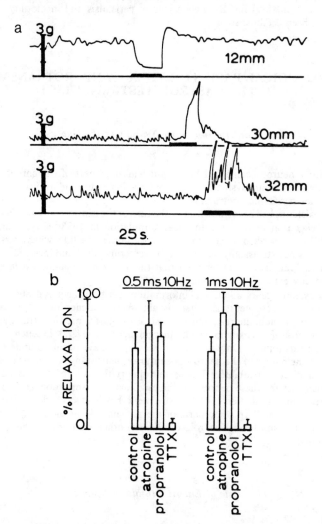

FIGURE 1. (A) Representative rabbit internal anal sphincter and rectal circular muscle strips. The internal anal sphincter strip (upper tracing) spontaneously maintains high resting tone and relaxes during electrical stimulation (1 msec, 10 Hz). Rectal strips (lower tracings) contract with varying latency after the beginning of the stimulus train. The stimulus train is shown by the thick horizontal bar. The distances in millimeters represent the distance of the strips from the outermost margin of the anal canal.

(B) Internal anal sphincter relaxation is blocked by tetrodotoxin (TTX) ($10^{-6} M$), but not by atropine or propranolol at the same molar concentration. Data represent mean ± SEM of four strips from four animals.

to look at a dysfunction of inhibitory neurons as a possible cause. Thus in order to imply a role of VIP in motility disorders in the GI tract, it is necessary to establish that VIP is a neurotransmitter, and that a defect of VIPergic innervation is present in those diseases that may be caused by lack or excess of inhibitory innervation. Decreased VIPergic innervation has been demonstrated in esophageal achalasia and in Hirschprung's disease, and is suspected in infantile pyloric stenosis. Conversely, increased VIPergic innervation may occur in some forms of diabetes.

Requirements of Neurotransmitters

For a substance to be a neurotransmitter, it must be contained and released from nerves to interact with the effector organ. Proving this point for any candidate substance may be difficult, as the synaptic space is small, the amount of neurotransmitter released minute, the time of presence in the synaptic space is short, and the neurotransmitter may be degraded or sequestered very rapidly. As it is difficult to determine directly what happens in the synaptic space, several less direct but experimentally verifiable criteria have been proposed to indicate that a substance may be a neurotransmitter.[7,18]

The criteria essentially are that the substance be detected in prejunctional neurons and in presynaptic terminals, released in measurable amounts from neurons in response to stimulation, and, when exogenously applied, should elicit responses similar to those elicited by neural stimulation.

None of these conditions, by themselves, are sufficient or even strictly necessary in order to establish a substance as a neurotransmitter. For instance, while presence in neurons and identity of effects are technically verifiable, demonstrating release is not always easy, as the amounts released may be small, and the even smaller quantity of peptide that escapes the receptors may be bound in the tissue or inactivated before diffusing into the perfusate in detectable amounts. Nevertheless, if sufficient material is released to escape and be detected, it must be decided whether it is the one responsible for the effect under investigation. Neural, that is electrical, stimulation of nerve trunks *in vivo* or field stimulation of tissue *in vitro* results in stimulation of a multiplicity of neurons and may release not only the neurotransmitter responsible for the effect under investigation, but also other transmitters that may be unrelated. Similarly, presence in neurons and identity of effects, by themselves, are not sufficient criteria, as multiple peptides are present in neurons, and their relative importance may be difficult to establish. In practice, as noted by Furness and Costa,[6] the criteria used in transmitter identification are empirical. Clues that accumulate over time lead to the hypothesis that a substance is a neurotransmitter, and the hypothesis may remain on trial for a long time.

The case for a neurotransmitter may be considerably strengthened if it can be shown that specific antagonists of the candidate substance antagonize the physiologic function of interest. For instance, *in vitro* contraction of the cat esophagus in response to field stimulation is abolished by atropine.[9] This finding strongly supports a role of cholinergic neurons in esophageal contraction. Conversely, the finding that propranolol, in doses that block relaxation induced by isoproterenol, does not affect LES relaxation in response to neural stimulation[8] excludes the possibility that LES relaxation may be mediated through β-adrenergic receptors.

Because of rapid advances in the discovery of new peptides, however, specific and selective antagonists are not always available. Less than ideal tools are often employed in order to show that the effects of neural stimulation and of the substances under investigation are blocked by the same interventions. Antisera and specific antagonists have been used to block relaxation induced both by exogenous VIP and by neural stimulation. These techniques have limitations that will be discussed in the following sections.

VIP as Neurotransmitter

Presence in Enteric Neurons

The presence of VIP-like immunoreactive material in the gastrointestinal tract has been extensively demonstrated and is discussed elsewhere in this symposium. It is generally agreed that in the gastrointestinal tract VIP is present only in neurons[19,20] that innervate circular muscle as well as mucosa and is especially rich in gastrointestinal sphincters.[21] VIPergic neurons contain other peptides, which include PHI,[22–25] neuropeptide Y (NPY),[24] and galanin,[26] but not necessarily all at the same time. The simultaneous presence of multiple peptides in the same neurons voids the argument that any one peptide may not be a neurotransmitter if its effect does not exactly mimic the effect of neural stimulation, since it is reasonable to expect that neural stimulation may cause release of more than one peptide, and produce results that are due to the interaction of multiple substances, rather than to any one single agent. Although VIP and PHI are unique in relaxing circular smooth muscle of the gut,[10–15] it is entirely possible that other inhibitory peptides yet to be discovered may also play a role in gut relaxation.

Release During Neural Stimulation

Electrical stimulation of the vagus and pelvic nerves,[27–31] as well as *in vitro* field stimulation of esophageal,[11] gastric,[13] and colonic[14] tissue result in measurable release of VIP. There is no evidence that the peptide plays a hormonal role, and the increase over basal levels reflects overflow of material released from neurons. The release is blocked by tetrodotoxin[14] and by the ganglionic antagonist hexamethonium, indicating that the pathway regulating the release involves cholinergic ganglionic transmission, coupled to a VIP-containing neuron. It therefore appears that VIP release is regulated by a mechanism similar to the one regulating gut relaxation.[8] In other organ systems it has been shown that VIP is coreleased with PHI,[32–34] and it is possible that the same may happen in the gut. Other peptides may also be released, but no evidence for this is yet available.

Inhibition by Antisera

In the body of the esophagus, lower esophageal sphincter, and internal anal sphincter preincubation in VIP antiserum, in concentrations sufficient to inhibit relaxation in response to ED_{50} VIP, results in reduction in relaxation in response to electrical (neural) stimulation (FIG. 2). It is apparent from the figure that preincubation in antiserum results only in partial block of relaxation induced by neural stimulation. This is not surprising as the antiserum at the concentrations used is only capable of inhibiting the half-maximal concentration of VIP, and higher concentrations of antiserum, after two hours' incubation, will affect the ability of the muscle to remain tonically contracted. A long period of incubation is required to insure that the large immunoglobulin molecule will diffuse through the tissue into the synaptic space. A

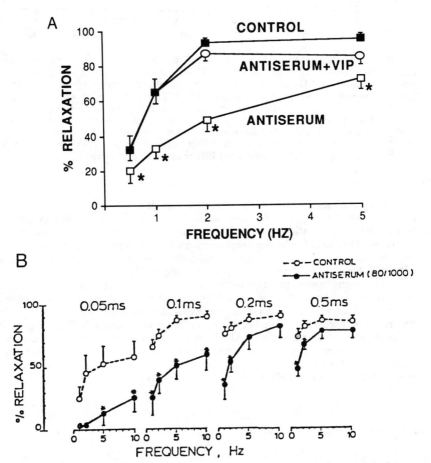

FIGURE 2. (A) Response of cat esophageal strips, precontracted by bethanecol (10^{-5} M), to electrical stimuli (0.4 msec, 0.5-5 Hz, supramaximal voltage) before and after incubation in Krebs' solution containing 5% VIP antiserum, or 5% VIP antiserum neutralized by 3×10^{-7} M VIP. Data shown represent means ± SEM of 13 strips from four animals.

(B) Response of rabbit internal anal sphincter strips to stimulus durations of 0.05 to 0.5 msec and 1 to 10 Hz frequency, before and after a two-hour incubatin in Krebs' solution containing 8% VIP antiserum. Data shown represent mean ± SEM of five strips from five animals for each experiment. Asterisks denote statistically significant differences from control. VIP antiserum has a similar effect on the lower esophageal sphincter.

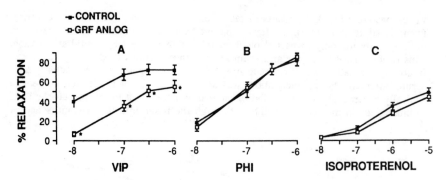

FIGURE 3. The GRF analogue (N-Ac-Tyr^1,D-Phe^2)-GRF(1-29)--NH$_2$ (10-5 M) inhibits cat LES relaxation induced by exogenous VIP (**A**, 17 strips from four animals). It does not affect relaxation induced by PHI (**B**, 13 strips from three animals) or by isoproterenol (**C**, 17 strips from four animals), a β-adrenergic agent that, like VIP and PHI, activates adenyl cyclase. Asterisks denote statistically significant differences from control. These data are consistent with the view that this GRF analogue does not operate on intracellular mechanisms responsible for inactivation of adenyl cyclase. The GRF analogue has been previously shown to prevent binding of VIP to VIP receptors. Furthermore, this GRF analogue is specific for VIP receptors, as it does not affect PHI-mediated relaxation, and PHI receptors may be different.

second problem inherent with use of antisera as peptide antagonists derives from their relatively slow binding.[35] As the time required for the peptide-receptor binding is short, a high concentration of antiserum must be used in order to obtain measurable effects. We have used the largest concentration of antiserum that had no effect of its own. It was serendipitous that this concentration was generally sufficient to block ED$_{50}$ VIP. Because the block is incomplete, it is impossible to determine whether VIP is the only neurotransmitter. The antiserum produces more complete inhibition for short stimuli and low frequencies, and it has been shown that maximum VIP release in the portal circulation occurs when the vagus is stimulated with 0.2-msec, 8-Hz pulses.[28] It is therefore possible that at higher frequencies enough VIP is released to escape the slow binding antiserum. Alternatively, at higher frequencies and durations different neurotransmitters may be released that would not be affected by VIP antiserum. At least for the LES there is evidence that relaxation may be mediated not only by VIP but also by PHI.[15]

Inhibition by Receptor Antagonists

Growth hormone releasing factor (GRF) and VIP analogues have been used to antagonize VIP-receptor binding. VIP and PHI are members of the secretin-glucagon family and are structurally related to GRF. They exhibit structural homology and cross-react with varying affinity with their homologues' receptors.[36–39] GRF interacts with VIP receptors in human and rat gut epithelial cells[40,41] and in rat pancreatic membranes.[42] Nevertheless, in the rat anterior pituitary VIP and GRF receptors are distinct entities, since the GRF analogue (N-Ac-Tyr^1,D-Arg^2)-GRF$_{1-29}$-NH$_2$ antagonizes GRF-induced stimulation of adenylate cyclase without affecting VIP-induced stimulation.[43] Conversely, (4Cl-D-Phe[6],Leu[17])-VIP antagonizes VIP-stimulated amylase release in dispersed pancreatic acinar cells and short-circuit current changes in a colonic tumor cell line but has no effect on GRF-stimulated release of growth hormone from cultured rat adenohypophyseal cells.[44]

The GRF analogue (N-Ac-Tyr[1],D-Phe[2])-GRF$_{1-29}$-NH$_2$, has been shown to behave like a VIP receptor antagonist in rat pancreatic plasma membranes.[42] A similarity between VIP and GRF receptors may be the underlying reason for this. In fact GRF and GRF analogues have been shown to interact with VIP reactors in pancreatic acinar cells,[42] in lung parenchymal membranes,[39] and in intestinal epithelial cells.[38]

FIGURE 3 shows that the GRF analogue (N-Ac-Tyr[1], D-Phe[2])-GRF$_{1-29}$-NH$_2$ caused a significant reduction in LES relaxation in response to VIP, but had no effect on relaxation in response to PHI or isoproterenol. Incubation in the GRF analogue also caused a small but significant reduction in relaxation in response to electrical stimulation (0.1 and 0.2 msec, 1-5 Hz), as shown in FIGURE 4, whereas incubation in the solvent (acetic acid) had no effect whatsoever. Increasing the duration of the stimuli above 0.2 msec reduced the inhibition caused by the GRF analogue. At 0.4- and 0.8-msec stimulus duration, the reduction in relaxation was no longer significant.

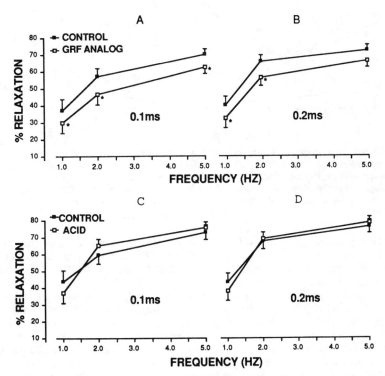

FIGURE 4. (N-Ac-Tyr[1],D-Phe[2])-GRF-(1-29)-NH$_2$ (10-5 M) causes a small reduction in cat LES relaxation induced by electrical stimulation (1-5 Hz 1 msec [**A**], and 1-5 Hz 2 msec [**B**]). Asterisks denote statistically significant differences (15 strips from four animals). Longer duration stimuli completely surmounted the inhibition caused by the GRF analogue (not shown). The solvent alone (0.1 N acetic acid) had no effect on relaxation (**C-D**, 18 strips from two animals).

Although the GRF analogue inhibits relaxation induced both by electrical stimulation and by VIP, it has no effect on relaxation induced by PHI and by isoproterenol. The implication of these findings are as follows: Since isoproterenol is known to stimulate adenyl cyclase through receptor-activated GTP-dependent G_s proteins, and since the GRF analogue has no effect on isoproterenol-induced relaxation, these data are consistent with the GRF analogue preventing binding of VIP to receptors on smooth muscle cells, rather than directly inhibiting the adenyl cyclase pathway activated by these receptors. As the receptor is never reached by VIP the adenyl cyclase pathway remains inactive, and the GRF analogue does not have any effect on the subsequent G_s protein activation and GTP hydrolysis, or any of the steps subsequent to receptor binding.

The fact that the GRF analogue inhibits VIP- but not PHI-induced relaxation suggests that there are some conformational differences in VIP and PHI receptors permitting the GRF analogue to recognize one (VIP) but not the other (PHI) receptor,

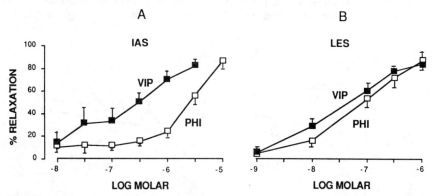

FIGURE 5. Dose-response relationships for VIP and PHI in rabbit internal anal sphincter (**A**) and cat LES circular muscle (**B**). Each data point represents mean ± SEM of at least 10 strips from five animals. Responses to VIP and PHI are not affected by TTX at a concentration that completely abolishes response to electrical stimulation (not shown). This finding is consistent with these peptides having a direct effect on muscle through receptors located on the smooth muscle cells.

and that, perhaps, GRF and VIP receptors may have closer similarities than GRF and PHI receptors. On the other hand VIP and PHI receptors must be similar, as PHI tachyphylaxis reduces relaxation induced both by VIP and by PHI (unpublished observations), and both VIP and PHI displace [125I]VIP bound to Molt 4b lymphoblasts[45] and to a GH3 rat pituitary tumor cell line.[46] Because of this very similarity between VIP and PHI receptors, and the fact that VIP, PHI, and other agonists are equally capable of binding to either one, it has been previously difficult to distinguish between VIP- and PHI-preferring receptors. However, the fact that the GRF analogue blocks the effect of exogenous VIP, but not of PHI, on the LES strongly suggests that there are indeed differences between one type of receptor and the other.

Unfortunately this antagonist is weak, resulting in a small percent of inhibition in the response to exogenously added agonists, and an even smaller reduction in the inhibition of relaxation in response to electrical stimulation. Because of the weakness of the antagonism, clear-cut conclusions, as would result if complete inhibition were obtained, cannot be reached. Nevertheless, it is worth noting that the GRF analogue inhibits the relaxation more effectively in response to exogenous VIP than to electrical stimulation. The reasons for this difference are not entirely clear, but a possible explanation is that VIP may not be the only neurotransmitter responsible for relaxation of the LES. In fact we know that LES relaxation may be mediated both by VIP and by PHI (see following). Furthermore *in vitro* electrical stimulation of the LES causes an increase in cyclic GMP,[47] whereas VIP and PHI do not. While no guanyl cyclase-activating neurotransmitter is presently known to exist in the LES, the presence of some as yet unknown substance that may be released by electrical stimulation cannot be excluded. Atrial natriuretic factor (ANF) is the only endogenous agent presently known to activate guanyl cyclase through receptor-operated mechanisms. ANF, however, has not been demonstrated in the LES, and exogenous ANF has a weak effect on *in vitro* LES smooth muscle (unpublished observations).

In conclusion, these data are consistent with the view that although VIP and PHI may both be involved in LES relaxation, there are some differences between VIP and PHI receptors that allow the GRF analogue to interfere with one type of receptors (VIP) but not with the other (PHI). It is possible that VIP and PHI may be but two of multiple agonists mediating LES relaxation, and that other as yet unidentified agents may be involved.

PHI as a Neurotransmitter in the LES

PHI and VIP have strong sequence homology. They are thought to be formed by cleavage of a common prepro-hormone chain,[48] are present together in numerous central and peripheral neurons,[22–25,49–53] and are coreleased by some tumors,[32] cerebral cortex,[33] and salivary glands.[54] Although they have similar effects in a variety of experimental preparations, their mode of interaction is unclear. VIP is generally more potent than PHI (FIG. 5a). PHI, however, is more potent than VIP in some preparations including the rat anterior pituitary and hemipituitaries[53] and perfused stomach.[55] In the female urogenital tract and in the lower esophageal sphincter (FIG. 5b) VIP and PHI are essentially equipotent.

PHI is present in high concentration in the distal esophagus. FIGURE 6 shows PHI concentration in homogenates of muscularis propria, containing circular and longitudinal muscle as well as myenteric plexus. LES and esophagus contain high concentrations of PHI, similar to that found in rat,[56] pig,[56] and cat cerebral cortex (unpublished observations), and comparable to CCK concentration in the cortex.[57]

PHI neutralization by a highly specific PHI antiserum inhibits LES response to neural stimulation. Two hours' incubation in Krebs' solution that contained 5 or 10% PHI antiserum diminishes the LES relaxation in response to electrical stimulation (FIG. 7). The reduction is not potentiated by increasing antiserum concentration from 5 to 10%, suggesting that 5% antiserum is sufficient to produce a maximal block of relaxation induced by release of endogenous PHI. Maximum PHI block, however, does not completely abolish relaxation. This is consistent with release of other neurotransmitters (such as VIP) by electrical stimulation.

The reduction in response to neural stimulation is due to PHI immuno-suppression since the antiserum is highly specific for PHI. FIGURE 8 shows that incubation in 10% PHI antiserum does not affect relaxation induced by exogenous VIP. The same concentration of antiserum almost completely blocks the relaxation induced by 10^{-6} M porcine PHI (not shown). This is consistent with the antiserum being specific for PHI and lacking cross reactivity with VIP as previously shown.[56]

These data are consistent with the finding that multiple peptides may be contained in the same neurons. For instance VIP, PHI, and NPY are found in intramural neurons in the small intestine[22] and in the stomach.[25] It is therefore reasonable to presume that more than one neurotransmitter may be involved in mediating any one physiologic function. In the LES, not only VIP[9,10] but also PHI may be a neurotransmitter mediating relaxation, since both are present in the LES region, both relax the LES by direct effect, and block of either VIP or PHI by preincubation in antiserum results in significant reduction in relaxation induced by the respective peptides, and a parallel reduction in relaxation induced by neural stimulation.

Other regulatory peptides may act as inhibitory neurotransmitters in the enteric

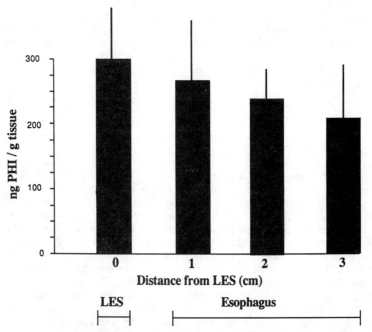

FIGURE 6. PHI concentration in ng/g tissue wet weight as determined by radioimmunoassay. The PHI radioimmunoassay and the immuno-neutralization experiments were performed with a highly selective antiserum against porcine PHI.[56] Cat LES and esophagus contain high concentrations of PHI, comparable to that found in rat,[56] pig,[56] and cat cerebral cortex.

system. It is not possible at this time, and it may not be for a long time, to produce a complete list of peptides occurring in the gut autonomic innervation. It would not be surprising to discover that other and new peptides may be involved with VIP and PHI in mediating relaxation in the gut.

DISEASES OF THE ENTERIC INHIBITORY NEURONS

At the present time a selective absence or dysfunction of VIP (or PHI) containing neurons has not been conclusively demonstrated to be the underlying cause of any

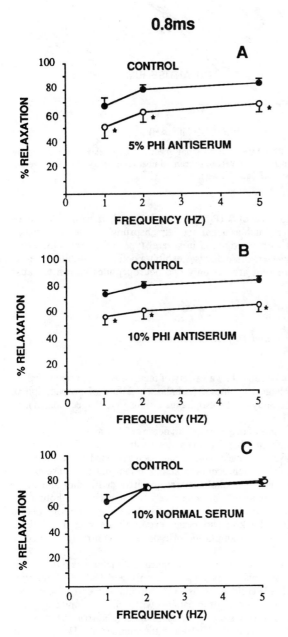

FIGURE 7. Response of cat LES strips to electrical stimulation (0.8 msec, 1-5 Hz) after a two-hour incubation in Krebs' solution containing 5% (**A**) or 10% (**B**) PHI antiserum, or 10% normal serum, obtained before immunization (**C**). Each data point represents the mean ± SEM of eight strips from three animals (**A**), 14 strips from four animals (**B**), and nine strips from three animals (**C**). Asterisks denote statistically significant differences from control. The reduction in relaxation after incubation in 5% antiserum was significant at all frequencies and durations tested (**A**). The reduction was not potentiated by increasing antiserum concentration to 10% (**B**). Incubation in 10% normal serum had no effect on relaxation at frequencies of 2 Hz or greater (**C**). At 1 Hz the slight reduction in relaxation subsequent to incubation in normal serum may be due to some binding of neurotransmitters (VIP, PHI, or possibly others) to serum proteins.

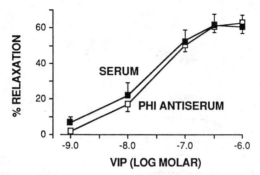

FIGURE 8. Incubation in 10% PHI antiserum does not affect cat LES relaxation induced by exogenous VIP. The same concentration of PHI antiserum almost completely blocks the relaxation induced by 10^{-6} M porcine PHI (not shown).

specific motility disorder. Absence of VIP-containing neurons, however, has been noted in some motility disorders, such as achalasia, Hirschsprung's disease or Chagas' disease, which are associated with a reduction in several types of neural cells. From a functional point of view, however, these diseases exhibit a defect of inhibitory neural input, and VIP and PHI at present are the only two neuropeptides known to cause relaxation in gut muscle.

Achalasia and Diffuse Esophageal Spasm

Esophageal dysphagia may be caused by a variety of factors. Among them is failure of opening of the lower esophageal sphincter (achalasia), failure of propagation of organized peristalsis along the body of the esophagus (diffuse esophageal spasm), or combinations of both.

In patients with achalasia, signs of degeneration in nerve cell bodies of the myenteric plexus and a reduction in their number has been demonstrated.[58] A feature differentiating achalasia from diffuse esophageal spasm has been reported to be increased sensitivity to cholinergic agents,[59] which occurs in achalasia but not in diffuse esophageal spasm. A concurrent reduction in cholinesterase-positive cell bodies and nerve fibers in the esophagus has been reported for achalasia.[60] In the cat acetylcholine has been shown to be responsible for the contraction that follows the inhibitory period caused by electrical stimulation.[9] Lack of cholinergic excitatory neurons in achalasia may be partly responsible for reduced amplitude of esophageal contraction noted in this disease.

As VIP may play a role in mediating lower esophageal sphincter relaxation,[10,11] it is reasonable to expect that achalasia may entail not only a defect of cholinergic neurons but also a defect of VIPergic neurons. VIP-containing nerves have been examined in the distalmost 5 cm of esophagus in patients with achalasia, and compared with similar specimens obtained during surgery for esophageal or gastric carcinoma.[61] In the achalasia patients the concentration of VIP and the number of VIP-containing nerve fibers were greatly reduced, and sometimes completely absent, when compared to the carcinoma patients. The pathologic significance of reduced VIP neurons has clear functional significance, as LES relaxation is likely to be mediated, at least in part, through these neurons. A possible role of PHI in achalasia has not been examined.

In the case of diffuse esophageal spasm, little morphologic information is available concerning a possible VIPergic defect, and we can only speculate about what may happen if VIP neurons are absent or damaged. In the cat esophagus,[9] as in the rat colon,[14] VIP plays an inhibitory role in mediating the descending relaxation, while the peristaltic contraction that follows is mediated by excitatory cholinergic neurons in the cat esophagus[9] or cholinergic and tachykinin-containing neurons in the rat colon.[14] In the human esophagus it has similarly been shown that cholinergic neurons may mediate esophageal contraction during peristalsis since the cholinergic antagonist atropine reduces the amplitude of esophageal peristaltic waves and increases their latency.[62] These findings suggest that the interplay of excitatory and inhibitory neurons determines both the length of descending relaxation (which is related to the speed of propagation of the peristaltic wave) and the amplitude of the peristaltic contraction. The motility changes occurring in diffuse esophageal spasm are consistent with a defect of inhibitory innervation, resulting in an imbalance between inhibitory and excitatory neural input, as they consist of high-amplitude simultaneous contraction. The contractions are simultaneous because the period of descending inhibition is extremely short throughout the esophagus (FIG. 9). They may be of high amplitude as inhibitory

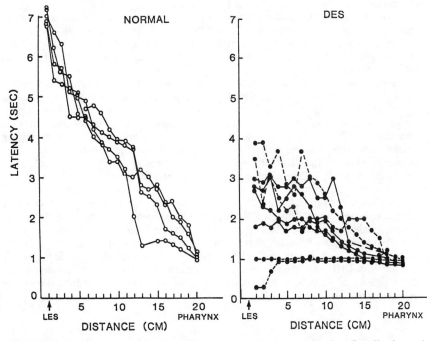

FIGURE 9. Latency, measured in seconds, as the interval between initiation of swallowing and contraction at a given location in the human esophagus, is shown as a function of distance from the LES, measured in centimeters. In the normal esophagus the peristaltic sweep reaches the distalmost esophagus in five to seven seconds. In patients with diffuse esophageal spasm (DES), this time interval is reduced to 0.2-4 seconds. Continuous or interrupted lines connect measurements obtained in the same individual.

innervation is damaged and excitatory, presumably cholinergic innervation dominates. As VIP is likely to be an inhibitory neurotransmitter in the body of the esophagus, a defect of VIPergic innervation could produce the same motility defects that are observed in patients with esophageal spasm. Unfortunately esophageal specimens from patients with esophageal spasm are not readily available and this issue may remain speculative.

Hirschsprung's Disease

Hirschsprung's disease results in obstruction of the distalmost portion of the gastrointestinal tract subsequent to a congenital absence of ganglion cells. In virtually all cases the aganglionic area extends proximally from the anal sphincter and involves varying amounts of colon. A murine model of distal colonic aganglionosis was first described in 1973,[63] and recent embryological studies suggest that the terminal segment of the colon in this model cannot be colonized by precursors of enteric neurons.[64] The area that is consistently aganglionic is located in the distal 2-3 mm of gut, while the constricted region often extends through a distal 6-8 mm transitional area. This lack of exact correlation between the area of aganglionosis and the constricted segment is recognized in humans with Hirschsprung's disease.[65]

FIGURE 10a shows relaxation, followed by contraction of the distalmost 2 mm of mouse colon in vitro. Relaxation reflects inhibition of the internal anal sphincter in response to neural stimulation, while the "off" contraction may be due to presence of rectal fibers in the specimen. Because of the minute size of the specimen, pure anal sphincter fibers are hard to separate.

In the aganglionic colon relaxation is absent. Although in this particular preparation, we have not tried to establish the VIPergic nature of the inhibitory neurons, as we did in the rabbit,[12] it is likely that VIP-containing neurons may, at least in part, mediate relaxation in the mouse, and that the absence of these neurons may be responsible for the lack of relaxation in the aganglionic colon. Lack of VIP-containing neurons has been demonstrated in this animal model[66] and is associated with super-sensitivity to VIP (FIG. 10b). In man the innervation of the aganglionic colon has been examined.[67-70] VIP-containing nerve cell bodies, fibers, and endings have been demonstrated in both the submucosal and myenteric plexus of the ganglionic segment and normal colon. In the aganglionic colon no VIP neurons were found in either plexus. Enkephalin and substance P containing fibers were also reduced, and possibly other peptides may also be lacking. Of these, however, only VIP causes relaxation. PHI-containing fibers have not been examined. In the internal anal sphincter of rabbit, however, PHI is less potent than VIP by one order of magnitude (FIG. 5a), and it is possible that PHI may play a lesser role in producing relaxation. Alternatively, the lesser potency of the porcine PHI used in this experiment may derive from differences between rabbit and porcine PHI.

Chagas' Disease

This disease is caused by infestation with the parasite trypanosoma Cruzi which, by an unknown mechanism, causes degeneration of intrinsic neurons. This denervation

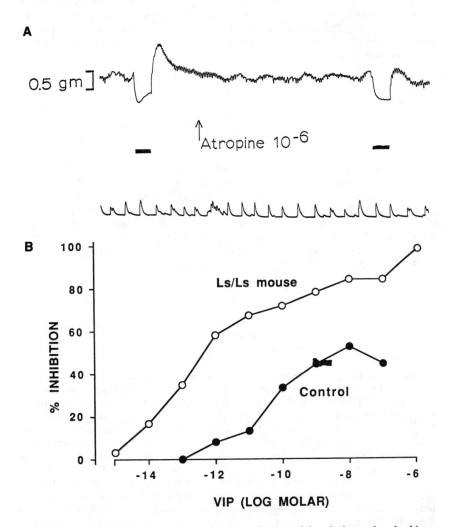

FIGURE 10. (A) The distalmost 2 mm of mouse colon, containing the internal anal sphincter, relaxes in response to electrical stimulation (top tracing). The relaxation is followed by a contraction occurring at the end of the stimulus, shown by the thick horizontal bars. The contraction is mediated by cholinergic neurons as it is abolished by atropine, and may be due to the presence of some rectal fibers in the specimen. The relaxation, like relaxation of the rabbit internal anal sphincter, is neurally mediated, and is most likely mediated by VIP-releasing neurons. In the Ls/Ls congenital mouse model of Hirschsprung's disease, both relaxation and contraction are absent (lower tracing).

(B) The Ls/Ls preparation is supersensitive to VIP, exhibiting relaxation at lower VIP doses than the normal littermate.

results in development of megaesophagus or megacolon, with results similar to the ones associated with esophageal achalasia or Hirschsprung's disease. In rectal biopsies from patients with Chagas' disease, low levels of peptidergic innervation and peptide content were found,[71,72] with VIP being one of the peptides present in reduced concentration and in fewer neurons.

Pyloric Stenosis

A number of theories have been presented concerning the cause of pyloric stenosis, and several investigators have focused on the innervation of the pylorus,[73–76] with the view that pyloric stenosis may be the equivalent of pyloric achalasia. Results have been contradictory. Only recently the occurrence, distribution, and relative frequency of some peptide-containing neurons has been examined.[77] In some patients with hypertrophic pyloric stenosis, enkephalin neurons were reduced or absent, and VIP neurons were reduced in the circular muscle, but increased in numbers in the myenteric plexus. The significance of these findings is at present unclear.

Diabetic Neuropathy

Symptoms of autonomic neuropathy are of clinical concern in diabetes. In the gastrointestinal tract, these include impairment of gastric emptying, diarrhea, and constipation. Changes in the gut innervation and their relationship to motility changes have not been examined in any detail in humans. A rat model of streptozotocin-induced diabetes has been used to study changes in autonomic innervation secondary to diabetes.[78,79] Increased VIP content has been noted in the small intestine and colon. Increased VIP per centimeter of gut in the small intestine was due to increased intestinal mass, perhaps secondary to gut distension, while increase in the colon was due to both increase in bowel mass and increased VIP concentration per gram of tissue.[79] While it is possible that these changes may contribute to the symptoms of gastrointestinal dysfunction occurring with diabetes, their functional significance is far from clear at this time.

Crohn's Disease

Increases in the thickness of VIP-containing nerve fibers and in VIP content of gut wall have been reported in patients with Crohn's disease.[80,81] These increases are mostly associated with the mucosa and the submucosal plexus but occasionally extend transmurally. The significance of these changes is unclear.

CONCLUSION

VIP is likely to be a neurotransmitter mediating descending relaxation in the gastrointestinal tract, as well as sphincter relaxation, and PHI may be a cotransmitter, at least in some parts of the gut. A defect of neurons containing and releasing these peptides may be the underlying cause of some gut motility disorders. The involvement of other, as yet unknown neurotransmitters, however, cannot be excluded.

REFERENCES

1. LANGLEY, J. N. 1898. On inhibitory fibers in the vagus for the end of the esophagus and the stomach. J. Physiol. (London) **23:** 407-414.
2. BAYLISS, W. M. & E. H. STARLING. 1899. The movements and innervation of the small intestine. J. Physiol. (London) **24:** 99-143.
3. BAYLISS, W. M. & E. H. STARLING. 1900. The movements and innervation of the large intestine. J. Physiol. (London) **26:** 107-118.
4. BAYLISS, W. M. & E. H. STARLING. 1901. The movements and innervation of the small intestine. J. Physiol. (London) **26:** 125-138.
5. LANGLEY, J. N. & R. MAGNUS. 1904. Some observations on the movement of the intestine before and after degenerative section of mesenteric nerves. J. Physiol. (London) **33:** 34-51.
6. FURNESS, J. B. & M. COSTA. 1982. Identification of gastrointestinal neurotransmitters. *In* Mediators and Drugs in Gastrointestinal Motility. G. Bertaccini, Ed. **1:** 382-462. Springer-Verlag. Berlin-Heidelberg-New York.
7. FURNESS, J. B. & M. COSTA. 1982. Enteric inhibitory nerves and VIP. *In* Vasoactive Intestinal Peptide. S. I. Said, Ed.: 391-406. Raven Press. New York.
8. GOYAL, R. K. & B. W. COBB. 1981. Motility of the pharynx, esophagus, and esophageal sphincters. *In* Physiology of the Gastrointestinal Tract. L. R. Johnson, Ed.: 359-391. Raven Press. New York.
9. BEHAR, J., V. GUENARD, J. H. WALSH & P. BIANCANI. 1988. Vasoactive intestinal peptide and acetylcholine: Neurotransmiters of cat esophagus. In press.
10. GOYAL, R. K., S. RATTAN & S. SAID. 1980. VIP as a possible neurotransmitter of non-cholinergic, non-adrenergic inhibitory neurones. Nature **288:** 378-380.
11. BIANCANI, P., J. H. WALSH & J. BEHAR. 1984. Vasoactive intestinal polypeptide: A neurotransmitter for lower esophageal sphincter relaxation. J. Clin. Invest. **73:** 963-967.
12. BIANCANI, P., J. WALSH & J. BEHAR. 1985. Vasoactive intestinal peptide: A neurotransmitter for relaxation of the internal anal sphincter. Gastroenterology **89:** 867-874.
13. GRIDER, J. R., M. B. CABLE, S. I. SAID & G. M. MAKHLOUF. 1985. Vasoactive intestinal peptide as a neural mediator of gastric relaxation. Am. J. Physiol. **248:** G73-78.
14. GRIDER, J. R. & G. M. MAKHLOUF. 1986. Colonic peristaltic reflex: Identification of vasoactive intestinal peptide as a mediator of descending relaxation. Am. J. Physiol. **251:** G40-45.
15. BIANCANI, P., M. C. BEINFELD, C. HILLEMEIER & J. BEHAR. 1987. Peptide Histidine Isoleucine: A Second Neurotransmitter for Lower Esophageal Sphincter Relaxation. In press.
16. BURLEIGH, D. E., A. D'MELLO & A. G. PARKS. 1979. Responses of isolated human internal anal sphincter to drugs and electrical field stimulation. Gastroenterology **84:** 409-417.
17. PENNINCKX, F. M., J. H. MEBIS & R. P. KERREMANS. 1982. The recto-anal reflex in cats analyzed *in vitro* Scand. J. Gastroenterol. **17**(Suppl. 71): 147-149.
18. FAHRENKRUG, J. 1982. VIP as a neurotransmitter in the peripheral nervous system. *In* Vasoactive Intestinal Peptide. S. I. Said, Ed.: 361-371. Raven Press. New York.

19. LARSSON, L. I., J. M. POLAK, R. BUFFA, F. SUNDLER & E. SOLCIA. 1979. On the immunocytochemical localization of the vasoactive intestinal polypeptide. J. Histochem. Cytochem. **27:** 936-938.
20. REINECKE, M., P. SCHLUTER, N. YANAIHARA & W. G. FORSSMAN. 1981. VIP immunoreactivity in enteric nerves and endocrine cells of the vertebrate gut. Peptides 2(Suppl. 2): 149-156.
21. ALUMETS, J., J. FAHRENKRUG, R. HAKANSON, O. B. SCHAFFALITZKY DE MUCKADELL, F. SUNDLER & R. UDDMAN. 1979. A rich VIP nerve supply is characteristic of sphincters. Nature **280:** 155-156.
22. BISHOP, A. E., J. M. POLAK, Y. YIANGOU, N. D. CHRISTOFIDES & S. R. BLOOM. 1984. The distribution of PHI and VIP in porcine gut and their co-localization to a proportion of intrinsic ganglion cells. Peptides (Fayetteville) **5:** 255-259.
23. CHRISTOFIDES, N. D., J. M. POLAK & S. R. BLOOM. 1984. Studies on the distribution of PHI in mammals. Peptides (Fayetteville) **5:** 261-266.
24. EKBLAD, E., R. HAKANSON & F. SUNDLER. 1984. VIP and PHI coexist with an NPY-like peptide in intramural neurones of the small intestine. Regul. Peptides **10:** 47-55.
25. EKBLAD, E., M. EKELUND, H. GRAFFNER, R. HAKANSON & F. SUNDLER. 1985. Peptide containing nerve fibers in the stomach wall of rat and mouse. Gastroenterology **89:** 73-85.
26. MELANDER, T., T. HOKFELT, A. ROKAEUS, J. FAHRENKRUG, K. TATEMOTO & V. MUTT. 1985. Distribution of galanin-like immunoreactivity in the gastro-intestinal tract of several mammalian species. Cell Tissue Res. **239:** 253-270.
27. FAHRENKRUG, J., H. GALBO, J. J. HOLST & O. B. SCHAFFALITZKY DE MUCKADELL. 1978. Influence of the autonomic nervous system on the release of vasoactive intestinal polypeptide from the porcine gastrointestinal tract. J. Physiol. (London) **280:** 405-422.
28. FAHRENKRUG, J., U. HAGLUND, M. JODAL, O. LUNDGREN, L. OLBE & O. B. SCHAFFALITZKY DE MUCKADELL. 1978. Nervous release of vasoactive intestinal polypeptide in the gastrointestinal tract of cats: Possible implications. J. Physiol. (London) **284:** 291-305.
29. BLOOM, S. R. & A. V. EDWARDS. 1980. Effects of autonomic stimulation on the release of vasoactive intestinal peptide from the gastrointestinal tract in the calf. J. Physiol. (London) **299:** 437-452.
30. PEDERSON, R., T. O'DORISIO, B. HOWE, C. MCINTOSH, M. MUELLER, J. BROWN & S. CATALANO. 1981. Vagal release of ir-VIP and ir-gastrin from the isolated perfused rat stomach. Mol. Cell Endocrinol. **23:** 225-231.
31. ANDERSSON, P. O., S. R. BLOOM & J. JARHULT. 1983. Colonic motor and vascular responses to pelvic nerve stimulation and their relation to local peptide release in the cat. J. Physiol. (London) **334:** 293-307.
32. BLOOM, S. R., N. D. CHRISTOFIDES, J. DELAMARTER, G. BUELL, E. KAWASHIMA & J. M. POLAK. 1983. Diarrhoea in vipoma patients associated with cosecretion of a second active peptide (peptide histidine isoleucine) explained by a single coding gene. Lancet **2**(8360): 1163-1165.
33. KORCHAK, D. M., K. GYSLING & M. C. BEINFELD. 1985. The subcellular distribution of PHI (peptide histidine isoleucine amide)-27-like peptides in rat brain and their release from rat cerebral cortical slices. J. Neurochem. **44:** 255-259.
34. LUNDBERG, J. M., J. FAHRENKRUG, O. LARSON & A. ANGGARD. 1984. Corelease of vasoactive intestinal polypeptide and peptide histidine isoleucine in relation to atropine-resistant vasodilatation in cat submandibular salivary gland. Neurosci. Lett. **52:** 37-42.
35. PANDIAN, M. R., A. HORVAT & S. SAID. 1982. Radioimmunoassay of VIP in blood and tissue. *In* Vasoactive Intestinal Peptide. S. I. Said, Ed.: 35-50. Raven Press. New York.
36. COUVINEAU, A., M. ROUSSET & M. LABURTHE. 1985. Molecular identification and structural requirement of vasoactive intestinal peptide (VIP) receptors in the human colon adenocarcinoma cell line HT-29. Biochem. J. **231:** 139-143.
37. DEHAYE, J. P., J. CHRISTOPHE, F. ERNST, P. POLOCZEK, P. VAN BOGAERT. 1985. Binding of *in vitro* vasoactive intestinal peptide on isolated acini of rat parotid gland. Arch. Oral Biol. **30:** 827-832.
38. LABURTHE, M., A. COUVINEAU, C. ROUYER-FESSARD. 1986. Study of species specificity in growth hormone releasing factor (GRF) interaction with vasoactive intestinal peptide

(VIP) receptors using GRF and intestinal VIP receptors from rat and human: Evidence that Ac-Tyr^{1}hGRF is a competitive VIP antagonist in the rat. Mol. Pharmacol. **29:** 23-27.

39. SCHACHTER, M., K. E. DICKINSON, C. M. MILES & P. S. SEVER. 1986. Characterization of high affinity VIP receptors in human lung parenchyma. FEBS Lett. **199:** 125-129.

40. LABURTHE, M., B. AMIRANOFF, N. BOIGE, C. ROUYER-FESSARD, K. TATEMOTO & L. MORODER. 1983. Interaction of GRF with VIP receptors and stimulation of adenylate cyclase in rat and human intestinal epithelial membranes. Comparison with PHI and secretin. FEBS Lett. **159:** 89-92.

41. LABURTHE, M., A. COUVINEAU, C. ROUYER-FESSARD & L. MORODER. 1985. Interactions of PHM, PHI and 24-glutamine PHI with human VIP receptors from colonic epithelium: Comparison with rat intestinal receptors. Life Sci. **36:** 991-995.

42. WAELBROECK, M., P. ROBBERECHT, D. H. COY, J. C. CAMUS, P. DE NEEF & J. CHRISTOPHE. 1985. Interaction of growth hormone releasing factor (GRF) and 14 GRF analogues with vasoactive intestinal peptide (VIP) receptors of rat pancreas. Discovery of (N-Ac-Tyr^1,D-Phe^2)-GRF(1-29)NH$_2$ as a VIP antagonist. Endocrinology **116:** 2643-2649.

43. ROBBERECHT, P., D. H. COY, M. WAELBROECK, M. L. HAIMAN, P. DE NEEF, J. C. CAMUS & J. CHRISTOPHE. 1985. Structural requirements for the activation of rat anterior pituitary adenylate cyclase by growth hormone releasing factor (GRF): Discovery of (N-Ac-Tyr^1,D-Arg^2)-GRF(1-29)-NH$_2$ as a GRF antagonist on membranes. Endocrinology **117:** 1759-1764.

44. PANDOL, S. J., K. DHARMSATHAPHORN, M. S. SCHOEFFIELD, W. VALE & J. RIVIER. 1986. Vasoactive intestinal peptide receptor antagonist [4Cl-D-Phe^6,Leu^{17}]VIP. Am. J. Physiol. **250:** G553-557.

45. O'DORISIO, M. S., C. L. WOOD, G. D. WENGER & L. M. VASSALO. 1985. Cyclic AMP-dependent protein kinase in Molt 4b lymphoblasts: Identification by photoaffinity labeling and activation in intact cells by vasoactive intestinal polypeptide (VIP) and peptide histidine isoleucine (PHI). J. Immunol. **134:** 4078-4086.

46. WOOD, C. L., M. S. O'DORISIO, L. M. VASSALO, W. B. MALARKEY & T. M. O'DORISIO. 1985. Vasoactive intestinal peptide effects on GH3 pituitary tumor cells: High affinity binding, affinity labeling, and adenylate cyclase stimulation. Comparison with peptide histidine isoleucine and growth hormone releasing factor. Regul. Pept. **12:** 237-248.

47. TORPHY, T. J., C. F. FINE, M. BURMAN, M. S. BARNETTE & H. S. ORMSBEE, III. 1986. Lower esophageal sphincter relaxation is associated with increased cyclic nucleotide content. Am. J. Physiol. **251**(Gastrointest. Liver Physiol. 14): G786-G793.

48. ITOH, N. K., K. OBATA, N. YANAIHARA & H. OKAMOTO. 1983. Human preprovasoactive intestinal polypeptide contains a novel PHI-27-like peptide, PHM-27. Nature **304:** 547-549.

49. CHRISTOFIDES, N. D., Y. YANGOU, P. J. PIPER, M. A. GHATEI, M. N. SHEPPARD, K. TATEMOTO, J. M. POLAK & S. R. BLOOM. 1984. Distribution of peptide histidine isoleucine in the mammalian respiratory tract and some aspects of its pharmacology. Endocrinology **115:** 1958-1963.

50. GRUNDITZ, T., R. HAKANSON, G. HEDGE, C. RERUP, F. SUNDLER & R. UDDMAN. 1986. Peptide histidine isoleucine amide stimulates tyroid hormone secretion and coexists with vasoactive intestinal polypeptide in intrathyroid nerve fibers from laryngeal ganglia. Endocrinology **118:** 783-790.

51. LUNDBERG, J. M., J. FAHRENKRUG, T. HOHFELT, C. R. MARTLING, O. LARSON & K. TATEMOTO. 1984. Coexistence of peptide HI (PHI) and VIP in nerves regulating blood flow and bronchial sooth muscle tone in various mammals including man. Peptides (Fayetteville) **5:** 593-606.

52. SAMSON, W. K., M. D. LUMPKIN, J. K. MCDONALD & S. M. MCCANN. 1983. Prolactin-releasing activity of porcine intestinal peptide (PHI-27). Peptides (Fayetteville) **4:** 817-819.

53. WERNER, S., A. L. HULTING, T. HOKFELT, P. ENEROTH, K. TATEMOTO, V. MUTT, L. MARODER & E. WUNSCH. 1983. Effect of the peptide PHI 27 on prolactin release in vitro. Neuroendocrinology **37:** 176-478.

54. LUNDBERG, J. M., J. FAHRENKRUG, O. LARSON & A. ANGGARD. 1984. Corelease of vasoactive intestinal polypeptide and peptide histidine isoleucine in relation to atropine-resistant vasodilatation in cat submandibular salivary gland. Neurosci. Lett. **52:** 37-42.

55. SCHUSDZIARRA, V., R. SCHMID, H. BENDER, M. SCHUSDZIARRA, J. RIVIER, W. VALE & M. CLASSEN. 1986. Effect of vasoactive intestinal peptide, peptide histidine isoleucine and growth hormone releasing factor-40 on bombesin like immunoreactivity, somatostatin and gastrin release from the perfused rat stomach. Peptides **7:** 127-133.

56. BEINFELD, M. C., D. M. KORCHAK, B. L. ROTH & T. L. O'DONOHUE. 1984. The distribution and chromatographic characterization of PHI (peptide histidine isoleucine amide)-27-like peptides in the rat and porcine brain. J. Neurosci. **212:** 51-57.

57. BEINFELD, M. C., D. K. MEYER, R. L. ESKAY, R. T. JENSEN & M. J. BROWNSTEIN. 1981. The distribution of cholecystokinin immunoreactivity in the central nervous system of the rat as determined by radioimmunoassay. Brain Res. **212:** 51-57.

58. MISIEWICZ, J. J., S. L. WALLER, P. P. ANTHONY & J. W. P. GUMMER. 1969. Achalasia of the cardia: Pharmacology and histopathology of isolated cardiac sphincteric muscle from patients with and without achalasia. Q. J. Med. **149:** 17-30.

59. KRAMER, P. & F. J. INGELFINGER. 1951. Esophageal sensitivity to mecholyl in cardiospasm. Gastroenterology **19:** 242-254.

60. ADAMS, C. W. M., E. A. MARPLES & J. R. TROUNCE. 1960. Achalasia of the cardia and Hirschsprung's disease. the amount and distribution of cholinesterases. Clin. Sci. **19:** 473-481.

61. AGGESTRUP, S., R. UDDMAN, F. SUNDLER, J. FAHRENKRUG, R. HAKANSON, H. RAHBEK SORENSEN & G. HAMBRAEUS. 1983. Lack of vasoactive intestinal polypeptide nerves in esophageal achalasia. Gastroenterology **84:** 924-927.

62. DODDS, W. J., J. DENT, W. J. HOGAN & R. C. ARNDORFER. 1981. Effect of atropine on esophageal motor function in humans. Am. J. Physiol. **240:** G290-296.

63. WEBSTER, W. 1973. Embryogenesis of the enteric ganglia in normal and in mice that develop congenital aganglionic megacolon. J. Embriol. Exp. Morphol. **30:** 573-585.

64. ROTHMAN, T. P. & M. D. GERSHON. 1984. Regionally defective colonization of the terminal bowel by the precursors of enteric neurons in lethal spotted mutant mice. Neuroscience **12:** 1293-1311.

65. LAVERY, I. C. 1984. The surgery of Hirschsprung's disease. Surg. Clin. North Am. **63(1):** 161-175.

66. VAILLANT, C., A. BULLOCK, R. DIMALINE & G. J. DOCKRAY. 1982. Distribution and development of peptidergic nerves and gut endocrine cells in mice with congenital aganglionic colon and their normal littermates. Gastroenterology **82:** 291-300.

67. BISHOP, A. E., G. L. FERRI, L. PROBERT, S. R. BLOOM & J. M. POLAK. 1982. Peptidergic nerves. Scand. J. Gastroenterol. (Suppl.) **71:** 43-59.

68. BISHOP, A. E., J. M. POLAK, B. D. LAKE, M. G. BRYANT & S. R. BLOOM. 1981. Abnormalities of the colonic regulatory peptides in Hirschsprung's disease. Histopathology **5:** 679-688.

69. TSUTO, T., H. OKAMURA, K. FUKUI, H. L. OBATA, H. TERUBAYASHI, N. IWAY, S. MAJIMA, N. YANAIHARA & Y. IBATA. 1982. An immunohistochemical investigation of vasoactive intestinal polypeptide in the colon of patients with Hirschsprung's disease. Neurosci. Lett. **34:** 57-62.

70. TSUTO, T., H. OKAMURA, K. FUKUI, H. L. OBATA, H. TERUBAYASHI, J. YANAGIHARA, N. IWAY, S. MAJIMA, N. YANAIHARA & Y. IBATA. 1985. Immunohistochemical investigation of gut hormones in the colon of patients with Hirschsprung's disease. J. Ped. Surg. **20:** 266-270.

71. LONG, R. G., A. E. BISHOP, A. J. BARNES, R. H. ALBUQUERQUE, O. J. O'SHAUGHNESSY, G. P. McGREGOR, R. BANNISTER, J. M. POLAK & S. R. BLOOM. 1980. Neural and hormonal peptides in rectal biopsy specimens from patients with Chagas' disease and chronic autonomic failure. Lancet **1(8168 Pt 1):** 559-62.

72. LONG, R. G., R. H. ALBUQUERQUE, A. E. BISHOP, J. M. POLAK & S. R. BLOOM. 1980. The peptidergic system in Chagas's disease [proceedings]. Trans. R. Soc. Trop. Med. Hyg. **74:** 273-274.

73. BELDING, H. & J. V. KERNOHAN. 1953. Morphologic studies of the myenteric plexus and

musculature in the pylorus with special reference to the changes in hypertrophic pyloric stenosis. Sug. Gynecol. Obstet. **97:** 322-334.

74. SPITZ, L. & C. E. KAUFFMAN. 1975. The neuropathological changes in congenital hypertrophic pyloric stenosis. S. Afr. J. Surg. **13:** 239-242.

75. FRIESEN, S. R., J. O. BOLEY & D. R. MILLER. 1956. The myenteric plexus of the pylorus: Its early normal development and its changes in hypertrophic pyloric stenosis. Surgery **39:** 21-29.

76. JONA, J. Z. 1978. Electron microscopic observations in infantile hypertrophic pyloric stenosis. J. Ped. Surg. **13:** 17-20.

77. MALMFORS, G. & F. SUNDLER. 1986. Peptidergic innervation in infantile hypertrophic pyloric stenosis. J. Ped. Surg. **4:** 303-306.

78. BALLMANN, M. & J. M. CONLON. 1985. Changes in the somatostatin, substance P and vasoactive intestinal polypeptide content of the gastrointestinal tract following streptozotocin-induced diabetes in the rat. Diabetologia **28:** 355-358.

79. BELAI, A., J. LINCOLN, P. MILNER, R. CROWE, A. LOESCH & G. BURNSTOCK. 1985. Enteric nerves in diabetic rats: Increase in vasoactive intestinal polypeptide but not substance P. Gastroenterology **89:** 967-976.

80. BISHOP, A. E., J. M. POLAK, M. G. BRYANT, S. R. BLOOM & S. HAMILTON. 1980. Abnormalities of vasoactive intestinal polypeptide-containing nerves in Crohn's disease. Gastroenterology **79:** 853-860.

81. O'MORAIN, C., A. E. BISHOP, G. P. McGREGOR, A. J. LEVI, S. R. BLOOM, J. M. POLAK & T. J. PETERS. 1984. Vasoactive intestinal peptide concentrations and immunocytochemical studies in rectal biopsies from patients with inflammatory bowel disease. Gut **25:** 57-61.

Vasoactive Intestinal Peptide as a Regulator of Exocrine Function and as a Possible Factor in Cystic Fibrosis[a]

PETER HEINZ-ERIAN AND SAMI I. SAID

Department of Medicine
University of Illinois College of Medicine and
West Side Veterans Administration Medical Center
Chicago, Illinois 60680

Considerable evidence suggests that normal exocrine function may be regulated in part by neuropeptides present in nerves supplying exocrine glands.[1] One of these neuropeptides, the vasoactive intestinal polypeptide (VIP), stands out as a likely regulator of normal exocrine function and as a possible factor in the pathogenesis of cystic fibrosis (CF).

VIP AND EXOCRINE FUNCTION

Localization

VIP-containing nerves richly supply all exocrine organs, including sweat, lacrimal, salivary, bronchial, and Brunner's glands, pancreas, and glands of the genito-urinary tract.[2-6] These nerves are localized around both acini and ducts and are in close relationship to epithelial cells.[7] In many neurons, VIP coexists, and is coreleased, with acetylcholine.[8,9]

Actions

1. VIP promotes blood flow to all exocrine organs[9,10] and potentiates cholinergic secretory activity on saliva[9] and sweat secretion.[11]
2. VIP stimulates water secretion by small and large intestine,[12,13] pancreas,[14,15] bronchial tree,[16] and lacrimal,[17] salivary,[18,19] and sweat glands.[11]

[a]Supported by National Institutes of Health Grant HL-30450, and by research funds from the Veterans Administration and from Sarkeys Foundation.

3. VIP enhances the transport of chloride in the intestine[12,13] and airways,[16] and of bicarbonate in the pancreas.[14,15]
4. VIP also augments macromolecular (enzyme) secretion by salivary,[18] lacrimal,[17] tracheobronchial[20] and Brunner's glands,[21] and pancreatic acini,[22] where it potentiates the secretory response to CCK.[23,24]

Receptors

VIP binds to specific membrane receptors on all exocrine structures, including human sweat glands,[25] as well as on intestinal and bronchial epithelium.[26-28] The VIP binding to these receptors leads to the accumulation of cyclic AMP,[25] which probably mediates the biological effects of the peptide. VIP receptors have been localized immunocytochemically, on the basis of increased cAMP levels, in submucosal serous and mucous glands of the ferret airways,[29] in ciliated and basal cells of tracheal epithelium of dog,[29] and, more recently, in human sweat gland secretory coils.[30] Use of autoradiographic techniques demonstrates VIP uptake sites on bronchial epithelium[31] and smooth muscle,[7] as well as on human sweat gland ducts.[32]

THE EXOCRINOPATHY OF CYSTIC FIBROSIS PARALLELS A POSTULATED VIP DEFICIENCY

Some of the major features of cystic fibrosis appear to parallel what might be expected from a lack of the peptide, judging from its known biological effects (TABLE 1).

IS VIP DEFICIENCY A FACTOR IN THE PATHOGENESIS OF CYSTIC FIBROSIS?

These observations suggested to us that some of the exocrine dysfunction of cystic fibrosis may be due to a deficiency of VIP biological activity.[39,40] Such a "deficiency" could result from one or more of these mechanisms: deficient biosynthesis, impaired receptor binding, neutralization of the active peptide by antibody or inhibitor, or excessive degradation.

Several recent observations in cystic fibrosis patients suggest that VIP metabolism may be altered, and that this alteration may play a significant role in the pathogenesis of the disease:

1. VIP-immunoreactive nerve fibers and nerve terminals, normally present around sweat gland acini and ducts, are deficient from both sites in cystic fibrosis.[41]
2. Plasma VIP levels are moderately higher in cystic fibrosis patients than in normal control subjects of comparable age.[32]

3. VIP-binding antibodies in plasma are detectable more commonly and at higher titers in cystic fibrosis than in normal subjects.[42]

The deficient VIP innervation of sweat glands in cystic fibrosis first raised the possibility that impaired VIP biosynthesis may be a primary defect in cystic fibrosis. The finding that the human VIP gene is located on a different chromosome (GP21-6QTER[43]) from that of the CF gene (7CEN-Q22[44,45]) is strongly against this possibility, however.

It is still possible that a "deficiency" of VIP could explain some of the exocrine abnormalities of CF, especially the decreased water secretion by epithelial surfaces and the chloride impermeability in sweat gland ducts. The lack of VIP-immunoreactive nerves in sweat glands, coupled with the elevated plasma VIP levels in CF, may represent "depletion" of the peptide due to exaggerated postsynaptic release, in an effort to overcome a dysfunction at or beyond the receptor level. This possibility remains to be tested.

TABLE 1. Features of Cystic Fibrosis Consistent with VIP Deficiency

CF Abnormality	Relationship to VIP
1. Generalized exocrine dysfunction.	
	VIP present in all glands.
2. Decreased Cl^- permeability,[33,34] increased sweat NaCl content.	
	VIP increases Cl^- movement.
3. Decreased H_2O content in exocrine secretions.	
	VIP stimulates H_2O secretion.
4. Elevated potential difference across sweat duct and respiratory epithelia.[35,36]	
	VIP reduces PD in submandibular gland.[37]
5. Decreased pancreatic H_2O and HCO_3.[38]	
	VIP stimulates pancreatic H_2O and HCO_3 secretion.

QUESTIONS TO BE ANSWERED

In order to establish and define the possible link between VIP and cystic fibrosis, several questions need to be answered, including these: Does VIP alter sweat composition (especially Cl^- content), in addition to promoting its secretion, in normal subjects? How does VIP affect sweat secretion or its composition in CF patients? Is VIP a major regulator of Cl^- permeability in normal sweat gland ducts and airway epithelial cells? Can VIP reduce the Cl^- impermeability of epithelial surfaces in CF? and Is the failure of Cl^- channels to open in CF epithelial cells[46-51] related to a defective response to VIP?

REFERENCES

1. HÖKFELT, T., O. JOHANSSON, A. LJUNGDAHL, J. M. LUNDBERG & M. SCHULTZBERG. 1980. Peptidergic neurones. Nature **284:** 515-521.
2. HÖKFELT, T., M. SCHULTZBERG, J. M. LUNDBERG, J. FUXE, V. MUTT, J. FAHRENKRUG & S. I. SAID. 1982. Distribution of vasoactive intestinal polypeptide in the central and peripheral nervous systems as revealed by immunocytochemistry. In Vasoactive Intestinal Peptide. S. I. Said, Ed.: 65-90. Raven Press. New York.
3. WHARTON, J., J. M. POLAK, M. G. BRYAND, S. VAN NOORDEN, S. R. BLOOM & A. G. E. PEARSE. 1979. Vasoactive intestinal polypeptide (VIP)-like immunoreactivity in salivary glands. Life Sci. **25:** 273-280.
4. UDDMAN, R., J. FAHRENKRUG, L. MALM, J. ALUMETS, R. HÅKANSON & F. SUNDLER. 1980. Neuronal VIP in salivary glands: Distribution and release. Acta Physiol. Scand. **110:** 31-38.
5. DEY, R. D., W. A. SHANNON & S. I. SAID. 1981. Localization of VIP-immunoreactive nerves in airways and pulmonary vessels of dogs, cats and human subjects. Cell Tiss. Res. **220:** 231-238.
6. ALM, P., J. ALUMETS, R. HÅKANSON & F. SUNDLER. 1977. Peptidergic (vasoactive intestinal peptide) nerves in the genitourinary tract. Neuroscience **2:** 751-754.
7. DEY, R. D. & S. I. SAID. 1985. Lung peptides and the pulmonary circulation. In The Pulmonary Circulation and Acute Lung Injury. S. I. Said, Ed.: 101-122. Futura Publishing Co. Mount Kisco, NY.
8. LUNDBERG, J. M., T. HÖKFELT, M. SCHULTZBERG, K. UVNÄS-WALLENSTEN, C. KOHLER & S. I. SAID. 1979. Occurrence of VIP-like immunoreactivity in certain cholinergic neurons of the cat: Evidence from combined immunohistochemistry and acetylcholinesterase staining. Neuroscience **4:** 1539-1559.
9. LUNDBERG, J. M., A. ÄNGGÅRD, J. FAHRENKRUG, T. HÖKFELT & V. MUTT. 1980. Vasoactive intestinal polypeptide in cholinergic neurons of exocrine glands: Functional significance of coexisting transmitters for vasodilation and secretion. Proc. Natl. Acad. Sci. USA **77:** 1651-1655.
10. SHIMIZU, T. & N. TAIRA. 1979. Assessment of the effects of vasoactive intestinal peptide (VIP) on blood flow-through and salivation of the dog salivary gland in comparison with those of secretin, glucagon and acetylcholine. Br. J. Pharmacol. **65:** 683-687.
11. SATO, K. & F. SATO. 1987. Effect of VIP on sweat secretion and cAMP accumulation in isolated simian eccrine glands. Am. J. Physiol. **253:** R935-R941.
12. SCHWARTZ, C. J., D. V. KIMBERG, H. E. SHERRIN, M. FIELD & S. I. SAID. 1972. Vasoactive intestinal peptide (VIP): Stimulation of adenylate cyclase and active electrolyte secretion in intestinal mucosa. J. Clin. Invest. **54:** 536-544.
13. KREJS, G. J. & J. S. FORDTRAN. 1980. Effect of VIP infusion on water and ion transport in the human jejunum. Gastroenterology **78:** 772-727.
14. SAID, S. I. & V. MUTT. 1972. Isolation from porcine intestinal wall of a vasoactive octacosapeptide related to secretin and to glucagon. Eur. J. Biochem. **28:** 119-204.
15. MAKHLOUF, G. M. & S. I. SAID. 1975. The effect of vasoactive intestinal peptide (VIP) on digestive and hormonal function. In Gastrointestinal Hormones. J. C. Thompson, Ed.: 599-610. The University of Texas Press. Austin, TX.
16. NATHANSON, I., J. H. WIDDICOMBE & P. J. BARNES. 1983. Effect of vasoactive intestinal peptide on ion transport across dog tracheal epithelium. J. Appl. Physiol. **55:** 1844-1848.
17. DARTT, D. A., A. K. BAKER, C. VAILLANT & P. E. ROSE, 1984. Vasoactive intestinal peptide stimulation of protein secretion from rat lacrimal gland acini. Am. J. Physiol. **247:** G502-G509.
18. Ekström, J., B. Mansson & G. TOBIN. 1982. Vasoactive intestinal peptide induces salivary secretion in the rat. J. Physiol. **332:** 76P.
19. INOUE, Y. & T. KANNO. 1982. Secretory effects of vasoactive intestinal polypeptide (VIP), adrenaline and carbachol in isolated lobules of the rat parotid gland. Biomed. Res. **3:** 384-389.
20. PEATFIELD, A. C., P. J. BARNES, C. BRATCHER, J. A. NADEL & B. DAVIS. 1983. Vasoactive

intestinal peptide stimulates tracheal submucosal gland secretion in ferret. Am. Rev. Respir. Dis. **128:** 89-93.

21. KIRKEGAARD, P., J. M. LUNDBERG, S. S. POULSEN, P. S. OLSEN, J. FAHRENKRUG, T. HÖKFELT & J. CHRISTIANSEN. 1981. Vasoactive intestinal polypeptidergic nerves and Brunner's gland secretion in the rat. Gastroenterology **81:** 872-878.

22. CHRISTOPHE, J. & P. ROBBERECHT. 1982. Effect of VIP on the exocrine pancreas. *In* Vasoactive Intestinal Peptide. S. I. Said, Ed.: 235-252. Raven Press. New York.

23. MAKHLOUF, G. M., W. M. YAU, A. M. ZFASS, S. I. SAID & M. BODANSZKY. 1978. Comparative effects of synthetic and natural vasoactive intestinal peptide on pancreatic and biliary secretion and on glucose and insulin blood levels in the dog. Scand. J. Gastroenterol. **104:** 499-501.

24. COLLEN, M. J., G. SUTLIFF, Z. PAN & J.D. GARDNER. 1982. Postreceptor modulation of action of VIP and secretin on pancreatic enzyme secretion by secretagogues that mobilize cellular calcium. Am. J. Physiol. **242:** G423-G428.

25. HEINZ-ERIAN, P., S. PAUL & S. I. SAID. 1986. Receptors for vasoactive intestinal peptide on isolated human sweat glands. Peptides **7(1):** 151-154.

26. AMIRANOFF, B. & G. ROSSELIN. 1982. VIP receptors and control of cyclic AMP production. *In* Vasoactive Intestinal Peptide. S. I. Said, Ed.: 307-322. Raven Press. New York.

27. BINDER, H. J., G. F. LEMP & J. D. GARDNER. 1980. Receptors for vasoactive intestinal peptide and secretin on small intestinal epithelial cells. Am. J. Physiol. **238:** G190-G196.

28. ROBBERECHT, P., P. CHATELAIN, P. DE NEER, J.-C. CAMUS, M. WAELBROECK & J. CHRISTOPHE. 1981. Presence of vasoactive intestinal peptide receptors coupled to adenylate cyclase in rat lung membranes. Biochim. Biophys. Acta **678:** 76-82.

29. LAZARUS, S. C., C. B. BASBAUM, P. J. BARNES & W. M. GOLD. 1986. Mapping of VIP receptors by use of an immunocytochemical probe for the intracellular mediator cyclic AMP. Am. J. Physiol. **251:** C115-119.

30. TAINIO, H. 1987. Cytochemical localization of VIP-stimulated adenylate cyclase activity in human sweat glands. Br. J. Dermatol. **116:** 323-328.

31. LEROUX, P., H. VAUDRY, A. FOURNIER, S. ST.-PIERRE & G. PELLETIER. Characterization and localization of vasoactive intestinal peptide receptors in the rat lung. Endocrinology **114:** 1506-1512.

32. SAID, S. I. & P. HEINZ-ERIAN. 1988. VIP and exocrine function: Possible role in cystic fibrosis. *In* Cellular and Molecular Basis of Cystic Fibrosis. G. Mastella & P. M. Quinton, Eds.: 355-361. San Francisco Press. San Francisco, CA.

33. QUINTON, P. M. 1983. Chloride impermeability in cystic fibrosis. Nature **301:** 421-422.

34. KNOWLES, M., J. GATZY, & R. BOUCHER. 1983. Relative ion permeability of normal and cystic fibrosis nasal epithelium. J. Clin. Invest. **71:** 1410-1417.

35. KNOWLES, M., J. GATZY & R. BOUCHER. 1981. Increased bioelectric potential difference across respiratory epithelia in cystic fibrosis. New Engl. J. Med. **305:** 1489-1495.

36. QUINTON, P. M. & J. BIJMAN. 1983. Higher bioelectric potentials due to decreased chloride absorption in the sweat glands of patients with cystic fibrosis. New Engl. J. Med. **308(20):** 1185-1189.

37. DENNIS, G. J. & J. A. YOUNG. 1978. Modification of salivary duct electrolyte transport in rat and rabbit by physalaemin, VIP, GIP and other enterohormones. Pfluegers Arch. **376:** 73-77.

38. GASKIN, K. J., P. R. DURIE, M. COREY, P. WEI & G. G. FORSTNER. 1982. Evidence for a primary defect of pancreatic HCO_3^- secretion in cystic fibrosis. Pediatric Res. **16:** 554-557.

39. MATSUZAKI, Y., Y. HAMASAKI & S. I. SAID. 1980. Vasoactive intestinal peptide: A possible transmitter of non-adrenergic relaxation of guinea pig airways. Science **210:** 1252-1253.

40. SAID, S. I. 1982. Vasoactive peptides in the lung, with special reference to vasoactive intestinal peptide. Exp. Lung Res. **3:** 343-348.

41. HEINZ-ERIAN, P., R. D. DEY, M. FLUX & S. I. SAID. 1985. Deficient vasoactive intestinal peptide innervation in the sweat gland of cystic fibrosis patients. Science **229:** 1407-1408.

42. PAUL, S., P. HEINZ-ERIAN & S. I. SAID. 1985. Increased levels of autoantibody to vasoactive intestinal peptide in cystic fibrosis. Clin. Res. **33:** 82A.

43. GOZES, I., R. AVIDOR, Y. YAHAV, D. KATZNELSON, C. M. CROCE & K. HUEBNER. 1987. The gene encoding vasoactive intestinal peptide is located on human chromosome 6p21 →6qter. Hum. Genet. **75**: 41-44.
44. KNOWLTON, R. G., O. COHEN-HAGUENAUER, N. VAN CONG, J. FREZAL, V. A. BROWN, D. BARKER, J. C. BRAMAN, J. W. SCHUMM, L. TSUI, M. BUCHWALD & H. DONIS-KELLER. 1985. A polymorphic DNA marker linked to cystic fibrosis is located on chromosome 7. Nature **318**: 380-382.
45. WAINWRIGHT, B. J., P. J. SCAMBLER, J. SCHMIDTKE, E. A. WATSON, L. HAI-YANG, M. FARRALL, H. J. COOKE. H. EIBERG & R. WILLIAMSON. 1985. Localization of cystic fibrosis locus to human chromosome 7cen-q22. Nature **381**: 380-382.
46. WIDDICOMBE, J. H., M. J. WELSH & W. E. FINKBEINER. 1985. Cystic fibrosis decreases the apical membrane chloride permeability of monolayers cultured from cells of tracheal epithelium. Proc. Natl. Acad. Sci USA **82**: 6167-6171.
47. WELSH, M. J. 1986. An apical-membrane chloride channel in human tracheal epithelium. Science **232**: 1648-1650.
48. COTTON, C. U., M. J. STUTTS, M. R. KNOWLES, J. T. GATZY & R. C. Boucher. 1987. Abnormal apical cell membrane in cystic fibrosis respiratory epithelium. J. Clin. Invest. **79**: 80-85.
49. FRIZZELL, R. A. 1987. Cystic fibrosis: A disease of ion channels. Trends Neurosci. **10**: 190-193.
50. KUHAR, M. J. 1985. Receptor localization with the microscope. *In* Neurotransmitter Receptor Binding. 2nd Ed. H. I. Yamamura *et al.*, Eds.: 153-175. Raven Press. New York.
51. LI, M., J. D. McCANN, C. M. LIEDTKE, A. C. NAIRN, P. GREENGARD & M. J. WELSH. 1988. Cyclic AMP-dependent protein kinase opens chloride channels in normal but not cystic fibrosis airways epithelium. Nature **331**: 358-360.

VIP$_{1-12}$ Is a Ligand for the CD$_4$/ Human Immunodeficiency Virus Receptor

PAOLA SACERDOTE

Department of Pharmacology
University of Milan
Milan, Italy

MICHAEL R. RUFF AND CANDACE B. PERT

Clinical Neuroscience Branch
National Institute of Mental Health
Bethesda, Maryland 20892

INTRODUCTION

Viruses may utilize unique and specific cell surface recognition molecules as their initial attachment sites. We have recently described and characterized the distribution of one such receptor in the brain, the surface molecule CD$_4$ (or T4), a differentiation antigen present on T lymphocytes, macrophages, and other cells.[1] The binding of the virus to this specific receptor is important in infectivity and pathogenesis of the human immunodeficiency virus (HIV), the etiologic agent of AIDS.[2,3] We have identified a five amino acid sequence (TTNYT) of the HIV external glycoprotein molecule, GP120, which is responsible for viral binding to the T4 molecule, and is able to prevent human T cell infectivity.[4] The pentapeptide had been shown to have potent human monocyte chemotactic activity through its binding to the T4 molecule.[5] Analyzing the VIP sequence,[6] we realized that the five amino acid sequence of position 7-11, TDNYT, shows strong homology with the pentapeptide TTNYT, suggesting that VIP also could bind the T4 molecule. Utilizing the *in vitro* human monocyte chemotaxis method, we characterized the interactions existing between the VIP molecule and the T4 receptor.

METHODS

Chemotaxis was performed as previously described.[7] Briefly, human peripheral blood was obtained from healthy volunteers and mononuclear cells separated by sedimentation over Ficoll-Paque. The cells were resuspended in modified Eagle's medium and diluted to a final concentration of one million monocytes per milliliter.

574

TABLE 1. Sequence Homology

VIP_{1-28}	H S D A L F <u>T D N Y T</u> R L R K Q M A M K K Y L N S V L N
VIP_{1-12}	H S D A L F <u>T D N Y T</u> R
VIP_{10-28}	<u>Y T</u> R L R K Q M A M K K Y L N S V L N
	<u>T D N Y T</u>
	<u>T T N Y T</u>

The assay was performed using a 48-well micro-chemotaxis chamber, a 5-μm pore polycarbonate filter separating the upper and lower compartment: Cells were placed in the upper compartments and chemoattractant peptides in the lower one. After a 90-minute incubation at 37°C, the migrated cells adherent to the distal part of the filter were quantified microscopically by an optical image-analyzer. Data are presented as stimulation index, the ratio of migrating cells in the test compared to cells in buffer alone; as positive control, migration to the chemotactic peptide fMLP was assessed (migration index = 9-11 at 10^{-8} M).

RESULTS AND DISCUSSION

We examined the chemotactic activity of the VIP fragments and the synthetic peptides shown in TABLE 1. Intact VIP was active in inducing chemotaxis, EC_{50} of 10^{-10} M; VIP_{1-12} was slightly less active, while VIP_{10-28} was considerably less active, eliciting a low chemotactic response even at 10^{-8} M. The peptide sequence TTNYT was more potent than VIP and, most interestingly, the chemotactic activity of the synthetic peptide TDNTY, EC_{50} of 10^{-11}, was comparable to that of VIP_{1-12} (TABLE 2). The agonistic activity on the T4 receptor is shown by the ability of OKT4A, a monoclonal antibody directed against T4,[5] to block VIP-induced chemotaxis. VIP-induced chemotaxis was specifically inhibited by 0.01 μg/ml of OKT4A, while chemotaxis by the control peptide fMLP was not affected. At a higher OKT4 dose, non-specific inhibition of fMLP chemotaxis was also present (TABLE 3). These data suggest that both VIP and the peptide sequence TTNYT induce chemotaxis by binding the T4 receptor.

TABLE 2. Human Monocyte Chemotaxis Activity of Various VIP Fragments and Synthetic Peptides

Fragment or Peptide	Chemotaxis Index			
	$10^{-12}M$	$10^{-11}M$	$10^{-10}M$	$10^{-9}M$
VIP_{1-28}	1.8	3	3.2	3
VIP_{1-12}	1.8	2.5	2.9	2.6
VIP_{10-28}	1.5	1.8	1.7	2
TDNYT	1.3	1.75	2.7	2.6
TTNYT	2	3.2	4	3.2

TABLE 3. Inhibition of VIP Chemotaxis by OKT4A[a]

OKT4A (μg/ml)	VIP 10^{-9}	VIP 10^{-10}	VIP 10^{-11}	fMLP 10^{-8}
0.01	100	100	100	23
0.1	100	100	93	70

[a] Inhibition of VIP chemotaxis by OKT4A, monoclonal antibody against T4. Two different concentrations of the OKT4A were added to the lower compartment of the chemotaxis chamber together with VIP. Data are expressed as percent inhibition: $1 - $ (experimental $-$ background / control $-$ background) $\times$ 100.

In order to provide additional evidence in support of this hypothesis, we performed chemotaxis experiments studying the possible additive effect of VIP and TTNYT on human monocyte chemotaxis. If these molecules had intrinsic chemotactic action on the same receptor, no additive biological response could be observed, while additivity should be observed in the presence of a structurally unrelated peptide like cholecystokinin (CCK), which has been shown to have potent receptor-mediated chemotaxis.[7]

When both VIP and TTNYT were included together in the lower chamber, no higher chemotactic response was observed than with TTNYT alone, while when CCK and TTNYT were added together a higher chemotactic response was elicited (TABLE 4). TTNYT and VIP, working through the identical receptor, are causing the same population of cells to migrate, while TTNYT and CCK attract different populations of cells by acting through their respective, independent receptors.

A further test of the hypothesis that VIP and TTNYT act through the identical receptor was to compare cross-desensitization. Desensitization of the TTNYT receptor could be achieved by incubating the cells for 30 minutes at 37°C in the presence of 10^{-10} M of TTNYT. A possible mechanism for this effect has been shown to be down-regulation of the number of receptors available for further ligand binding and biological activity.[8] We performed chemotaxis studies using monocytes where the TTNYT receptor was desensitized. As expected, TTNYT-pretreated cells had diminished chemotaxis to TTNYT (TABLE 5). Desensitization was also observed with intact VIP and VIP$_{1-12}$, while the chemotactic activity of the control peptide fMLP was not impaired after preincubation of monocytes with TTNYT, ruling out the possibility of a non-specific modulation of receptors. These data indicate that the TTNYT receptor and the VIP$_{1-12}$ receptor on monocytes, that is, the T4 molecule, are the same.

An analysis of the immunologic abnormalities of AIDS and the immunologic effects of VIP reveals many striking similarities. In AIDS patients the T lymphocytes

TABLE 4. TTNYT and VIP Are Agonists for the Same Receptor[a]

Peptide	10^{-12}	10^{-11}	10^{-10}	10^{-9}
TTNYT	3.15	3.55	4.55	3.3
TTNYT + 10^{-10} M VIP	3.4	3.2	4.1	3.95
TTNYT + 10^{-10} M CCK	4*	4.3*	5.1*	3

[a] When included together in the lower chamber, TTNYT and CCK show an additive effect (*$p < 0.05$), while TTNYT and VIP do not.

TABLE 5. TTNYT Desensitization[a]

	Chemotaxis Index	
Peptide	Control Cells	TTNYT-Desensitized Cells
10^{-11} M TTNYT	5	2
10^{-11} M VIP_{1-28}	4.2	1.9
10^{-11} M VIP_{1-12}	3.8	1.95

[a] Chemotactic activity of various peptides to human monocytes incubated for 30 minutes in the presence of 10^{-10} TTNYT.

show a decreased proliferative response to mitogens such as concanavalin A and especially PHA.[9] VIP has been shown to inhibit the proliferative response of T lymphocytes to PHA.[10] Also in AIDS patients a paradoxical polyclonal B cell activation with elevated serum immunoglobulin levels is observed, and VIP increases B cell production of IgG, IgM, and IgA.[9,11] AIDS patients also have deficits in NK cell activity and a further immunological action of VIP is inhibition of NK function.[9,12]

These observations reveal a novel activity of VIP associated with the NH_2-terminal TDNYT sequence. In contrast, the COOH-terminal VIP_{10-28} was much less active in promoting chemotaxis, in agreement with numerous other studies in many systems showing low intrinsic activity of this peptide. The basic amino acids in position 14 and 15[6] represent a natural cleavage site in the VIP molecule, suggesting a possible role of VIP as a prohormone.[14] Shorter fragments of VIP that can be easily generated by enzymatic action and that contain the core active TDNYT sequence, such as VIP_{1-14} or 1-12, are likely candidates as endogenous ligands for the T4. The profound immunosuppression of AIDS patients is not easily explained by direct virus infection; in fact it has been demonstrated that polyclonal B-cell activation and the inhibition of T lymphocyte proliferation in AIDS patients is at least in part due to an enormous amount of viral proteins (mainly GP120) in the blood.[13] These observations lead us to envision a system where an ectopic production of a VIP-like hormone by a viral source, in the form of GP120 or its degradation fragments, can contribute to the AIDS immunodeficiency. This new aspect could eventually lead to a new therapeutic approach to AIDS.

REFERENCES

1. HILL, J. M., W. L. FARRAR & C. B. PERT. 1986. Psychopharmacol. Bull. **22**: 686-689.
2. DAGLEISH, A. G., P. C. BEVERLY, P. R. CLAPHAM, D. H. CRAWFORD, M. F. GREAVE & R. A. WEISS. 1984. Nature **312**: 763-766.
3. KLATZMAN, D., E. CHAMPAGNE, S. CHAMARET, J. GRUEST, D. GUETARD, T. HERCEND, J. C. GLUCKMAN & L. MONTAGNIER. 1985. Nature **312**: 767-768.
4. PERT, C. B., J. M. HILL, M. R. RUFF, R. M. BERMAN, W. G. ROBEY, L. O. ARTHUR, F. W. RUSCETTI & W. L. FARRAR. 1986. Proc. Natl. Acad. Sci. USA **83**: 9254-9258.
5. RUFF, M. R., B. M. MARTIN, E. I. GINNS, W. L. FARRAR & C. B. PERT. 1987. FEBS Lett. **211**: 17-22.
6. MUTT, V. & S. I. SAID. 1974. Eur. J. Biochem. **15**: 518-519.
7. SACERDOTE, P., M. R. RUFF & C. B. PERT. 1988. Peptides **9**: 29-34.
8. SNYDERMAN, R., C. D. SMITH & M. W. VERGHESE. 1985. Leukocyte Biol. **40**: 785-800.

9. LANE, M. C. & A. S. FAUCI. 1985. Annu. Rev. Immunol. **3:** 2640-2644.
10. STANITZ, A. M., D. BEFUS & J. BIENENSTOCK. J. Immunol. **133:** 152-156.
11. OTTAWAY, C. D. & G. R. GREENBERG. 1984. J. Immunol. **132:** 417-423.
12. DREW, P. A. & J. C. SHEARMAN. 1985. Aust. J. Exp. Biol. Med. Sci. **63:** 313-318.
13. BODANSZKY, M., A. BODANSZKY, S. S. DESHMANE, J. MARTINEZ & S. I. SAID. 1979. Bioorg. Chem. **8:** 399-407.
14. MANN, D. L., F. LaSANE, M. POPOVIC, L. O. ARTHUR, G. W. ROBEY, W. A. BLATTNER & M. J. NEWMAN. 1987. J. Immunol. **138:** 2640-2644.

Vasoactive Intestinal Polypeptide Increases Inositol Phospholipid Breakdown in the Rat Superior Cervical Ganglion

S. AUDIGIER,[a] C. BARBERIS, AND S. JARD

Centre INSERM-CNRS de Pharmacologie Endocrinologie
Montpellier, France

Immunohistochemical studies have revealed the presence of vasoactive intestinal polypeptide (VIP) in nerve fibers of the rat superior cervical ganglion (SCG).[1,2] Furthermore, this polypeptide induces the depolarization of ganglionic cells and selectively enhances the muscarinic slow excitatory postsynaptic potential.[3-5] Besides their similar electrophysiological effects, acetylcholine (Ach) and VIP stimulate the activity of tyrosine hydroxylase (TyrOHase).[6,7] Since the activation of TyrOHase by Ach might result from its action on the phosphatidylinositol (PI) turnover, VIP-induced stimulation of this enzyme could be mediated through the same second messenger.

The effect of VIP on the PI metabolism was investigated in isolated rat SCG. The ganglia were removed and prelabeled with [^{3}H]myoinositol for two hours at 37°C. They were rinsed, preincubated with 10 mM LiCl for 20 minutes, and stimulated with the different agonists for 20 minutes. The incubations were terminated by perchloric acid and processed as previously described.[8] The results were expressed as the ratio of the radioactivity found in inositol phosphates to that found in phosphatidylinositides (PIs). Under these conditions, VIP induced a fivefold increase of the PI breakdown; the stimulation was concentration dependent, saturable, and half of the maximal response was achieved at 1 μM of VIP (FIG. 1). The removal of extracellular calcium ions or the addition of tetrodotoxin did not alter the response induced by VIP (FIG. 2), suggesting a direct action on ganglionic cells mediated by a specific receptor for VIP or a structurally related peptide. Such a related peptide is not a member of the VIP family since none of them were able, even at concentrations higher than 10 μM, to produce any increase in PI breakdown (FIG. 1).

The inactivity of the peptides from the VIP family on PI turnover suggests that SCG contains low-affinity VIP receptors coupled to PI breakdown for which VIP itself or an as yet unidentified peptide might be the endogenous ligand.

---

[a] Present address: Laboratory of Molecular and Cellular Neuroscience, Rockefeller University, 1230 York Avenue, New York, NY 10021.

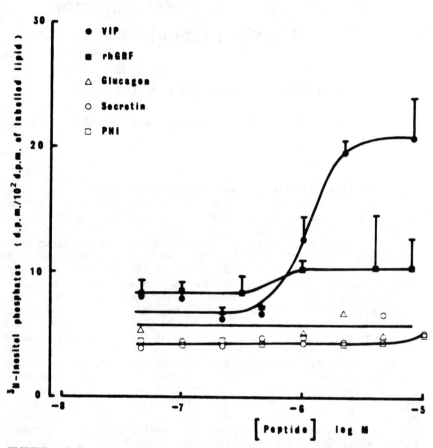

FIGURE 1. Concentration-dependent effect of VIP and peptides of the VIP family on inositol lipid breakdown in rat superior cervical ganglia. The experiments were performed as described in the text. Results are means ± SD of three determinations.

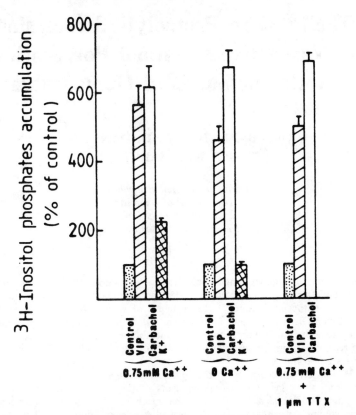

FIGURE 2. Effect of calcium removal and tetrodotoxin (TTX) on VIP-induced inositol phosphate accumulation. Isolated ganglia were labeled as described in the text. When present, 1 μM TTX was added during the preincubation with LiCl. The ganglia were stimulated with VIP (40 μM), carbachol (1 mM) or K$^+$ (50 mM) for 20 minutes in the appropriate medium. The values represent the means $\pm$ SD of three independent determinations.

REFERENCES

1. HOKFELT, T., L. G. ELFVIN, M. SCHULTZBERG, K. FUXE, S. I. SAID, V. MUTT & M. GOLDSTEIN. 1977. Neuroscience **2:** 885-896.
2. HEYM, C., M. RENECKE, E. WEIKE & W. G. FORSSMANN. 1984. Cell. Tissue Res. **235:** 411-418.
3. MO, N. & N. J. DUN. 1984. Neurosci. Lett. **52:** 19-23.
4. KAWATANI, M., M. RUTIGLIANO & W. C. DE GROAT. 1985. Science **229:** 879-881.
5. KAWATANI, M., M. RUTIGLIANO & W. C. DE GROAT. 1987. Neurosci. Lett. **73:** 59-64.
6. IP, N. Y., C. K. HO & R. E. ZIGMOND. 1982. Proc. Natl. Acad. Sci. USA **79:** 7566-7569.
7. HORWITZ, J., S. TSYMBALOV & R. L. PERLMAN. 1984. J. Pharmacol. Exp. Ther. **229(2):** 577-582.
8. BONE, E. A., P. FRETTEN, S. PALMER, C. J. KIRK & R. H. MICHELL. 1984. Biochem. J. **221:** 803-811.

The *in Vitro* Proteolytic Processing of Vasoactive Intestinal Polypeptide by Rat Spinal Cord Homogenate

G. F. BARBATO,[a,b] F. JORDAN,[c] AND
B. R. KOMISARUK [b]

[b]*Institute of Animal Behavior and*
[c]*Department of Chemistry*
Rutgers University
Newark, New Jersey 07102

The proteolytic breakdown of neuropeptides is of considerable interest from the aspect of both activation of precursor polypeptides and degradation of released transmitter. Subsequent to the elucidation of the sequence of vasoactive intestinal polypeptide (VIP),[1] Staun-Olsen *et al.*[2] and Fahrenkrug *et al.*[3] observed that VIP was degraded less than 10% by brain synaptosomes, liver membrane, and uterine muscle membrane during receptor assays. To our knowledge, the proteolytic products of VIP in biological systems are not known.

VIP is highly concentrated in the spinal cord[4] appearing to increase in concentration from the cervical to sacral segments of the cord.[5] Concomitant with our investigations of VIP as a mediator of spinal mechanisms of analgesia (Komisaruk *et al.*, this volume), we investigated the proteolytic degradation of VIP in the spinal cord.

MATERIALS AND METHODS

Tissue Preparation

The spinal cord and cerebral cortex were removed from 250–350-g ovariectomized rats ($n = 12$). Each tissue sample was weighed, frozen on dry ice, and stored at $-80°C$. Membrane-bound enzymes were isolated by homogenizing each tissue sample in 1 mg/10 μl 10 mM sodium phosphate buffer (pH = 7.2; 0.3% Brij) and centrifuged at $27,000 \times g$ for 60 minutes at 4°C. The supernatant was discarded and the pellet resuspended in the same amount of buffer and recentrifuged. A 100 μl-aliquot was brought to pH 2.0 using 30% TCA (trichloroacetic acid), in order to inactivate any

---

[a]Address for correspondence: Guy F. Barbato, Ph.D., Department of Poultry Science, The Pennsylvania State University, 213 William L. Henning Building, University Park, PA 16802.

enzymes, and assayed on HPLC to act as a blank control. Three 100-μl samples were incubated for 75 minutes at 37°C with 25 nmoles of VIP. TCA was added to the samples and the resulting fragments were separated by HPLC. For the inhibitor studies, spinal cord homogenates ($n = 3$) were incubated in the presence of various peptidase inhibitors, each at a concentration of 10 mM. After 75 minutes, TCA was added to the samples and prepared for analysis by HPLC.

HPLC Methodology

All samples were prepared for application to an ODS, C_{18}, 3μ, reversed-phase column (15 $\times$ 0.46 cm; Phenomenex, Rancho Palos Verdes, CA) through the use of a C_{18} SepPak cartridge.[6] Peptides and peptide fragments were eluted using a TEAP (triethylamine phosphate) mobile phase,[7] using an LDC gradient HPLC with exponential control (e = 2), detected at 214 nm, and collected with an LKB fraction collector. Each fraction containing a UV-absorbing peak was divided into aliquots and was subjected to one of two chemical protocols: (1) gas-phase acid hydrolysis, for determination of amino acid composition, and (2) manual Edman degradation, for determination of the NH_2-terminal amino acid. All amino acid analyses were quantitatively and qualitatively identified using precolumn OPA (*o*-phthalaldehyde) derivatization (fluorescent detection) and separation for PTH (phenylthiohydantoin) derivatives of the NH_2-terminal amino acid (UV detection at 269 nm). Each of these assays utilized a 10 $\times$ 0.3 cm, ODS, C_{18}, 3μ, reversed-phase Chromegabond column (ES Industries, NJ), with the appropriate mobile phase, in conjunction with a Beckman 421 gradient HPLC. These data allowed us to identify scissile bond(s) subject to degradation under these conditions.

RESULTS AND DISCUSSION

Incubation of VIP with cerebral cortex homogenate produced a large number of fragments at a 15% conversion of starting material, suggesting multiple, nondiscriminating degradative pathways. In contrast, 37% degradation of VIP by spinal cord homogenate led to the formation of only four major peaks (FIG. 1). Amino acid composition of the cleavage products is shown in TABLE 1. Each fragment was produced by specific cleavage on the carboxy side of a tyrosine residue (Tyr[10] and Tyr[22]).

The degradation of VIP by spinal cord homogenate was completely inhibited by metallo-endopeptidase inhibitors (EDTA and 1,10-phenanthroline). Leupeptin and Traysylol exhibited a small degree of inhibition (15% and 20%, respectively) under the same conditions. Phenylmethanesulfonyl fluoride, bacitracin, and pepstatin did not inhibit VIP degradation (< 3% degradation). Therefore a metallo-endopeptidase(s) is likely to be involved with the degradation of VIP. This is a previously unreported, highly specific, degradative pathway of VIP.

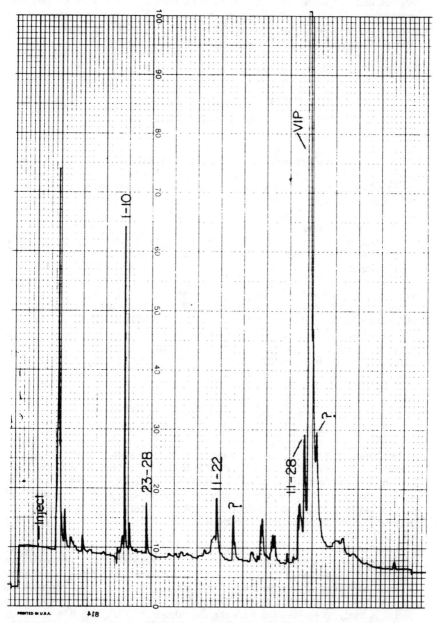

FIGURE 1. Chromatographic profile of the peptide fragments produced by incubation of VIP with spinal cord homogenate (25 nmole VIP + 5 μg homogenate protein). Chromatogram was obtained using an LDC gradient HPLC and Phenomenex 3μ, C_{18}, ODS 15 × 0.46 column. Mobile phase: A = 50 mM sodium phosphate, 0.3% TEA, pH = 3.0; B = 40% A + 60% acetonitrile. Gradient: 5-95% B in 50 minutes, 0.9 ml/min, e = 2.

TABLE 1. Amino Acid Composition of the Purified Degradative Products of VIP from Spinal Cord Homogenate[a]

Fragment	Mole/Mole Peptide									
	1 HIS -	2 SER -	3 ASP -	4 ALA -	5 VAL -	6 PHE -	7 THR -	8 ASP -	9 ASN -	10 TYR -
1–10	0.94	0.98	1.17	1.00	0.93	0.98	0.94	1.17	1.17	0.99
11–22	—	—	—	—	—	—	—	—	—	—
11–28	—	—	—	—	—	—	—	—	—	—
23–28	—	—	—	—	—	—	—	—	—	—

Fragment	Mole/Mole Peptide									
	11 THR -	12 ARG -	13 LEU -	14 ARG -	15 LYS -	16 GLN -	17 MET -	18 ALA -	19 VAL -	20 LYS -
1–10	—	—	—	—	—	—	—	—	—	—
11–22	0.76	0.92	1.00	0.97	0.86	1.12	0.89	0.98	0.97	0.86
11–28	0.81	0.93	0.98	0.93	0.91	1.00	0.93	0.99	0.95	0.91
23–28	—	—	—	—	—	—	—	—	—	—

Fragment	Mole/Mole Peptide							
	21 LYS -	22 TYR -	23 LEU -	24 ASN -	25 SER -	26 ILE -	27 LEU -	28 ASN-NH$_2$
1–10	—	—	—	—	—	—	—	—
11–22	0.86	0.99	—	—	—	—	—	—
11–28	0.91	0.99	0.98	1.10	0.99	1.01	0.98	1.10
23–28	—	—	1.00	0.91	0.97	0.95	1.00	0.91

[a] GLN and ASN were determined as GLU and ASP, respectively. Total recovery amounted to 87 ± 4%; AAA replicates, CV = 8.7%.

REFERENCES

1. MUTT, S. & S. I. SAID. 1974. Eur. J. Biochem. **42:** 581.
2. STAUN-OLSEN, P. B., B. OTTESEN, P. D. BARTELS, M. H. NIELSEN, S. GAMMELTOFT & J. FAHRENKRUG. 1982. J. Neurochem. **39:** 1242.
3. FAHRENKRUG, J., S. GAMMELTOFT, P. STAUN-OLSEN, B. OTTESEN & A. SJOQUIST. 1983. Peptides **4:** 133.
4. ANAND, P., S. J. GIBSON, G. P. MCGREGOR, M. A. BLANK, M. A. GHATEI, A. J. BACARESE-HAMILTON, J. M. POLAK & S. R. BLOOM. 1983. Nature **305:** 143.
5. GIBSON, S. J., J. M. POLAK, P. ANAND, J. A. BLANK, J. F. B. MORRISON, J. S. KELLY & S. R. BLOOM. 1984. Peptides **5:** 201.
6. BENNETT, H. P. J. 1983. J. Chromatogr. **266:** 501.
7. RIVIER, J. 1978. J. Liq. Chromatogr. **1:** 343.

Vasoactive Intestinal Polypeptide Given Intrathecally Increases the Secretion of Oxytocin and Vasopressin in Rats

B. BARDRUM,[a,b] B. OTTESEN,[c] J. FAHRENKRUG,[b]
AND A-R. FUCHS[d]

[a] Institute of Medical Physiology C
[b] Department of Clinical Chemistry
Bispebjerg Hospital and
[c] Department of Obstetrics and Gynecology
Hvidovre Hospital
University of Copenhagen
Copenhagen, Denmark

[d] Department of Obstetrics and Gynecology
Cornell University Medical College
New York, New York 10021

Vasoactive intestinal polypeptide (VIP) immunoreactivity has been localized within the hypothalamo-neurohypophyseal system[1,2] suggesting a role for VIP in the release of oxytocin (OT) and vasopressin (AVP). Previous experiments supporting this hypothesis have been performed in cat and rat.[3,4] Therefore, we have studied the effect of intrathecally administered VIP on plasma OT, plasma AVP, and plasma VIP in 60 rats.

VIP was administered either intrathecally in the anterior horn of the lateral ventricle in doses increasing from 0.3 pmol/kg/min to 3 nmol/kg/min or intraarterially in stepwise increasing doses from 30 to 3000 pmol/kg/min for five minutes. Six animals were used for control infusion and six animals were used for each concentration of VIP tested. Blood samples were drawn from the vena cava in the time period of -15 minutes until 90 minutes. The injection of VIP was given at t = 0 minutes. Controls received 0.9% NaCl with 0.5% HSA. A dose-dependent rise in plasma AVP occurred at 15 minutes with a threshold dose of 300 pmol/kg/min and maximum levels (33.9 $\pm$ 8.9 μU/ml) at 3 nmol/kg/min. The threshold dose for OT release was the same, 300 pmol/kg/min and maximum levels were significantly higher (96.1 $\pm$ 14.7 μU/ml OT); furthermore the response in plasma OT was prompt and reached significant values at t = $+5$ minutes, whereas the plasma AVP reached significant values 15 minutes after VIP infusion. In comparison to VIP given intraarterially,[4] plasma OT reached 10 times higher values when given intrathecally, whereas plasma AVP reached the same maximum in the two experimental setups. Plasma VIP was also tested, and when administered intrathecally the level of plasma VIP reached only 5% of the plasma VIP level compared to intraarterial administration.

586

The stimulatory effect of VIP on the posterior pituitary hormones OT and AVP confirms the previous results obtained in cat and rat.[3,4] The rapid onset of at least the level of plasma OT and the relatively low plasma VIP level when administered intrathecally, favors the hypothesis of central stimulation of neuropituitary hormone release rather than stimulation of peripheral receptors. Although the site of action of VIP has not been established, these data support the hypothesis that endogenous VIP participates in the release mechanism of neuroendocrine hormones.

REFERENCES

1. OKAMURA, H. *et al.* 1986. Biomed Res. **7(4)**: 295-299.
2. ROSTENE, W. H. 1984. Prog. Neurobiol. **22**: 103-129.
3. OTTESEN, B. *et al.* 1984. Endocrinology **115**: 1648-1650.
4. BARDRUM, B. *et al.* 1987. Life Sci. **40**: 169-173.

Neurogenic Vasoactive Intestinal Peptide Dilation in a Resistance Artery[a]

JOHN A. BEVAN

Department of Pharmacology
University of Vermont
Burlington, Vermont 05405

Although there are remarkable species differences, studies show that vasoactive intestinal peptide immunoreactive (VIP-IR) perivascular axons are found in most organ systems.[1] The regional vascular bed surveyed in most detail is the head of the cat. VIP-IR perivascular fibers are absent from the major arteries in the neck, but are found often in extreme density in these arteries supplying just about all cephalic tissues.[2] In the cat cerebral and lingual arteries, all criteria to establish VIP as a neurotransmitter have been satisfied. The peptide is present in the artery wall in the vesicles[3] found in predominantly perivascular fibers. It is released through a Ca^{2+}-dependent process and is a potent vasodilator with a time course of action similar to the response to a nerve stimulation. Neuro-vasodilation is inhibited selectively by antiserum to VIP. The extent of neuro-vasodilation is related to the density of innervation.[4,5] The peptide is presumably inactivated by nonspecific protease activity. Finally, there is considerable direct and indirect evidence that excludes other putative vasodilator transmitters. In some, but not all, arteries acetylcholine (Ach) is also released by field stimulation.

The studies described above were carried out on a middle-sized muscular artery, a vessel that contributes relatively little to the control of peripheral resistance. More recently we have been investigating VIP-related dilation in small branches (100-200 μ O.D.) of the lingual arteries that have a high density of VIP innervation. A nonadrenergic tetrodotoxin-sensitive, frequency-dependent dilation after sympathetic block can be seen in these vessels whether the development of tone is spontaneous or induced pharmacologically (FIG. 1). As in the parent vessel dilation is often reduced with atropine and is relatively slow in onset with a slow recovery. Pretreatment with ouabain ($10^{-5}M$) very significantly attenuates this dilation.

The microinjection of small volumes of physiological salt solution into the lumen of the resistance artery also causes dilation. The dilation is large and can be markedly attenuated by ouabain. The dilation is presumably in response to an increase in shear stress. Both dilator mechanisms summate.

VIP released in response to central command would relax directly vascular smooth muscle, and this relaxation would be expected to lead to an increase in flow with resultant flow-induced dilation. Because both processes are influenced by ouabain, at least part of the intracellular mechanisms are the same. Lingual resistance arteries show the capacity to develop intrinsic myogenic basal tone, presumably in response

[a]Supported by United States Public Health Service Grant HL 32383.

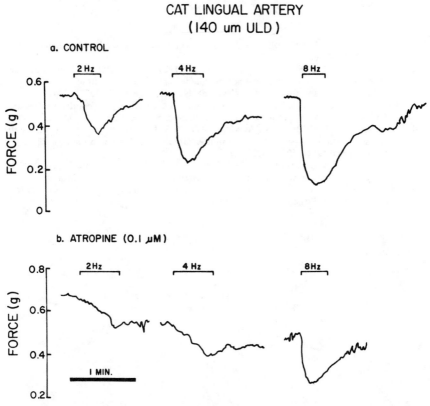

FIGURE 1. Effect of atropine on the tetrodotoxin-sensitive dilation of a small branch of the cat lingual artery to electrical field stimulation. The artery is mounted in a resistance vessel myograph in Krebs saline solution at 37°C equilibrated with 95% oxygen and 5% Co_2. Tone has been increased with $PGF_{2\alpha}$ (3×10^{-7}).

to stretch.[6] Dilation of the blood vessel when intramural pressure remains constant would be associated with an increase in tangential stress, the physiologic stimulus to the myogenic response. Thus, the final diameter of the resistance artery achieved as a consequence of the increased dilator nerve traffic would be the result of at least three interactive processes.

The VIP dilator system over the long term is an economical one. Dilation can be distinguished with dilator tonic nerve activity of approximately 0.1 Hz and is appropriate for one in which the transmitter is not conserved.

Presumptive evidence has been accumulated from *in vivo* studies for VIP transmission in a variety of organs. However, due to the complexity of the biological preparations used in these studies, a definitive source for the VIP was not established with complete certainty. This must be sought, as in this study, using isolated blood vessels. However, the evidence is extremely suggestive that VIP is an important vasodilator transmitter in many organs.

REFERENCES

1. BEVAN, J. A. & J. E. BRAYDEN. 1987. Non-adrenergic neural vasodilator mechanisms. Circ. Res. **60:** 309-326.
2. GIBBINS, I. L., J. E. BRAYDEN & J. A. BEVAN. 1984. Perivascular nerves with immuno-reactivity to vasoactive intestinal polypeptide in cephalic arteries of the cat: Distribution, possible origins and functional implications. Neuroscience **13(4):** 1327-1346.
3. LEE, T. J.-F., A. SAITO & I. BEREZIN. 1984. Vasoactive intestinal polypeptide-like substance: The potential transmitter for cerebral vasodilation. Science **224:** 898-901.
4. BEVAN, J. A., G. M. BUGA, M. A. MOSKOWITZ & S. I. SAID. 1986. *In vitro* evidence that vasoactive intestinal peptide is a transmitter of neurovasodilation in the head of the cat. Neuroscience **19(2):** 597-604.2.
5. BRAYDEN, J. E. & J. A. BEVAN. 1986. Evidence that vasoactive intestinal polypeptide (VIP) mediates neurogenic vasodilation of feline cerebral arteries. Stroke **17:** 1189-1192.
6. HWA, J. J. & J. A. BEVAN. 1986. Stretch-dependent (myogenic) tone in rabbit ear resistance arteries. Am. J. Physiol. **250:** H87-H95.

Postprandial Portal Venous Blood Flow and Portal Plasma Vasoactive Intestinal Peptide in Man

CARL HOLM, BJÖRN BIBER,[a] BENGT GUSTAVSSON,
IAN MILSOM, AND OLA WINSÖ

Östra Hospital
University of Gothenburg
Gothenburg, S-416 85 Sweden

JAN FAHRENKRUG

Bispebjerg Hospital
Copenhagan, Denmark

Postprandial portal blood flow (PBF) has previously been studied in animal models, but data thus far accumulated in man are scarce. Experimental data indicate that local intestinal neurogenic mechanisms and specific neurogenic transmitters are involved in the postprandial splanchnic hyperemic response.[1] Subsequently, much interest has been focused on the role of vasoactive intestinal peptide (VIP) in the regulation of intestinal blood flow. Current reports suggest that VIP is a neurotransmitter in the noncholinergic, nonadrenegic vasodilation in the intestinal mucosa in the cat.[2] VIP-containing nerve fibers have been demonstrated in the wall of the portal vein in several species and may participate in the regulation of PBF.[3] The aim of this study was to investigate postprandial PBF and postprandial portal VIP.

MATERIALS AND METHODS

A new application of the continuous thermodilution technique was used for measurements of PBF, as previously described and evaluated in our laboratory.[4,5] Following umbilico-portal cannulation, a thermodilution catheter (o.d. F 8 = 2.6 mm, length 82 cm) was passed into the main branch of the portal vein (in a direction against the blood stream) during elective cholecystectomy in seven patients. Blood samples for analysis of portal plasma VIP concentrations[6] were drawn through the indicator injection lumen of the thermodilution catheter. The catheter was left in its intraportal

[a] Address for correspondence: Björn Biber, M.D., Ph.D., Department of Anesthesiology, Östra Hospital, University of Gothenburg, Gothenburg, S-416 85 Sweden.

position for measurements of PBF and portal plasma VIP before and after alimentation on the second postoperative day. The protocol included measurements at baseline during olfactory-visual stimulation and at 15 and 30 minutes after alimentation.

RESULTS

PBF was 914 ± 211 ml·min^{-1} (mean $\pm$ SE) at baseline and remained essentially unchanged (915 ± 165 ml·min^{-1}) after a four-min olfactory-visual stimulation. PBF increased to 1475 ± 228 ml·min^{-1} at 15 minutes postprandially and to 1138 ± 226 ml.min^{-1} at 30 minutes postprandially (FIG. 1). Portal plasma VIP concentrations did not change significantly from baseline (14.1 ± 2.7 pmol·l^{-1}) throughout the

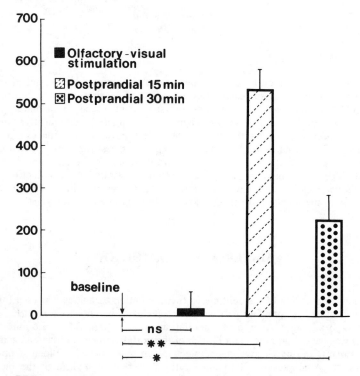

FIGURE 1. Changes in mean portal venous blood flow. Vertical lines indicate SEM; $n = 7$, ** $= p < 0.01$; * $= p < 0.05$; ns = not significant. Absolute values are given at the bottom.

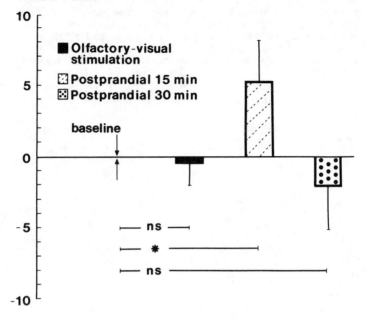

CHANGE IN VIP TRANSPORT
IN THE PORTAL VEIN
PMOL • MIN $^{-1}$

VIP TRANSPORT
(pmol·min^{-1})   8.3 ± 3.0   8.0 ± 2.6   12.5 ± 3.5   7.0 ± 2.0

FIGURE 2. Changes in mean VIP transport. Vertical lines indicate SEM; $n = 7$; * = $p <$ 0.05; ns = not significant. Absolute values are given at the bottom.

protocol. Portal VIP transport (product of PBF and portal whole blood VIP concentration) amounted to 8.3 ± 3.0 pmol·min^{-1} at baseline and increased significantly to 12.5 ± 3.5 pmol·min^{-1} 15 minutes postprandially (FIG. 2).

CONCLUSION

Concomitant postprandial increases in PBF and portal VIP transport were demonstrated. We suggest this reflects an increased release of VIP into the preportal vascular system. Our data agree with the concept that postprandial splanchnic hyperemia is, at least partly, elicited through VIP-related control mechanisms.

REFERENCES

1. BIBER, B. 1973. Acta Physiol. Scand. Suppl. **401:** 1-31.
2. SJÖQVIST, A., *et al.* 1983. Acta Physiol. Scand. **119:** 69-76.
3. JÄRHULT, J., *et al.* 1982. Cell Tissue Res. **221:** 617-624.
4. HÄGGMARK, S., *et al.* 1982. Scand. J. Clin. Lab. Invest. **42:** 315-321.
5. BIBER, B., *et al.* 1983. Scand. J. Gastroenterol.: 233-239.
6. FAHRENKRUG, J. & O. SCHAFFALITZKY DE MUCKADELL. 1977. J. Lab. Clin. Med. **89:** 1379-1388.

Regulation of Activity-Linked Neuronal Survival by Vasoactive Intestinal Peptide

DOUGLAS E. BRENNEMAN

Laboratory of Developmental Neurobiology
National Institute of Child Health and Human Development
Bethesda, Maryland 20892

A fundamental characteristic of the mammalian nervous system is the overproduction of neurons during development.[1] During the course of maturation, the number of neurons is reduced by mechanisms that involve electrical activity and perhaps substances derived from both target cells and glia. Such a process undoubtedly entails extensive communication between various types of cells to ensure that the appropriate neurons survive to form the "correct" neuronal networks. Previous work has suggested that neuropeptides play a role in determining neuronal survival during development in culture and that vasoactive intestinal peptide may supply one means of neuron-glia communication that results in the increased availability of glia-derived trophic substances necessary for neuronal survival.[2]

Dissociated spinal cord cultures from the fetal mouse have been used as a model system to study the effects of activity and glia-derived trophic substances on neuronal survival. Investigations of the molecular basis of activity-related regulation of neuronal survival have indicated that vasoactive intestinal peptide can increase the survival of neurons during a critical two-week period when 50% of the neurons normally die. Electrical activity has two apparent influences on this action of VIP: (1) The survival-promoting action of VIP is observed after the blockade of electrical activity, and (2) the spontaneous release of endogenous VIP from neurons is prevented by treatment with tetrodotoxin.[3] Significant increases in neuronal survival were observed with low concentrations (10^{-12} to 10^{-10} M) of VIP whereas amounts greater than 10^{-9} M produced an attenuation of this action (FIG. 1). Chronic treatment of spinal cord cultures with substances (VIP antiserum and VIP_{10-28}) that interfere with the action of VIP produced neuronal cell death similar in amount to that produced by electrical blockade (FIG. 2). After cotreatment with tetrodotoxin (TTX), closely homologous peptides (PHI-27, GRF, secretin) showed either no effect on neuronal survival or were far less potent. Addition of PHI-27 and GRF to electrically active cultures produced significant neuronal cell death. The neuronal deficits resulting from PHI-27 treatment could be prevented by cotreatment with VIP.

Mechanistic studies of VIP action on neuronal survival have revealed that nonneuronal cells were involved. By manipulating the cellular composition of spinal cord cultures, it was found that VIP stimulation of astroglia resulted in an increased availability of a trophic substance necessary for neuronal survival. Thus, VIP may have a developmental role in mediating neuron-glia interactions that are important to the determination of nervous system structure.

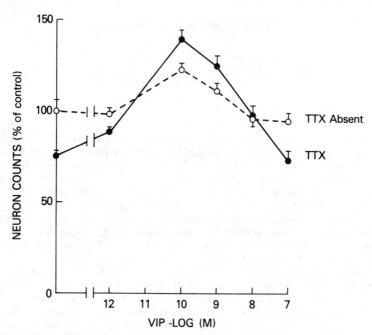

FIGURE 1. Neuronal cell counts from dissociated spinal cord-dorsal root ganglion cultures treated VIP alone ○ or VIP plus TTX ●. Additions to the cultures were made on day nine after plating. Nutrient medium was completely changed before the various treatments. After five days of exposure to the peptide, cultures were fixed with 2.5% glutaraldehyde (60 min, 25°C) followed by 0.15 M sodium cacodylate. Cell counts for day-14 control cultures were between 1500 and 2000 cells per 100 fields. Each point is the mean of six to eight determinations from two experiments.

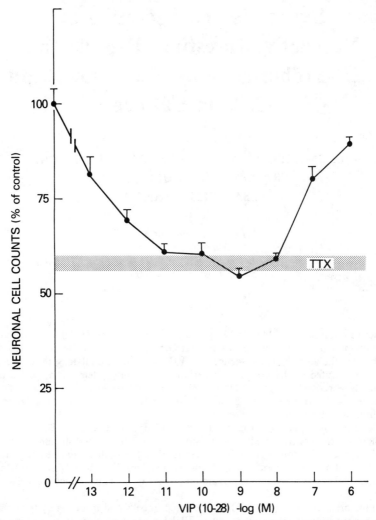

FIGURE 2. Neuronal cell counts after chronic treatment with VIP_{10-28}. This carboxy-terminal fragment of VIP has been shown to inhibit VIP-stimulated cAMP levels. The VIP fragment was added to the cultures 24 hours after plating. Treatment was continued until day 13 when the cells were fixed for counting. The shaded area indicates the cell counts from cultures treated with TTX alone in sister cultures during the same test period. Each point is the mean of four to six cultures dishes.

REFERENCES

1. BERG, D. K. 1982. Cell death in neuronal development. *In* Neuronal Development. N. Spitzer, Ed.: 297-331. Plenum Press. New York.
2. BRENNEMAN, D. E. & L. E. EIDEN. 1986. Proc. Natl. Acad. Sci. USA **83:** 1159-1162.
3. BRENNEMAN, D. E., L. E. EIDEN & R. E. SIEGEL. 1985. Peptides **6(Suppl. 2):** 35-39.

Synthesis and Secretion of Vasoactive Intestinal Peptide and VIP-Prohormone by Fetal Rat Brain Cells in Culture

L. CACICEDO,[a,b] M. J. LORENZO,[b] M. T. DE LOS
FRAILES,[b] S. REICHLIN,[c] AND
F. SANCHEZ FRANCO[b]

[b]Hospital Ramon y Cajal
Madrid, Spain
[c]Department of Medicine New England Medical Center Hospital
Boston, Massachusetts 02111

Vasoactive intestinal peptide (VIP) is a 28 amino acid polypeptide widely distributed in the peripheral nervous system; its highest concentration is in the cerebral cortex and the hypothalamus.[1,2] The evidence that VIP is a neuromodulatory substance has been demonstrated in the central and peripheral nervous system.[3] The factors that regulate its secretion have not been well established. We have investigated the synthesis and secretion of VIP by fetal rat brain cells in primary cultures and its regulation by membrane active stimuli.

The cortex was removed from fetal rats at 17 days of gestation. The cells were mechanically dispersed, plated at a density of 5×10^6 cells/dish and grown in minimum essential medium, 10% horse serum, 10% fetal calf serum, penicillin (100 U/ml), streptomycin (0.25 μg/ml), glucose (6 g/l), insulin (80 mU/ml), and 2mM glutamine. VIP was measured by radioimmunoassay in acid extracts of cells and media.

Immunoreactive VIP (IR-VIP) was detected in cells and media as early as three days after planting. The concentration of IR-VIP increased steadily to a maximum of approximately threefold between days 12 and 18, when production reached an average value of 17 ng/mg DNA per dish (TABLE 1). Chromatographic characteristics of the IR-VIP of both the cell extracts and the media were determined using a Sephadex G-50 column eluted with acetic acid 0.1 N, 0.025% BSA buffer. The IR-VIP from the cell extracts eluted in two forms, one corresponding to VIP_{1-28} and a large one that probably represents prohormone. Exposure to potassium in the presence of 2.5 mM calcium resulted in a significant stimulation of IR-VIP release rising from basal values of 117 $\pm$ 13 (pg/dish) to values of 287 $\pm$ 17 and 370 $\pm$ 35 after stimulation with 30 and 56 mM K^+, respectively. Simultaneous addition of 20 μM verapamil, a

[a] Address for correspondence: Lucinda Cacicedo, Servicio de Endocrinologia, Hospital Ramon y Cajal, 28034 Madrid, Spain.

Ca^{2+} channel blocker, completely reversed the response (256 ± 11 to 174 ± 13 pg/ dish).

These results indicate that fetal brain cerebrocortical cells established in primary culture can synthesize VIP. The finding of a larger form of IR-VIP corresponds with similar findings for other neuropeptides in cultured rat cerebral neurons.[4] IR-VIP release can be stimulated by membrane depolarization and is dependent on calcium entry into the cells, as previously shown in brain synaptosomal fractions.[5] Evidence supporting VIP as a neurotransmitter has been provided.[3] Our results are compatible with the view that VIP is an endogenous cerebrocortical neuromodulator.

TABLE 1. IR-VIP Content of Cultured Cerebrocortical Cells and Media at Different Times after Planting[a]

Days in Culture	Media	Cells (ng/mg DNA/dish)	Total (Cells + Media)
4	4.06 ± 0.35	2.27 ± 0.12	6.33 ± 0.48
7	3.29 ± 0.146	1.88 ± 0.1	5.18 ± 0.24
11	7.19 ± 0.84	4.3 ± 0.9	11.5 ± 0.81
17	10.6 ± 1.0	13.9 ± 1.1	24.5 ± 0.18
19	5.9 ± 0.53	9.0 ± 0.9	15.0 ± 1.12
22	7.2 ± 0.54	10.0 ± 1.6	17.2 ± 1.2

[a] Each value represents mean $\pm$ SEM of four dishes.

REFERENCES

1. SAID, S. I. & V. MUTT. 1970. Science **169:** 1217-1218.
2. SAID, S. I. & R. N. ROSENBERG. 1976. Science **192:** 907-908.
3. ROSSELIN, G., M. MALETTI, J. BESSON & W. ROSTENE. 1982. Mol. Cell. Endocrinol. **27:** 243-260.
4. DELFS, J., R. ROBBINS, J. L. CONNOLLY, M. DICHTER & S. REICHLIN. 1980. Nature **283:** 676-677.
5. EMSON, P. C., J. FAHREKRUG, O. B. SCHAFFALITZKY DE MUCKADELL, T. M. JOSSEL & L. L. IVERSEN. 1978. Brain Res. **143:** 174-178.

Vasoactive Intestinal Peptide Receptor Activity in Intestinal Cells Isolated from Human Fetuses with Cystic Fibrosis

Comparison with the Liver[a]

E. CHASTRE,[b] S. EMAMI,[b] W. BAWAB,[b] D. FAGOT,[b]
H. BODÉRÉ,[b] F. MULLER,[c] A. BOUÉ,[d] G. ROSSELIN,[b]
AND C. GESPACH, [b]

[b]INSERM U.55, Hôpital St. Antoine
75571 Paris Cédex 12, France

[c]Laboratoire de Biochimie
Hôpital Ambroise Paré
92104 Boulogne Cédex, France

[d]INSERM U.73
Château de Longchamp
75016 Paris, France

Cystic fibrosis (CF) is an inherited genetic disorder of the exocrine-eccrine glands that is characterized by a generalized epithelial dysfunction involving an alteration in fluid and electrolyte secretions. It is estimated to occur in 1:2000 live births in Western Europe and North America. Although the genetic locus of CF has been located on chromosome 7, the biochemical basis of the disease is not yet known.[1] The gastrointestinal symptoms remain the prominent features of CF and can be detected during fetal life in humans.[2] Prenatal diagnosis in human fetuses at 17-19 weeks of gestation was achieved by detection of a decreased activity of intestinal microvillar enzymes in amniotic fluid and meconium ileus.[2,3] Since VIP has been shown to promote water and chloride secretions in several tissues such as intestine,[4] a defect of the VIP receptor-adenylate cyclase system may be related to the pathogenesis of CF during fetal life. This view is consistent with the presence of functional and specific VIP receptors in intestinal epithelial cells isolated from human fetuses at 18-23 weeks of gestation.[5] We therefore compared VIP receptor activity and molecular forms in intestine (a target of the disease) and liver (a control tissue) from human fetuses with CF or other inherently lethal disorders.

[a]This work was supported in part by a grant to C. G. from l'Association Française de Lutte contre la Mucoviscidose (AFLM).

METHODS

Diagnosis of CF was performed in human fetuses at 17 to 20 weeks of gestational age.[3] Plasma membrane-enriched particles were obtained for measurements of VIP receptor activity ([^{125}I]VIP binding, adenylate cyclase activation), as described in Gespach *et al.*[5] Determination of the molecular components of the VIP receptor in intestine and liver was performed according to minor modifications of the technique previously described.[6]

RESULTS AND DISCUSSION

TABLE 1 shows that the efficacy S/B (stimulation over basal value) of VIP on the intestinal adenylate cyclase was significantly reduced from 6.1-fold (± 1.1) in control fetuses, to 2.7-fold (± 0.4) in human fetuses with CF ($p < 0.05$). The potency K_a and the S/B ratios for sodium fluoride and forskolin were also reduced in CF, but the values were not significantly different from controls. In contrast, the functional characteristics of the VIP receptor-adenylate cyclase in liver (K_a and S/B ratios) showed no detectable alteration in CF. The same observation was made for the activation by glucagon and the adenylate cyclase activators, sodium fluoride and forskolin. In intestinal membranes, half-maximal inhibition of [^{125}I]VIP binding (2×10^{-11} M) by native VIP was observed at concentrations $IC_{50} = 4.3 \pm 1.2 \times 10^{-10}$ M and $2.9 \pm 0.5 \times 10^{-10}$ M VIP in control and CF fetuses, respectively ($n = 4$). In liver membranes, these respective IC_{50} values were obtained at 1.3 ± 0.4 and $2.3 \pm 1 \times 10^{-10}$ M VIP ($n = 3$-6). Three major bands of [^{125}I]VIP covalently linked to intestinal membrane proteins were observed with apparent molecular masses of 69, 35, and 13 kDa in human fetal intestine with CF (FIG. 1, lane A). At 10^{-7} M, VIP inhibited almost completely the labeling of the 69-kDa protein (lane B). Similar results have been obtained in the human colonic epithelium.[6] In adult intestine, three bands of 63 kDa (the high-affinity VIP binding site), 30 kDa (the low-affinity VIP binding site) and 16 kDa (nonspecific [^{125}I]VIP binding component) are identified.[6] However, the labeling of the low-affinity VIP binding site (35-kDa protein) was not reduced by 10^{-7} M VIP in CF intestine (lane B).

The results presented here indicate that differences exist in the functional characteristics of the VIP receptor in intestinal epithelial membranes prepared from human fetuses with CF. It is therefore possible that the VIP receptor-adenylate cyclase complex might be involved in the pathological states of CF in intestine and other exocrine organs bearing this transduction system. This work will be extended and completed by: (1) comparisons of the density and affinity of the [^{125}I]VIP binding sites (Scatchard analyses); (2) determination of the molecular components of the VIP receptor in human intestinal membranes from control and CF fetuses; (3) measurements of the VIP content and determination of its biologically active forms in the submucosa; and (4) examination of other messengers (IP_3-Ca^{2+} translocation) and hydro-ionic secretions regulated by VIP.[7]

TABLE 1. Adenylate Cyclase Activity in Intestinal Epithelial Cells and Liver Isolated from Human Fetuses with Cystic Fibrosis or Other Lethal Diseases[a]

Tissues	K_a	Adenylate Cyclase				n
		VIP/B	GLU/B	NaF/B	FK/B	
Intestine						
Control	$1.4 \times 10^{-10} M$	6.1 ± 1.1	—	10.3 ± 1.7	28.8 ± 7.9	5-6
CF	$7.4 \times 10^{-10} M$	2.7 ± 0.4^b	—	5.7 ± 1.2	10.9 ± 2.8	5
Liver						
Control	$6.7 \times 10^{-10} M$	1.7 ± 0.3	3.7 ± 0.9	5 ± 1.5	8.7 ± 0.3	4-5
CF	$4.5 \times 10^{-10} M$	1.9 ± 0.2	3.7 ± 0.7	7.4 ± 1.8	11 ± 2.2	4-5

[a] Plasma membrane preparations were incubated with 10 different concentrations of VIP in intestine (10^{-11}-$3 \times 10^{-7} M$) and nine different concentrations of glucagon in liver (10^{-10}-$10^{-6} M$). The action of sodium fluoride ($10^{-2} M$ NaF) and forskolin ($4 \times 10^{-5} M$ FK) was also investigated. The criteria to compare the functional characteristics of hormone–receptor interactions are the efficacy (ratio of stimulated to basal AC activity: S/B) and the potency, that is, the apparent half-maximal activation of the enzyme by a given peptide (K_a values). Values shown are means ± SEM of four to six experiments performed in duplicate.

[b] Significantly different from the corresponding control value, $p < 0.05$.

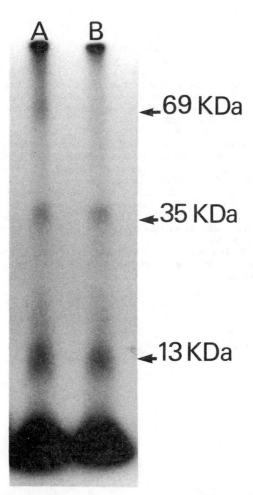

FIGURE 1. Molecular identification of the [^{125}I]VIP binding proteins in intestinal epithelial membranes from human fetuses with cystic fibrosis. For cross-linking studies, intestinal membranes were incubated in the presence of $2 \times 10^{-10}M$ [^{125}I]VIP alone (lane A) or in combination with $10^{-7}M$ VIP (lane B). The VIP receptor was then covalently linked with [^{125}I]VIP after treatment with the bifunctional reagent DSP. This was followed by solubilization with SDS and migration of the complex on polyacrylamide gel electrophoresis.

ACKNOWLEDGMENTS

We thank Miss M. Le Hein for her secretarial assistance and AFLM for the research grant (1986-1987).

REFERENCES

1. KNOWLTON, R. G., O. COHEN-HAGUENAUER, N. VAN CONG, J. FRÉZAL, V. A. BROWN, D. BARKER, J. C. BRAMAN, J. W. SCHUMM, L. C. TSUI, M. BUCHWALD & H. DONIS-KELLER. 1985. A polymorphic DNA marker linked to cystic fibrosis is located on chromosome 7. Nature **318**: 380-382.
2. CARBARNS, N., C. GOSDEN & D. J. H. BROCK. 1983. Microvillar peptidase activity in amniotic fluid; possible use in the prenatal diagnosis of cystic fibrosis. Lancet **i**: 329-331.
3. MULLER, F., S. BERG, J. C. FROT, J. BOUÉ & A. BOUÉ. 1985. Prenatal diagnosis of cystic fibrosis. I. Prospective study of 51 pregnancies. Prenatal Diagn. **5**: 97-108.
4. SAID, S. 1986. Vasoactive intestinal peptide (review article). J. Endocrinol. Invest. **9**: 191-200.
5. GESPACH, C., E. CHASTRE, S. EMAMI & N. MULLIEZ. 1985. Vasoactive intestinal peptide receptor activity in human fetal enterocytes. FEBS Lett. **180**: 196-202.
6. COUVINEAU, A. & M. LABURTHE. 1985. The human vasoactive intestinal peptide receptor: Molecular identification by covalent cross-linking in colonic epithelium. J. Clin. Endocrinol. Metab. **61**: 50-55.
7. CHASTRE, E., W. BAWAB, C. FAURE, S. EMAMI, F. MULLER, A. BOUÉ & C. GESPACH. 1988. Vasoactive intestinal peptide (VIP) and VIP receptors in human fetuses with cystic fibrosis. Submitted.

Immunohistochemical Localization of Vasoactive Intestinal Peptide in the Dogfish Rectal Gland

STUART R. CHIPKIN, JEFFREY S. STOFF,
AND NEIL ARONIN

Divisions of Endocrinology and Renal Medicine
University of Massachusetts Medical School
Worcester, Massachusetts 01605

Vasoactive intestinal peptide (VIP) has been shown to increase chloride secretion from the rectal gland of the spiny dogfish, *Squalus acanthias,* by a cyclic AMP-mediated Na^+, K^+-ATPase mechanism.[1] VIP-stimulated chloride ion secretion is completely inhibited by somatostatin.[2] Localization of the peptides that affect chloride secretion in the dogfish rectal gland is not known. We therefore studied by immunohistochemistry the localization of immunoreactive VIP (IR-VIP) and immunoreactive somatostatin (IR-SS) in this model system of ion transport.

Rectal glands perfused with 30 ml of either buffered 5% acrolein or 4% paraformaldehyde containing 0.1% glutaraldehyde were sectioned (20 μm) on a vibratome and processed for immunohistochemistry by either avidin-biotin complex (ABC) or peroxidase anti-peroxidase (PAP) methods using VIP antiserum (Immunonuclear, Stillwater, MN) at a dilution of 1:800. The somatostatin antiserum (a gift from Dr. G. Nilaver, University of Oregon Health Sciences Center, Portland, OR) was used at 1:300 dilution with 0.5% Triton X-100. Processed tissues were either mounted with gelatin for light microscopy, or prepared for electron microscopy by treatment with 2% osmium tetroxide (one hour) and uranyl acetate (two hours) and then embedded in epon. Ultrathin sections were cut serially and mounted on formvar-coated slot grids.

All shark rectal glands processed for immunohistochemistry demonstrated staining for IR-VIP. When synthetic VIP (100 μg/ml) was used to preabsorb the VIP antibody, all immunoreactivity was lost. Rectal glands perfused with acrolein demonstrated more nerve fiber staining than those perfused with paraformaldehyde/glutaraldehyde.

By light microscopy, axons containing IR-VIP had beaded swellings along the lengths of fibers. Thick fibers containing IR-VIP originated from the supporting mesentery of the rectal gland and traversed the fibromembranous capsule. Within the capsule, fibers were observed to form multiple branches. While some of these branching fibers followed the contour of the outer portion of the gland, other axons entered the parenchyma of the gland.

Axons within the parenchyma were generally of smaller diameter than those in the capsule (FIG. 1). These small axons coursed through the interstitial space between tightly packed secretory tubules. Fibers containing IR-VIP were frequently observed alongside of the epithelial cells that surrounded secretory tubules.

Ultrastructural examination confirmed that IR-VIP-containing fibers were surrounded by connective tissue and were not myelinated. Nerve fibers containing IR-VIP were observed within connective tissue upon entering the fibromembranous capsule. Connective tissue was also noted close to axons as they branched and entered the parenchyma. Bouton terminals containing IR-VIP were identified along thick nerve fibers within the fibromembranous capsule as well as along smaller diameter fibers located throughout the parenchyma. Within the nerve terminals, vesicles of different diameters were observed. Reaction product was present primarily in dense-core vesicles (60-120 nm). The presence of vesicles without reaction product was also noted. Electron micrographs documented that IR-VIP-containing fibers were in close proximity to cells surrounding the secretory tubules (FIG. 2). Nerve terminals were consistently located along the basal aspect of the peritubular cells away from the tubular lumen.

The pattern of staining with IR-SS antiserum was markedly different from that of IR-VIP. Light microscopy for IR-SS revealed few, very lightly stained fibers that contained reaction product. These axons were thinner and had smaller beaded swellings when compared to the staining pattern for IR-VIP. The distribution of IR-SS nerves was similar to that of IR-VIP. Evidence of fibers was found along the fibromembranous capsule and within the parenchyma of the rectal gland.

Because the staining for IR-SS nerves was sparse compared to IR-VIP, the amount of IR-SS in the shark rectal gland was determined by radioimmunoassay (with the assistance of Dr. M. Flint Beale, Massachusetts General Hospital, Boston, MA). After being homogenized, acid extracted, lyophilized, and reconstituted in buffer, shark rectal gland was found to contain approximately 200 pg IR-SS/mg protein. Dilutions of the extracted immunoreactive material ran parallel in radioimmunoassay to somatostatin standard.

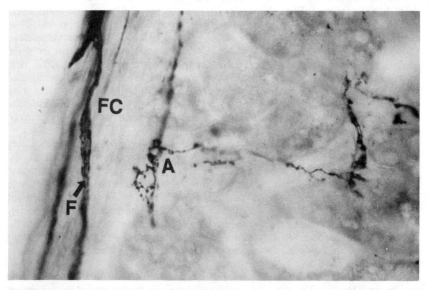

FIGURE 1. Light-microscopic view of a longitudinal section of shark rectal gland. Thick fibers (F) containing IR-VIP can be seen within the fibromembranous capsule (FC). A smaller diameter axon (A) containing IR-VIP courses through the parenchyma. Original magnification × 40; reduced by 15%.

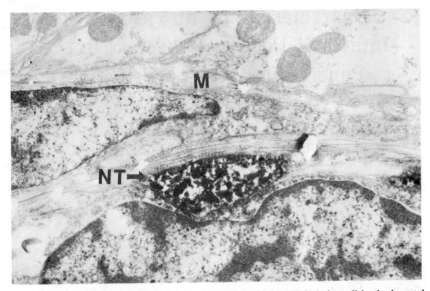

FIGURE 2. Electron micrograph of the basolateral aspect of a peritubular cell in shark rectal gland. Adjacent to the cell membrane (M) is a nerve terminal (NT) containing IR-VIP. Vesicles containing reaction product are present within the nerve terminal. Connective tissue matrix is also visible. Original magnification × 14,310; reduced by 15%.

VIP-like immunoreactivity was clearly demonstrable in nerve fibers throughout the shark rectal gland at both the light and ultrastructural levels. This anatomic evidence strongly supports the hypothesis that a component of VIP activity within the shark rectal gland is neurally mediated. In the shark rectal gland, VIP enhances the transport of chloride ions from the blood into the peritubular cell.[3] Once within the peritubular cell, chloride ions diffuse down an electrical gradient into the tubular lumen. The site of neural activation of this system is unknown.

In conclusion, the dense staining of numerous fibers for IR-VIP and the localization of the terminals near the tubule cells provide evidence that the VIP actions on chloride transport in the shark rectal gland are neurally mediated. The sparse fiber staining for IR-SS raises the possibility that somatostatin, or a somatostatin-like peptide, may be released from nerve terminals within the gland. Whether the sparse fiber labeling accounts for all of the VIP-like or SS-like material present in the rectal gland is unknown. Work is in progress in this laboratory to elucidate the origins of the peptide containing fiber network in this gland.

REFERENCES

1. STOFF, J. S., R. ROSA, P. HALLAC, P. SILVA & F. H. EPSTEIN. 1979. Hormonal regulation of active chloride transport in the dogfish rectal gland. Am. J. Physiol. **237:** F138-F144.
2. SILVA, P., J. S. STOFF, D. R. LEONE & F. H. EPSTEIN. 1985. Mode of action of somatostatin to inhibit secretion by shark rectal gland. Am. J. Physiol. **249:** R329-334.
3. SILVA, P., J. S. STOFF, M. FIELD, L. FINE, J. N. FORREST & F. H. EPSTEIN. 1977. Mechanism of active chloride secretion by shark rectal gland: Role of Na^+-K^+-ATPase in chloride transport. Am. J. Physiol. **233:** F298-F306.

Characterization of Vasoactive Intestinal Peptide Receptors in the Pancreatic AR 4-2J Cell Line

MICHAL SVOBODA, PATRICK ROBBERECHT,
FRANÇOISE GOMEZ, JACQUES WINAND, AND
JEAN CHRISTOPHE

Department of Biochemistry and Nutrition
School of Medicine
Université Libre de Bruxelles
B-1000 Brussels, Belgium

The AR 4-2J cell line derives from azaserine-induced hyperplastic nodules of the rat exocrine pancreas. Treatment of this cell line by dexamethasone induces *in vitro* a more highly differentiated phenotype and increases the number of pancreozymin (CCK) receptors with little change in receptor affinity.[1] In this study, we characterized the vasoactive intestinal peptide (VIP) receptors of this cell line.

AR 4-2J cells (kindly provided by Dr. Vaysse, INSERM, U 151, Toulouse, France) were grown in Dulbecco's modified Eagle's medium enriched with 10% fetal bovine serum. Cells were harvested by very mild trypsinization.

COMPETITIVE INHIBITION OF SPECIFIC [^{125}I]VIP BINDING

On Crude Membranes

Dispersed AR 4-2J cells were washed in phosphate-buffered saline (PBS: 10 mM phosphate buffer, pH 7.4, 145 mM NaCl, 5 mM KCl) then disrupted by sonication (3 × 5 sec, 120 W) in buffer A made of 20 mM Tris-Cl (pH 7.5) enriched with 0.25 M sucrose and a protease inhibitor mix (1 mM EDTA, 1 mg/ml bacitracin, 0.1 mg/ml soybean trypsin inhibitor, and 1 mM phenylmethylsulfonyl fluoride). The lysate was centrifuged for five minutes at 500 g and the supernatant centrifuged for 30 minutes at 50,000 g. The pellet was homogenized in buffer A to a 5 mg protein/ml concentration and stored in liquid nitrogen until use.

Crude membranes (100 μg proteins) were incubated with 0.2 nM [^{125}I]VIP in 50 mM Tris-maleate buffer (pH 7.5), 2 mM MgCl$_2$, 0.5% bovine serum albumin, 500 units/ml Trasylol (Bayer), and 0.2 mg/ml bacitracin, in a final volume of 0.12 ml. Binding equilibrium was attained after 15 minutes at 37°C, and membranes were separated by rapid filtration on glass fiber filters Whatman GF/C previously soaked in 0.3% polyethyleneimine.

The IC_{50} was 0.3 nM for VIP, 5 nM for PHI, 70 nM for helodermin, and 150 nM for secretin. Similar affinities were observed in membranes from control and differentiated cells (after two days in the presence of 20 nM dexamethasone) but a twofold increase in the binding capacity occurred after differentiation (not shown).

On Intact Cells

The same potency sequence for [^{125}I]VIP binding competition was observed in suspended intact trypsinized cells but IC_{50} values were higher: 7 nM for VIP, 100 nM for PHI, and 1000 nM for secretin, suggesting sensitivity of [^{125}I]VIP binding to intracellular nucleotides.

CHEMICAL CROSS-LINKING OF [^{125}I]VIP

The molecular properties of VIP receptors were studied by [^{125}I]VIP cross-linking to membranes and to intact cells still attached to the culture dish well. We compared six double agents: bis(2-(succinimidooxycarbonyloxy)ethyl)sulfone (BSCOCOES) gave the best cross-linking yield, in both membranes (FIG. 1) and intact cells (FIG. 2) as revealed by SDS-PAGE autoradiography. SDS-PAGE was performed on 5-20% T gradient, 2.7% polyacrylamide gels (80 $\times$ 80 $\times$ 1.5 mm) using the discontinuous system of Laemmli.[2] Dried gels were autoradiographied with Kodak AR films in X-Omatic cassettes equipped with regular intensifying screens.

In membranes (FIG. 1), the two main specifically cross-linked peptides had a M_r of 60K and 30K, when tested on 5-20% gradient polyacrylamide gel under reducing conditions. In some membranes cross-linking revealed the added specific labeling of a high-M_r smearing material (in the 130-180K range). The main 60K-labeled peptide migrated with a higher relative velocity (+5%) under nonreducing conditions, suggesting the presence of intramolecular disulfide bridges in the native peptide. However, the velocity of the native bovine serum albumin standard was also higher than that of reduced albumin (and this time by 15-20%), suggesting that the folding of native VIP receptors depends less heavily on disulfide bridges than that of albumin.

The labeling of the cross-linked peptides was competitively suppressed by 1 μM VIP, PHI, and helodermin, and diminished by 1 μM secretin. The IC_{50} of their labeling inhibition by VIP was comparable to the IC_{50} value of VIP on [^{125}I]VIP reversible binding, suggesting that the cross-linked radioactive bands correspond to VIP receptors.

In intact cells (i.e., cells still attached to their growth surface) the M_r of [^{125}I]VIP cross-linked peptides depended on the mode of cell solubilization (FIG. 2). After direct solubilization in the well, the major cross-linked radioactivity, under reducing conditions, migrated as a smear of 130-180K but a 60K peptide was also detectable. In contrast, the solubilization of cross-linked cells detached by mild trypsinization gave mainly 60K and 30K labeled peptides. This indicates that VIP receptors in intact attached cells were in a high-M_r complex and that a mild treatment, such as that used for cell passage, sufficed to cleave this complex to 60K and 30K receptor peptides.

The high-M_r smear could represent the association and cross-linking of the VIP receptor with other membrane component(s) such as N_s. Couvineau et al.[3] have indeed demonstrated that solubilized liver VIP receptors remain partly associated to N_s. In addition, they obtained a labeled 150K peptide after cross-linking solubilized VIP receptors to N_s. El Battari et al.[4] similarly observed a 120K species in human colonic adenocarcinoma. Association of VIP receptors with N_s was also demonstrated in lung.[5] Our cross-linking experiments were performed at 0°C so that the noncovalent association of VIP receptors with N_s and/or other components should preexist before cross-linking in intact AR 4-2J pancreatic cells. Alternatively, the 160K smear corresponded to native VIP receptors highly sensitive to cleavage as described by Nguyen et al.[6] for native 80K liver VIP receptors.

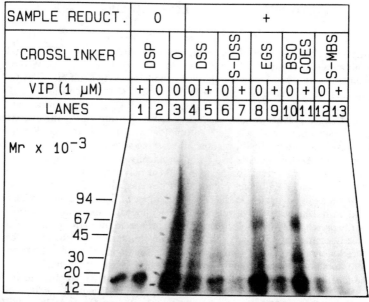

FIGURE 1. Covalent labeling of rat AR 4-2J membranes by [^{125}I]VIP induced with six cross-linkers. Crude membranes (2 mg protein) of dexamethasone-pretreated AR 4-2J cells were incubated with 0.2 nM [^{125}I]VIP for 15 minutes at 37°C in the absence or presence of 1 μM VIP. Washed membranes homogenized in 1.2 ml 50 mM phosphate buffer (pH 7.5) then distributed in six aliquots. Cross-linking was induced by adding 2 μl of 0.1 M double agent in dimethylsulfoxide. After 10 minutes at 0°C, 5 μl 1 M ethanolamine was added. Proteins were precipitated by acetone. SDS-PAGE analysis was performed on 5-20% polyacrylamide (80 × 80 × 1.5 mm) gels with sample reduction in lanes 4 to 13. Autoradiography was conducted for one week at −70°C.

Abbreviations: BSOCOES, bis(2-(succinimidooxycarbonyloxy)ethyl)sulfone; DSP, dithiobis(succinimidylpropionate); DSS, disuccinimidyl suberate; EGS, ethylene glycolbis(succinimidylsuccinate); SANAH, N-succinimidyl-6-(4′azido-2′-nitrophenylamino) hexanoate; S-DSS, bis(sulfosuccinimidyl)suberate; S-MBS, m-maleimidobenzoylsulfosuccinimide ester.

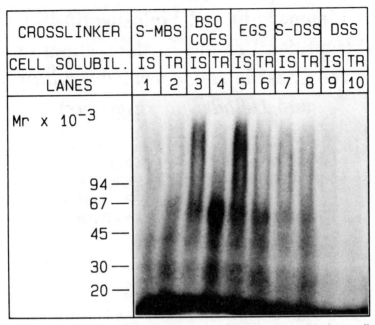

CROSSLINKER	S-MBS		BSO COES		EGS		S-DSS		DSS	
CELL SOLUBIL.	IS	TR	IS	TR	IS	TR	IS	TR	IS	TR
LANES	1	2	3	4	5	6	7	8	9	10

FIGURE 2. Covalent labeling of rat AR 4-2J cells by [^{125}I]VIP induced with six cross-linkers. Cells grown in a 24-well dish were cross-linked by the indicated double agents added at a 1 mM final concentration. Cross-linked cells were solubilized directly in the well (*in situ*, IS) or after mild trypsinization (TR) as follows:

(a) Cross-linking of [^{125}I]VIP was performed on subconfluent cells incubated at 37°C in a cell culture medium containing 0.5 nM [^{125}I]VIP (0.25 ml per well). Attached cells were washed and overlayed with 0.2 ml of PBS containing 1 mM cross-linker. After 10 minutes at 0°C, 20 μl of 0.1 M ethanolamine was added and the attached cells were washed and either solubilized *in situ* or after mild trypsinization.

(b) *In situ* solubilization: 0.2 ml Tris-Cl 10 mM (pH 7.5), 5 mM MgCl$_2$, and 20 μg/ml DNAse I were added to the well and cells were disrupted by sonication (3 × 5 sec of 90 W). After an incubation of 15 minutes at 0°C the cell lysate was precipitated by 0.8 ml acetone and submitted to electrophoresis.

(c) Solubilization after mild trypsinization. One drop of standard Gibco trypsin-EDTA solution (0.5 mg/ml trypsin) was added to each well. After five minutes at 8°C, cells were suspended in ice-cold PBS and pelleted by centrifugation. Pellets were lysed and submitted to electrophoresis.

Autoradiography of dried gels (80 × 80 × 1.5 mm) was conducted for two weeks at −70°C.

REFERENCES

1. LOGSDON, C. D. 1986. J. Biol. Chem. **261:** 2096-2101.
2. LAEMMLI, U. K. 1970. Nature **227:** 680-685.
3. COUVINEAU, A., B. AMIRANOFF & M. LABURTHE. 1986. J. Biol. Chem. **261:** 14482-14489.
4. EL BATTARI, A., J. LUIS, J. M. MARTIN, J. FANTINI, J. M. MULLER, J. MARVALDI & J. PICHON. 1987. Biochem. J. **242:** 185-191.
5. PAUL, S. & S. I. SAID. 1987. J. Biol. Chem. **262:** 158-162.
6. NGUYEN, T. D., J. A. WILLIAMS & G. M. GRAY. 1986. Biochemistry **25:** 361-368.

Helodermin and Helospectin-like Peptides Present in the Venom of the Lizards *Heloderma horridum* and *Heloderma suspectum*

ANDRÉ VANDERMEERS, YASSIR BOUNJOUA,
MARIE-CLAIRE VANDERMEERS-PIRET, PHILIPPE
GOURLET, ANNICK CAUVIN, PATRICK
ROBBERECHT, AND JEAN CHRISTOPHE

Department of Biochemistry and Nutrition
School of Medicine
Université Libre de Bruxelles
B-1000 Brussels, Belgium

Having previously isolated helodermin, the major VIP-like peptide from the venom of *Heloderma suspectum*,[1,2] we explored all VIP-like peptides in the venom of another lizard of the Helodermatidae family, *Heloderma horridum*, as well as any minor form in the venom of *Heloderma suspectum*. The purification of the active material was monitored by its capability to stimulate adenylate cyclase activity in rat pancreatic plasma membranes and by its cross-reactivity with radioimmunoassays for helodermin and PHI.[3]

Six (VIP-PHI)-like peptides (PHH 1-6 with ranking order based on increasing hydrophobicity) were purified to homogeneity from the venom of *Heloderma horridum:* four major forms (PHH 1, 2, 5, and 6) and two minor forms (PHH 3 and 4; FIG. 1). All peptides cross-reacted in radioimmunoassays for helodermin and, surprisingly, for PHI but not for VIP. They yielded only four fragments (T1 to T4) after trypsin digestion (TABLE 1) as the arginine-proline bound between positions 34 and 35 could not be hydrolyzed by trypsin. T1, T2, and T3 showed the same retention time by reverse-phase HPLC and the same amino acid composition; the differences were confined to T4, the COOH-terminal sequence.[3] PHH 5 and 6 were found to be identical to helospectins I and II described by Parker *et al.*[4] PHH 1 and 3 probably resulted from a secondary modification of PHH 5 (helospectin I), while PHH 2 and 4 derived from PHH 6 (helospectin II). Thus, the VIP-like peptides previously called helospectins by Parker *et al.*[4] and their derivatives are in fact typical of *Heloderma horridum* venom. By contrast, helodermin is absent in *Heloderma horridum* venom.

Eight VIP-like peptides were isolated from the venom of *Heloderma suspectum* (PHS 1, 2, 3, 4, 5a, 5b, 6a, and 6b) the ranking order depending on increasing hydrophobicity. We confirmed that helodermin (PHS 6a) is the major VIP-like peptide in this venom. Three minor forms, PHS 3, 4, and 5a, were related to helodermin and were purified to homogeneity (FIG. 2). None of them cross-reacted in a PHI radioimmunoassay. Each of them generated five tryptic fragments (T1 to T5) like helodermin

(TABLE 1). The differences were confined to T5, the COOH-terminal sequence of the molecule.[3]

In addition to this subclass of four helodermin-like peptides, a second subclass of four helospectin-like peptides (PHS 1, 2, 5b, and 6b) was also detected in small amounts in *Heloderma suspectum* venom thanks to their cross-reactivity in the PHI radioimmunoassay (FIG. 2). Each member represented about 5% of the total bioactive

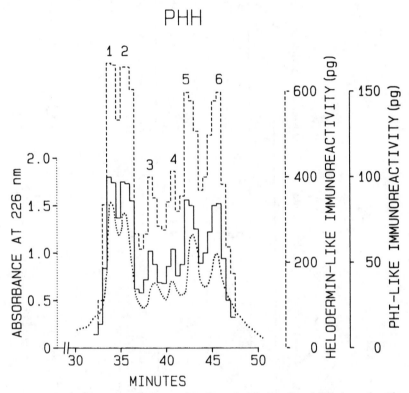

FIGURE 1. HPLC profile of VIP-like peptides from the Mexican lizard *Heloderma horridum.* The sample was the pooled active material eluted from a semipreparative column Supelcosil LC-8-DB (1 × 25 cm) starting from the crude venom.[3] The column was a Supelcosil LC-308 (0.46 × 25 cm) eluted with solvent A (0.25 *M* H₃PO₄-triethylamine at pH 3.0) and solvent B (CH₃CN/H₂O in a 4 : 1 ratio) using a linear gradient (30-32%) of B in 45 minutes at 30°C. Flow rate 0.8 ml/min. Absorbance recorded at 226 nm (.....). Helodermin-like (_ _ _) and PHI-like (_____) immunoreactivities were assayed by using, respectively, 0.01 μl and 0.3 μl aliquots of each fraction.

material. PHS 1 and 2 were already pure after RP-HPLC. PHS 5b and 6b were further separated, respectively, from PHS 5a and PHS 6a (i.e. helodermin) by ion-exchange HPLC on a Mono S HR 5/5 column (data not shown).

PHS 1, 2, 5b, and 6b exhibited, respectively, the properties of PHH 1, 2, 5, and 6 from *Heloderma horridum,* that is, (a) they all yielded four fragments after trypsin digestion, and (b) they coeluted by reverse-phase chromatography (PHS1 with PHH1,

TABLE 1. The Five Tryptic Fragments (T1-T5) and Four Tryptic Fragments (T1-T4) Obtained with Helodermin and Helospectins, Respectively[a]

Peptide	1	5	10	15	20	25	30	35	40
	< - - - - T1 - - - - - >	< - - T2 - - >	< - - T3 - - >	< - - T4 - - - >	< - - T5 - - - >				
Helodermin[b]	H-S-D-A-I-F-T-E-E-Y-S-K-L-L-A-K-L-A-L-Q-K-Y-L-A-S-I-L-G-S-R-T-S-P-P-P-*								
Helospectin I[c]	H-S-D-A-T-F-T-A-E-Y-S-K-L-L-A-K-L-A-K-L-A-L-Q-K-Y-L-E-S-I-L-G-S-T-S-P-R-P-P-S-S								
	< - - - - T1 - - - - - >	< - - T2 - - >	< - - T3 - - >	< - - - - - - - T4 - - - - - - - - >					

[a] Differences between the amino acid sequences are represented by bars. Abbreviations: ALA, A; ARG, R; ASP, D; GLN, Q; GLU, E; GLY, G; HIS, H; ILE, I; LEU, L; LYS, K; NH$_2$, *; PHE, F; PRO, P; SER, S; THR, T; TYR, Y.

[b] According to Hoshino et al.[2] and corrected for positions 8 and 9.[3]

[c] According to Parker et al.,[4] helospectin II is identical to helospectin I except that it lacks serine 38.

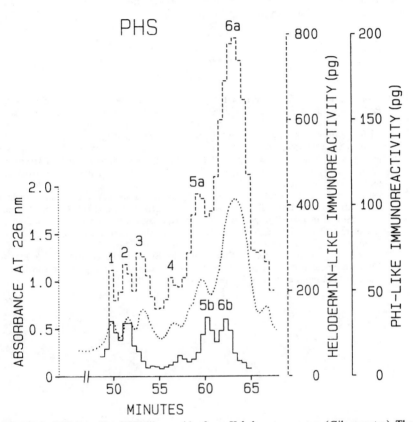

FIGURE 2. HPLC profile of VIP-like peptides from *Heloderma suspectum* (Gila monster). The sample was the pooled active material eluted from a semipreparative column Supelcosil LC-8-DB (1 × 25 cm) starting from crude *Heloderma suspectum* venom.[3] Two columns of Supelcosil LC-308 (0.46 × 25 cm) were coupled and eluted with solvent A (0.1% TFA, 28% CH₃CN) and solvent B (0.1% TFA, 32% CH₃CN) using a concave gradient (0-50%) of B in 80 minutes at 25°C. Flow rate 0.8 ml/min. Absorbance recorded at 226 nm (.....). Helodermin-like (_ _ _ _) and PHI-like (_____) immunoreactivities were assayed by using 0.01 μl and 0.3 μl aliquots of each fraction.

PHS2 with PHH2, etc.) indicating the probable identity between the second group of (minor) PHS peptides from *Heloderma suspectum* and the corresponding PHH peptides from *Heloderma horridum*.

In both venoms, all VIP-like peptides were equally potent and efficient when tested for: (a) their ability to occupy VIP as well as secretin receptors in rat pancreatic membranes and VIP receptors in rat liver membranes, and (b) the ensuing activation of adenylate cyclase in both membrane preparations.[3]

REFERENCES

1. VANDERMEERS, A., M. C. VANDERMEERS-PIRET, P. ROBBERECHT, M. WAELBROECK, J. P. DEHAYE, J. WINAND & J. CHRISTOPHE. 1984. Purification of a novel pancreatic secretory factor (PSF) and a novel peptide with VIP- and secretin-like properties (helodermin) from Gila monster venom. FEBS Lett. **166:** 273-276.
2. HOSHINO, M., C. YANAIHARA, Y. M. HONG, S. KISHIDA, Y. KATSUMARU, A. VANDERMEERS, M. C. VANDERMEERS-PIRET, P. ROBBERECHT, J. CHRISTOPHE & N. YANAIHARA. 1984. Primary structure of helodermin, a VIP-secretin-like peptide isolated from Gila monster venom. FEBS Lett. **178:** 233-239.
3. VANDERMEERS, A., P. GOURLET, M. C. VANDERMEERS-PIRET, A. CAUVIN, P. DE NEEF, J. RATHE, M. SVOBODA, P. ROBBERECHT & J. CHRISTOPHE. 1987. Chemical, immunological and biological properties of vasoactive intestinal peptide-peptide histidine isoleucinamide (VIP-PHI)-like peptides extracted from the venom of two lizards (*Heloderma horridum* and *Heloderma suspectum*). Eur. J. Biochem. **164:** 321-327.
4. PARKER, D. S., J. P. RAUFMAN, T. O'DONOHUE, M. BLEDSOE, H. YOSHIDA & J. J. PISANO. 1984. Amino acid sequences of helospectins, new members of the glucagon superfamily, found in Gila monster venom. J. Biol. Chem. **259:** 11751-11755.

Colocalization of Vasoactive Intestinal Peptide- and Substance P-Containing Nerves in Cat Airways[a]

RICHARD D. DEY

Department of Anatomy
West Virginia University Medical Center
Morgantown, West Virginia 26506

The lung is supplied with autonomic nerve fibers that partially regulate airway function. At least two neuropeptides, vasoactive intestinal peptide (VIP) and substance P (SP), are present in nerves of the respiratory system.[1,2] VIP may be a neurotransmitter for nonadrenergic relaxation of bronchial smooth muscle,[3] while release of SP from nerve fibers may be responsible for noncholinergic contraction of bronchial smooth muscle.[4] The purpose of this paper is to show that VIP and SP are stored together in the same nerve fibers and nerve cell bodies in the lung.

METHODS

The colocalization procedure used in this study has been described recently.[5] Cryostat sections of fixed cat airways were incubated in combined primary antiserum (rabbit antiSP antiserum and mouse antiVIP monoclonal antibodies; diluted 1:100), rinsed, incubated in combined secondary antiserum (fluorescein-labeled goat anti-rabbit IgG and rhodamine-labeled goat anti-mouse IgG). The sections were viewed with a fluorescence microscope using filters for selective visualization of fluorescein or rhodamine.

RESULTS

SP and VIP were colocalized in nerve fibers around bronchial smooth muscle (FIG. 1, a and b) and in close association with submucosal glands. Only SP-containing fibers were present in the airway epithelium. Colocalization of VIP and SP was also observed in nerve cell bodies that comprised the intrinsic airway ganglia (FIG. 2, a and b).

[a] This work was supported by Grant #G158 from the American Heart Association, Texas Affiliate, by NIH-BRSG Grant #2 S07 RR05433-24, and by the West Virginia University Medical Corporation.

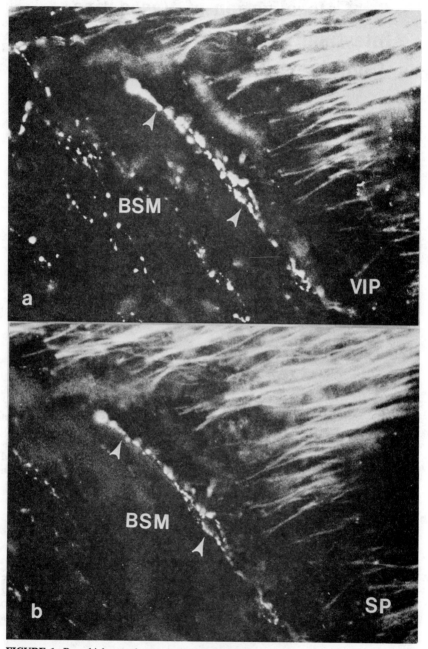

FIGURE 1. Bronchial smooth muscle (BSM) of cat lung showing colocalization of VIP (**a**) and SP (**b**) in the same nerve fibers (arrows). Magnification × 275.

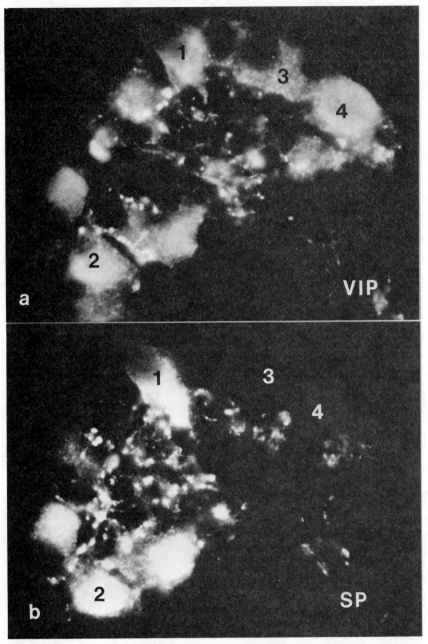

FIGURE 2. Intrinsic airway ganglion showing VIP-containing (a) and SP-containing (b) nerve cell bodies. Neurons numbered 1 and 2 contain both VIP and SP, while neurons numbered 3 and 4 contain only VIP. Magnification × 450.

DISCUSSION

The results demonstrate that VIP and SP are colocalized in nerve fibers supplying the airways and in nerve cell bodies that comprise the intrinsic airway ganglia. Although the significance of colocalization is not known, it is of interest that VIP and SP have almost exactly opposite actions in the airways. The release of VIP[3] and SP[4] from nerves in the airways by electrical field stimulation suggests that both peptides may act as neurotransmitters. Thus, control of airway function may be regulated by the simultaneous or sequential release of VIP and SP from the same nerve fiber.

REFERENCES

1. DEY, R. D., W. A. SHANNON, JR. & S. I. SAID. 1981. Localization of VIP-immunoreactive nerves in airways and pulmonary vessels of dogs, cats, and human subjects. Cell Tissue Res. 220: 231-238.
2. LUNDBERG, J. M., T. HOKFELT, C.-R. MARTLING, A. SARIA & C. CUELLO. 1984. Substance P-immunoreactive sensory nerves in the lower respiratory tract of various mammals including man. Cell Tissue Res. 235: 251-261.
3. MATSUZAKI, Y., Y. HAMASAKI & S. I. SAID. 1980. Vasoactive intestinal peptide: A possible transmitter of non-adrenergic relaxation of guinea pig airways. Science 210: 1252-1253.
4. LUNDBERG, J. M., A. SARIA, E. BRODIN, S. ROSELL & F. FOLKERS. 1983. A substance P antagonist inhibits vagally induced increase in vascular permeability and bronchial smooth muscle contraction in the guinea pig. Proc. Natl. Acad. Sci. USA 80: 1120-1124.
5. WESSENDORF, M. W. & R. P. ELDE. 1985. Characterization of an immunofluorescence technique for the demonstration of coexisting neurotransmitters within nerve fibers and terminals. J. Histochem. Cytochem. 33: 984-994.

Amino Acid Sequence of a Biologically Active Vasoactive Intestinal Peptide from the Elasmobranch *Scyliorhinus canicula*

R. DIMALINE,[a] JANICE YOUNG,[b] D. T. THWAITES,[a]
CAROLINE M. LEE,[a] AND M. C. THORNDYKE [c]

[a]*Physiological Laboratory*
University of Liverpool
Liverpool, L69 3BX, United Kingdom
[b]*ICI Pharmaceuticals*
Macclesfield, Cheshire, United Kingdom
[c]*Department of Zoology*
Royal Holloway and Bedford New College
University of London
London, United Kingdom

Identical octacosapeptide vasoactive intestinal peptides (VIPs) occur in pig, man, cow, and rat, while guinea pig and chicken VIP have four amino acid substitutions. Immunochemical studies suggested that the COOH-terminus of VIP from elasmobranch differs from that of other species,[1] and in order to examine structure-activity relationships and the phylogeny of VIP, we have isolated and sequenced this peptide from the dogfish, *Scyliorhinus canicula*. The peptide was isolated from acid extracts of intestine using gel filtration, ion-exchange chromatography, and reversed-phase HPLC. Microsequence and amino acid composition analyses were performed on intact peptide and fragments produced by cleavage with cyanogen bromide (1% wt/vol CNBr, 25°C, six hours). Overlapping sequence data indicated an octacosapeptide differing from porcine VIP at residues 11, 13, 23, 26, and 28 (FIG. 1); it is of interest that three of these (13, 26, and 28) are also substituted in chicken VIP. To determine if the COOH-terminal alanine residue was amidated, intact *Scyliorhinus* VIP was digested with carboxypeptidase Y, and derivatized with phenylisothiocyanate. Reversed-phase HPLC of the phenylthiocarbamyl derivatives yielded unequivocal identification of alanine amide, and no free alanine.

Dogfish	H S D A V F T D N Y S R I R K Q M A V K K Y I N S L L A
Pig	T L L I N
Chicken	F L V T

FIGURE 1. Amino acid sequences of dogfish (*Scyliorhinus*), pig, and chicken VIPs in single-letter notation. Human, rat, and bovine VIPs are identical to that of pig. All COOH-terminal residues are amidated.

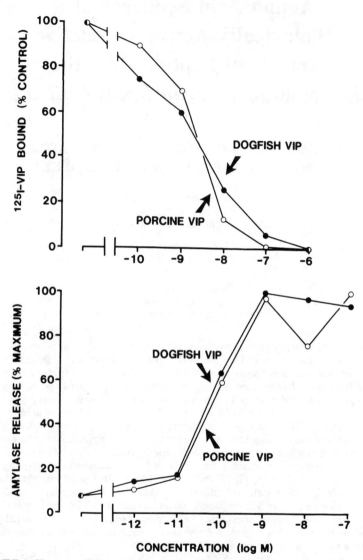

FIGURE 2. Upper panel. Example of a receptor binding study. Monoiodinated VIP (60 pM) was incubated with guinea pig dispersed pancreatic acini in the presence of porcine (open circles) or dogfish (closed circles) VIP (10^{-6}-10^{-10} M). Binding is expressed as percent [^{125}I]VIP saturably bound in the absence of unlabeled VIP. Nonspecific binding, determined in the presence of 10^{-6} M VIP, was subtracted in all cases. Each point was determined in triplicate.

Lower panel. Example of an amylase release experiment. Porcine (open circles) or dogfish (closed circles) VIP was incubated with guinea pig dispersed pancreatic acini in the presence of 5 mM theophylline. Amylase release was estimated using the Phadebus reagent (Pharmacia, Uppsala, Sweden).

Dispersed acini from guinea pig pancreas were prepared by collagenase digestion according to published methods.[2] Incubation of porcine VIP and *Scyliorhinus* VIP (10^{-8} to 10^{-12} M) with acinar suspensions stimulated amylase release in a dose-dependent manner (FIG. 2). In four separate experiments the mean concentration of porcine VIP for half-maximal amylase secretion was 3.4×10^{-11} M compared with 3.5×10^{-11} M for *Scyliorhinus* VIP. When monoiodinated porcine VIP was incubated with dispersed pancreatic acini, inclusion of unlabeled porcine or *Scyliorhinus* VIP (10^{-6} to 10^{-10} M) inhibited label binding dose dependently (FIG. 2). In three separate experiments the mean concentration of porcine VIP for half-maximal inhibition of radiolabel binding was 3.8×10^{-9} M, compared with 4.3×10^{-9} M for *Scyliorhinus* VIP.

CONCLUSIONS

Dogfish (*Scyliorhinus*) VIP differs from porcine VIP at five residues and from chicken VIP at four residues. It has full potency for binding to mammalian pancreatic VIP receptors and eliciting amylase secretion. Residues prone to substitution (13, 26, and 28) are presumably unimportant biologically; in particular, the identity of the amidated COOH-terminal residue is not crucial. Elsewhere, the molecule is highly conserved.

REFERENCES

1. DIMALINE, R., M. C. THORNDYKE & J. YOUNG. 1986. Isolation and partial sequence analysis of elasmobranch VIP. Reg. Peptides **14:** 1-10.
2. PEIKIN, S. R., A. J. ROTTMAN, S. BATZRI & J. D. GARDNER. 1978. Kinetics of amylase release by dispersed acini prepared from guinea pig pancreas. Am. J. Physiol. **235:** E743-E749.

PreproVIP-Derived Peptides in Man and Rat

R. DIMALINE AND LYNNE VOWLES

MRC Secretory Control Group
Physiological Laboratory
University of Liverpool
Liverpool L69 3BX, United Kingdom

JANICE YOUNG

Imperial Chemical Industries PLC
Pharmaceuticals Division
Macclesfield, Cheshire, United Kingdom

After the signal sequence, preproVIP contains five functional domains[1,2]; these are, an NH_2-terminal flanking peptide (NFP, preproVIP$_{22-80}$), PHI/M, a bridging peptide, VIP itself, and a COOH-terminal flanking peptide (CFP, preproVIP$_{156-170}$; FIG. 1). Several studies have indicated that the two biologically active peptides, VIP and PHI/M, are not always produced in equimolar quantities. In order to study biosynthetic processing of preproVIP, we raised antisera to the NFP and CFP, using short synthetic peptides that in both cases excluded the extreme COOH-terminal basic residue, which may be removed during processing (FIG. 1). The synthetic peptides were also used for radiolabeling and as radioimmunoassay standards. In acid extracts of the rat gastrointestinal tract, concentrations of NFP-like immunoreactivity (NFP-LI) were

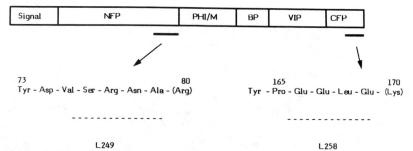

FIGURE 1. Schematic diagram of preprovasoactive intestinal peptide. NFP, NH_2-terminal flanking peptide; BP, bridging peptide; CFP, COOH-terminal flanking peptide. Synthetic peptides below were used for antibody production; in both cases the COOH-terminal basic residues of NFP and CFP were excluded. Phe 164 of preproVIP (CFP) was substituted by Tyr. Broken lines indicate specificities of antisera L249 (NFP) and L258 (CFP).

TABLE 1. Concentrations of PreproVIP-Derived Peptides in Acid Extracts of Rat Brain and Gastrointestinal Tract

	Peptide Concentration (pmol/g)[a]		
Tissue	NH$_2$-Terminal Flanking Peptide	VIP	COOH-Terminal Flanking Peptide
Brain	34.5 ± 5.7	28.2 ± 4.8	7.6 ± 1.2
Gastric corpus	79.0 ± 5.5	45 ± 10.3	14.7 ± 2.6
Gastric antrum	152.5 ± 25.9	80 ± 7.9	58.3 ± 5.6
Duodenum	138.1 ± 25.9	117.7 ± 9.0	18.5 ± 3.0
Jejunum	210.9 ± 18.3	167.3 ± 11.7	25.5 ± 3.9
Ileum	158.0 ± 24.5	187.2 ± 24.4	16.2 ± 2.0
Colon	149.8 ± 11.0	76.8 ± 9.8	15.3 ± 2.2

[a] Values are mean ± standard error; $n = 6$.

generally similar to those of VIP (estimated using an NH$_2$-terminal antiserum), while CFP-LI concentrations were five- to tenfold lower (TABLE 1). However, in both gastric corpus and small intestine, the concentrations of CFP-LI could be increased about fivefold by digestion with carboxypeptidase B, indicating that the extreme COOH-terminal lysine residue of preproVIP is not normally removed. In contrast, human stomach and large intestine contained high concentrations of CFP-LI without prior enzymic digestion, suggesting *in vivo* processing of the COOH-terminal lysine.

CFP from human antral muscle was isolated by a combination of gel filtration, ion-exchange chromatography and reversed-phase, high-performance liquid chromatography. Preliminary microsequence data indicated the structure (Ser)-Ser-Glu-Gly-Glu-Ser-Pro-Asp-Phe-Pro-Glu-Glu-Leu_____, which corresponds to residues 156-168 predicted from the cDNA sequence of human preproVIP.

In both rat and man, NFP exists in several molecular forms, whose pattern of expression is tissue specific; a smaller and less hydrophobic molecule predominated in rat intestine, while a larger peptide was found in the stomach. Isolation and sequence analysis of the gastric and intestinal NFP should reveal the nature of the alternative processing that underlies their production. Tissue-specific differences in NFP distribution have also been observed by immunohistochemistry; in particular a subpopulation of VIP-containing neurons was identified in rat stomach, but not intestine, that did not react with NFP antisera.[3]

CONCLUSION

The COOH-terminal flanking peptide of prepro-VIP, predicted from cDNA sequencing, is produced and stored in the human antrum. However, antisera to both NFP and CFP reveal tissue- and species-specific differences in precursor processing that may not be evident using antisera to VIP and PHI. Digestion with carboxypeptidase B indicates that in man, but not rat, the COOH-terminal lysine residue of preproVIP may normally be removed *in vivo*. In the rat the NH$_2$-terminal flanking peptide differs in structure between stomach and intestine.

REFERENCES

1. ITOH, N., K.-I. OBATA, N. YANAIHARA & H. OKAMOTO. 1983. Human preprovasoactive intestinal polypeptide contains a novel PHI-27-like peptide, PHM-27. Nature **304:** 547-549.
2. NISHIZAWA, M., Y. HAYAKAWA, N. YANAIHARA & H. OKAMOTO. 1985. Nucleotide sequence divergence and functional constraint in VIP precursor mRNA evolution between human and rat. FEBS Lett. **183:** 55-59.
3. RAYBOULD, H. E. & R. DIMALINE. 1987. Antibodies to fragments of provasoactive intestinal peptide reveal subpopulations of vasoactive intestinal peptide containing neurons in the rat gut. Neuroscience **20:** 201-208.

Vasoactive Intestinal Peptide

A Possible REM Sleep Factor

RENÉ DRUCKER-COLÍN,[a] OSCAR PROSPÉRO-GARCÍA,
RUY PÉREZ-MONTFORT, AND MARÍA T. PACHECO

Departamento de Neurociencias
Instituto de Fisiología Celular
Universidad Nacional Autónoma de México
México, D.F.

The search for sleep factors was initiated at the turn of this century by Legendre and Pieron who demonstrated hypogenic properties of cerebrospinal fluid (CSF) obtained from sleep-deprived dogs. Since then, several factors of peptidic nature have been suggested to have a role in regulating sleep. Most such peptides, however, seem to restrict their effects to slow-wave sleep.[1,2] Recently, our laboratory and others have shown that vasoactive intestinal peptide (VIP) produces a small increase of REM sleep in normal cats and rats[3] and that this effect is independent of brain temperature.[4] It has been suggested that more dramatic effects would be observed if a putative sleep factor is administered at times when sleep does not predominate.[5] We have thus tested the effects of the administration of several substances on cats pretreated with two consecutive injections of 400 mg/kg of PCPA, 24 hours apart. This treatment induces severe insomnia that peaks at hours 48 to 56 after the first injection. Thus, at hour 48, cats were injected into the fourth ventricle with CSF obtained from normal cats, CSF from 24-hour REM sleep-deprived (SD) cats (half of this CSF was heated for 15 minutes at 94°C and also injected), CSF from SD cats simultaneously treated with chloramphenicol (CAP), VIP (200 ng), and pancreozymin-8 (CCK-8; 100 ng). The results showed that REM sleep was restored in cats treated with CSF from sleep-deprived cats, with VIP, and with CCK-8[6,7] (FIG. 1). Additionally, it was observed that VIP increased the frequency of REM periods, while CCK-8 increased mainly the duration of each REM period (TABLE 1). These results suggest that the CSF of sleep-deprived cats contains a REM sleep factor that is thermolabile, sensitive to CAP, and may contain VIP and/or CCK-8. Considering that CCK-8 behaves quite differently from VIP, it is conceivable that both peptides control REM sleep through two different neural control mechanisms that may be synergistic. In order to test whether these peptides elicit a synergistic response, we administered them together (200 ng of VIP and 100 ng of CCK-8 in 100 ml of saline) to cats pretreated with PCPA. The results showed that frequency and duration of REM sleep epochs induced by this combination were higher than when each peptide was injected alone. In order to obtain further evidence for the VIP effects, PCPA-pretreated cats were injected with either VIP (200 ng) or CSF (100 μl) each incubated with 10 μl of anti-VIP. These

[a] Address for correspondence: Dr. René Drucker-Colín, Instituto de Fisiología Celular, Universidad Nacional Autónoma de México, Apartado Postal 70-600, 04510 México, D.F.

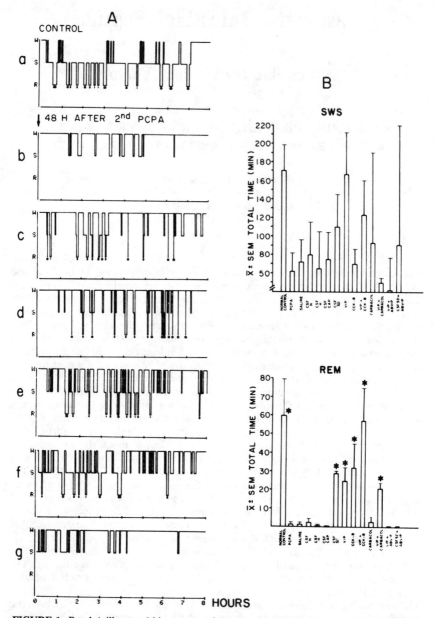

FIGURE 1. Panel A illustrated hipnograms of the sleep-wake cycle of cats during eight hours after the second injection of PCPA: (**a**) Effects of PCPA only; (**b**) After 100 μl i.v.t. injection of CSF obtained from 24-hour REM sleep-deprived cats; (**c**) i.v.t. injection of 200 ng/100 μl of VIP; (**d**) i.v.t. injection of 100ng/100μl of CCK-8; (**e**) i.v.t. injection of a 100 μl solution containing 200 ng of VIP and 100 ng of CCK-8; (**f**) i.v.t. injection of 100 μl of CSF SD incubated with 10 μl of AbVIP. Panel **B** shows the mean ± SEM of total time spent in SWS and REM sleep under all conditions. * ($p < 0.01$).

TABLE 1. Mean ± SEM of Different Treatments on Sleep Parameters of PCPA-Pretreated Insomniac Cats

Treatment	(n)	Waking (min)	SWS (min)	REM (min)	Duration of REM Epochs (min)	Frequency of REM Epochs	REM Latency (min)
Normal control	(10)	248.58 ± 30.4	171 ± 27	60 ± 19	6.2 ± 0.5	9.8 ± 1.06	51.24 ± 16.22
Control PCPA	(10)	415.92 ± 19.7	62.55 ± 20	1.43 ± 0.8	0.66 ± 0.43	0.3 ± 0.2	344.36 ± 73.03
Control saline	(10)	406.33 ± 24	72.27 ± 24	1.3 ± 0.9	0.69 ± 0.44	0.4 ± 0.3	438.09 ± 29.04
Cats receiving CSF N	(5)	398 ± 31	79.5 ± 35	2.5 ± 1.8	0.9 ± 0.7	1.4 ± 0.6	333 ± 134
Cats receiving CSF H	(5)	414 ± 40	65.5 ± 40	0.5 ± 0.4	0.2 ± 0.1	2.2 ± 1.9	380 ± 204
Cats receiving CSF CAP	(5)	405 ± 29	75 ± 29	0	0	0	480
Cats receiving CSF SD	(5)	342 ± 38	110 ± 35	28 ± 2.3	1.8 ± 0.3	18.6 ± 8	139 ± 100
Cats receiving VIP	(5)	288 ± 50	167 ± 45	25 ± 7	2.3 ± 0.9	12.2 ± 2.1	111 ± 76
Cats receiving CCK-8	(10)	377.01 ± 26.72	70.43 ± 16.2	32.6 ± 12.7	4.27 ± 1.0	7.8 ± 1.5	88.86 ± 17.69
Cats receiving VIP + CCK-8	(4)	298.85 ± 43.51	123.48 ± 36.26	57.65 ± 17.07	5.56 ± 1.1	10.5 ± 2.8	90.37 ± 58.38
Cats receiving Carbacol	(3)	383.7 ± 95.7	93.3 ± 97.1	2.8 ± 3.5	0.86 ± 0.7	1 ± 1.2	338 ± 175
Cats receiving VIP + carbacol	(2)	408.1 ± 8.2	50.3 ± 5.3	21.4 ± 2.7	3.2 ± 0.7	7.5 ± 0.7	21.7 ± 17
Cats receiving VIP + Ab VIP	(2)	445.9 ± 43.59	34.08 ± 43.59	0	0	0	0
Cats receiving LCF SD + Ab VIP	(2)	388.64 ± 129.20	91.36 ± 129.19	0	0	0	0

results showed that the anti-VIP antibodies blocked the REM-inducing effects. In addition we tested the effects of injecting VIP into the fourth ventricle while simultaneously giving carbachol (4 μg in 1 μl) into pontine cells and observed a decrement of the effects of VIP. These latter experiments suggest that the REM-enhancing properties of VIP may not indirectly involve a cholinergic effect. A complementary study determined VIP's effects on the sleep-wake cycle of cats with lesions of the basal forebrain area. Cats were rendered partially insomniac by the lesion (50% or less of the total time of a normal cat's sleep). Ten days after the lesion, VIP was administered into the fourth ventricle. Results showed that VIP normalized REM sleep epochs for 24 to 48 hours, but that after this period insomnia was restored.

In conclusion, these experiments suggest that VIP may be a powerful REM sleep factor, probably involved in its triggering mechanisms, while CCK-8 may be involved in the maintenance of this state of sleep.

ACKNOWLEDGMENTS

We wish to acknowledge the aid of Mrs. Ma. Teresa Torres for typing the manuscript.

REFERENCES

1. URSIN, R. 1984. Exp. Brain Res. Suppl. **8:** 118-132.
2. WAUQUIER, A., J. M. GAILLARD, J. M. MOUTI & M. RADULOVACKI. 1985. Sleep: Neurotransmitters and Neuromodulators. Raven Press. New York.
3. DRUCKER-COLÍN, R., F. BERNAL-PEDRAZA, F. FERNÁNDEZ-CANCINO & A. OKSENBERG. 1984. Peptides **5:** 837-840.
4. OBAL, F., JR., G. SARY, P. ALFALDI, G. RUBICSEK & F. OBAL. 1986. Neurosci. Lett. **64:** 236-240.
5. INOUÉ, S., K. UCHIZONO & H. NAGASAKI. 1981. TINS **5:** 218-220.
6. PROSPÉRO-GARCÍA, O., M. MORALES, G. ARANKOWSKY-SANDOVAL & R. DRUCKER-COLÍN. 1986. Brain Res. **385:** 169-173.
7. PROSPÉRO-GARCÍA, O., T. OTT & R. DRUCKER-COLÍN. 1987. Neurosci. Lett. **78:** 205-210.

Release of Vasoactive Intestinal Peptide in Response to Suckling

MAUD ERIKSSON, TOMAS HÖKFELT, BRANKA
PROSLONCEC, AND KERSTIN UVNÄS-MOBERG

Department of Pharmacology and Histology
Karolinska Institutet
104 01 Stockholm, Sweden

The aim of this study was to investigate whether vasoactive intestinal peptide (VIP), known to be involved in the control of many secretory processes, also may participate in the regulation of milk secretion. We therefore measured VIP levels in venous blood following suckling in lactating animals and women and VIP levels were also measured following oxytocin infusion and mammary nerve stimulation.

Immunohistochemistry studies were performed to visualize VIP immunoreactivity in the nipple of lactating rat.

METHODS

Blood samples were drawn from a peripheral vein during suckling in dogs and pigs and breast feeding in women. In cows blood samples were drawn from both mammary and jugular vein during machine milking and following bolus injection of oxytocin (10 IE). In rats blood samples were collected by decapitation after a 10-minute-long suckling period. Samples were drawn from the jugular vein in anesthetized rats and in connection with oxytocin infusions (0.22 and 2.2 nmol/kg/hr) and mammary nerve stimulations (5 V, 5 Hz, 0.2 msec). VIP levels in plasma were determined by the radioimmunoassay described by Fahrenkrug *et al.*[1]

Indirect immunohistochemistry according to Coons and collaborators[2] was performed on the mammary gland and nipple from lactating rats.

RESULTS

TABLE 1 shows the results of analysis of venous blood samples during suckling.

Oxytocin infusion or injection and mammary nerve stimulation raised VIP levels to about the same extent as following suckling.

After incubation with VIP antiserum, fluorescent nerve fibers were observed in the nipple of the rat. The fibers were mainly localized in smooth muscle around the ductus lactipherus.

DISCUSSION

We suggest that the elevation of VIP seen during suckling in dogs, rats, pigs, cows, and women is due to an increased release of the peptide caused by suckling-related activation of somatosensory neurons. The fact that VIP levels were found to rise after low-intensity afferent electrical stimulation of the mammary nerves supports this assumption. The origin of VIP released can not be established by these experiments, but we propose that VIP neurons from several sources are activated and contribute to the VIP released in response to suckling. The fact that in cows the levels of VIP was higher in the mammary vein than in the jugular vein following stimulation suggest that VIP is also released from the mammary gland. The VIP released in response to suckling may be secondary to previously released oxytocin. However, since VIP can be released in response to vagal nerve activation and since the vagal nerves are activated by suckling,[3] a part of the VIP release occurring in response to suckling may be due to vagal release of gastrointestinal VIP.

It is known that during milk ejection the alveolar contraction caused by oxytocin is paralleled by dilatation of the ductuli[3] to allow expression of milk. Since VIP, which relaxes smooth muscle, was demonstrated by immunohistochemical methods around the ductus lactipherus, we suggest that VIP may be involved in milk ejection.

TABLE 1. VIP Levels (pM) in Peripheral Venous Blood during Suckling

Subject	(n)	Basal Level	Peak Level	
Dog	(10)	15 (5-20)	44 (18-72)	(median [range])
Rat	(9)	12 ± 3	88 ± 23	(mean ± SEM)
Pig	(4)	25 ± 10	52 ± 5	(mean ± SEM)
Cow	(4)			
Mammary vein		12 ± 4	31 ± 9	(mean ± SEM)
Jugular vein		10 ± 3	21 ± 7	(mean ± SEM)
Women	(15)	6 (5-10)	14 (8-24)	(median [range])

REFERENCES

1. FAHRENKRUG, J. & O. B. SCHAFFALITSKY DE MUCKADELL. 1977. Radioimmunoassay of vasoactive intestinal polypeptide (VIP) in plasma. J. Lab. Clin. Med. **80:** 1379-1388.
2. COONS, A. H. 1958. Fluorescent antibody methods. *In* General Cytochemical Methods. J. F. Danielli, Ed.: 399-422. Academic Press. New York.
3. UVNÄS-MOBERG, K. 1983. Release of gastrointestinal peptides in response to vagal activation induced by electrical stimulation, feeding and suckling. J. Auton. Nerv. Syst. **9:** 141-155.
4. COWIE, A. T. & J. TINDAL. 1971. *In* The Physiology of Lactation.: 137-282. Edward Arnold Ltd. London, England.

Vasoactive Intestinal Peptide Protects Against HCl-Induced Pulmonary Edema in Rats

HUSSEIN D. FODA, TOMOAKI IWANAGA, LE-WEN
LIU, AND SAMI I. SAID [a]

Department of Medicine
University of Oklahoma Health Sciences Center and
Veterans Administration Medical Center
Oklahoma City, Oklahoma 73190

Acute, diffuse lung injury, leading to catastrophic respiratory failure, often complicates septic shock, extensive trauma, drug overdose, and acid aspiration. The hallmark of this condition is damage to the pulmonary capillary endothelium and alveoli, resulting in increased pulmonary vascular permeability and pulmonary hypertension, both leading to pulmonary edema.[1]

Despite advances in the understanding of this condition, its outcome remains grave, and more effective means of preventing or reducing it are urgently needed. Pretreatment with several pulmonary vasodilators that increase cyclic AMP level, including isoproterenol, terbutaline, PGI_2, and theophylline, was recently reported to reduce the severity of lung injury in animal models.[2,3]

In this study, we investigated the possible protective effect of vasoactive intestinal peptide (VIP) in an experimental model of acute lung injury produced by instillation of 0.2 M HCl in rat lungs.

METHODS

Adult Sprague-Dawley rats were anesthetized with pentobarbital, intubated through a tracheostomy, and ventilated by a Harvard respirator at 6.5 ml/kg body weight tidal volume that was held constant throughout the experiment. The chest was opened and the heart and lung exposed but left in place. Heparin (500 units) was injected into the inferior vena cava. A catheter was placed into the left atrium through the atrial appendage, and another catheter was inserted into the pulmonary artery through a right ventricular incision. The lungs were perfused with Krebs solution containing 4% albumin, at 37°C. Initial perfusion pressure was kept at 8-10 cm H_2O (usually at a flow rate of 30 ml/kg·min^{-1}). Peak airway pressure (P_{AW}) and pulmonary arterial (perfusion) pressure (P_{PA}) were measured continuously by pressure transducers.

[a] Address for Correspondence: Sami I. Said, M.D., Department of Medicine, University of Illinois, P.O. Box 6998, Chicago, IL 60680.

At the end of the experiment the right lung was ligated and removed, then weighed (wet weight) and dried in a 70°C oven until serial weights were constant (dry weight). A small sample (0.5 g) was removed from the left lung, quick-frozen in liquid nitrogen, homogenized, and stored in −70°C until assayed for cyclic AMP.[4]

The animals were divided into three groups, each comprising six rats: (a) a saline control group that received saline (2 ml/kg) intratracheally and was observed for 60 minutes; (b) a HCl alone group, in which 0.2 M HCl (2 ml/kg) was instilled intratracheally, followed by a 60-minute observation period; and (c) a VIP pretreatment group, in which VIP, 1 $\mu g/kg \cdot min^{-1}$, was perfused beginning 10 minutes before acid instillation and continued for the balance of the experiment (60 min).

RESULTS

Control animals showed little or no change in P_{AW} or P_{PA}. With HCl alone, P_{AW} increased immediately and continued to rise for the rest of the hour reaching five times basal value. Mean P_{PA} increased by 68%, and the wet/dry lung weight ratio increased by 74% (from 6.91 to 12.05).

In the VIP-pretreated group the P_{AW} was attenuated by 79% ($p < 0.01$), the P_{PA} initially increased by 16% but then returned back to basal value within 30 minutes ($p < 0.01$) (FIG. 1), and the lung wet/dry weight ratio was attenuated by 52% ($p = 0.004$) (FIG. 2).

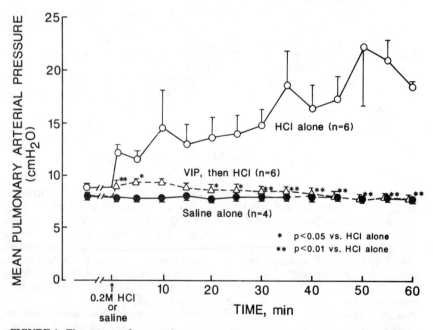

FIGURE 1. Time course of mean pulmonary arterial pressure after intratracheal instillation of 2 ml/kg physiological saline or of 2 ml/kg 0.2 M HCl, with or without pretreatment with VIP (1 $\mu g/kg$ body wt·min^{-1}). Values are means ± SEM. Pretreatment with VIP prevented the increase in pulmonary artery pressure caused by HCl injection (*$p < 0.05$, **p 0.01).

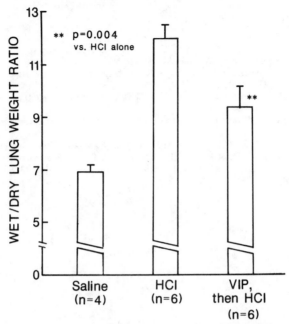

FIGURE 2. Wet/dry (W/D) lung weight ratio after intratracheal administration of 2 ml/kg physiological saline or of 2 ml/kg 0.2 M HCl, with or without pretreatment with VIP (1 μg/kg body wt·min^{-1}). Values are means ± SEM. VIP attenuated the increase in W/D due to acid injury by 52% (**$p = 0.004$).

Pulmonary levels of cAMP were decreased by 34% with acid only. This decrease was reversed with pretreatment with VIP ($p < 0.05$).

CONCLUSIONS

These experiments demonstrate that VIP protects against HCl-induced pulmonary edema, pulmonary hypertension, and increased airway pressure in perfused rat lungs. The mechanism(s) of this protective effect of VIP are uncertain but may include the stimulation of cyclic AMP production in the lung and the induction of vasodilation. Vasodilation alone is unlikely to be the principal mechanism as at least some pulmonary vasodilators, such as sodium nitroprusside, do not protect against injury.[5] Another means by which VIP may protect the lung is by inhibiting the release of mediators of injury; VIP has been found to inhibit mast cell degranulation[6] and PAF-induced release of leukotrienes.[7]

The above observations suggest that VIP may be useful in the prevention and management of acute, diffuse lung injury.

REFERENCES

1. SAID, S. I. 1985. *In* The Pulmonary Circulation and Acute Lung Injury. S. I. Said, Ed.: 3-10. Futura Publishing Co., Inc. Mt. Kisco, NY.
2. MIZUS, I., W. SUMMER, I. FRANKLIN, J. R. MICHAEL & G. H. GURTNER. 1985. Am. Rev. Respir. Dis. **131:** 256-259.
3. TOKIOKA, H., O. KOBYASHI, Y. OHTA, J. WAKABAYASHI & F. KOSAKA. 1985. Intensive Care Med. **11:** 61-64.
4. BROOKER, G., J. F. HARPER, W. L. TERASAKI & R. D. MOLAN. 1979. Adv. Cyclic Nucleotide Res. **10:** 1-34.
5. BROTZ, P. J., T. J. K. TOUNG, S. PEMUTT & J. L. CAMERON. 1983. Surgery **94:** 95-99.
6. UNDEM, B. J., E. C. DICK & C. K. BUCKNER. 1983. Eur. J. Pharmacol. **88:** 247-249.
7. DI MARZO, V., J. R. TIPPINS & H. R. MORRIS. 1986. Biochem. Int. **13:** 933-942.

Release of Vasoactive Intestinal Peptide during Hyperdynamic Sepsis in Conscious, Awake Dogs

MICHELE FUORTES, MARION A. BLANK,
THOMAS W. POLLOCK, BEVERLY A. PAZUR,
MARVIN A. McMILLEN, BERNARD M. JAFFE, AND
THOMAS M. SCALEA

Department of Surgery
SUNY Health Science Center at Brooklyn
Brooklyn, New York 11203

Vasoactive intestinal peptide (VIP) is known to be a potent vasodilator and hypotensive peptide[1] and has been reported previously to be a likely mediator during hypodynamic septic shock in anesthetized animals.[2,3] These studies showed a release of VIP after infusion of endotoxin, but this way of inducing sepsis caused a sharp drop in blood pressure. Other authors have shown a release of VIP from the gut after intestinal ischemia.[4] It is possible, therefore, that VIP secretion is just a secondary response of the gut to hypoperfusion and does not play a primary role in the hemodynamics of septic shock. In this study we investigated the release of VIP in awake, conscious dogs in a model of sepsis that is hyperdynamic, *not* hypotensive, similar to the pattern of sepsis seen in humans.

METHODS

Under general anesthesia (pentobarbital 30 mg/kg and halothane 0.5%) a Swan-Ganz catheter was placed in the pulmonary artery and an arterial catheter was placed in the aorta via the carotid artery in nine mongrel dogs (17.6 ± 3.7 kg). Following 48 hours of recovery and with the animals awake, basal hemodynamic measurements (systemic and pulmonary blood pressure, heart rate, cardiac output) were taken and blood samples from the pulmonary artery and aorta collected for radioimmunoassay for VIP. Sepsis was then induced by implanting an intraperitoneal fibrin clot (fibrinogen 0.5%, thrombin 1000 U), containing live *E. coli* (0.9×10^9 organisms/kg body weight). All measurements and blood samples were taken every day for five days. Blood samples were collected into tubes containing aprotinin, centrifuged, and the plasma decanted and stored at $-20°C$ until radioimmunoassay for VIP.[5] The VIP-like immunoreactivity in the plasma was characterized by chromatography on Sephadex G-50 superfine gel.

RESULTS

Twenty-four hours after induction of sepsis all dogs showed significantly increased heart rate (HR), cardiac index (CI), and decreased peripheral vascular resistances (SVRI), but no change in mean arterial pressure (MAP); all blood cultures were positive for *E. coli*. Pulmonary arterial VIP concentration was significantly increased from 3.6 ± 0.4 pmol/l to 7.6 ± 2.1 pmol/l (TABLE 1). The significant increase in pulmonary arterial VIP concentration noted 24 hours following induction of sepsis was no longer present after 48 hours although HR and CI remained significantly elevated and SVRI significantly decreased.

TABLE 1. Concentrations of VIP and Hemodynamic Parameters during Hyperdynamic Sepsis

	HR (beats/min)	MAP (mmHg)	CI (1/min/m²)	SVRI (dyne·sec/cm⁵·m²)	VIP (pmol/l) (pulm. artery)	VIP (pmol/l) (aorta)
Basal	98 ± 7	106.2 ± 2.3	4.6 ± 0.2	1,779 ± 86	3.6 ± 0.4	3.7 ± 0.4
Day 1	123 ± 5[b]	96.7 ± 4.3	6.8 ± 0.5[b]	1,115 ± 111[c]	7.6 ± 2.1[b]	6.7 ± 2.2
Day 2	112 ± 5	100.8 ± 5.1	5.1 ± 0.3[b]	1,515 ± 85[b]	5.3 ± 1.1	4.7 ± 0.9
Day 3	112 ± 5	95.0 ± 2.7	5.6 ± 0.4[b]	1,339 ± 97[b]	4.7 ± 0.6	4.7 ± 0.6
Day 4	111 ± 5	101.5 ± 3.7	5.3 ± 0.1[b]	1,467 ± 80[b]	5.1 ± 1.0	4.5 ± 0.9
Day 5	109 ± 6	104.9 ± 3.5	5.4 ± 0.5	1,503 ± 132	5.0 ± 1.4	5.2 ± 1.9

[a] Results expressed as mean ± SE.
[b] $p < 0.05$ versus basal, Student's *t*-test, Bonferroni method.
[c] $p < 0.01$ versus basal, Student's *t*-test, Bonferroni method.

CONCLUSION

Our results show that during the first 24 hours of sepsis VIP was released without a concomitant drop in blood pressure. This suggests that during septic shock VIP is released not because of hypotension, but by a direct mechanism, although redistribution of splanchnic blood flow is still a possibility. More difficult is to establish whether VIP is the major mediator of the low SVRI in sepsis, or just one of a group of mediators. The hypothesis that it plays a major role as a vasodilator and is responsible for the drop in vascular resistance is contradicted in our experiments by the finding that vascular resistance remains significantly lower at days two and three while VIP has already returned to basal levels. Therefore VIP may be an early mediator in the onset of hyperdynamic sepsis, but other mediators are likely to be responsible for maintenance of the septic state.

REFERENCES

1. SAID, S. I. & V. MUTT. 1970. Potent peripheral and splanchnic vasodilator peptide from normal gut. Nature **225:** 863-864.
2. REVHAUG, A., I. LYGREN, T. I. LUNDGREN, O. K. ANDERSON, P. G. BURHOL & K. E. GIERCKSKY. 1985. Increased plasma levels of vasoactive intestinal peptide in pigs during endotoxinaemia. Eur. Surg. Res. **17:** 75-82.
3. FREUND, H., A. M. EBEID & J. E. FISCHER. 1981. An increase of vasoactive intestinal peptide levels in canine endotoxin shock. Surg. Gynecol. Obstet. **152:** 604-606.
4. MODLIN, I. M., S. R. BLOOM & S. MITCHELL. 1978. Plasma vasoactive intestinal polypeptide (VIP) levels and intestinal ischaemia. Experientia **34:** 535-536.
5. MITCHELL, S. J. & S. R. BLOOM. 1978. Measurement of fasting and postprandial VIP in man. Gut **19:** 1043-1048.

Vasoactive Intestinal Peptide Stimulation of Feline Renal Adenylate Cyclase

Inhibitory Effects of (4Cl-D-Phe⁶, Leu¹⁷)VIP[a]

NINA M. GRIFFITHS,[b] J. RIVIER,[c] AND
N. L. SIMMONS[b]

[b]Department of Physiological Sciences
The Medical School
Framlington Place
Newcastle upon Tyne, United Kingdom NE2 4HH

[c]Peptide Biology Laboratory
Salk Institute
San Diego, California 92138

Vasoactive intestinal peptide (VIP) has been shown to influence renin release and promote Na output.[1,2] VIP regulation of glomerular and tubular cell function is most likely to be mediated by stimulation of adenylate cyclase (AC) activity.[3] Recently, a selective, competitive peptide antagonist[4] of VIP, which does not inhibit the actions of related agonists on secretin, GRF, or glucagon receptors, has been introduced. This has allowed the confirmation of specific physiological responses to VIP mediated by VIP receptors coupled to adenylate cyclase in several cell types.[4] In order to demonstrate that VIP may have specific physiological actions in renal tissue, rather than pharmacological actions via related receptors, we have examined the effect of (4Cl-D-Phe⁶,Leu¹⁷)VIP upon agonist-stimulated AC activity in plasma membranes isolated from feline cortical and medullary tissue.

VIP ($1\mu M$) typically stimulated AC activity 4.1 ± 0.23 (SD, $n = 3$) and 3.1 ± 1.2 (SD, $n = 3$) -fold over basal levels in feline cortical and medullary membranes, respectively. Feline material gave the largest quantitative response to VIP compared with other species examined (guinea pig, rabbit, mouse, and rat). That VIP is capable of stimulating medullary AC is indicative that VIP-responsive elements are not confined to glomeruli. Related hormones to VIP, PHI, glucagon, and secretin all increased AC activity, but to a lesser degree than VIP (FIG. 1). Half-maximal stimulation (EC_{50}) of AC by VIP was 9.1 ± 5.8 nM (SD, $n = 3$), comparable to AC stimulation in intestinal enterocyte plasma membranes,[5] while that for glucagon (15 ± 3.5 nM, SD, $n = 3$) was similar to that observed in isolated microdissected rat nephron tubule segments.[6] Secretin and PHI were less effective in stimulating AC activity with EC_{50}

[a]This work was supported by the National Kidney Fund (U.K.). The Physiological Society (U.K.) and the Wellcome Trust provided further financial assistance to NMG.

values of 25 and 63 nM, respectively. The antagonist, (4Cl-D-Phe^6,Leu^{17})VIP had no agonist activity up to 10 μM (FIG. 1).

When tested at 10 μM, (4Cl-D-Phe^6, Leu^{17})VIP effectively antagonized the action of VIP on AC shown by a shift in the dose-response curve to the right and an increase in the apparent EC$_{50}$ to 91 ± 26 nM (FIG. 2). A similar right-shift was observed with PHI. (4Cl-D-Phe^6,Leu^{17})VIP was without significant effect on the glucagon or secretin EC$_{50}$ values. Similar data was obtained for plasma membranes derived from outer (red) medulla (not shown).

This data is consistent with the existence of a specific VIP stimulation of AC in feline renal plasma membranes. PHI is also capable of stimulating AC activity via the VIP receptor but is of lower affinity.

Glucagon and secretin stimulation of AC activity is distinct from that mediated by VIP. Whether glucagon and secretin stimulation of AC activity is via a common receptor is not known.

ACKNOWLEDGMENTS

We are grateful to Professor Mutt for kindly donating the VIP and PHI.

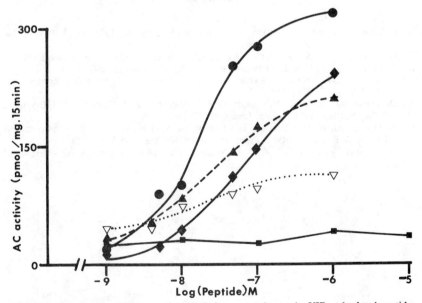

FIGURE 1. Stimulation of feline renal cortical plasma membranes by VIP and related peptides. (●) VIP, (◆) PHI, (▲) glucagon, (▽) secretin, (■) (4Cl-D-Phe^6, Leu^{17})VIP. Data from a single representative preparation. Each data point was determined in triplicate, duplicate samples for each replicate being assayed for cAMP. Feline plasma membranes were prepared according to the method of Boumendil-Podevin and Podevin.[7] Cortical and red medullary tissue was dissected from decapsulated kidneys. Homogenization was in sucrose Tris-Hepes pH 7.4 containing PMSF and EDTA. Plasma membranes were then prepared by differential centrifugation and stored at −90°C until used. AC activity was measured as previously described.[3]

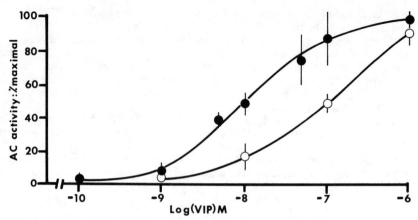

FIGURE 2. Effect of (4Cl-D-Phe⁶,Leu¹⁷)VIP on VIP-stimulated AC. (●) VIP alone, (○) VIP plus 10 μM (4Cl-D-Phe⁶,Leu¹⁷)VIP. Details as in FIGURE 1.

REFERENCES

1. PORTER, J. P., T. N. THRASHER, S. I. SAID & W. F. GANONG. 1985. Am. J. Physiol. **246:** F84-89.
2. ROSA, R. M., P. SILVA, J. S. STOFF & F. H. EPSTEIN. 1985. Am. J. Physiol. **249:** E494-497.
3. GRIFFITHS, N. M. & N. L. SIMMONS. 1987. J. Physiol. (London) **387:** 1-17.
4. PANDOL, S. J., K. DHARMSATHAPHORN, M. S. SCHOEFFIELD, W. VALE & J. RIVIER. 1986. Am. J. Physiol. **250:** G553-557.
5. DHARMSATHAPHORN, K., V. HARMS, D. J. YAMASHIRO, R. J. HUGHES, H. J. BINDER & E. M. WRIGHT. 1983. J. Clin. Invest. **71:** 27-35.
6. BAILLY, C., M. IMBERT-TEBOUL, D. CHABARDES, A. HUS-CITHAREL, M. MONTEGUT, A. CLIQUE & F. MOREL. 1980. Proc. Natl. Acad. Sci. USA **77:** 3422-3424.
7. BOUMENDIL-PODEVIN, E. F. & R. A. PODEVIN. 1983. Biochim. Biophys. Acta **735:** 86-94.

Vasoactive Intestinal Peptide-Containing Nerve Fibers in Bone and Periosteum May Be Adrenergic

ESTHER L. HILL AND ROBERT ELDE

Department of Cell Biology and Neuroanatomy
University of Minnesota
Minneapolis, Minnesota 55455

Vasoactive intestinal peptide (VIP) increases bone resorption *in vitro*[1] and VIP receptors have been characterized in an osteoblastic cell line.[2] VIP-immunoreactive nerve fibers have been demonstrated in bone and periosteum of several species, suggesting a possible role for VIP in neuronal regulation of bone metabolism. In pig, VIP-immunoreactive fibers innervating bone and periosteum originate from cell bodies in sympathetic chain ganglia.[3] The distribution of VIP in sympathetic postganglionic cells and whether these VIP-immunoreactive cells are adrenergic, cholinergic, or neither is unknown.

In contrast, calcitonin gene-related peptide (CGRP) has been shown to inhibit bone resorption *in vitro*[4,5] and, at high doses, to reduce plasma calcium levels *in vivo*.[5] This peptide, like VIP, circulates at levels too low to evoke hormonal responses from bone. Since nerve fibers may release high concentrations of neuropeptides into small tissue areas, we sought to determine if CGRP fibers, like VIP fibers, exist in bone and periosteum.

This study attempted to (1) establish the extent of VIP-containing cell bodies and fibers in the sympathetic chain of the pig, (2) determine the possible coexistence of VIP and dopamine-β-hydroxylase (DβH, an adrenergic marker), and (3) demonstrate VIP- and CGRP-immunoreactive fibers in rat periosteum.

Four- to eight-week-old pigs were perfused with Zamboni's fixative. Alternate serial cryostat sections of cervical and paravertebral sympathetic ganglia at all levels and immersion-fixed periosteum from fresh 200-g rat long and flat bones were incubated in primary rabbit antisera directed against VIP or DβH. Whole mounts were also incubated in a rabbit antiserum directed against CGRP. Tissue was then incubated with FITC-labeled goat anti-rabbit IgG and photographed on a fluorescence microscope.

VIP-immunoreactive cells were most evident in thoracic sympathetic chain ganglia, with some cells in cervicothoracic and lumbar ganglia. VIP-immunoreactive fibers occurred in all ganglia and in both interganglionic connectives and rami. The density of immunoreactive fibers varied from infrequent fibers in vertebral and lumbar ganglia to dense networks in stellate and thoracic ganglia. The majority of neurons throughout the sympathetic chain were DβH-immunoreactive, but with varying intensities. In several cells in thoracic ganglia, it was possible to demonstrate the coexistence of VIP- and DβH-immunoreactivity in the same cell body (FIG. 1). Coexistence occurred preferentially in cells DβH-immunostained at moderate intensity. VIP- and CGRP-immunoreactive fibers were found in rat periosteum (FIG. 2). The extent, origin, and possible role of these fibers in focal bone remodeling is presently under investigation, as is the possibility that norepinephrine acts synergistically with VIP upon bone cells.

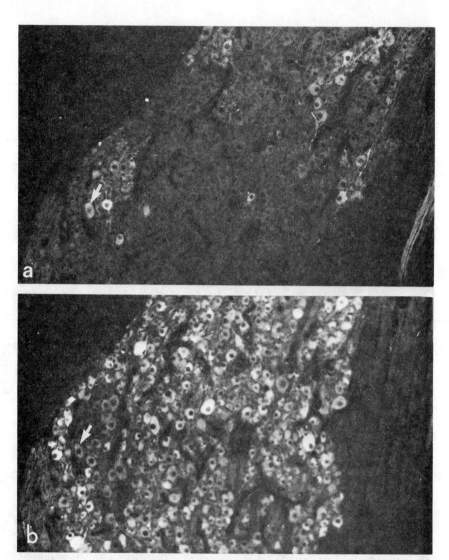

FIGURE 1. Immunofluorescence micrographs of adjacent 4-μ sections of midthoracic chain ganglia of pig stained for VIP (a) or DβH (b). VIP staining occurs in small clusters of cells, while DβH immunoreactivity can be seen in the majority of principal ganglion cells. Note that DβH immunoreactivity occurs at varying intensities. Arrows indicate a cell moderately DβH-immunostained in which coexistence of VIP- and DβH-immunoreactivity can be seen.

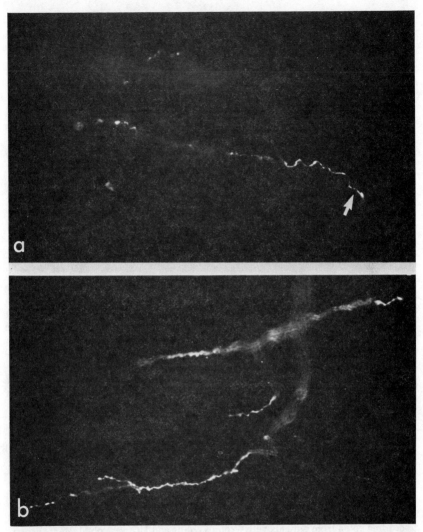

FIGURE 2. Immunofluorescence micrographs of rat periosteal whole mounts. In (a) a VIP-immunoreactive fiber in mandibular periosteum can be seen. Arrow indicates collateral of perivascular fiber that extends into periosteal tissue. Fibers in (b), from tibia periosteum, are CGRP-immunoreactive.

REFERENCES

1. HOHMANN, E. L., L. LEVINE & A. H. TASHJIAN, JR. 1983. Endocrinology **112:** 1233-1237.
2. HOHMANN, E. L. & A. H. TASHJIAN, JR. 1984. Endocrinology **114:** 1321-1325.
3. HOHMANN, E. L., R. P. ELDE, J. A. RYSAVY, S. EINZIG & R. L. GEBHARD. 1986. Science **232:** 868-871.
4. D'SOUZA, S. M., I. MACINTYRE, S. I. GIRGIS & G. R. MUNDY. 1986. Endocrinology **119:** 58-61.
5. ROOS, B. A., J. A. FISCHER, W. PIGNAT, C. B. ALANDER & L. G. RAISZ. 1986. Endocrinology **118:** 46-51.

Colonic Vasoactive Intestinal Peptide-Containing Nerves in Crohn's Disease and Ulcerative Colitis[a]

TIMOTHY R. KOCH,[b] LISA GO, J. AIDAN CARNEY,
AND VAY LIANG W. GO

Gastroenterology Unit and Department of Pathology
Mayo Clinic and Foundation
Rochester, Minnesota 55905

Morphological studies of Crohn's disease have described neural abnormalities in the bowel that include irregular, tortuous nerve bundles (termed "neuromatous lesions"[1]) and autonomic nerve axonal necrosis and proliferation.[2] Studies of vasoactive intestinal peptide (VIP) in ulcerative colitis (UC) and Crohn's disease are of interest because of the proposed regulatory function of VIP on mucosal secretion,[3] smooth muscle relaxation,[4] and proliferation of and immunoglobulin synthesis by lymphocytes.[5] Hyperplasia of VIP-containing colonic nerves has been previously purported to be evidence for the diagnosis of Crohn's disease.[6] In this study, colonic concentrations of VIP were determined by radioimmunoassay and VIP-containing neural structures in UC and Crohn's colitis were examined by immunocytochemistry.

METHODS

Permission for human studies was granted by the Mayo Clinic Institutional Review Board on December 6, 1984. Grossly and histologically normal descending colon and descending colon from patients with Crohn's colitis and UC were obtained at surgery. The mucosal-submucosal layer was removed by microdissection; VIP was extracted into 0.1 N HCl, followed by neutralization and specific radioimmunoassay.[7] Small transmural sections from each colonic specimen were incubated for 20 hours at 4°C in Zamboni's fixative.[8] Following processing, sections were immunostained for VIP by the indirect immunoperoxidase method of Nakane, using rabbit antibody 4823.[7] Immunoreactivity was extinguished by preadsorption of antibody 4823 with porcine VIP.

[a]Supported by a research award in clinical gastroenterology from the American College of Gastroenterology. T. R. K. is recipient of a Career Development Award from the National Foundation for Ileitis & Colitis.

[b]Address for correspondence: Timothy R. Koch, M.D., Department of Physiology, Guggenheim 801, Mayo Clinic, Rochester, MN 55905.

RESULTS

In both ascending colon and descending colon, concentrations of immunoreactive VIP were significantly decreased in the mucosal-submucosal layer from Crohn's colitis and UC compared to normal colon (FIG. 1). Concentrations of VIP were lowest in patients with UC (FIG. 1).

In the mucosal-submucosal layer of normal colon ($n = 6$), immunoreactive VIP

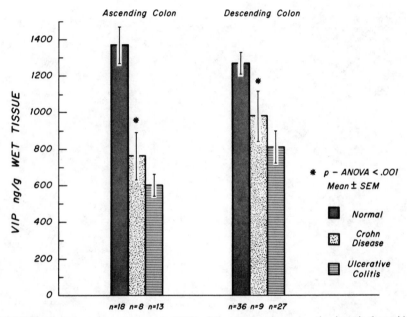

FIGURE 1. Concentrations (mean ± SEM) of immunoreactive vasoactive intestinal peptide (VIP) determined by radioimmunoassay in the mucosal-submucosal layer of human colon. Significantly decreased mean concentrations of VIP were found in Crohn's colitis and ulcerative colitis in both the ascending colon and the descending colon compared to histologically normal colon (one-way analysis of variance: p-ANOVA < 0.001).

was localized within nerve cell bodies in the submucosal plexus and within nerve fibers in the lamina propria mucosae, the muscularis mucosae, and the submucosa. In the mucosal-submucosal layer of colon from patients with Crohn's colitis ($n = 7$) and UC ($n = 7$), immunoreactive VIP was again localized within submucosal nerve cell bodies (FIG. 2). By contrast, VIP was identified within the muscularis mucosae in only one patient with Crohn's colitis and in no patients with UC, and within the lamina propria mucosae in four patients with Crohn's colitis and in five patients with UC. However, immunoreactive VIP was identified within submucosal neuromatous lesions in four patients with Crohn's colitis and in three patients with UC (FIG 2).

SUMMARY

Decreased mucosal-submucosal VIP in patients with Crohn's colitis and UC was associated with diminished staining of VIP-containing nerve fibers in the lamina propria mucosae and the muscularis mucosae. The localization of VIP within neuromatous lesions suggests that secondary regeneration of VIPergic nerves occurs in Crohn's colitis and UC. Abnormalities of VIP-containing nerves that were diagnostic of Crohn's disease were not identified. Alteration of VIP-containing nerves in Crohn's colitis and UC may contribute to the pathophysiology of these colonic diseases.

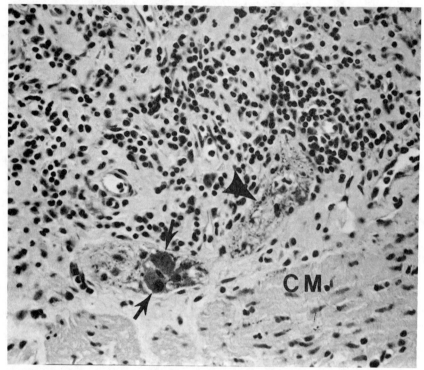

FIGURE 2. Immunoreactive vasoactive intestinal peptide (VIP) in descending colon from a patient with Crohn's colitis localized by an indirect immunoperoxidase stain. The large arrowhead demonstrates immunoreactive VIP within a submucosal neuromatous lesion. The small arrows demonstrate immunoreactive VIP within the cytoplasm of submucosal nerve cell bodies. CM: circular smooth muscle layer (magnification × 400).

REFERENCES

1. ANTONIUS, J. I., F. E. GUMP, R. LATTES & M. LEPORE. 1960. Gastroenterology **38:** 889-905.
2. DVORAK, A. M., J. E. OSAGE, R. A. MONAHAN & G. R. DICKERSIN. 1980. Human Pathol. **11:** 620-634.

3. BOIGE, N., A. MUNCK & M. LABURTHE. 1984. Peptides **5:** 379-383.
4. COUTURE, R., J. MIZRAHI, D. REGOLI & G. DEVROEDE. 1981. Can. J. Physiol. Pharmacol. **59:** 957-964.
5. STANISZ, A. M., D. BEFUS & J. BIENENSTOCK. 1986. J. Immunol. **136:** 152-156.
6. O'MORAIN, C., A. E. BISHOP, G. P. MCGREGOR, A. J. LEVI, S. R. BLOOM, J. M. POLAK & T. J. PETERS. 1984. Gut **25:** 57-61.
7. YAKSH, T. L., E. O. ABAY, II & V. L. W. GO. 1982. Brain Res. **242:** 279-290.
8. STEFANINI, M., C. DEMARTINO & L. ZAMBONI. 1967. Nature **216:** 173-174.

Analgesia Produced by Vasoactive Intestinal Peptide Administered Directly to the Spinal Cord in Rats[a]

BARRY R. KOMISARUK, CYNTHIA BANAS,
STEPHEN B. HELLER, BEVERLY WHIPPLE,
GUY F. BARBATO, AND FRANK JORDAN

Institute of Animal Behavior and Department of Chemistry
Rutgers-the State University of New Jersey
Newark, New Jersey 07102

This laboratory has identified and characterized a specific sensory stimulus that produces a powerful suppression of sensory and motor responses to noxious stimulation in rats and humans.[1-3] Vaginal mechano-stimulation (VS) totally blocks withdrawal reflex responses to intense noxious (foot pinch or radiant heat) stimulation,[4] differentially blocks the response of single neurons in the somatosensory thalamus to noxious (pinch) stimulation but not to innocuous (brushing the fur) stimulation,[1] and elevates pain thresholds but not tactile thresholds in women.[2] This is evidence that VS produces analgesia, not anesthesia. VS increases firing rate activity in the pelvic nerve[5] and the VS effect in rats persists after complete spinal transection.[4] The neuropeptide vasoactive intestinal peptide (VIP) is present in the pelvic nerve dorsal root ganglion[6] and is concentrated in the spinal cord sites of the primary sensory terminals of the pelvic nerve.[7-10] This evidence led us to hypothesize that in response to VS, VIP is released from pelvic nerve terminals into the spinal cord and there triggers analgesia. To test this hypothesis, we administered VIP directly to the spinal cord and measured its effect on pain thresholds in rats. In a second experiment, we determined whether or not the effect of VIP is opiate-mediated by pretreating the rats with naloxone. Naloxone-independent analgesia produced by administration of VIP to the periaqueductal gray has been reported.[11]

METHODS

Rats were ovariectomized and prepared at least one week before testing with a PE10 intrathecal (i.t.) catheter inserted to the lumbar level of the spinal cord. In the first experiment VIP (5 µg, 500 ng, 250 ng, 50 ng, or 0) dissolved in 5 µl saline was

[a]This study was supported by Public Health Service Grant NS 22948-01 (to BRK) and funds from the Charles and Johanna Busch Foundation, Rutgers University. This is publication number 482 from the Institute of Animal Behavior.

injected i.t. ($n = 10$ rats/group). Two measures of analgesia were used: first, tail flick latency (TFL) to radiant heat was determined immediately and at five-minute intervals up to 30 minutes post-i.t. injection. All animals also received a baseline TFL test immediately before the drug injection. In the second experiment, VIP (5 µg or 2.5 µg) dissolved in 5 µl saline was injected in combination with naloxone (10 mg/kg i.p., 30 min before VIP) or saline, i.p. Controls received saline i.t. or naloxone i.p. only ($n = 11$/group in each of these six groups). TFL was determined in the same sequence as in Experiment 1. Second, vocalization threshold to tail shock was determined, by using an ascending/descending method of limits (stimulation parameters: 100-msec trains of 60-Hz square waves at three-second intervals ranging from 0.01 to 0.3 mA using a Coulbourn computer-controlled constant current stimulator). Electrodes were blunt 18-ga SS needles coated with electrode gel and taped to the midsection of the tail 2 cm apart. The advantage of this test over TFL is that the motor apparatus utilized in the vocalization response (lower brain stem) is more remote from the site of i.t. drug administration (lumbar region) than in the case of the TFL test. Consequently, after i.t. drug administration, an increase in vocalization threshold is probably a more valid indicator of antinociception or analgesia than is an elevation of TFL, since the former is less likely to be confounded by possible motor effects of the drug. Data were analyzed using ANOVA with subsequent paired comparisons tests.

RESULTS

Experiment 1: Effect of VIP on Tail Flick Latency

VIP (5 µg) significantly increased tail flick latency (TFL) by more than 120% over preinjection baseline TFL within three minutes postinjection (FIG. 1). Significant elevation of TFL persisted for 10 minutes. At lower doses (500 ng and 250 ng), significant TFL elevation was observed that was of lower magnitude and shorter duration (FIG. 1). At the lowest dose tested (50 ng) and in the saline control group, no significant TFL elevation was observed.

Experiment 2: Effect of VIP + Naloxone on Tail Flick Latency and Vocalization Threshold

Naloxone HCl (10 mg/kg) was injected i.p. 30 minutes before i.t. injection of VIP (5 µg or 2.5 µg). Control groups received only saline, naloxone, or VIP alone at these doses. The VIP (5 µg and 2.5 µg) groups showed TFLs that were significantly greater (60-62% above baseline) than those in the saline or naloxone-only groups (1-6% above baseline) within three minutes postinjection. The naloxone + VIP groups (TFLs 18-49% greater than baseline) did not differ significantly from the VIP-only groups. TFL in the VIP (5 µg, but not 2.5 µg) + naloxone group was significantly greater than TFL in the saline group. At 15 and 20 minutes the VIP 5 µg group was significantly higher than the saline group (FIG. 2a).

In a second nociceptive threshold test, VIP (5 μg) significantly elevated vocalization threshold to tail shock at 3-10 minutes and 20 minutes post-i.t. injection (FIG. 2b). At 5 and 10 minutes the VIP 5 μg group was also significantly elevated over the VIP (5 μg) + naloxone group.

CONCLUSIONS

1. Spinal administration of VIP produces analgesia as measured by TFL and tail shock-induced vocalization tests.

2. VIP may produce analgesia by an action on both opioid and nonopioid-modulated pain pathways since naloxone was more effective in antagonizing the analgesic effect of VIP on the vocalization threshold test than on the TFL test.

3. It may be speculated that vaginal stimulation normally releases VIP from terminals of the pelvic nerve into the spinal cord, where the VIP triggers an analgesia-producing mechanism.

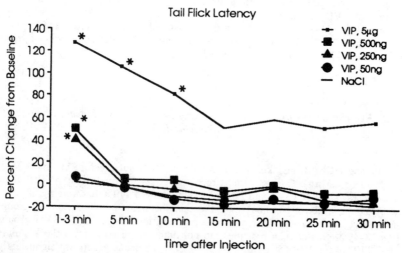

FIGURE 1. Intrathecal administration of VIP increases tail flick latency. *Compared to the saline group, $p < 0.05$ Duncan test.

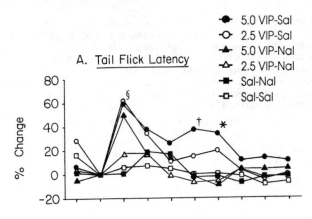

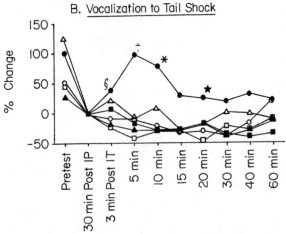

FIGURE 2. (**A**) Effect of naloxone on VIP-induced increase in tail flick latency. §VIP 5.0, 2.5 > □■ ($p < 0.05$, Duncan test). †VIP 5.0 > □ ($p < 0.05$, Duncan test). *VIP 5.0 > □ ($p < 0.05$, t-test).

(**B**) Effect of naloxone on VIP-induced elevation of vocalization threshold. 5.0 VIP greater than: §□ only ($p < 0.05$, t-test); †all group ($p < 0.05$, Duncan test); *all groups except △ ($p < 0.05$, Duncan test); ★□△○ ($p < 0.05$, Duncan test).

REFERENCES

1. KOMISARUK, B. R. & J. WALLMAN. 1977. Brain Res. **137:** 85-107.
2. WHIPPLE, B. & B. R. KOMISARUK. 1985. Pain **21:** 357-367.
3. KOMISARUK, B. R. & B. WHIPPLE. 1986. Ann. N.Y. Acad. Sci. **476:** 30-39.

4. KOMISARUK, B. & K. LARSSON. 1971. Brain Res. **35:** 231-235.
5. PETERS, L. C., M. B. KRISTAL & B. R. KOMISARUK. 1987. Brain Res. **408:** 199-204.
6. KAWATANI, M., J. NAGEL & W. C. DE GROAT. 1986. J. Comp. Neurol. **249:** 117-132.
7. BASBAUM, A. I. & E. J. GLAZER. 1983. Somatosensory Res. **1:** 69-82.
8. NADELHAFT, I. 1983. Soc. Neurosci. Abstr. **9:** 293.
9. MORGAN, C., I. NADELHAFT & W. C. DE GROAT. 1981. J. Comp. Neurol. **201:** 415-440.
10. ANAND, P., S. J. GIBSON, G. P. MCGREGOR, M. A. BLANK, M. A. GHATEI, A. J. BACARESE-HAMILTON, J. M. POLAK & S. R. BLOOM. 1983. Nature **305:** 143-145.
11. SULLIVAN, T. L. & A. PERT. 1981. Soc. Neurosci. Abstr. **7:** 504.

Production of Biologically Active Secretin in *E. coli*

H. OLSSON,[a] P. LIND,[a] C. HENRICHSON,[a]
B. ÖSTERLÖF,[a] G. POHL,[a] G. KLEIN,[b] H. JÖRNVALL,[c]
V. MUTT,[c] M. UHLÈN,[d] AND M. LAKE[a]

[a]*KabiGen AB*
S-112 87 Stockholm, Sweden
[b]*Skandigen AB*
S-111 43 Stockholm, Sweden
[c]*Karolinska Institutet*
S-104 01 Stockholm, Sweden
[d]*Royal Institute of Technology*
S-100 44 Stockholm, Sweden

Secretin is a peptide hormone 27 amino acids in length and amidated in the carboxy terminus. It is produced in the intestinal mucosa, and its main action is the stimulation of the secretion of the pancreas. The complete amino acid sequence of human secretin has recently been determined,[1] and a precursor to porcine secretin has been identified.[2] It is extended with the three amino acids Gly-Lys-Arg at the carboxy terminus and exhibits a biological activity comparable to the amidated form.[2] The enzyme systems for amidation are not present in *E. coli,* so we have circumvented the amidation by extending the carboxy-terminal end of human secretin with the three amino acids Gly-Lys-Arg. A gene for human secretin extended with Gly-Lys-Arg was designed based on the determined amino acid sequence[1] and the codon usage of *E. coli.* The synthetic gene was cloned into the expression vector with the codon for methionine between the fusion partner and the secretin (FIG. 1). The methionine made it possible to cleave the fusion protein with CNBr, giving active secretin.

    E. coli strain RW308 was transformed with the expression vector and secretin was produced and secreted into the medium as a fusion protein where the fusion partner (fragment ZZ) was a synthetic IgG binding fragment (FIG. 1). After fermentation the medium was filtered and an IgG affinity chromotography step was carried out. The fusion protein was freeze dried, dissolved in formic acid, and cleaved with CNBr. The IgG portion was removed by a second IgG affinity chromotography step. The secretin was further purified by gel filtration and reversed-phase HPLC.

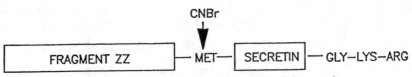

FIGURE 1. Schematic representation of the fusion protein.

The purity of the secretin peak from HPLC was analyzed by amino acid analysis and the results confirmed that the composition of the precursor secretin was in accordance with the desired composition. The biological activity of the produced variant of secretin was compared to extracted porcine secretin in a cat model.[3] The pancreas of the cat was dissected *in situ*. Samples and references were injected into the bloodstream and the secretion from the pancreas was collected. The volume was determined and the secrete was analyzed for alkali content.[3]

The data (FIG. 2) showed that precursor secretin exhibits biological activity. The activity of human "precursor" secretin was at least 80% of the activity of porcine secretin.

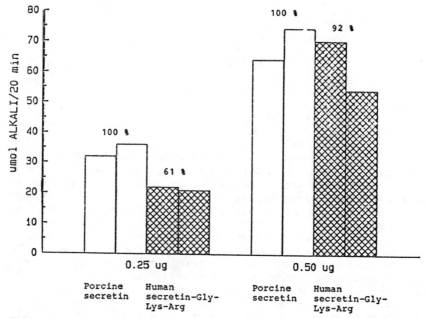

FIGURE 2. Comparison of the biological activity between porcine secretin and human Gly-Lys-Arg extended secretin analyzed in cat.

REFERENCES

1. CARLQVIST, M., H. JÖRNVALL, G. FORSSMAN, L. THULIN, C. JOHANSSON & V. MUTT. 1985. Human secretin is not identical to the porcine/bovine hormone. IRCS Med. Sci. **13:** 217-218.
2. GAFVELIN, G., M. CARLQVIST & V. MUTT. 1985. A proform of secretin with high secretin-like bioactivity. FEBS Lett. **184.2:** 347-352.
3. JORPES, J. E. & V. MUTT. 1966. On the biological assay of secretin. The reference standard. Acta Physiol. Scand. **66:** 316-325.

Vasoactive Intestinal Peptide and Secretin Receptors in Rat Brain

Localization and Second Messenger Production[a]

TERRY W. MOODY, REINA GETZ,
ROBERT T. FREMEAU, JR., AND
MARGARET M. SHAFFER

Department of Biochemistry
The George Washington University School of Medicine and Health
Sciences
Washington, D.C. 20037

Vasoactive intestinal peptide (VIP), a 28 amino acid peptide, and secretin, a 27 amino acid peptide, may function as neuromodulators in the CNS. These peptides are structurally similar in that they share nine sequence homologies and eight of the nine are in the NH_2-terminal half of the peptide. In spite of these sequence similarities, two distinct central nervous system VIP[1,2] and secretin[3] receptors have been identified using brain homogenate. In particular, VIP receptors bind VIP with high and secretin with low affinity, whereas secretin receptors bind secretin with high affinity and VIP with low affinity. Here the regional distribution of VIP and secretin receptors and the effects of VIP and secretin on second messenger (cAMP) production were compared.

Receptors were localized using binding studies as described previously.[2,3] For secretin receptors, [^{125}I]secretin was radiolabeled and bound to rat brain homogenates using a centrifugation assay. For VIP receptors, [^{125}I]VIP was radiolabeled and bound to rat brain homogenate using a centrifugation assay as well as rat brain slices using *in vitro* autoradiographic techniques.[4] The density of secretin receptors was greatest in the cerebellum (8.7 fmol/mg protein); intermediate in the cortex, striatum, hippocampus, thalamus, and hypothalamus; and lowest in the midbrain and medulla pons. In contrast, using [^{125}I]VIP, the density of VIP receptors was high in the cortex, striatum, hippocampus, and thalamus but not the cerebellum or medulla pons. Thus the regional distribution of secretin and VIP receptors is different. Using *in vitro* autoradiographic techniques, high densities of VIP receptors were present in the dentate gyrus, pineal gland, supraoptic and suprachiasmatic nuclei, superficial gray layer of the superior colliculus, and the area postrema. Moderate grain densities were present in the olfactory bulb and tubercle, cerebral cortex, nucleus accumbens, caudate putamen, interstitial nucleus of the stria terminalis, paraventricular thalamic nucleus, medial amygdaloid nucleus, subiculum, and medial geniculate nucleus. Thus, VIP receptors are discretely distributed in the mammalian CNS.[4-6]

[a] This research is supported by National Science Foundation Grant BNS 8500552.

657

Previous studies indicated that VIP receptors are tightly coupled to the enzyme adenylate cyclase.[7-10] Here rat cortex slices were prepared and the cAMP levels determined by radioimmunoassay.[11] TABLE 1 shows that VIP and secretin, but not bombesin (10 μM), elevated the cAMP levels nine- and threefold relative to controls. Secretin$_{5-27}$ (25 μM) had no effect on the basal cAMP levels but reversed the cAMP increase caused by secretin but not VIP (TABLE 1). Because secretin$_{5-27}$ inhibits cAMP caused by secretin but not VIP, it may prefer secretin relative to VIP receptors. This was verified by binding assays where secretin$_{5-27}$ inhibited specific binding of [^{125}I]secretin but not [^{125}I]VIP. The K_i for secretin$_{5-27}$ binding to secretin receptors was 400 nM. Thus secretin$_{5-27}$ may function as a central secretin receptor antagonist.

In summary, both secretin and VIP receptors are present in the central nervous system and utilize the second messenger cAMP. The receptors are distinct, however, a conclusion that is based on their unique regional distribution and different binding pharmacology.

TABLE 1. Effects of Peptides on Cyclic AMP Production[a]

Peptide	cAMP Concentration (pmol/mg protein)
None	54 ± 4
VIP (10 μM)	471 ± 53
Secretin (10 μM)	155 ± 6
Bombesin (10 μM)	50 ± 5
Secretin$_{5-27}$ (25 μM)	49 ± 6
VIP + Secretin$_{5-27}$	514 ± 48
Secretin + Secretin$_{5-27}$	58 ± 7

[a] Rat frontal cortex was dissected and chopped into 230-μm slices. The slices were preincubated in Krebs-Ringer bicarbonate buffer at 37°C for 10 minutes and after changing the buffer two times, the brain slices (1 mg protein) were placed in Krebs-Ringer bicarbonate buffer that contained 10 mM theophylline. Peptides were then added and after a 20-minute incubation the reaction was stopped by boiling. An aliquot was removed and the cAMP determined by radioimmunoassay.[10] The mean value ± SD of six determinations is indicated.

REFERENCES

1. ROBBERECHT, P., P. DE NEEF, M. LAMMENS, M. DESCHODT-LANCKMAN & J. P. CHRISTOPHE. 1978. Eur. J. Biochem. 90: 147-154.
2. TAYLOR, D. P. & C. B. PERT. 1979. Proc. Natl. Acad. Sci. USA 76: 660-664.
3. FREMEAU, R. T., R. T. JENSEN, C. G. CHARLTON, R. L. MILLER, T. L. O'DONOHUE & T. W. MOODY. 1983. J. Neurosci. 3: 1620-1625.
4. SHAFFER, M. M. & T. W. MOODY. 1986. Peptides 7: 283-288.

5. BESSON, J. M., DUSSAILANT, J. C. MARIE, W. ROSTENE & G. ROSSELIN. 1984. Peptides
     5: 339-340.
6. DESOUZA, E. B., H. SEIFERT & M. J. KUHAR. 1985. Neuroci. Lett. **56:** 113-120.
7. DESCHODT-LANCKMAN, M., P. ROBBERECHT & J. P. CHRISTOPHE. 1977. FEBS Lett. **83:**
     76-80.
8. KERWIN, R. W., S. PAY, K. D. BHOOLA & C. J. PAYCOCK. 1980. J. Pharm. Pharmacol.
     32: 561-566.
9. QUICK, M., L. L. IVERSON & S. R. BLOOM. 1978. Biochem. Pharmacol. **27:** 2209-2213.
10. ETGEN, A. M. & E. T. BROWNING. 1983. J. Neurosci. **3:** 2487-2493.
11. FREMEAU, R. T., L. Y. KORMAN & T. W. MOODY. 1986. J. Neurochem. **46:** 1947-1955.

Design, Synthesis, and Analysis of Secondary Structure Based Vasoactive Intestinal Peptide Analogues

GARY F. MUSSO, THOMAS C. RYSKAMP,
SARASWATHI PATTHI, SALLY PROVOW, AND
GÖNÜL VELIÇELEBI

The Salk Institute Biotechnology/Industrial Associates, Inc.
La Jolla, California 92037

Vasoactive intestinal polypeptide (VIP) is a 28 amino acid peptide initially isolated and characterized from porcine gut tissue.[1] VIP has strong sequence homology with several closely related peptides including glucagon, secretin, growth hormone releasing factor (GRF), porcine peptide histidine isoleucine (PHI), human PHI (PHM), and gastric inhibitory peptide (GIP).[2] It is proposed that the biologically active conformation of these peptides can be understood in terms of the "amphiphilic helical hypothesis."[3,4] Using this approach, a series of VIP analogues have been designed, synthesized, and characterized for VIP-like properties. Five analogues, ranging from 28 to 68% homology with mammalian VIP, were designed to test this hypothesis. Model 1 was designed to be a helical peptide analogue of VIP in the region from 6-28 with minimal sequence identity to VIP. Models 2 and 3 were variants of Model 1 in which the pairs of basic residues were scrambled so as to separate them in the linear sequence, yet retain similar spatial presentation when in a helical conformation. Since the amphiphilic helical structure has two surfaces, one hydrophobic and one hydrophilic, Models 4 and 5 were designed to analyze the specific structural requirements of each domain. Model 4 was a hybrid utilizing the hydrophobic surface of Model 1 and the hydrophilic surface of VIP. In Model 5, the amino acids chosen for the respective domains were the inverse of those used in Model 4.

The peptides were synthesized by solid-phase peptide synthesis and purified by preparative HPLC. Analytical HPLC and amino acid analysis confirmed the homogeneity, purity, and proper composition of the analogues.

The ability of the analogues to behave as VIP agonists were assessed by their ability to interact specifically with VIP receptors on rat lung membranes (FIG. 1)[5] and to stimulate amylase release in dispersed guinea pig acini (FIG. 2).[6] Comparison of results obtained with Models 4 and 5 indicated that the integrity of the hydrophobic surface of the VIP sequence was essential for specific binding to VIP receptors with high affinity. From the data obtained for Model 1, it appeared that radically redesigned analogues could still effectively compete for specific binding to lung membrane receptors, but displayed much weaker potency in stimulating amylase secretion. Further experiments are being conducted to determine if Model 1 is a weak VIP agonist or a strong antagonist.

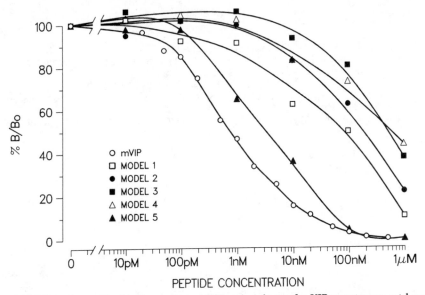

FIGURE 1. Competitive binding profiles of VIP and analogues for VIP receptors on rat lung membranes. All data is expressed in terms of specific VIP binding with 100% being in the absence of competing ligand and 0% being in the presence of 10^{-6} M mammalian VIP.

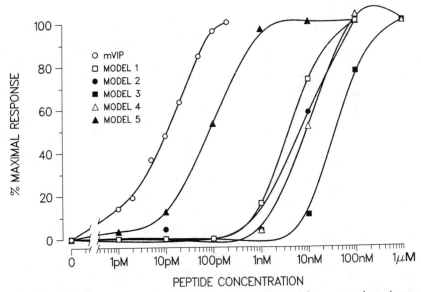

FIGURE 2. Stimulation of amylase release effected by VIP and analogues on guinea pig pancreatic acini. All data has been normalized so that basal release is that amount of amylase released with no stimulating ligand and 100% maximal response is the plateau value achieved by each of the ligands. In all cases, maximal release effected by each peptide was within 10% of that caused by VIP.

REFERENCES

1. SAID, S. I. & V. MUTT. 1970. Science **169:** 1217-1218.
2. BODANSKY, M., Y. KLAUSNER & S. I. SAID. 1973. Proc. Natl. Acad. Sci. USA **70:** 382-384.
3. KAISER, E. T. & F. J. KEZDY. 1984. Science **223:** 249-255.
4. KAISER, E. T. & F. J. KEZDY. 1983. Proc. Natl. Acad. Sci. USA **80:** 1137-1143.
5. LEROUX, P., H. VAUDRY, A. FOURNIER, S. ST. PIERRE & G. PELLETIER. 1984. Endocrinology **114:** 1506-1512.
6. PEIKEN, S. R., A. J. ROTTMAN, S. BATZRI & J. D. GARDNER. 1978. Am. J. Physiol. **235:** E743-E749.

Vasoactive Intestinal Peptide Receptors in Human Platelet Membrane

Characterization of Binding and Functional Activity

N. ERCAL, M. S. O'DORISIO, A. VINIK, T. M.
O'DORISIO, AND M. KADROFSKE

Departments of Physiology, Pediatrics, and Medicine
The Ohio State University
Columbus, Ohio 43210
and
Department of Medicine
University of Michigan
Ann Arbor, Michigan

Vasoactive intestinal peptide (VIP) mediated inhibition of platelet aggregation has been demonstrated in rabbit platelets.[1] While the mechanism by which VIP inhibits aggregation is thought to be via a specific receptor linked to adenylate cyclase, platelet receptors for VIP have not yet been demonstrated. The current studies were designed to test whether VIP regulates aggregation in human platelets and to determine whether specific, high-affinity VIP receptors are expressed on platelet membranes.

MATERIALS AND METHODS

Membrane Preparation

Platelet-rich plasma was isolated from peripheral blood of normal human subjects. Platelets were disrupted in lysis buffer (10 mM Tris, 5 mM EDTA, pH 7.4) with a polytron. Plasma membranes were isolated by differential centrifugation[2] and stored in Buffer A (20 mM Hepes, 150 mM NaCl, 2 mM MgCl$_2$, 5 mM EDTA, 1 mM-β-mercaptoethanol, 50 μg/ml phenylmethyl sulfonyl fluoride, pH 7.4).

[^{125}I]VIP Binding Studies

Membranes (200 μg protein) were incubated at 17°C with 100-150 pM [^{125}I]VIP (SA = 647 Ci/g), in the absence or presence of competing unlabeled peptide, in a final volume 0.5 ml. Membrane-bound [^{125}I]VIP was separated from free by filtration through Whatman GF/C filters presoaked in 0.3% polyethylenimine as described by O'Dorisio *et al.*[3] Time course and temperature studies demonstrated steady-state binding from 30 to 90 minutes at 17°C. The percentage of total counts bound to membrane protein ranged from 18% to 31% with 61% to 82% of bound ligand representing specific binding. Specific binding increased linearly with increasing concentration (50 to 500 μg) of membrane protein. Kinetic parameters were determined by a nonlinear computer-assisted fit of the competitive binding data.[4]

Platelet Aggregation Studies

Peripheral blood was obtained from healthy volunteers and slowly dispensed into 5-ml polystyrene tubes containing citrate (4.5 ml blood + 0.5 ml citrate). Platelet-rich plasma was prepared by centrifuging citrated blood at 25°C for six minutes at 400 × g. Platelet-poor plasma was obtained by recentrifuging the blood specimen 10

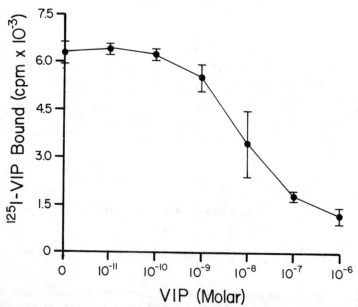

FIGURE 1. Competitive binding of [^{125}I]VIP to platelet membranes. 200 μg of membrane protein was incubated with 100 pM [^{125}I]VIP in the presence of indicated concentrations of unlabeled VIP for 45 minutes at 17°C. Computer-assisted fit of 12 competitive binding experiments was used to calculate affinity constants (K_D) and maximum number of binding sites (B_{max}).

TABLE 1. Effect of VIP on Platelet Aggregation[a]

Agent	Percent Transmission
ADP	80.5 ± 7
ADP + VIP	83.2 ± 5
PAF	75.8 ± 4.1
PAF + VIP	38.1 ± 2

[a] VIP-mediated inhibition of platelet aggregation using platelet-rich plasma from three healthy volunteers. Platelets were stirred in siliconized glass cuvettes for 60 seconds in the presence or absence of 1 μM VIP before addition of PAF or ADP. Values are mean ± SD for three experiments.

minutes at 1500 × g. Aliquots of platelet-rich plasma were stirred in siliconized glass cuvettes in a Bio/Data platelet aggregation profiler, Model PAP-3. PAF (1-alkyl-2-acetyl-glycero-3-phosphorylcholine) was purchased from Sigma and dissolved in modified Tyrode's solution[5] containing 5 mg/ml bovine serum albumin. VIP was dissolved in Tyrode's solution containing 0.5% BSA and 0.005% bacitracin. Platelet-rich plasma was incubated 60 seconds with or without VIP before addition of PAF or ADP.

RESULTS AND CONCLUSIONS

The specific binding (total bound [^{125}I]VIP minus label bound in the presence of 1 μM unlabeled VIP) increased linearly with membrane protein concentration. Computer analysis of the data from 12 separate experiments demonstrated a single class of high-affinity binding sites with a mean dissociation constant (K_D) of 23 ± 6.3 nM (FIG. 1). PHI, glucagon, and GHRF competed less effectively for [^{125}I]VIP binding sites, exhibiting K_Ds of 254 ± 51, 441 ± 21 and 135 ± 73 nM, respectively.

VIP effects on platelet aggregation were investigated as shown in TABLE 1. VIP inhibited PAF-induced platelet aggregation by 50%. PAF is a potent platelet aggregating agent.[6] This phospholipid has been shown to inhibit cyclic AMP accumulation in intact platelets and to inhibit adenylate cyclase activity in membranes of rabbit and human platelets.[7] VIP stimulates adenylate cyclase in intact platelets[1] and thus VIP-mediated inhibition of PAF-induced platelet aggregation may result from the opposing effects of VIP and PAF on adenylate cyclase.

In summary, platelet membranes have been shown to possess receptors for vasoactive intestinal polypeptide (VIP). Competitive binding experiments using 200 μg membrane protein demonstrated a K_D of 23 ± 6.3 nM for [^{125}I]VIP with a B_{max} of 3.9 ± 1.1 nM. The binding of [^{125}I]VIP to platelet membranes is highly specific; the homologous peptides, PHI, GHRF, and glucagon, have lower affinity than VIP. VIP antagonizes platelet aggregation induced by platelet-activating factor, but not ADP-induced aggregation. These results suggest that human platelets possess functional VIP receptors that modulate platelet aggregation.

REFERENCES

1. Cox, C. P., J. Linden & S. I. Said. 1984. VIP elevates platelet cyclic AMP (cAMP) levels and inhibits *in vitro* platelet activation induced by platelet-activating factor (PAF). Peptides **5:** 325-328.
2. Baenziger, N. L. & P. W. Majerus. 1974. Isolation of human platelets and platelet surface membranes. Methods Enzymol. **31:** 149.
3. O'Dorisio, M. S., T. M. O'Dorisio, C. L. Wood, J. C. Bresnahan, M. S. Beattie & L. B. Campolito. 1988. Characterization of vasoactive intestinal peptide receptors in nervous and immune systems. Ann. N.Y. Acad. Sci. This volume.
4. Akera, T. & V. J. K. Cheng. 1977. A simple method for the determination of affinity and binding site concentration in receptor binding studies. Biochem. Biophys. Acta **470:** 412-423.
5. Farr, R. S., C. P. Cox, M. L. Wordlow & R. Jorgensen. 1980. Preliminary studies of an acid-labile factor (ALF) in human sera that inactivates platelet-activating factor (PAF). Clin. Immunol. Immunopathol. **15:** 318-330.
6. Chignard, M., J. P. Le Couedic, M. Tence, B. B. Vargaftig & J. Beneviste. 1979. The role of platelet activating factor in platelet aggregation. Nature (London) **279:** 799-800.
7. Haslam, R. J. & M. Vanderwell. 1982. Inhibition of platelet adenylate cyclase by 1-0-alkyl-2-0-acetyl-sn-glycerl-3-phosphorylcholine (PAF). J. Biol. Chem. **257:** 6879-6885.

The Glycoprotein Nature of the Vasoactive Intestinal Peptide Binding Site

Role of Carbohydrates in VIP Binding on HT 29-D4 Cells[a]

A. EL BATTARI, J. LUIS, J. M. MARTIN, J. FANTINI,
J. M. MULLER, J. MARVALDI, AND J. PICHON

Institut de Chimie Biologique
UA CNRS 202
Université de Provence
F-13331 Marseille Cedex 3, France

AFFINITY CHROMATOGRAPHY OF VIP BINDING PROTEIN ON IMMOBILIZED LECTIN COLUMN

[^{125}I]VIP specifically bound to HT 29-D4 cell monolayers was cross-linked to its binding site with disuccnimidylsuberate as previously described.[1] Cells were then treated with 1% NP 40 and solubilized material applied to a wheat germ agglutinin (WGA)-sepharose column. Forty-three percent of the applied radioactivity was retained by the lectin and could be eluted from the column with 0.5 M N-acetyl-glucosamine (FIG. 1a). Eluted fractions were analyzed by SDS-PAGE. Autoradiographic patterns (FIG. 1b) showed that these fractions contained the M_r 67,000 and M_r 120,000 polypeptides previously characterized in intact HT 29 cells.[1]

DEGLYCOSYLATION AND DESIALILATION OF VIP-BINDING PROTEINS

To further analyze the glycoprotein nature of the VIP-binding complex, we treated the solubilized cross-linked material with endo-β-acetyl-glucosaminidase F (Endo F). Autoradiographic analysis of material treated with the enzyme show that the major M_r 67,000 component is converted to a M_r 47,000 component after 4 or 12 hours of

[a]Supported by CNRS UA 202, INSERM Grant CRE 847006 and ARC Grant 6187.

667

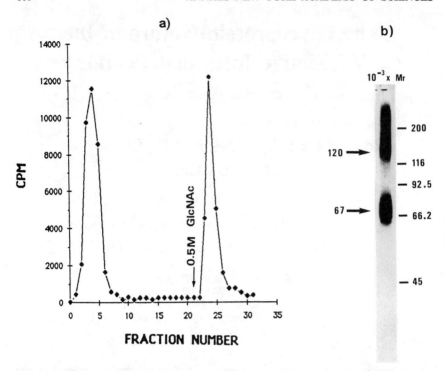

FIGURE 1. Affinity chromatography of VIP-binding protein on WGA-sepharose column. [^{125}I]VIP affinity-labeled cells were incubated for two hours at 4°C in 50 mM Hepes, pH 7.5, 160 mM NaCl, 1 mM MgCl$_2$, 1 mM CaCl$_2$, 150 mM phenylmethanesulphonyl fluoride, 2 mM benzamidine, 12 μM leupeptin (buffer A) containing 1% NP 40. Solubilized material was run through a WGA-sepharose column equilibrated with buffer A containing 0.1% NP 40. (**a**) Bound material was eluted with 0.5 M N-acetylglucosamine (GlcNAc). (**b**) Eluted material was precipitated with trichloroacetic acid and analyzed by SDS/PAGE and autoradiography. Migration of M_r standards is indicated on the right.

treatment (FIG. 2, lanes a & b). With the same conditions the minor M_r 120,000 component is converted to a M_r 100,000 species. The major M_r 47,000 cleavage product was also obtained after treatment of solubilized material with trifluoromethane-sulfonic acid (not shown). On the other hand, neuraminidase treatment of cell monolayers or incubation of solubilized material with chlorhydric acid leads to a slight increase in the electrophoretic mobility of the M_r 67,000 species that corresponds to the removal of approximately 10 sialic acid residues per polypeptide accounting for 3 K_d (results not shown).

EFFECTS OF LECTINS AND INHIBITORS OF PROTEIN GLYCOSYLATION ON VIP BINDING TO HT 29-D4 CELLS

FIGURE 3 shows that WGA, which interacts with sialic acid and N-acetyl-D-glucosamine, inhibits the binding of VIP, whereas succinyl-WGA (S-WGA), which does not interact with sialic acid,[2] does not inhibit VIP binding. On the other hand Concavalin A (Con A), which interacts with mannose, does not affect VIP binding. Thus sialic acid probably plays a role in [^{125}I]VIP binding to cells.

Inhibitors of glycosylation, which act at different stages during the process of glycoprotein maturation, also inhibit the binding of [^{125}I]VIP to HT 29-D4 cells (TABLE 1). It remains to be seen whether these inhibitions result from a defect in glycosylation of surface VIP receptors or from the absence of a receptor from the cell surface in drug-treated cells. Either route is possible depending on the action of the drug.

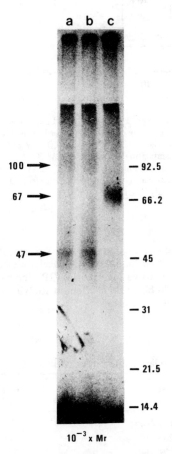

FIGURE 2. Endo F treatment of VIP-binding proteins. [^{125}I]VIP affinity-labeled cells were solubilized in 0.1 *M* sodium phosphate buffer, pH 6.1, containing 5 m*M* EDTA, 1% 2-mercaptoethanol, and 0.1% SDS. Sample was boiled for two minutes; NP 40 was then added up to 1%. To 100 μl of the mixture 10 μl of Endo F provided as a 50% (vol/vol) glycerol/25 m*M* EDTA solution (a gift of Drs. J. Elder & S. Alexander, Scipps Clinic, La Jolla CA) were added. Incubation was carried out as described by Elder and Alexander.[3] Samples were analyzed by SDS/PAGE. (**a**) and (**b**) treatment with Endo F for 12 hours and four hours, respectively. (**c**) incubation for 12 hours without enzyme.

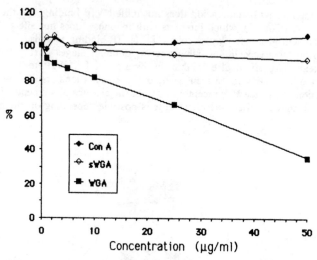

FIGURE 3. Effects of lectins on [¹²⁵I]VIP binding. HT 29-D4 cell monolayers were incubated at 4°C for three hours with increasing concentrations of lectins in binding buffer (DME medium pH 7.3, 1% BSA, 0.1% bacitracin, 15 mM Hepes, 150 mM phenylmethanesulphonyl fluoride, 2 mM benzamidine, 12 μM leupeptin) containing 1 mM CaCl₂ and 1 mM MgCl₂ for incubation with WGA and S-WGA, and containing 1 mM CaCl₂ and 0.5 mM MnCl₂ for incubation with Con A. Monolayers were then washed three times with ice-cold NaCl/Pi/BSA and [¹²⁵I]VIP binding performed as previously described.[4]

From these data we conclude that: (1) The VIP receptor from intact HT 29-D4 cells is a glycoprotein with an N-linked oligosaccharide side chain containing sialic acid. (2) Sialic acid seems to be involved in VIP binding. (3) Use of inhibitors of protein glycosylation could be a valuable tool in studying the role of glycosylation in VIP binding and in receptor metabolism.

TABLE 1. Effect of Glycosylation Inhibitors on [¹²⁵I]VIP Binding[a]

Preincubation with	Percent Inhibition of [¹²⁵I]VIP Binding
Tunicamycin (1 μg/ml)	47
Glucosamine (20 mM)	42
Swainsonine (1 μg/ml)	33
Monensin (1 μg/ml)	60
Control	0

[a] HT 29-D4 cell monolayers were preincubated at 37°C for 18 hours in the presence of 10% FCS supplemented medium containing the indicated concentration of inhibitors. [¹²⁵I]VIP binding was performed as previously described.[4]

REFERENCES

1. MULLER, J. M., J. LUIS, J. FANTINI, B. ABADIE, F. GIANNELLINI, J. MARVALDI & J.
    PICHON. 1985. Eur. J. Biochem. **151:** 411-417.
2. JOSHI, S. S., J. D. JACKSON & J. G. SHARP. 1985. Cancer Detect. Prev. **8:** 237-245.
3. ELDER, J. H. & S. ALEXANDER. 1982. Proc. Natl. Acad. Sci. USA **79:** 4540-4544.
4. LUIS, J., J. M. MULLER, B. ABADIE, J. M. MARTIN, J. MARVALDI & J. PICHON. 1986.
    Eur. J. Biochem. **156:** 631-636.

Localization of Vasoactive Intestinal Peptide Binding Sites in Rat Pancreatic Islets by Computer-Assisted Analysis of Electron Microscopy Video-Autoradiographs

ANNY ANTEUNIS,[a] ANY ASTESANO,[a] GILLES
HEJBLUM,[a] JEAN-CLAUDE MARIE,[a] BERNARD
PORTHA,[b] AND GABRIEL ROSSELIN [a]

[a]Hôpital Saint-Antoine
INSERM U.55
Saint-Antoine 75012 Paris, France
[b]Laboratoire de Physiologie du Développement
Université de Paris VII, 75005 Paris, France

The VIPergic signal coming from alimentary tract might be communicated to the endocrine pancreas through the peptidergic afferent innervation of islets.[1,2] On the other hand, *in vitro* studies on isolated pancreases have shown that VIP perfused at low concentrations stimulates the release of insulin,[3–5] glucagon,[3–5] somatostatin,[6] and PP.[7] We showed previously the presence of VIP receptors in pancreatic beta cells.[8] Further quantitative studies of VIP receptors, after pancreatic perfusion of 1×10^{-9} M mono-[^{125}I]VIP for four minutes at 37°C was performed using computer-assisted analysis of video-autoradiographs. The ultrastructural quantitation of the labeling was realized as described by Hejblum *et al.* in this volume. The biological samples were randomly selected from four rats, three islets per rat and four fields per islet (one field = 14,400 μm^2). The normalized specific activity (percent of corrected grains/volume density) computed for each type of endocrine cell was 2.57, 2.57, 2.44, and 0.87 for the A, PP, D, and beta cells, respectively, whereas the background labeling was as low as 0.16. The total number of corrected grains was of 2,318 and the total volume density was estimated on 4,680 points. Ultrastructural analysis of the cellular grain distribution on beta cells further shows a prevalence of labeling on the cell surface with a normalized specific activity of 3.60 as compared to 0.99 for the intracellular vesicles (endosomes, multivesicular bodies, and Golgi elements). Our results show the presence of specific binding sites in beta, A, PP, and D cells and indicate that VIP might directly stimulate the secretion of the corresponding hormones. The detection of specific receptors for VIP on the different endocrine cells at VIP concentrations that are compatible with those released at the peri-insular VIP nerve endings substantiates the hypothesis that VIP has a physiological role and acts as a neuroregulator involved in the local control of the endocrine pancreas function.

REFERENCES

1. LARSSON, L. I., J. FAHRENKRUG, J. J. HOLST & D. B. SCHAFFALITZKY DE MUCKADELL. 1978. Life Sci. **22:** 773-780.
2. BISHOP, A. E., J. M. POLAK, I. C. GREEN, M. G. BRYANT & S. R. BLOOM. 1980. Diabetologia **18:** 73-78.
3. BATAILLE, D., C. JARROUSSE, N. VAUCLIN, C. GESPACH & G. ROSSELIN. 1977. *In* Glucagon, Its Role in Physiology and Clinical Medicine. P. P. Foa *et al.,* Eds.: 255-269. Springer-Verlag. New York.
4. SCHEBALIN, M., S. I. SAID & G. M. MAKLHOUF. 1977. Am. J. Physiol. **232:** E197-E200.
5. JENSEN, S. L., J. FAHRENKRUG, J. J. HOLST, O. V. NIELSEN & O. B. SCHAFFALITZKY DE MUCKADELL. 1978. Am. J. Physiol. **235:** E387-E391.
6. IPP, E., E. DOBBS & R. H. UNGER. 1978. FEBS Lett. **90:** 76-78.
7. ADRIAN, T. E., S. R. BLOOM, K. HERMANSEN & J. IVERSEN. 1978. Diabetologia **14:** 413-417.
8. ANTEUNIS, A., G. HEJBLUM, A. ASTESANO, J. C. MARIE, D. HUI BON HOA, M. KERGOAT, B. PORTHA & G. ROSSELIN. 1986. C. R. Acad. Sci. Paris. **303:** 357-360.

A Computer-Assisted Analysis of Ultrastructural Autoradiographs Applied to the Localization of Vasoactive Intestinal Peptide Binding Sites in Pancreatic Acini

GILLES HEJBLUM,[a] ANNY ANTEUNIS,[a] ANY
ASTESANO,[a] JEAN-CLAUDE MARIE,[a] BERNARD
PORTHA,[b] AND GABRIEL ROSSELIN [a]

[a]Unité de Recherches sur les Peptides Neurodigestifs et le Diabète
INSERM U.55, Centre de Recherches Paris-St. Antoine
75571 Paris, Cedex 12, France

[b]Laboratoire de Physiologie due Développement
Université Paris VII
75005 Paris, France

The presence of vasoactive intestinal peptide (VIP) receptors in rat acinar cells was directly demonstrated after perfusion of isolated pancreas with 1 nM mono-[^{125}I]VIP for four minutes at 37°C. Ultrastructural autoradiographs were analyzed from four rats, four samples per rat, 10 fields per sample (a field = 7225 μm^2). Because of the radiation spread, a grain cannot be directly assigned to the underlying ultrastructural compartment.[1] The analysis therefore included a correction for cross-fires between the compartments considered. Furthermore, the data were normalized to the compartment volume densities (Vvs) in order to assess an objective comparison of the labeling of the different compartments considered. The analysis was computer-assisted. Images of sections observed in a JEOL 1200-EX electron microsope were digitized using a direct connection of a Kontron SEM-IPS image analyzer with the scanning transmission mode of the electron microscope. Images were analyzed using our own programs,[2] which are based on the method initially described by Blackett & Parry[3] as modified by Downs & Williams.[4] Vvs estimates were obtained by the point counting method according to the general stereological principles.[5] The total number of observed grains amounted to 1001, and a total of 2055 points were counted to estimate Vvs. Acinar cells were partitioned in three compartments: plasma membrane and microvilli (SURF), vesicular system including endosomes, Golgi and phagosomes (VGP), and the other cell structures (OS). The percent disintegrations per Vv (NSA) were finally calculated and allow an objective comparison between the different compartments labeled. NSA amounted to (mean ± SEM) 11.7 ± 2.4, 1.13 ± 0.24, 0.5 ± 0.03, 0.15 ± 0.03 for SURF, VGP, OS, and background, respectively. Most of the bound

VIP is located at the cell surface, whereas no significant internalization is observed in our experimental conditions. The presence of specific VIP receptors on acinar cells as well as on islets β cells[6] suggests that both exocrine and endocrine pancreas are subjected to the same type of regulation by neuro-acinar and neuro-insular VIPergic complexes.

REFERENCES

1. SALPETER, M. M., H. C. FERTUCK & E. E. SALPETER. 1977. J. Cell Biol. **72:** 161-173.
2. HEJBLUM, G., A. M. DOWNS & J. P. RIGAUT. 1986. Acta Stereol. **5:** 245-249.
3. BLACKETT, N. M. & D. M. PARRY. 1973. J. Cell Biol. **57:** 9-15.
4. DOWNS, A. M. & M. A. WILLIAMS. 1978. J. Microsc. **114:** 143-156.
5. WEIBEL, E. R. 1979. Stereological Methods, Vol 2: Practical Methods for Biological Morphometry. Academic Press Inc. New York.
6. ANTEUNIS, A., G. HEJBLUM, A. ASTESANO, J. C. MARIE, D. HUI BON HOA, M. KERGOAT, B. PORTHA & G. ROSSELIN. 1986. C. R. Acad. Sci. (Paris) **303:** 357-360.

Human Lung Cancer Cell Lines Have Vasoactive Intestinal Peptide Receptors[a]

MARGARET M. SHAFFER,[b] LOUIS Y. KORMAN,[c]
ROBERT T. JENSEN,[d] ZHI CHAO ZHOU,[d] DESMOND
N. CARNEY,[e] AND TERRY W. MOODY [b,f]

[b]Department of Biochemistry
The George Washington University School of Medicine and Health
Sciences
Washington, D.C. 20037

[c]Gastroenterology Section
Veterans Administration Medical Center
Washington, D.C. 20422

[d]Digestive Disease Branch
National Institute of Digestive and Kidney Disease
Bethesda, Maryland 20205

[e]NCI-Navy Medical Oncology Branch
National Cancer Institute and
National Naval Medical Center
Bethesda, Maryland 20814

Vasoactive intestinal peptide (VIP) is biologically active in numerous organs including the lung. In the lung endogenous VIP is present in nerves supplying airway smooth muscle as well as glands and pulmonary vessels.[1] VIP is a potent bronchodilator in man and other species and relaxes pulmonary vascular smooth muscle.[2-4] These biological effects caused by VIP may be mediated by the receptors that have been detected in the normal lung.[5,6] By means of *in vitro* autoradiographic techniques, these receptors have been localized to the alveoli and the epithelium of the rat lung and the pulmonary artery smooth muscle and alveolar walls of the normal human lung.[6,7] Recently, VIP receptors were characterized in the malignant lung using a large cell carcinoma cell line.[8] Here, we investigated whether or not VIP receptors were present in other human lung cancer cell lines.

Small-cell lung cancer (SCLC), adenocarcinoma, squamous cell carcinoma, and large-cell carcinoma cell lines were cultured in a serum-free Hites medium (RPMI-

[a]This research is supported in part by National Cancer Institute Grants CA-33767 and CA-42306.

[f]Send correspondence to: Dr. T. Moody, Department of Biochemistry, The George Washington University Medical Center, 2300 Eye Street, N.W., Washington, D.C. 20037.

TABLE 1. VIP Receptor Density in Human Lung Cancer Cell Lines[a]

Lung Cancer Cell Line	VIP Receptor Density (fmol/mg Protein)	
SCLC	1.0–9.3	(23/25)
Adenocarcinoma	1.6	(1/3)
Large cell carcinoma	0.4–12.0	(2/2)
Squamous cell carcinoma	1.2	(1/1)

[a] The number in parentheses indicates the number of cell lines that tested positive for VIP receptors relative to the number of cell lines examined. For SCLC, 23 of 25 cells lines tested positive and specific [^{125}I]VIP binding ranged from 1 to 9.3 fmol/mg protein using 0.4 nM [^{125}I]VIP. For adenocarcinoma and squamous cell carcinoma, one cell line tested positive and the concentration of VIP receptors was 1.6 and 1.2 fmol/mg, respectively. For large cell carcinoma, two cell lines tested positive and the VIP receptor density was 0.4 and 12.0.

1640 containing 10^{-8} M hydrocortisone, 5 μg/ml bovine insulin, 10 μg/ml human transferrin, 10^{-8} M β-estradiol, and 3×10^{-8} M Na$_2$SeO$_3$) or a serum-supplemented medium (RPMI-1640 containing 10% heat-inactivated fetal bovine serum). Two days after a medium change, the cells were harvested by centrifugation at 1,000 $\times$ g for 10 minutes. The cells were resuspended in Hites medium and used in receptor binding studies. One $\times$ 10^6 cells were placed in buffer (Hites medium that contained 1% bovine serum albumin and 0.5 mg/ml bacitracin). The cells were incubated with 50,000 cpm of [^{125}I]VIP (1100 Ci/mmol) in the absence or presence of 1 μM unlabeled VIP; the total volume was 200 μl. The cells were pelleted for one minute in a Beckman microfuge B and the pellet that contained bound peptide rinsed twice in buffer. Protein was determined using the method of Lowry *et al.*[9]

TABLE 1 shows that most of the cell lines examined bound [^{125}I]VIP with high affinity at 37°C. Large-cell carcinoma cell line CALU-6 bound VIP best (12.0 pmol/mg protein). Low levels of binding were also detected in one other large-cell carcinoma cell line, one of three adenocarcinoma cell lines and one squamous cell carcinoma cell line. Twenty-three of 25 SCLC cell lines bound radiolabeled VIP with high affinity. Because SCLC cell line NCI-N592 bound VIP well (9.3 pmol/mg protein), its binding was further characterized.

[^{125}I]VIP bound to membranes derived from cell line NCI-N592 in a reversible and time-dependent manner. Radiolabeled VIP bound with high ($K_d = 1.3$ nM) and moderate ($K_d = 39$ nM) affinity to two classes of sites (B$_{max}$ = 88 and 1160 fmol/mg protein). Pharmacology studies indicated that the order of peptide potency was VIP > PHI > secretin. Biochemical studies indicated that [^{125}I]VIP was cross-linked to a protein of 42,000 daltons using disuccinimidylsuberate. These data indicate that protein VIP receptors may be present on SCLC cells.

Previously, we determined that VIP elevates cAMP levels in certain SCLC cells.[10] In particular, VIP (1 μM) elevated the cAMP levels approximately fourfold in two different SCLC cell lines. Also, VIP, secretin, and PHI increased the secretion rate of bombesin-like peptides from SCLC cell *in vitro* and secretin infusion elevated the plasma levels of bombesin-like peptides sevenfold in patients with extensive SCLC. Hypersecretion of bombesin-like peptides may account for some paraneoplastic syndromes associated with SCLC such as anorexia.

Bombesin-like peptides are made in and secreted from SCLC cells. When released these bombesin-like peptides may interact with cell surface receptors and stimulate growth of SCLC. Therefore, bombesin-like peptides can function as SCLC autocrine growth factors.[11] It remains to be determined if VIP alters the growth of lung cancer.

REFERENCES

1. LEY, R. D., W. A. SHANNON & S. I. SAID. 1981. Cell Tissue Res. **220:** 231-238.
2. MORICE, A. H., R. J. UNWIN, P. S. SEVER & N. DALTON. 1984. Lancet i: 457-458.
3. DIAMOND, L., J. L. SZAREK, M. N. GILLESPIE & R. J. ALTIERE. 1983. Am. Rev. Respir. Dis. **128:** 827-832.
4. SAID, S. I., ED. 1982. Vasoactive Intestinal Peptide. Raven Press. New York.
5. CHRISTOPHE, J., P. CHATELAIN, G. TATON, M. DELHAYE, M. WAELBROECK & P. ROBBERECHT. 1986. Peptides 2(Supp. 2): 253-258.
6. LEROUX, P., H. VAUDRY, A. FOURNIER, S. ST. PIERRE & G. PELLETIER. 1984. Endocrinology **114:** 1506-1512.
7. LEYS, K., A. H. MORICE, O. MADONNA & P. S. SEVER. 1984. FEBS Lett. **199:** 198-202.
8. LABURTHE, M., C. BIOSSARD, G. CHEVALIER, A. ZWEIBAUM & G. ROSSELIN. 1981. Regul. Peptides **2:** 219-230.
9. LOWRY, O. H., J. J. ROSEBROUGH, L. FARR & R. J. RANDELL. 1951. J. Biol. Chem. **193:** 265-275.
10. KORMAN, L. Y., D. N. CARNEY, M. L. CITRON & T. W. MOODY. 1986. Cancer Res. **46:** 1214-1218.
11. CUTTITTA, F., D. CARNEY, J. MULSHINE, T. MOODY, J. FEDORKO, A. FISCHLER & J. MINNA. 1985. Nature **316:** 823-825.

A Synthetic Peptide, L-8-K, and Its Antibody Both Inhibit the Specific Binding of Vasoactive Intestinal Peptide to Hamster Pancreatic Cancer Cells[a]

HARBANS SINGH,[b] ASHOK KUMAR,[c] COURTNEY M.
TOWNSEND, JR.,[b] ZAHIDA SAMAD,[b]
AND POMILA SINGH [b,d]

[b]Departments of Surgery and
[c]Human Biological Chemistry
The University of Texas Medical Branch and
Shriners-Burns Institute
Galveston, Texas 77550

In preliminary studies we have observed the presence of vasoactive intestinal peptide (VIP) receptors (R) ($\sim$ 6 fmoles/10^6 cells) on a hamster pancreatic cancer cell line (H_2T cells, developed in our laboratory; unpublished data). [^{125}I]VIP, covalently cross-linked to VIP-R on H_2T cells by disuccinimidyl suberate, was solubilized and subjected to gel electrophoresis by the method of Laemmli.[1] Two molecular species of VIP-R with molecular weights of 63,000 and 93,000 were identified. Both were specific for the VIP family of peptides and demonstrated the highest binding affinity for VIP > secretin > growth hormone-releasing factor. The VIP-R on H_2T cells demonstrated no appreciable binding for glucagon, cholecystokinin (CCK), or insulin. A synthetic peptide, L-8-K (Leu-Met-Tyr-Pro-Thr-Tyr-Leu-Lys), on the other hand, was found to specifically bind [^{125}I]VIP (15-25%) in an ELISA test, with less than 1% binding for [^{125}I]gastrin-17-I and [^{125}I]BH-CCK-8-SO$_4$. In these studies, we have examined if L-8-K and its antibody (L-8-K-Ab, developed in the rabbit) inhibit the binding of VIP to H_2T cells, and if the inhibition is specific for VIP.

[a]Supported by grants from the National Institutes of Health (CA 38651 and RCDA CA 00854) and a grant from the American Cancer Society (PDT-220).

[d]Address for correspondence: Pomila Singh, Ph.D., Associate Professor, Department of Surgery, The University of Texas Medical Branch, Galveston, Texas 77550.

METHODS AND RESULTS

We have used [^{125}I]VIP (NEN) as the labeled ligand in our studies. Unlabeled peptides were from Peninsula (Belmont, CA). H$_2$T cells, 48 hours postculture, were scraped with a rubber policeman and suspended in Hank's balanced salt solution plus 0.1% BSA, at a concentration of 10^6 cells/ml. The relative inhibition of [^{125}I]VIP to H$_2$T cells by VIP, L-8-K, and L-8-K-Ab was examined as described for insulin[2] (given in detail in the legend of FIG. 1) and is shown in FIGURE 1. As seen from the figure, both L-8-K and its Ab significantly inhibited the binding of [^{125}I]VIP to H$_2$T cells in a dose-dependent manner. The relative binding affinity (RBA) of L-8-K for inhibiting the binding of [^{125}I]VIP to VIP-R on H$_2$T cells was also determined by incubating the H$_2$T cells with [^{125}I]VIP (1 nmole) ± increasing concentration of VIP or L-8-K, or an increasing dilution of L-8-K-Ab. The RBA, calculated from the dose-response of percent inhibition of specific binding, was 56% for L-8-K compared to 100% for VIP. The ED$_{50}$ for the inhibition of total specific binding was 2×10^{-7} M for VIP, 3.8×10^{-6} M for L-8-K, and 1 : 550 final dilution for L-8-K-Ab. The specificity of L-8-K and L-8-K-Ab inhibition of VIP binding to H$_2$T cells was also measured (TABLE 1). Radiolabeled peptides ([^{125}I]VIP; [^{125}I]BH-CCK-8-SO$_4$, Amersham; [^{125}I]gastrin-17-I, prepared by us as previously published[3]; [^{125}I]^{4}Tyr-bombesin,

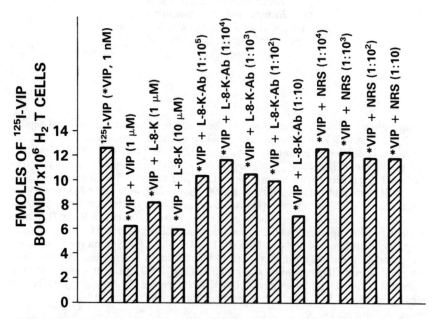

FIGURE 1. Relative inhibition of [^{125}I]VIP binding to H$_2$T cells by VIP, L-8-K, and L-8-K-Ab. H$_2$T cells were incubated with 1 nM [^{125}I]VIP/10^6 cells in the presence or absence of either VIP, L-8-K, L-8-K-Ab, or normal rabbit serum (NRS), at concentrations or dilutions indicated, for 30 minutes at 37°C. The cells were washed at the end of the incubation and the fmoles of [^{125}I]VIP remaining bound to the cells were plotted against the test substance used. The first bar to the left represents total VIP bound, the second bar represents the total nonspecifically bound VIP, and the difference is the specifically bound VIP.

TABLE 1. Specificity of L-8-K and L-8-K-Ab Inhibition of VIP Binding

Radiolabeled Peptide per Cell Type[a]	Unlabeled Homologous Peptide	Percent Inhibition of Specific Binding in the Presence of:					
		L-8-K		L-8-K-Ab			NRS[b]
		1 μM	10 μM	1 : 10	1 : 10^2	1 : 10^3	1 : 10
VIP/H$_2$T Cells	100	83 ± 3	95 ± 5	90 ± 2	44 ± 4	34 ± 3	10 ± 0.5
CCK/Guinea Pig Acini	100	<1.0	<1.0	10 ± 5	4 ± 2	<1.0	13 ± 1.3
Bombesin/ Guinea Pig Acini	100	10 ± 3	15 ± 4	8 ± 2	<1.0	<1.0	11 ± 4.0
Gastrin/MC-26 Cells	100	<1.0	<1.0	5 ± 0.5	<1.0	<1.0	9 ± 3.0

[a] In each case 5 × 10^6 cells were incubated with 1 nM of the radiolabeled peptide ± 1000 × excess unlabeled homologous peptide, and cells were washed at the end of the incubation and counted. In experiments using L-8-K and L-8-K-Ab, the radiolabeled peptide or the cells were preincubated with either L-8-K or L-8-K-Ab, respectively, for 15 minutes, before adding either the cells or the radiolabeled peptide.

[b] Normal rabbit serum.

prepared by us) at a concentration of 1 nM were incubated with either H$_2$T cells or guinea pig acini on MC-26 (mouse colon cancer) cells ± 1000 × excess homologous peptide for either 30 minutes at 30°C (CCK, bombesin, gastrin) or 120 minutes at 4°C (VIP), and the percent inhibition of specific binding determined in the presence or absence of L-8-K or its Ab. As seen from the table, both L-8-K and its Ab specifically inhibited the binding of only VIP to VIP-R on cancer cells, while L-8-K slightly inhibited the binding of bombesin to guinea pig acini.

DISCUSSION

The specific inhibition of VIP binding to VIP-receptors on H$_2$T cells by L-8-K and its antibody indicates that L-8-K may represent at least a part or all of the VIP-receptor binding site, and that the L-8-K-Ab probably blocks the VIP receptors, resulting in reducing binding of VIP. We plan to use the L-8-K-Ab for purifying the VIP receptors on the H$_2$T cells.

REFERENCES

1. LAEMMLI, U. K. 1970. Cleavage of structural proteins during the assembly of the head of bacteriophage T4. Nature **227:** 680-685.
2. FLIER, J. S., C. R. KAHN, D. B. JARRETT & J. ROTH. 1976. Characterization of antibodies to the insulin receptor. A cause of insulin-resistant diabetes in man. J. Clin. Invest. **58:** 1442-1449.
3. SINGH, P., B. RAE-VENTER, C. M. TOWNSEND, JR., T. KHALIL & J. C. THOMPSON. 1985. Gastrin Receptors in normal and malignant gastrointestinal mucosa. Age-associated changes in gastrin receptors. Am. J. Physiol. **249:** G761-G769.

Dopamine-Vasoactive Intestinal Peptide Interactions on Mixed GH-PRL Pituitary Adenomas

D. TATER, G. CHARPENTIER, M. KUJAS, G. BESSON,
G. ROSSELIN, AND J. P. BERCOVICI

Universitary Hospital
Brest, France
and
INSERM U. 55
Hôspital Saint-Antoine
Paris, France

Vasoactive intestinal peptide (VIP) was demonstrated to stimulate the secretion of prolactin in humans,[1] whereas the effect of VIP on GH release is not established.[2-4] We have previously observed that VIP can induce prolactin secretion in prolactinoma only after prior infusion of DA[5] (review in Rostène[6]). We have tested VIP-DA interactions in seven males patients suffering from mixed somatotroph and lactotroph cell pituitary adenomas (immunohistologically proven) and in nine matched controls.

STUDY PROTOCOL

Day 1: 75 μg of porcine VIP was injected i.v. for 12 minutes in all patients. Day 2: In patients with adenomas, DA (1 μg·kg·min) was infused i.v. for 240 minutes and saline was infused from t = 200-212 minutes. Day 3: DA was administered as on day two and VIP (75 μg/12 min) was infused instead of saline. Statistical analyses were performed with the Wilcoxon test.

RESULTS

No side effects of the drug infusions were observed. The plasma GH and prolactin concentrations ([GH] and [PRL]) of the control subjects significantly ($p < 0.05$) increased after VIP infusion from 3 to 9.0 and 6.0 to 15.8 ng/ml. *No effect of VIP on [GH] and [PRL] was observed in patients* (FIG. 1). At day two and three, the initial [GH] and [PRL] were identical, and upon DA infusion, exhibited a significant

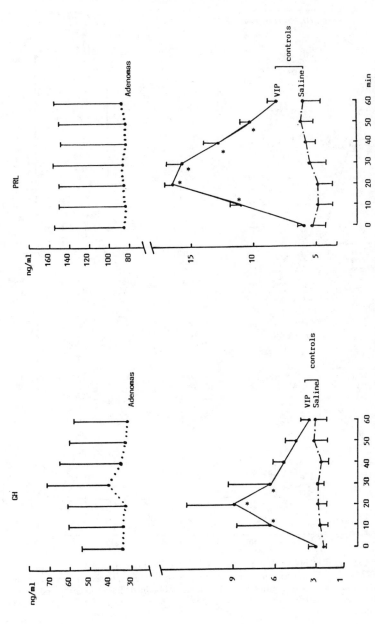

FIGURE 1. VIP effects on GH (**A**) and prolactin (**B**) secretion: ... in patients with GH and prolactin pituitary adenomas ($n = 7$); —— in controls ($n = 9$); -·- controls injected with saline. Asterisk indicates $p < 0.05$ versus hormone concentration at t = 0, and versus controls.

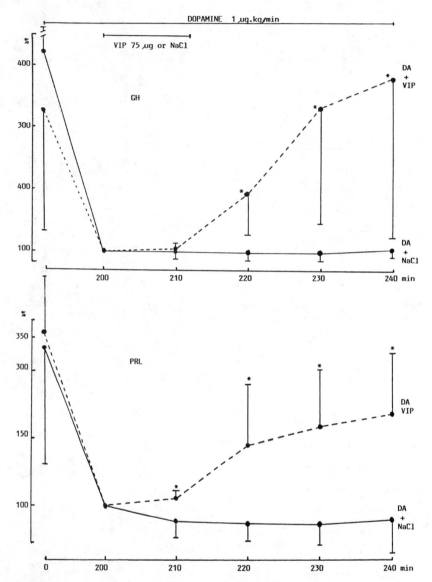

FIGURE 2. Evolution of plasma prolactin and GH concentrations during DA infusion, and either VIP (75 μg in 12 minutes) or saline injection. Results are expressed as percent of the hormone concentration at 200 minutes when the nadir is obtained. Basal values (−60, −30, −15, 0) were plotted. Asterisk indicates $p < 0.05$ versus hormone concentration at t = 200 and versus controls.

drop ($p < 0.05$) at 200 minutes from 29 to 9.0 ng/ml and from 83.6 to 31.2 ng/ml, respectively. After saline from t = 200-212 minutes, both hormones remained unchanged, whereas upon VIP infusion [GH] and [PRL] increased by 177 and 421% above their corresponding concentrations at 200 minutes (FIG. 2). The initial concentrations were recovered in six patients for GH and in one for prolactin.

DISCUSSION

In controls, the discrepancy between the GH responsiveness to VIP that we observed and those of other authors[3,4] could be related to the different route of VIP injection (i.v. versus i.m.). Our results demonstrate identical responsiveness to VIP and DA for all patients. In mixed pituitary adenomas, VIP is able to stimulate prolactin release only after prior infusion of DA, in agreement with our previous data on pure prolactinoma.[5] Furthermore we demonstrate here that DA might also exert an inhibitory tone on the VIP-induced release of GH by the mixed pituitary adenoma. The counteraction of VIP on the DA inhibition of the pituitary hormone is due to the presence of VIP or VIP-like receptors that are coupled to a stimulatory guanyl regulatory protein or Ns, whereas it is known that DA receptors, such as those in pituitary[7] are of the D2 type and inhibit adenylyl cyclase (review in Rosselin[8]). Further works will indicate the specificity of the receptor present in the mixed adenoma in regard to the VIP and the GRF action. Whatever is the type of receptor involved in the hormonal hypersecretion observed in these patients, a DA deficiency is also present, which might also play a role in the genesis of the mixed GH-prolactin adenoma, mostly if the GH- and prolactin-secreting cells derive from a single acidophilic stem cell.

REFERENCES

1. ROSSELIN, G., W. ROTSZTEJN, M. LABURTHE & P. M. DUBOIS. 1982. Is VIP a neuroregulator of a hormone? *In* Hormonally Action Brain Peptides. McKerns & Pantic, Eds. Plenum. New York.
2. VIJAYAN, E., W. K. SAMSON, S. I. SAID & S. M. MCCANN. 1979. Vasoactive intestinal peptide: Evidence for a hypothalamic site of action to release growth hormone, luteinizing hormone, and prolactin in conscious ovariectomized rats. Endocrinology **104:** 53-57.
3. CHIHARA, K., H. KAJI, N. MINAMITANI, H. KODAMA, T. KITA, B. GOTO, T. CHITA, D. H. COY & T. FUJITA. 1984. Stimulation of growth hormone by vasoactive intestinal polypeptide in acromegaly. J. Clin. Endocrinol. Metab. **58:** 81-86.
4. KATO, Y., A. SHIMATSU, N. MATSUSHITA, H. OHTA & H. IMURA. 1984. Role of vasoactive intestinal polypeptide (VIP) in regulating the pituitary function in man. Peptides **5:** 389-394.
5. TATER, D., G. CHARPENTIER, G. BESSON, G. ROSSELIN & J. P. BERCOVICI. 1983. Le VIP lève l'inhibition de la sécrétion de prolactine induite par la dopamine chez les sujets présentant un prolactinome. C. R. Acad. Sci. Paris **297:** 331-334.
6. ROSTÈNE, W. H. 1984. Neurobiological and neuroendocrine functions of the vasoactive intestinal peptide (VIP). Prog. Neurobiol. **22:** 103-129.
7. CARON, M. G., M. BEAULIEU, V. RAYMOND, B. GAGNÉ, J. DROUIN, R. J. LEFKOWITZ & F. LABRIE. 1978. Dopaminergic receptors in the anterior pituitary gland. J. Biol. Chem. **253:** 2244-2253.
8. ROSSELIN, G. 1986. The receptors of the VIP family peptides (VIP, secretin, GRF, PHI, PHM, GIP, glucagon, and oxyntomodulin). Specificities and identity. Peptides **7:** 89-99.

Vasoactive Intestinal Peptide Prevents Increase in Pulmonary Artery Pressure during Hypoxia in Newborn Lambs

P. L. TOUBAS,[a] K. C. SEKAR,[a] R. E. SHELDON,[a]
N. PAHLAVAN,[a] AND S. I. SAID[b]

[a]Department of Pediatrics and
[b]Department of Medicine
University of Oklahoma
Oklahoma City, Oklahoma 73190

We studied the effect of vasoactive intestinal peptide (VIP) on the pulmonary artery pressure flow and vascular resistance during normoxic and hypoxic ventilation in conscious newborn lambs. Three newborn lambs aged 4 to 14 days were implanted with pulmonary artery catheter (PA) and electromagnetic flow probe, aortic catheter, and inferior vena cava catheter (IVC) under general anesthesia. Platinum Grass electrodes were implanted subcutaneously to record heart rate (HR) and impedance respirations (RR). The following variables were continuously recorded after recovery (48 hours): HR, RR, mean pulmonary artery pressure and flow, and mean aortic pressure. The pulmonary vascular resistance was calculated. VIP was administered at doses of 0.67 and 1.35 μg/kg/min during normoxic and hypoxic respirations (9% FiO_2) in the conscious animal. The range of oxygen tension during 9% hypoxic ventilation was 20-37 Torr. A total of seven sets of experiments was performed. The results are given in TABLES 1 and 2.

TABLE 1. Results of VIP Administration at a Rate of 0.67 μg/kg/min[a]

Variable	Control	Hypoxia	Control	VIP	Control	VIP + Hypoxia
HR/min	150	225 ± 64[b]	161 ± 13	258 ± 14[b]	148 ± 23	225 ± 43[b]
RR/min	59 ± 18	59 ± 22	57 ± 18	69 ± 34	55 ± 21	76 ± 5.6[a]
AoP	80 ± 5	87 ± 3[c]	70 ± 10	50 ± 8.6[c]	72 ± 11	57 ± 10.6
PAP	13 ± 1	19 ± 5	14 ± 0.6	14 ± 3.2	14 ± 3	13 ± 3
PA flow	700 ± 141	900 ± 120[b]	667 ± 115	780 ± 150[b]	675 ± 114	837 ± 169[b]
PVR	18.5 ± 2	17.5 ± 3.5	21 ± 4.3	18 ± 5	18.3 ± 1.5	15 ± 1.7[c]

[a] Figures given represent the mean of four experiments. Abbreviations: HR, heart rate; RR, impedance respirations; AoP, aortic pressure; PAP, pulmonary artery pressure; PA, pulmonary artery; and PVR, pulmonary vascular resistance.
[b] $p < 0.01$.
[c] $p < 0.05$.

686

TABLE 2. Results of VIP Administration at a Rate of 1.35 μg/kg/min[a]

Variable	Control	Hypoxia	Control	VIP	Control	VIP + Hypoxia
HR/min	146 ± 6	241 ± 38[b]	149 ± 28	252 ± 35[c]	175 ± 35	280 ± 28[c]
RR/min	58 ± 16	115 ± 35[b]	68 ± 37	70 ± 39	65	100
AoP/torr	84 ± 27	90 ± 20	70 ± 26	51 ± 23[b]	70 ± 21	66 ± 16
PAP/torr	13.5 ± 2.1	21 ± 4[b]	18 ± 11	15 ± 4[b]	19 ± 7	20 ± 1
PA flow	833 ± 104	1050 ± 173[c]	675 ± 210	905 ± 241[c]	525 ± 35	505 ± 77
PVR (units)	18 ± 8.4	20 ± 10	23.3 ± 17	17 ± 7	33 ± 9	38 ± 3[b]

[a] Figures given represent the mean of three experiments. Abbreviations are the same as TABLE 1.

[b] $p < 0.05$.

[c] $p < 0.01$.

SUMMARY AND CONCLUSIONS

1. Hypoxic ventilation produced marked increases in heart rate, aortic and pulmonary pressure, pulmonary blood flow, and pulmonary vascular resistance.

2. VIP infusion alone (0.67 and 1.35 μg/kg/min) produced tachycardia and systemic hypotension at both administered doses.

3. Mild reduction in pulmonary artery pressure was observed with VIP infusion alone. Pulmonary blood flow increased and pulmonary vascular resistance decreased at both administered doses.

4. The administration of VIP during hypoxia (0.67 μg/kg/min) prevented the increase in pulmonary artery pressure, increased pulmonary blood flow, and decreased pulmonary vascular resistance.

5. These observations were not seen when VIP was administered (during hypoxia) at a dose of 1.35 μg/kg/min. This might be due to marked tachycardia observed at higher doses of VIP.

6. Arterial blood gases did not change significantly at both administered doses during normoxia and hypoxia.

Index of Contributors

689